# 1250
## Health-Care Questions
## Women Ask

1250

# Health-Care Questions Women Ask

### Joe S. McIlhaney, Jr., M.D.
### with Susan Nethery

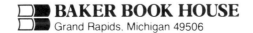
**BAKER BOOK HOUSE**
Grand Rapids, Michigan 49506

Scripture references identified as RSV are from the Revised
Standard Version, © 1946, 1952, 1971 by Division of Christian
Education of the National Council of the Churches of Christ
in the United States of America. Scripture references identi-
fied as NASB are from the New American Standard Version,
© 1960, 1962, 1963, 1968, 1971, 1972, 1973, 1975, 1977 by The
Lockman Foundation. Scripture references identified as LB are
from the Living Bible, © 1971 by Tyndale House Publishers.
Scripture references identified as KJV are from the King James
Version. Those identified as NIV are from the New International Version, © 1978 by New York International Bible
Society.

Several people and firms graciously allowed the use of their
material:

Excerpts from Sexual Freedom by V. Mary Stewart. © 1974
by Inter-Varsity Christian Fellowship of the USA and used by
permission of Inter-Varsity Press, Downers Grove, IL 60515.

Excerpt from "Hold the Eggs and Butter." in TIME, March
26, 1984, p. 56. Copyright 1984, Time, Inc. All rights reserved.
Reprinted by permission from TIME.

Excerpt from Preparing for Adolescence by Dr. James Dobson. Copyright 1978, Regal Books, Ventura, CA 93006. Used
by permission.

Excerpts from Journal of the American Medical Associa-
tion, Feb. 10, 1984, Vol. 251, No. 6, Copyright 1984 American
Medical Association, and July 9, 1982, Vol. 248, No. 2, p. 177,
Copyright 1982 by American Medical Association.

Excerpt taken from "Does Sex Education in Schools Help or
Hurt?" by Hans H. Neumann, M.D., in Medical Economics,
May 24, 1982. Copyright © 1982 by Medical Economics Com-
pany, Inc. at Oradell, N.J. 17649. Reprinted by permission.

The table, "Indicators of Possible Child Abuse," was taken
from Child Sexual Abuse: Recognition and Management, by
Donald W. Cox, M.D. in The Female Patient, Vol. 9, June 1984.

The quotation by Dr. Domeena C. Renshaw appeared in Vol. 8,
October 1983.

Excerpts from Solomon on Sex by Joseph C. Dillow.
Copyright 1977 by Joseph Dillow. Reprinted by permission of
Thomas Nelson Publishers, Inc.

Excerpt from Why I Afraid to Tell You Who I Am? by John
Powell, S. J. © 1969 Argus Communications, a division of
DLM Inc., Allen, TX 75002.

The Sexual Response Pattern illustration on p. 644 is
adapted from Human Sexual Response by Masters and
Johnson, Copyright 1966 by Little Brown and Company. Used
with permission of the publisher and Virginia Johnson.

Excerpts from Understanding Human Sexual Inadequacy
by Belliveau and Richter, copyright 1970 by Little Brown and
Company.

Excerpts from The Gift of Sex by Clifford and Joyce Penner,
p. 149, © 1981 by Word Books, Publishers, Waco, TX.

The chart on p. 567 is based on information applied by The
American College of Obstetricians and Gynecologists.

Quotations from Clinical Obstetrics and Gynecology by
Drs. Arnold, Anderson, and Sherline, Vol. 24, No. 2, June 1981,
used with permission of Lippincott/Harper & Row.

Excerpts from "Miscarriage: Bearing One Another's Bur-
dens" by Leslie Snodgrass in Stepping Stones, October, 1982.

Excerpts from The Joy of Being a Woman by Ingrid Trobisch,
© 1975 by Harper & Row.

Excerpts from Better Is Your Love than Wine by Banyolak
and Trobisch, © 1979 by Inter-Varsity Press.

Excerpt from The Hiding Place by John and Elizabeth Sherrill, © 1971 by Chosen Books.

Excerpts from Benign Diseases of the Vulva and Vagina by
Gardner and Kauffman, © 1981 by G. K. Hall.

Quotation from Dallas Times Herald, April 4, 1984.

To Marion, uncommonly gifted by God.

Marion's keen mind,
her wisdom,
her strength of character,
and her love for our Lord
have made
our first twenty-five years
as man and wife
a delightful journey.

# Contents

# Preface

In the years that I have been a practicing obstetrician-gynecologist, I have had the privilege of being many other things as well: the grateful husband of a wonderful woman, Marion; the devoted father of three fascinating girls: Lynne, Anne, and Caren; a founding member and board member of two great churches in Austin; and a friend of many fine men, women, and children.

Additionally, I have found myself in the position of being a source of medical information not only to my patients, but to all those other important people in my life: my family, the members of my church, my close friends. I consider the role of medical advisor a privilege—*and* an obligation.

God has allowed me to acquire a measure of education and wisdom. It is my responsibility as a Christian, and as a good steward of God's benevolence to me, to share those things he has given me with others.

My belief in the wisdom of God and his plan for each life will be evident—but not intrusive—throughout this book. I did not write the book this way to attempt to convince you to believe the way I do, but because my faith is a foundation for my life, both personal and professional.

A famous obstetrician-gynecologist wrote years ago that human beings were a "pure chance" combination of a random sperm and a random egg. This doctor wrote from his personal persuasion. That was okay for him. I, however, write from my own perspective because it is me.

This book is my sincere effort to provide you with information that will keep you from making wrong choices about your medical care and personal health. Bad decisions in this area can adversely affect you physically, mentally, and emotionally the rest of your life.

The principles discussed in this book can help you avoid physical problems that can lead to regret. Use intelligence and discretion not only in the physical area of your life, but in all areas of daily living.

The results of bad decisions may not bother you immediately, but they can start you down a road that will later lead to much unhappiness and ill health. Foresight is never easy, but with more knowledge, it can become less difficult. This book provides you with the information that will make right choices a little easier to reach. It presents in a clear, straightforward, and digestible way the necessary background information for arriving at the right decisions about medical care.

Although many of the concepts presented in this book are rather technical, every attempt has been made to make them interesting and easy to understand. The human body and how it functions is fascinating, as is the state of modern medical knowledge and technology.

I wish that you could go with me to medical seminars and meetings, that you could look with me through a laparoscope at the interior of a woman's abdomen, or that you could share with me the thrill of seeing a newly developing embryo. Although those things are not feasible for us to do together, I hope that it *is* possible, through this book, to share with you some of the excitement I have found in the practice of medicine.

My purpose, however, is not just to entertain you. Unless you have medical training, and even, perhaps, if you do, you need the information contained here. You may not need it now, but you or someone you love will need it at some time. You may not ever need all of it, but sooner or later you will be able to use most of it.

Susan Nethery has been my invaluable editor, assistant, and encourager in the writing of this book. She is a successful author in her own right and has written *One Year and Counting: Breast Cancer, My World and Me,* (Baker Book House, 1978), and *A Mother Shares: Perspectives on Parenting,* (Baker Book House, 1981). She was one of the top ten winners in the 1981 Texas Press Women's Communications Contest and was awarded The Texas

Baptist Communications Award for 1983. She lives in east Texas and I live in central Texas. In spite of the distance involved, we worked on this project with great enthusiasm, harmony, and enjoyment. Susan and I are first cousins. She is currently a homemaker, mother of four children, wife to her husband, Jim, and a free-lance writer.

We have written this book for you.

Joe S. McIlhaney, Jr.
April 1985

# Acknowledgments

This book is evidence of the truth of the proverb, "Plans fail for lack of counsel, but with many advisors they succeed" (Prov. 15:22, NIV). The counsel from many people, given to me over a period of many years, made it possible for me to write this book. While I cannot name all those people, I do want to mention several who had a particular impact on the book.

My wife, Marion, and my daughters Lynne, Anne, and Caren, whom I dearly love and from whom I have learned so much, provided the stimulus and encouragement needed to begin and complete the book. Marion and Lynne patiently read and reread the manuscript, reacted with sensitivity and insight, and eliminated many of my biases.

Gill Harber, John Calland, Bill Lucy, Bryan Newberry, Dwight Dow, members of the Wednesday Morning Bible Study Group, were enthusiastic about this writing at just the right times, as were Ron Bower, Bill Crocker, Jim Saxton, Edgar Perry, and Bill and Beverly Counts. Members of Grace Covenant Church and Westlake Bible Church, and their pastors Dick Flaten and Sid Buzzell, sustained me with their prayers and moral support.

My associates—Marion Stahl, Robert Fulmer, Jo Bess Hammer, and Jeff Youngkin—the most competent and caring group of obstetrician-gynecologists I know, generously and graciously allowed me time to work on this book. Marion, Jo Bess, and Jeff read initial drafts and made important recommendations for changes. Carlon Dyess, Pat Edwards, R.N., Charlotte Matthews, and Libbie Seaton, my excellent medical office staff, perceptively reacted to thoughts and ideas included in this book. Charlotte willingly spent hundreds of hours typing and retyping chapters and assisted in all the associated details.

Barbara Law, John Clare and Ted Edwards, M.D., helped to get the book started. Tammy Long provided precise recommendations for change. Clyde Danks, M.D., gave invaluable assistance on the chapter on breasts. Louigi Monteleone, M.D., made comments and corrections on the sections on bulimia and anorexia nervosa. Richard Baum, M.D., reviewed the section on fetal monitoring and the status of the newborn; Boone Powell, Jr. critiqued the section on health-care organizations. Phil Mockford and Barbara Spielman gave expert legal assistance. St. David's Community Hospital allowed Teresa White to photograph the hospital scenes which illustrate the labor and delivery chapter. Mike Levy sent a steady supply of resource materials. Robert Fulmer, M.D., furnished the ultrasound illustrations.

Several physicians at Baylor Medical School, Houston, had a special role in my training, especially chairmen of the department of OB/GYN Charles Flowers, M.D., and Ray Kaufman, M.D. Drs. Robert Franklin, Warren Jacobs, Jack Moore, and Stanley Rogers profoundly influenced me as I developed as a physician. My patients have asked many good questions during the years I have practiced. They gave the impetus to begin, continue, and complete the book.

Betty De Vries, Associate Editor at Baker Book House, has been an enthusiastic, driving force behind the completion of this project and has orchestrated hundreds of tasks and deadlines.

All the information contained in this book could be here but without Susan Nethery's touch it would not have been very palatable. Her work was more than a job; it was a labor of love. I thank her for her superb writing style, her tenacity, and for the pleasure of working with her.

For years I have felt that God wanted me to write this book, and it took God's supernatural influence in my life and schedule to make the dream a reality.

# Introduction

## You and Your Doctor

Throughout your life you will find it necessary to make decisions about your health, and sometimes these decisions will be matters of life and death. How will you make them? On what information will you base your choices? Will you have access to the knowledge you need at the time you need it? How will you know if your physician's advice is correct?

Consider for a moment some of the decisions you may already have had to make: Should I take birth-control pills? Is taking hormones after menopause a good idea for me? Is a hysterectomy really necessary for me? Am I too old to have a baby?

These are but a random sampling of some of the potentially life-changing decisions with which today's woman must deal. And, if you are like the majority of people, you must often base your decisions on inadequate information. Friends give you their opinions, but are they objective and factual? Newspaper and magazine articles may seem to have the answers, but are they comprehensive and accurate? Your doctor makes recommendations, but is he or she up on the latest information—and does he or she have biases?

If you have ever had to ask yourself these questions, this book is for you. The next time you have a question about your total health, I hope you will be able to find the answer—quickly and easily—within these pages. I hope, too, that after your physician suggests a course of action, you will look in this book for a "second opinion," to compare what he or she says with what other physicians think.

If you have a "bad" physician—one who is poorly informed, money-hungry, inflexible, too busy to talk to you, thoughtless, rude, prejudiced toward certain procedures, or who suffers from a doctor/God-complex—your need for this book is obvious.

If you have a "good" physician—someone you trust, who is fair and concerned for your welfare, offers options and alternatives, and tells you what you want to know—you *still* have a need for this book.

A good doctor will be using up-to-date and recently developed drugs and treatments that are new to you. This book will help you to understand those innovations. He or she will explain a procedure or use a word that—because of its unfamiliarity and/or your state of mind—may not stick in your head once you are out of the office. This book will help you recall what was said and perhaps clarify the physician's explanation. Even a good doctor is not always or instantly available for consultation. This book is.

Physicians often become frustrated because they find it difficult to explain medical situations and terminology to people who have limited medical knowledge. Patients are suspicious of physicians when they are bombarded from all sides with conflicting opinions and ideas. They have trouble knowing whether their doctor or the other information is correct.

The problem is a real one. Whether the lack of trust is based on the doctor's inability to communicate or on the patient's inability to understand, the problem is there and, this book addresses that dilemma.

## Selecting a Doctor

There is no handy ten-item checklist to use in finding the right doctor for you. Granted, books and magazines may have some tips for evaluating a doctor, and well-meaning friends can give you personal reactions. But a doctor/patient relationship is a private, sensitive area. It is your responsibility to be an informed, cooperative patient. Assuming your doctor has technical expertise and is well-trained and competent, you also have the right to be treated with honesty, compassion, and respect. An informed patient and a dedicated doctor can successfully combat, minimize, or alleviate almost all health problems.

Some of the basic factors involved in selecting and evaluating a doctor are discussed in this section. Search for a doctor you can trust and feel comfortable with, one you like and respect.

---

**1** **How can I establish good rapport with my doctor so that I am comfortable with him or her and feel free to discuss concerns?**

Communication can be a serious problem between physician and patient. Doctors usually feel a problem exists because patients do not ask enough questions of them and their staff. Patients usually feel doctors do not tell them the things they want to be told. The following suggestions may be helpful to minimize or alleviate a communication problem:

Find out if your doctor has a patient-information booklet available. It would probably include information about services, fees, office hours, and procedures. Be sure to read it and keep it in a handy place so you can refer to it.

Be straightforward and open in asking about fees. Disagreement or misunderstanding about fees is one of the major problems between patients and doctors. Physicians' fees are generally preset. The receptionist knows the prices, and you can ask before seeing the doctor what a certain service will cost.

Do, however, give your doctor a chance! It may be that he or she is quite willing to work with you on financial problems. You will certainly never know unless you discuss it together. One doctor I know has a patient who pays him a dollar a month for a procedure that he did on her. Although it will take her about twenty years to pay the total fee, he is satisfied with the arrangement and

does not even send her a bill. Most doctors will do this or, if they are aware that a patient has serious financial problems, will not even charge for a service if they know that the patient is diligently trying to get a job, for example. Problems develop when patients stop communicating with their physicians about bills. If you say nothing and just stop making payments on a bill, your doctor will assume that you are trying to avoid payment. If you need to stop paying on a bill for a few months for financial "breathing room," you should call your physician's office and let the bookkeeper know. Communication does a world of good.

Realize that your doctor may have personal quirks and idiosyncrasies, just as you do, that you may have to accept and work around. Don't expect your doctor to change medical or office policies to accommodate you. Talk about it together, but don't expect or demand change. It would probably be better to change doctors than to create friction that would make a good doctor/patient relationship impossible.

If you are intimidated by your doctor, or if you cannot remember everything you wanted to ask when you are in the office, make a list. A truly caring doctor will want to provide the answers you need concerning your medical care and will certainly want to know all the symptoms and problems you are experiencing to make a correct diagnosis.

If you are having obstetric care, be sure to get definite answers to the questions most important to you before you progress in your pregnancy. If there is going to be a conflict, it is better that you change doctors early rather than late. Such questions might include whether or not the doctor does home deliveries, what is his or her attitude toward "natural childbirth," if fathers are allowed in the delivery room, and so on.

If you are continually unhappy with your doctor and this is a real problem to you, change doctors. Unfortunately, some doc-

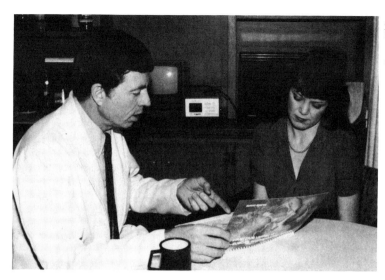

Communication between doctor and patient is vitally important.

tors do overcrowd their schedules, some do feel that certain patients cannot understand a clear explanation when it is given to them, and others do forget that a patient is not only paying for services rendered but also for time and information. Obviously a doctor will not always have the same amount of time or be in the same frame of mind each time a patient is in the office. A patient has to be flexible enough to understand that most doctors work on tight, unpredictable schedules. If, however, your doctor is consistently "short" with you, never attempts to explain a situation or diagnosis, and makes you feel as if you are taking up his or her valuable time, find another doctor.

Remember, what you are seeing the doctor for today may be minor but tomorrow's problem may be an emergency or major operation. If you must have surgery, is this the doctor you would want operating on you? If not, now is the time to change.

You should know the answers to the following questions whether you are a long-standing patient or a new one. If your physician does not have a patient-information booklet, ask the receptionist or other office staff.

What are the office hours?

When is the doctor in the office to see patients?

Does the doctor see patients by appointment or as they come in?

How do I reach the doctor?

What doctor (or doctors) are on call when my doctor is not available? What is the call schedule?

Is there a nurse I can see when the doctor is out of the office?

How often does the doctor like to see patients for routine examinations?

What obstetric or gynecologic problems does the doctor not take care of?

When will I be billed by outside professionals, such as a pathologist, radiologist, and so on?

When I call the office with a question, who will talk to me—the doctor, nurse, or someone else?

What is the usual charge for an office visit? A phone call? A prescription?

Will I be billed for charges, or must I pay at the time of the visit?

This is not an all-inclusive list, but it gives you an idea of the basic information you should have. I know of no physicians who would not willingly and eagerly provide this information to their patients.

You will also want to evaluate carefully your doctor's personality, views, and ethics. In all of these areas you should feel comfortable and compatible with him or her. If you have reason to question your doctor's level of training and knowledge or think he or she is not well organized, change doctors.

If you have any reason to suspect that your doctor is not ethical, change doctors. Physicians' ethics and morality cannot be isolated to one area of their lives or just to certain patients. If you know that your doctor has lied to you or to other patients, he or she has an ethical problem. If you know that a male doctor has become sexually involved with his patients, he obviously has a moral problem. If you know that the doctor has been charged with fraud by the IRS or by insurance companies, for example, or has been convicted for misuse of drugs, that same immorality may cause the doctor to be dishonest with you. In any of these cases, I would suggest that you switch doctors. This does not include a doctor who you believe has had an occasional error in morality or judgment, but one who is a flagrant violator of common ethics and morality.

It takes a great deal of personal discipline and integrity to be a good physician. It is too easy for a doctor to recommend an operation that is not really necessary, or to do a C-section instead of waiting two or three more hours for a normal delivery that would make him or her late for a tennis match. Doctors whose immorality and lack of integrity are publicly known (assuming that knowledge is accurate), are not as disciplined and ethical as they should be, and this can affect their medical judgment as they care for you.

If you want to be medically cared for in a way with which your doctor disagrees, don't get mad—change doctors. Do not try to educate your doctor or change his or her perspective. It will only cause tension and anger between the two of you. If you are unsure about the doctor's opinion in a matter that is important to you, ask directly.

Some patients want more communication than others, and your doctor should communicate to you the amount of information that you want to know. If your physician is not a good communicator, and you are a patient who wants a great deal of information, you should change doctors. If you try to force your doctor into more open and detailed communication, you are probably not going to do anything but cause frustration and friction between the two of you.

There are great variations in what physicians charge for their care. In our community, for instance, there is one doctor, not a gynecologist, who charges one thousand dollars more for a hysterectomy than any gynecologist I know. If you are uncomfortable about your physician's fees, you should call other physicians' offices and ask how much they charge. If your doctor is a great deal more expensive than others, then you can decide whether or not you want to change doctors. Higher charges do not necessarily mean that a doctor is better trained or better qualified to care for you.

I have known doctors who would dismiss a patient from their practice if that patient got a second opinion or even asked for one. If your doctor is one who objects to your getting a second opinion, he or she probably has something to hide or is insecure. You would be better off changing doctors.

Second opinions are much more common than they were in the past. Some insurance companies will not even pay for a surgical procedure unless the patient has two opinions about its necessity. I encourage people to get a second opinion any time they want to, whether they are my patients or patients of another doctor.

**2   Does it really help to change doctors? Don't they all band together and make decisions about medical care?**

There is no "medical union" whose rules doctors have agreed to obey. The American Medical Association has no program for telling doctors what to do, except to encourage sound ethics. Its energy is directed primarily toward lobbying governmental representatives. Besides, only about 50 percent of American physicians are members of the American Medical Association.

As far as "banding together" goes, it is highly unlikely that this could ever happen, because it is almost impossible to get even two doctors to completely agree on anything! The independence that gets physicians through the long, arduous medical training they undergo would prevent their integrating their knowledge that much.

Your physician is basically an independent person. Most doctors are probably well motivated, and they are most likely keeping up with modern medical advances and are quite competent to care for you. But, remember, you are competent too. You can understand what your doctor has to say if he or she will go to the trouble of explaining it in nontechnical terms.

**3   Is it possible that physicians and pharmaceutical houses do not want some medical situations to change, such as finding a cure for cancer, because it would hurt them financially?**

While doctors are not perfect, as a group they are intelligent, well-meaning, and concerned for their patients' best interests. There is no conspiracy of physicians to continue expensive medical therapy instead of accepting techniques that would cure, nor to continue particular medical policies and care that are outdated.

I read a statement recently in a non-medical organization's publication that urges physicians to use nutritional therapy to cure cancer. This group says:

> Incredible, isn't it? A forty percent to sixty percent link between nutrition and cancer—over twelve hundred Americans dying of the disease every day—and the medical establishment wants to "study the issue for ten more years." Why, you ask? Why such a promising area in cancer research and treatment given only token support by the medical establishment? I'll tell you why! From the doctors who treat cancer patients—to the pharmaceutical companies who make chemotherapy drugs—cancer is a multi-billion dollar a year industry. But, cancer prevention and cancer control through nutrition don't make money.

Statements of this type are also made concerning doctors. In most cases there are proper, valid, logical reasons for a doctor's opinion, and most doctors are not too eager to abandon tried and true procedures for every exciting new concept or treatment that comes along, nor should they be.

A patient's welfare is the primary concern of the overwhelming majority of physicians. Most doctors will listen to new, up-to-date information on providing better care for patients, and all will be happy beyond words when a cure for cancer is found.

**4   What new changes in medical care are being made available to patients? How do they affect my choice of health care professionals?**

Currently there are many sweeping changes in medical care. Changes are occurring so rapidly, in fact, that both you and your doctor may experience culture shock!

At the present time, particularly in larger cities, the most significant decision you might have to make is whether or not to join a health plan offered at your place of employment, as opposed to continuing to consult the doctor you have gone to in the past. The following situations are common.

The plan available at your place of work may be an HMO (health maintenance organization). If you join it, your health care will probably be less expensive than if you and your family continue going to the physicians that you have been using.

There are drawbacks, however. Many HMOs require that you see a general practitioner instead of a specialist, whether or not you want to do so. If the general practitioner thinks you should see a specialist, he or she will refer you to one. In the meantime, you may spend some frustrating hours with a less-experienced doctor when a specialist could have gotten the problem cleared up quite quickly. Also, HMOs may be less personal in their care than your own private physician.

One word of warning I have concerning the start-up of a new HMO in your community is that it will usually hire young, inexperienced physicians. The group is then without the older, seasoned physicians necessary to balance out a medical group. Because of this, I do not recommend joining a newly formed HMO immediately unless you have no other choice. Even then, talk to people who have used the group before you make the switch.

Another option sometimes available through your place of employment is an HMO provided by your personal doctors who have organized to compete with an "outside" HMO. For example, an insurance company came into our city, hired doctors and moved them here, and built offices for them. To meet this competition, our medical society set up a separate organization that any doctor already practicing in town could join. Consequently, most businesses here are now offering the choice of joining either the HMO brought in by the insurance company or the HMO which has been set up by the local physicians. The cost is about the same. The major advantage to patients signing up with the medical society HMO is that they may continue going to their original physicians. In this way they can go straight to a specialist when there is a need and be treated in their own physician's private office, even though they are HMO patients.

## Emergency Situations

**5  What should I know about emergency medical care and about obtaining medical care during non-office hours?**

Friends and patients frequently tell me of problems in obtaining adequate medical care for problems and emergencies that develop during non-office hours. Many of these problems develop as a result of not knowing how to take best advantage of the medical system and its resources.

There are three classifications of emergencies, and it is very important that you know the difference. If you go to a hospital emergency room with less than a true emergency, you will not only spend a great deal more money than is necessary, but you will also encounter a great deal of frustration and, possibly, anger. Emergency room personnel know almost immediately whether or not you have a true emergency, and they will take care of all true emergencies before they attend to you. This accounts for the many hours that are often spent waiting in emergency rooms. On the other hand, if you fail to go to an emergency room for proper medical attention for a true emergency, there may be serious, possibly fatal, consequences.

The three classifications of so-called emergencies are true emergencies, minor emergencies, and non-emergencies.

### A True Emergency

A true emergency is a life-threatening event, such as (but not limited to):

Serious injuries, unconsciousness, pain, and/or dangerous bleeding as a result of a motor vehicle accident

Lacerations that cause dangerous loss of blood

Life-endangering injuries

Sudden unconsciousness

Severe chest or abdominal pain (suffocating, oppressive chest pain located behind the breast bone can be very dangerous)

Sudden loss of blood flow to a leg causing it to turn white

Back pain that results from an injury or fall from a height

Hemorrhage from vagina, intestines, or lungs

In the event of a true emergency, go immediately to the nearest hospital emergency room. Transportation by ambulance or EMS will probably be necessary, and the personnel of such a service will notify the hospital that you are on the way. In other circumstances, someone should call the hospital or the doctor so that your arrival will be expected and the necessary staff and equipment will be on hand.

### A Minor Emergency

Although minor emergencies are not life-threatening, they are often frightening, are legitimately intolerable for very long, and do warrant a visit to a doctor. They do not necessitate an emergency room visit, except as a last resort.

A minor emergency often seems like a *major* emergency, however, especially if the person hurting is your child. The best thing to do, however, is to stay calm, determine the nature of the problem using the guidelines in this section, and proceed to get the medical care best suited to your needs.

These conditions are examples of minor emergencies:

Broken bones and severe sprains—hips, legs, and arms

Lacerations without dangerous blood loss

Abdominal or chest pain of moderate severity or less (chest pain of a sharp, sticking nature, even if in the left side of the chest, is usually not dangerous)

Fever

Inability to void

Insect bites and mild allergic reactions

If you determine that your medical situation is a minor emergency rather than a major one, call your doctor for advice as to the best course to follow. If you do not have a doctor, cannot reach your doctor, or the emergency occurs after office hours, follow the procedures outlined below.

### A Non-Emergency

Non-emergencies are neither life-threatening nor do they require immediate attention. They do, however, produce discomfort and pain (and often fear), and a doctor's advice should be sought.

Non-emergencies include:

Back pain

Mild abdominal pain

Minor sprains

Mild spotting and cramping during pregnancy

If you determine that the discomfort and pain you are having is of a non-emergency nature, you should call your doctor *if it occurs during office hours.* If it is after office hours, wait until the next morning to call.

### Medical Care During Non-Office Hours

If you do not have a personal physician, or if you are unable to reach your doctor, call a doctor you may have consulted for another problem (ophthalmologist; ear, nose, and throat doctor; gynecologist) and ask for a referral.

If you have a friend who is a physician, ask him or her for a referral.

If you have never seen a doctor in the town in which you now live, call a doctor from the town in which you lived previously and ask for a referral.

The doctor to whom you are referred will probably work you in, as all doctors expect that a few patients will need to be worked in each day.

In the event of a minor emergency after your doctor's regular office hours, call your health maintenance organization if you are a member of one. Otherwise, call your own doctor.

If you are unable to get the care you need, however, call a local minor emergency clinic and ask if they treat the kind of problem you have. If they do not, they will refer you to a physician or send you to a hospital emergency room.

Minor emergency clinics, available in many areas, are useful if you cannot otherwise obtain the services of a doctor. They are less expensive than hospital emergency rooms, and one normally does not have to wait to be seen.

In a complicated situation, however, they may not be able to provide the necessary care because they are essentially general practitioners of emergency medicine. They will often refer you to your own physician for an exam the following day.

Minor emergency centers do not generally have any continuing responsibility for your problem. Once they have seen you, they will expect you to receive ongoing care from another physician.

---

## An Afterword

I believe that the more access you have to facts and information, the better will you be able to understand medical situations. This clearer understanding will result in closer cooperation between you and your doctor and in better health for you.

Every attempt has been made to free the contents of this book of medical gobbledygook. Even difficult concepts and ideas can be explained to almost everyone if they are stated properly, in everyday language. Because medical information does not generally lend itself to cover-to-cover reading, I have chosen to use the above question-and-answer format throughout. These are questions my patients have asked me through the years and others that are only now being asked, in light of new advances in medical knowledge and procedures.

Each new chapter will begin with a concise but thorough survey of the information concerning one broad topic of female health concerns. This background material is followed by answers to specific questions in that area. Finally, some brief afterthoughts will serve as a postscript and commentary for the contents of the chapter.

There is a comprehensive index and a glossary of unfamiliar, new, or specialized words and procedures.

This book is not intended to take the place of a physician; it is an attempt to help you establish a better and more productive relationship with your doctor, so that your care will be the best that you can secure. A better-informed patient is a better-prepared patient. A better-informed patient will recover more quickly from—

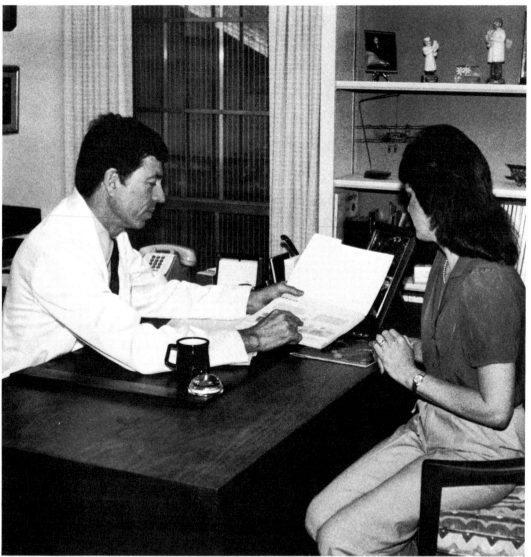

Teresa White

The more access you have to facts and information, the better will you be able to understand medical situations.

and be less frustrated by—the state of illness, uncertainty, or inde-cision she is experiencing.

If this book enlightens and entertains you, I will be pleased. If it assists you in acquiring information that will provide you with responsible, informed health care, I will have accomplished my goal. You *can* be a confident, knowledgeable woman, capable of making well-informed, sensible decisions concerning your body and its care.

# Part One

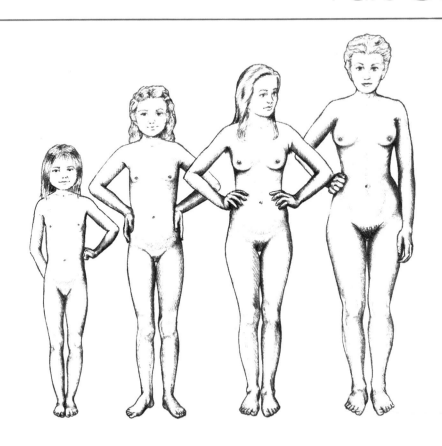

# The Female Body in Change

# 1

## Basic Anatomical Facts

Although most women today have reasonably good knowledge of the structure of their bodies, there remains a great deal of interesting and helpful information that the average woman does not know about her own physiology. Some of this is basic anatomy. Because patients frequently are confused about these anatomical facts, it is important to include some background information.

Lack of such knowledge can cause many problems for women. A woman cannot properly care for a body about which she is ignorant. A woman may be embarrassed by her sexuality if she is unaware of the beauty, purpose, and importance of her body's form and function. A lack of such understanding may also breed fears that only knowledge can dispel.

If you have never taken time to study your body, perhaps this is the time to do that. If you have felt uncomfortable in the past when reading books on this subject, or when looking at pictures of the female reproductive organs, perhaps the information in this chapter can help you shed that embarrassment. God made your body, including your sexual organs. If he had intended for your body to be secret and mysterious, he would not have made 50 percent of the bodies in the world just like yours!

You should not experience false modesty or embarrassment about using your God-created organs sexually. That's what they are for! All the babies ever born are a result of the proper use and function of these sexual organs. But God obviously designed them not only for procreation but for enjoyment—yours and your husband's. Being female is both a privilege and a joy. You have an amazing and fantastic body. As you learn more about its development, its intricate structure, and its function, you will be even more amazed at God's great creative genius.

Your body began changing the moment you were conceived, and it will continue to change until your death. There are four specific milestones in this process of change: birth, adolescence, the reproductive age, and postmenopause. These periods will be discussed in depth in the next four chapters. As you learn more about the parts of your body, you will see that although there is continual change, there are plateaus during these different phases.

One of the best ways to discover your body is to look at it! Reading books is enlightening, and looking at pictures is helpful, but the best way to learn is to look at yourself. Just looking can clear up many questions and misconceptions. For instance, some women (and some husbands) are unsure about the exact location of the clitoris, or about the relationship of the labia to the vagina, or about other specific aspects of a woman's body. The obvious solution is for such a woman to get a mirror, lie down on her back with her head propped up on a pillow, and study herself in the mirror. If she is married, she may want to include her husband in this most important learning session. If she is unsure about doing this herself, she should make an appointment with her doctor and have him or her identify the various parts of her visible anatomy.

This self-examination can involve more than just looking at one's external female organs. A plastic vaginal speculum can be bought at a drugstore and used at home. In this way with practice, and perhaps with her husband's help, a woman can see her vaginal walls and even her cervix. However, since this requires very good lighting and correct positioning, it might be more easily accomplished in a doctor's office. Doctors are not often asked to help in a learning process of this type, but most would be pleased to comply.

In addition to looking, feeling is a good way to learn about your body! I have often asked patients to explore up into their vaginas with their fingers, touching the cervix, feeling the vaginal walls, and so on. Most women are surprised to learn that there is so much room in there! Such personal exploration is useful when a young woman is learning to insert tampons and is also good preparation for using a diaphragm for contraception.

However, knowing about your body by looking and feeling is not enough. There has never been a time in the history of mankind

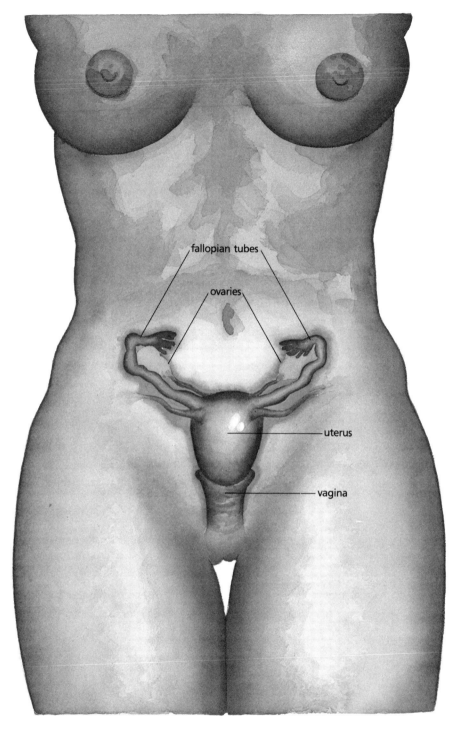

fallopian tubes

ovaries

uterus

vagina

**Reproductive Organs**

when both men and women have had as much sexual education and knowledge as they do today. You must also take care of your body properly and use it wisely. There is always a penalty for misusing and mistreating an intricate, finely tuned instrument, and your body is no exception to this rule.

A final step in the progression of knowledge leading to a more fulfilled life is a woman's acceptance of herself as she is. This self-acceptance involves not only acknowledging herself as a female but also joyfully recognizing the sexual and reproductive organs that she has been given. In the book *The Joy of Being a Woman* (New York: Harper & Row, 1975), Ingrid Trobisch speaks eloquently about self-acceptance. She says (pp. 1–5):

> Women will not be freed by trying to be like men. The challenge of liberation is more difficult. It is also more precious and rewarding. The key is that women accept themselves in their uniqueness as women.
> . . . The task of self-acceptance applies to men as well as women. It is hard work because it is not something with which we are born. We have to learn it during the course of life and the learning process is not easy. Just how difficult it is becomes clear when we ask ourselves the following questions: Have I accepted myself with my gifts? With my limitations? With my dangers? Have I accepted my age, my state of health, my economic situation? Have I accepted the way I look? Do I say "yes" to my marriage or to my being single? Above all, have I accepted my sexuality, my gender? Have I accepted my femininity or masculinity?
> A professional man in his best years was asked: "What is your secret? How do you live in such peace with yourself?" He answered without hesitation: "It is because my wife lives in harmony with herself." A husband can accept his masculinity only if his wife accepts her femininity. Living and accepting one's own gender is the greatest help which the sexes can give to each other. I cannot accept my partner unless I accept myself. I cannot love my partner unless I love myself.
> Jesus points to this secret when He commands us to love our neighbor not **instead** of ourselves, but **as** ourselves. In this way He makes self-love in the sense of self-acceptance the yardstick for our attitude toward our neighbor. . . .
> In Jesus Christ we are unconditionally accepted. In Jesus Christ we are unconditionally loved. In Him is the source from which any deficit of love in our lives can be filled. In Him is the source of power which can enable us to love and accept ourselves—and thus our neighbor. . . .
> Both men and women alike have to work on self-acceptance. It seems to me, though, that it is harder for a woman to accept herself than it is for a man.
> One reason is evidently in the conscious or unconscious discrim-

ination against women in our society. The other reason may be that in her life as a person, the woman is more related to her body than the man.

Her physical being is more complicated than that of a man. For him the sexual experience is simpler and more straightforward. His function in procreation is certainly less complicated than the event of conception. The experiences of a menstrual cycle, of pregnancy, birth, and breastfeeding remain foreign to a man. . . .

Therefore self-acceptance for a woman is to a greater degree physical self-acceptance. What she has to accept weighs heavier. Women who know themselves to be accepted by Christ are no exception in this struggle.

One reason why Christian women especially have such a hard time accepting themselves, including their bodies, is because the idea still prevails that the spiritual and mental areas of our lives are somehow closer to God, more pleasing to Him and more "Christian" than the physical realm. The Bible, which calls the body the "temple of the Holy Spirit" (I Corinthians 6:19), says the contrary: the more authentic our faith is, the more we are able to live in peace with our bodies. The more I succeed in accepting myself as a physical creature, the more I am able to live in harmony and peace with myself.

This is true also for my peace with God. I believe that the relationship I have to my body is reflected in my relationship to God. If I do not live in peace with my body, I do not live in peace with my Creator. . . .

I know from many conversations with women from all over the world that it is just their bodies which often make it difficult for them to accept themselves and to love themselves as women.

This is not only true for the married woman in the full flower of her years, but also the woman during and after menopause. It is just as true for the single woman and for the adolescent girl. Every woman has to learn anew in every phase of her life to understand what happens in her body biologically and to live in harmony with herself. . . .

It is a well-known fact today that spiritual conflicts can affect a person physically. But we have not yet drawn the opposite conclusion, namely, that physical conflicts can hinder and disturb our spiritual life. . . .

I agree with those women of today who underline the fact that "body education is core education. Our bodies are the physical bases from which we move out into the world; ignorance, uncertainty—even, at worst, shame—about our physical selves create in us an alienation from ourselves that keeps us from being the whole people that we could be."

(The portion of this last paragraph which is in quotation marks is from Boston Women's Health Book Collective, *Our Bodies, Ourselves—A Book for and About Women*, New York: Simon and Schuster, 1976, p. 13.)

The goal of this chapter is not pure anatomical knowledge, but rather anatomical knowledge as it contributes to self-acceptance. As we explain how the reproductive and sexual parts of a woman's body are put together, we will provide a general account of the physical makeup of the female body. This will be followed with a description of the different parts of a woman's anatomy, how they developed, and how they change through life.

## 6 What are my sexual and reproductive organs?

The sexual and reproductive parts of your body include the following: the vulva, the vagina, the uterus, the fallopian tubes, the ovaries, and the breasts. Our discussion of those major body parts will be broken up into several subtopics:

| | |
|---|---|
| vulva | vagina |
| mons pubis | hymen |
| labia | uterus |
| clitoris | cervix |
| vestibular bulbs | corpus of the uterus |
| urethral opening | fallopian tubes |
| Bartholin's glands | ovaries |
| anus | breasts |
| perineum | |

## External Female Sexual and Reproductive Organs

## 7 What is the vulva?

The vulva is the area of your body between your legs that can be seen when your legs are spread apart. This area serves as the entrance to the vagina, and the tissues here cover and protect the vagina and the opening from the bladder (the urethra). The vulva is comprised of several parts, which are discussed in the following questions.

## 8 What is the mons pubis?

The hair-covered area at the front of the vulva (mons veneris or mons pubis) is often called the pubic mound. This area is the most obvious part of a woman's genital area when she is standing or lying with her legs together; technically it is not part of the vulva but is its border on the front side of the body.

*Mons* is Latin for "mountain," and the protuberance of this area is obviously the reason for its name. This prominence is due to the fact that the pubic bone underlying this area is covered by a mound of fatty tissue. This fat serves as a cushion during intercourse, keeping pressure from the man's body from being applied directly against the woman's pubic bone.

It is normal for a woman's hair growth to be confined to the mons, but it is just as normal for it to extend up to her umbilicus (navel). If this hair growth does extend to the umbilicus and seems a problem to her, a woman can shave it off or use one of the depilatory creams that are available to dissolve the hair, using caution to avoid getting the cream on sensitive vulvar skin. This "excessive" hair growth is almost always due to "inheritance" from family members.

## 9 What are the labia?

The word *labia* comes from the Latin for "lips." A woman has labia majora (major lips) and labia minora (minor lips). The labia majora are the thicker lips on the outside of the vulva, and the outside margins of the labia majora mark the outer limits of what is considered the vulva. The labia majora have hair growth on the outside surfaces but not on their inner surfaces. The bulk of the labia majora consists of fat.

Inside the labia majora are the labia minora. These thin and sensitive folds of skin surround the entrance to the vagina. They have no hair growth. The labia minora of women who have not borne children are usually hidden by the labia majora; women who have had babies usually have labia minora that project beyond the labia majora. Even in virginal women, or in women who have not delivered babies, however, the labia minora may become enlarged by normal growth, or from manipulation or masturbation, and then project beyond the labia majora.

## 10 What is the clitoris?

The clitoris (klit'-or-is) is a small tube-shaped body of tissue that is about an inch long. If you spread your labia minora apart and look at the top (front) where they come together, just below the hair of the mons pubis, you will see the small hood that overlies the clitoris. The tip of the clitoris can normally be seen peeking out from under this hood. The urethra, or outlet of the bladder, is between the clitoris and vagina.

Since the tip of the clitoris is sensitive, gentle stimulation normally produces sexual arousal. The clitoris contains erectile tissue (tissue that can become engorged with blood) which causes the clitoris to become enlarged during sexual excitement.

Sexual stimulation of the clitoris does not always have to be directly applied to be effective. Because the labia minora form a hood over the clitoris, and because this hood is actually attached to the clitoris, movement of the labia minora will cause clitoral stim-

ulation. During intercourse, as the pressure of the man's penis causes movement of the labia minora, stimulation of the clitoris is produced, whether or not the clitoris is touched. The same results occur during foreplay when the man gently pulls and stimulates the labia minora. In this way he is stimulating both the labia minora and the clitoris.

It is interesting to note that once a woman has experienced orgasm and has established orgasm as her response to sexual activity, the presence of the clitoris is not absolutely necessary for achieving orgasm or sexual fulfillment. Consequently, if a woman develops a growth that requires surgical removal of the clitoris, she can continue to have satisfactory sexual responsiveness.

## 11 What are the vestibular bulbs?

These two accumulations of tissue are located under the skin just inside the labia minora (but still outside the hymen) on either side of the entrance to the vagina. These areas are important for sexual responsiveness and sensitivity. Like the clitoris, they contain erectile tissue that adds to the sexual sensitivity of the area. They also cause some protrusion of the vulva, making the vaginal tract longer during intercourse.

## 12 What is the urethra and where is the urethral opening?

The urethra is the tube through which urine flows out of the bladder. While lying on your back and using a mirror, the urethral opening or "meatus" can be seen just above the vaginal opening and just below the clitoris. If you spread your labia minora and look above the vagina, you can see the slightly puckered, vertical slit that marks the urethral opening.

# Female External Genitalia

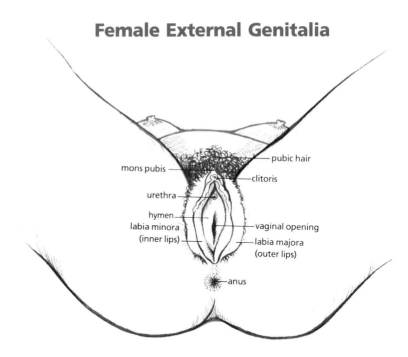

- mons pubis
- urethra
- hymen
- labia minora (inner lips)
- pubic hair
- clitoris
- vaginal opening
- labia majora (outer lips)
- anus

Because the urethra is located so close to the vaginal entrance and is therefore in the path of sexual stimulation, bladder infections connected with intercourse are fairly common. The urethra is very short. As the penis is pushing back and forth near the opening to the urethra, germs can enter the bladder through the urethra. Also, friction against the urethra and the urethral opening during intercourse can cause irritation of the urethra and burning during urination, even when there are no germs and infection involved.

## 13   What are Bartholin's glands?

There are two Bartholin's glands (vulvo-vaginal glands), one located on either side of the vaginal opening. Each has an opening on the surface, just outside the hymen and inside the labia minora. The glands produce mucoid, a slippery secretion. Although they probably secrete a small amount of mucus

all the time, during sexual excitement they produce a significant amount of mucoid material for lubrication. Abscess of the Bartholin's glands and Bartholin's gland cysts are fairly common among women. (See Q. 676–678.)

## 14   What is the anus?

The anus is located at the rear-most portion of the vulva. It is not actually part of the vulva but marks its rearward border. The anus is the opening at the lowest portion of the intestinal tract; it is from the anus that stool leaves the body. External hemorrhoids (dilated blood veins) often occur around the anal opening. Anal or rectal sex refers to the man's penis entering the rectum through the anus instead of being inserted into the vagina.

## 15   What is the perineum?

The perineum consists of the muscles that underlie the skin of the vulvar area. It is these muscles that keep the intestines from falling out of the body. It is also these muscles that are in part responsible for keeping the vagina from turning inside out. Finally, it is these muscles that a woman exercises when she does "Kegel's exercises" to tighten up the vagina and give better support to the rectum and bladder. (See Q. 703, 704.)

When doctors speak of the perineum being cut or lacerated, they are generally talking about the perineal body—the area under the skin that is between the anus and the vagina. It is through this perineal body that an episiotomy is done to prevent tears that often occur during delivery. When these tissues are cut or torn, they must be sewn back together. This repair prevents the vaginal opening from gaping open after healing and also helps keep the vaginal tissues from prolapsing (falling) outside the vagina.

## 16   What is the vagina?

The vaginal opening is below (behind) the urethra and above (in front of) the place where the labia majora and minora come together in front of the anus. The vagina is basically a tube about three and one-half inches long, and its walls are made up of three different layers. The first is a delicate lining called a mucous membrane. Next is a thin layer of muscle, and the third layer is strong connective tissue which provides most of the strength of the vaginal walls.

The vagina is normally closed and does not contain air, but if a woman has had several children her vagina may tend to gape open, allowing air inside. This is normal and is in no way harmful.

When a woman is in a standing position, the vagina points back up toward the upper part of the buttocks. This is why the vagina does not normally turn inside out; pressure from the abdomen tends to push the vagina back against the backbone and not down toward the outside of the body.

The vagina has three primary functions. First, it accommodates the penis during intercourse and, in so doing, receives the semen, providing it access to the opening of the uterus for sperm penetration. Second, the vagina serves as an important part of the birth canal through which a baby is delivered. Finally, the vagina serves as an outlet for the menstrual flow. It also provides a convenient place for tampons to absorb that menstrual flow, allowing most women to avoid the inconvenience of external protection.

Some women wonder whether their vagina is large enough for intercourse with a man who has a relatively large penis. The vagina is quite capable of stretching enough to allow intercourse, no matter what size the penis is. If a baby's head can get out through the vagina, then a man's penis can get in!

The front wall of the vagina is in contact with the urethra and the bladder, separated from them by only thin layers of tissue. The back wall of the vagina is in contact with the rectum, and, again, only thin layers of tissue separate them. The upper vaginal lining is continuous with the lining of the cervix (the mouth of the uterus). The cervix projects about an inch into the upper vagina.

Normally, a woman cannot see her vaginal walls without a speculum. However, if she has had children and her tissues are fairly relaxed, she may be able to observe these walls. To accomplish this she must use a mirror. Sitting with her legs spread apart, she must push as though she were going to have a bowel movement. In so doing, it might be possible to see the front and back walls of her vagina bulging down toward the opening as the labia spread apart.

Occasionally, with marked relaxation of the vaginal tissues, a woman will feel a bulge of tissue, about the size of a golf ball or a tennis ball or even larger, from her vagina. A woman with this problem needs to be checked by her physician. The problem of vaginal relaxation is not just relaxation of the vaginal tube itself. It is as much a problem of the organs surrounding the vagina (the bladder, rectum, and uterus) collapsing in on the walls of the vagina as it is of the stretching of the vaginal tissues. (If you have a problem with vaginal looseness, see Q. 699–704.)

## 17   What is the hymen?

The hymen is a ring of mucous membrane just inside the labia minora. If you are a virgin, you cannot see your vaginal opening without spreading the labia minora apart. Even then, your vagina will look almost totally closed because of the hymenal membrane.

Occasionally the hymen may be so thick as to require surgical incision to allow intercourse, although this is uncommon. Normally at first intercourse the hymen dilates by being both stretched and torn along its edges at several different points. After the first act of intercourse and for the rest of a woman's life, the small pieces of tissue that are the residual hymenal tags remain around the vaginal opening.

The normal openings that a woman has in her hymen before she starts having intercourse or using tampons can be of many different types. Most common is one central opening, but there can also be several smaller openings. Occasionally there is no opening at all. This, of course, prevents the flow of menstrual blood from the vagina. If a girl at the appropriate age has symptoms of menstruation (cramping, bloating) but does not have any menstrual flow she should see a physician immediately.

Tampons do not tear a girl's hymen since they are made small enough in diameter to go through the hymenal opening of a virgin. When a woman uses tampons for many months or years, the hymen does tend to stretch open a little. This is actually an ad-

vantage, since it allows the first pelvic examination to be more comfortable. A vaginal exam does not tear or break the hymen either, although it may stretch the opening a little bit. The instruments used are made small enough to allow a pelvic examination without damaging the hymen.

## Internal Female Sexual and Reproductive Organs

## 18   What is the uterus?

The uterus is made up of the cervix and the corpus. The cervix is the mouth of the uterus, and the corpus (or body) is the portion of the uterus that produces the menstrual flow and holds a baby during pregnancy. The uterus is normally about three and a half inches long and about the size of a woman's fist. About one-third of this length is the cervix, and the remaining two-thirds of it is the body of the uterus.

The bulk of the uterus is muscle, and the cavity of the uterus is lined by a delicate tissue called the endometrium. The outside of the body of the uterus is covered with the peritoneum, the lining that covers all the internal organs of the abdomen.

The uterus is located at the top of the vagina, between the bladder and the rectum. The bladder is attached to the lower part of the front of the uterus. When the uterus is removed at hysterectomy, or when a cesarean section is done, the bladder is normally detached from the uterus and pushed down. On the back side, the uterus is not attached to the rectum, but merely lies in front of it.

# 19  What is the cervix?

The cervix is the doorway of the uterus. It is through the cervical canal that sperm swim into the uterus for fertilization; it is through this opening that menstrual flow enters the vagina.

Since the mouth of the cervix is very small, it is impossible for a man's penis to go through it during intercourse, just as it is impossible for tampons to go through it. The cervix has the special capability, however, of expanding during delivery to allow a baby's head and body to leave the uterus. Even after delivering babies for many years, I continue to marvel at the tremendous elasticity of the cervix.

You can feel your cervix with your fingers by reaching inside your vagina. The cervix feels very much like your nose, with a small dimple in the middle! If you have had a baby, the size of your cervix may be more like that of your chin. The cervix feels firm, and the dimple in the middle is the opening into the uterus.

Although most of the uterus is muscle, the cervix is different, since 85 percent of it is made up of fibrous connective tissue. The lining of the cervix does not shed tissue and blood during menstruation as the lining of the uterus does, but it serves another important function: it produces mucus through which sperm can swim.

When the semen from a male's ejaculation comes in contact with a woman's cervix, the sperm swim out of the semen and into the cervical mucus. From there they go on up into the uterus. If the cervix did not produce this important mucus, it would be impossible for a woman to become pregnant in a normal fashion.

When your doctor does a Pap smear, he or she scrapes a spatula across the surface of the cervix, collecting cells for a pathologist to examine. The cervix is the second most common site of malignancy (cancer) in females, the first being the breast.

# 20  What is the corpus of the uterus?

The corpus of the uterus is its main body. There are three openings into the uterus: one from the cervix (at the lower end) and two from the fallopian tubes (at the upper corners on each side). The fallopian tube openings are quite small, but—with an instrument called a hysteroscope—a doctor can look through the cervix into the uterus and actually see them.

The uterus stays in position inside the body because ligaments are attached to various parts of the corpus. These ligaments, made of strong connective tissue that does not stretch easily, are much like the guy wires that hold television transmission towers in place.

Round ligaments come off the upper front part of the uterus on either side; uterosacral ligaments come from the lower back part of the uterus near the junction between the cervix and the corpus; cardinal ligaments come off the lower part of the uterus on either side, helping to support the upper vagina as well as the uterus; and utero-ovarian ligaments come off the uterus on either side, near where the round ligaments attach. It is from these utero-ovarian ligaments that the fallopian tubes and ovaries hang.

In spite of all these attached ligaments, the uterus is still a fairly mobile organ. After its enlargement and displacement during pregnancy, the uterus goes back down into the pelvis to resume its former position and smaller size when the pregnancy is over.

In past years, doctors have told patients that when their uterus was tilted back toward their backbone, they could experience problems with infertility, pain during intercourse, or some other "female" problem. This is untrue. One-third of all women have a uterus that is tilted back; two-thirds have a uterus tilting forward. It does not make any difference in which direction the uterus is tilting, and it is not unusual for a

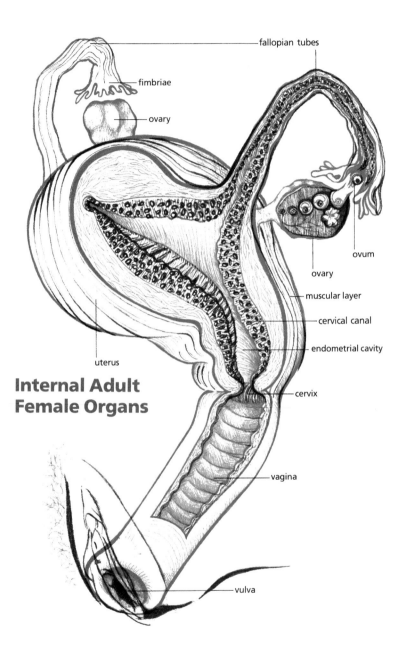

fallopian tubes

fimbriae

ovary

ovum

ovary

muscular layer

cervical canal

endometrial cavity

uterus

cervix

## Internal Adult
## Female Organs

vagina

vulva

woman to have a forward-tilting uterus one year and have it tilted back the next.

---

## 21   What are the fallopian tubes?

The fallopian tubes are two wormlike tubes attached to either side of the uterus at the upper corners. Each tube is about four and a half to five inches long.

The tubes serve one purpose—transporting eggs. Without the fallopian tubes, there is normally no way for fertilized eggs to reach the uterus. (See Q. 288–293.)

Fallopian tubes are muscle, the inner lining of which is a delicate mucous mem-

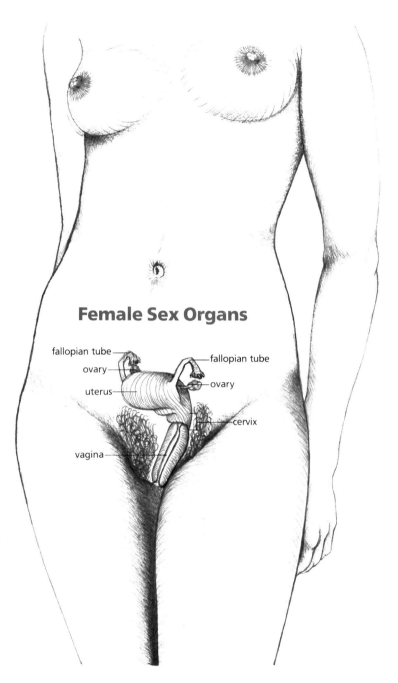

## Female Sex Organs

fallopian tube

ovary

uterus

fallopian tube

ovary

cervix

vagina

brane. The outer lining of the tubes is peritoneum, the same delicate lining that covers all organs inside the abdominal cavity.

The inner lining is specialized. The cells that line the fallopian tubes have little hair-like projections called cilia. The wavelike beating of these cilia produce a current of fluid which moves down the fallopian tube, providing the propulsion for the eggs to travel through the tube.

The outer diameter of the fallopian tubes

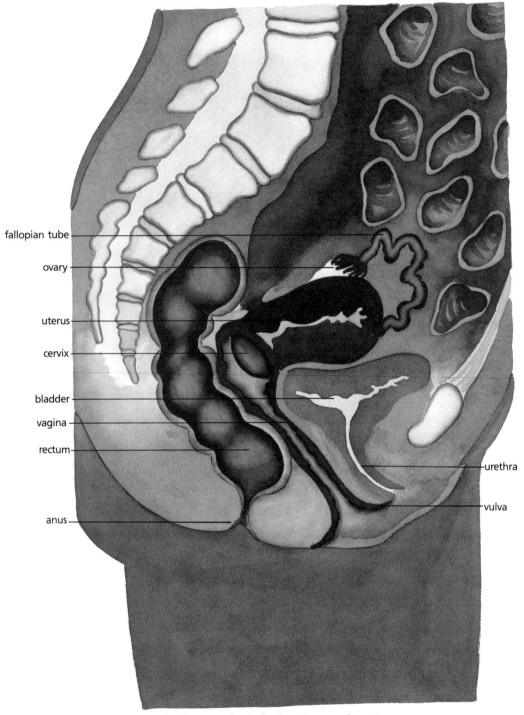

fallopian tube
ovary
uterus
cervix
bladder
vagina
rectum
anus
urethra
vulva

**Internal Adult Female Organs**

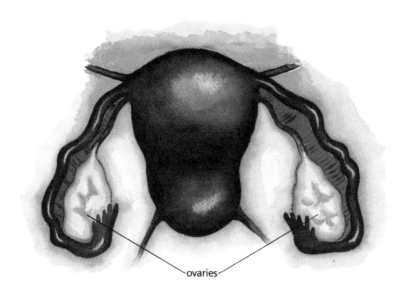

ovaries

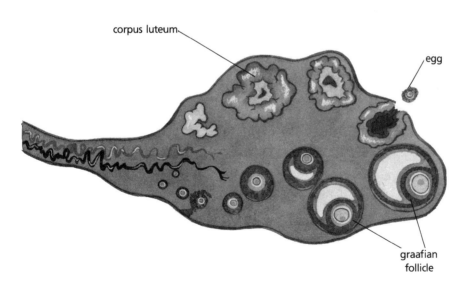

corpus luteum

egg

graafian
follicle

## The Ovary

is much like a medium-sized earthworm. It is soft and flaccid, like a relaxed worm! The inner diameter of the tube is very small, and the portion attached to the uterus is so small that only a thin thread could pass through. The outer half of the tube is only slightly larger.

At the tip end of the fallopian tube is a flowerlike structure called the fimbria. This acts as a "doorman," ushering the egg (ovum) from the ovary into the tube. The fimbria's "tentacles" are apparently capable of sensing from which part of the ovarian surface the egg is going to come; they move over that area of the surface of the ovary to pick up the egg as soon as it is exuded.

---

## 22   What are the ovaries?

Ovaries are the organs that are the source of a woman's eggs (ova) and her female hormones. They are located deep in the pelvis, behind the pubic bone. Incidentally, the ovaries are not straight back in your abdomen above your pubic bone; they are far deeper and lower in your body than that. I emphasize this because many women complain to their gynecologists about "pain in the ovaries" when, in fact, the pain they are having is much higher in the abdomen than the ovaries could possibly be located. This type of higher abdominal pain usually orginates in the intestines.

The ovaries, which are almond-shaped organs, are about one and a half inches by one inch by one-half inch. Upon examination, your ovaries, which are firm, can usually be felt by the doctor when he or she has two fingers in your vagina and the other hand feeling your abdomen externally. When your ovaries are pressed you will probably feel some pain.

Each ovary has two parts—the cortex and the medulla. The outer layer of the ovary is the cortex. In this layer are located all the eggs that a woman will ever have, since she is born with her entire lifetime supply. Each month as an egg ripens, it does so in a small cyst. As the egg matures in this cyst, ovulation occurs. Ovulation is the rupture of the cyst with consequent release of an egg.

The inner part of the ovary, the medulla, is responsible for producing female hormones, although not all the hormones are produced by the medulla. Some are produced by the cortex and some by the follicle from which an egg has developed.

As the blood supply to the ovaries comes from a woman's entire body rather than from the uterus, ovarian function is not affected by hysterectomy (removal of the uterus). The ovaries still continue producing normal amounts of hormones. The hormones produced by the ovary are poured into a woman's blood supply through blood vessels flowing toward the sides of the body and then go into larger blood vessels through which they spread to the rest of the body.

---

## The Breasts

---

## 23   What can you tell me about female breasts?

The female breast is the most visible part of female sexual and reproductive anatomy. As such, a woman's breasts are the focus of much attention, both cosmetically and sexually. Primarily, however, the female breasts were designed to nurture babies, and even in a society of meticulously prepared, nutritionally calculated infant formulas, mother's milk is still the best source of nutrition for a newborn infant.

Externally, the female breast is made up of a mound of tissue. In the center of this mound is the areola (areola mammae), a circular, darker colored area, approximately

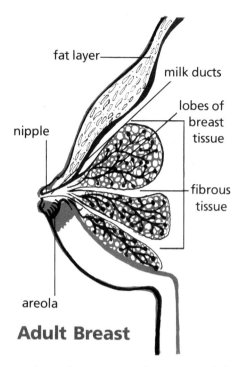

fat layer

milk ducts

lobes of breast tissue

nipple

fibrous tissue

areola

**Adult Breast**

one inch in diameter. In the center of the areola is the nipple. Around the nipple and in the areola are ten or fifteen oil glands called the glands of Montgomery. These glands, which are right under the skin, appear as small bumps in the areola. It is thought that secretions from these glands lubricate the nipple, helping to decrease the chance of dryness during nursing. There are also some small muscles in the areolar tissue that tend to make the nipple stiffen during nursing so that the baby can handle the nursing process more easily.

Sometimes a woman's nipples are elevated and sometimes they are depressed, or inverted. Either position is "normal," and nursing a baby is possible whether or not the nipple protrudes. Each of the fifteen or twenty milk-producing lobes of the breast empties via its own special duct through the end of the nipple. Before the duct reaches the nipple surface, however, there is an expansion called a *lactiferous sinus*. This widening of the ducts allows a sinus reservoir for the nursing process.

Beneath the areola and nipple is an area that is much softer than other areas of breast tissue, and this is normal. This softened area actually represents a decrease in the amount of supporting tissue because of the convergence in one place of all the ducts from the different portions of the breast.

A breast is essentially gland tissue; it is not just an accumulation of fat under a covering of skin. The gland portion of breast tissue is firm, just as a man's testicles are firm. This firm, normal breast tissue is covered over by fat. The fat is soft, and when one feels through the fat in palpating the breast, the nodularity of the lobules of breast tissue can be felt. When a woman is palpating her breasts and checking them for lumps, she is not particularly concerned with this firm, nodular tissue. She is looking for a more precise and well-defined marble of tissue that could represent a growth or a cancer.

The breast is supported by fascia, sheets of fibrous tissue which hold muscles and various body organs in place. The breast itself is contained in a fascial envelope that is attached to the chest wall to give the breast support. It extends down into the breast itself and separates the fifteen or twenty lobules of the breast from each other.

It is common for breasts to be asymmetrical (unequal in size or shape). Although a woman may be bothered by this, such asymmetry is quite normal and healthy. If a woman is quite upset about the problem, the solution is to have augmentation mammoplasty, an operation in which an implant is used to enlarge the breast. This is done by a plastic surgeon.

## How Female Organs Develop and Change

**24**  **How did my female organs develop?**

There are cells in an unborn baby's body that can develop into either male organs or female organs, as will be explained in chapter 6 on conception. Certain cells that could develop into female organs are suppressed if the baby is destined to be a male. Similarly, cells that could develop into male organs are suppressed if the baby is going to develop into a female.

If a baby is genetically determined to be a girl, the initially bisexual group of cells will develop into female organs. The group of cells that are definitely female will develop further and the cells that are definitely male will be suppressed. If the baby will be a male, the bisexual group of cells will develop into specific male organs. The group of "male" cells will be stimulated, while the group of "female" cells in his body will be suppressed. This process is internal until about the eleventh or twelfth week of pregnancy, when it becomes possible to tell externally whether a baby will be a boy or a girl.

The group of initially neutral cells are precursors to what are called "homologous structures" in the male and female. These homologous structures, which come from the same neutral tissue in the embryo, include the following groups:

| Female | Male |
| --- | --- |
| clitoris | penis |
| labia majora | scrotum |
| labia minora | corpus spongiosum (a tissue that encloses the urethra in the penis) |
| periurethral gland (small glands in the woman that empty near the opening of the urethra) | prostate |

The female organs that develop from the group of cells that are definitely "feminine"

(mullerian duct cells) are the fallopian tubes, the uterus, and the upper portion of the vagina. The organs in the male that develop from cells that are definitely "male" (wolffian duct cells) are the vas deferens, the epididymis, and the seminal vesicles.

The gonads or sex organs have their future determined by the chromosomes that the baby received at fertilization. This is discussed in chapter 6.

It is difficult to comprehend that all of the tissues that make up all of the organs of the human body develop from a single fertilized egg cell! This cell splits into several other cells, becoming a slightly irregular ball of cells by the fourth day of life. From that clump the cells develop into a flat, platelike disk by the seventeenth day of life. This small flat organism, about a twenty-fifth of an inch across, is made up of three different layers: the endoderm, the mesoderm, and the ectoderm. These three types of tissue give rise to either entire organs or parts of organs. The ectoderm, for instance, gives rise to skin; the mesoderm produces the muscles and skeleton and blood-vessel system; and the endoderm provides the lining of the intestine. Major portions of the genital organs come from the mesoderm, but part of the genital system comes from both the endoderm and the ectoderm.

The development of a baby is a miracle in itself. The young embryo starts as a small disk, elongates, and develops small prominences, grooves, and folds; a new human being develops from this amorphous accumulation of cells!

---

**25** How does the vulva develop in the fetus?

The vulva of the developing baby does not assume its characteristic appearance until the tenth or eleventh week of intrauterine life. This is the very earliest that the sex of a baby can be differentiated. The vulvar struc-

# Development of Genitalia in the Fetus

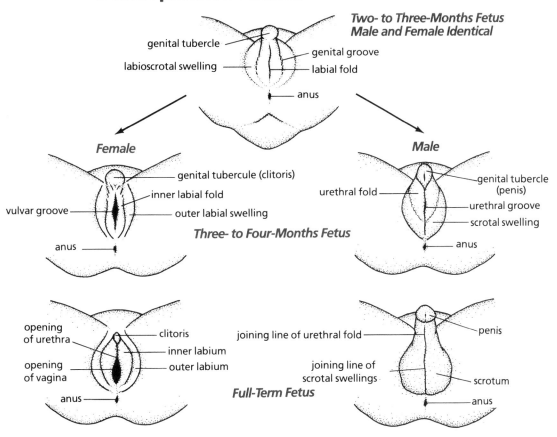

**Two- to Three-Months Fetus
Male and Female Identical**

genital tubercle
labioscrotal swelling
genital groove
labial fold
anus

**Female**

genital tubercule (clitoris)
inner labial fold
vulvar groove
outer labial swelling
anus

**Three- to Four-Months Fetus**

**Male**

genital tubercle (penis)
urethral fold
urethral groove
scrotal swelling
anus

opening of urethra
clitoris
inner labium
opening of vagina
outer labium
anus

joining line of urethral fold
joining line of scrotal swellings
penis
scrotum
anus

**Full-Term Fetus**

tures begin formation during the fifth week of embryonic life. At this time the genital tubercle—a small protuberance near the tail end, front side, of the embryo—first appears. This genital tubercle, and the labioscrotal folds that develop on either side of the unborn baby's body, evolve from the cloacal membrane.

During the sixth and seventh week of intrauterine life, the genital tubercle enlarges to form a protuberance which eventually becomes the phallus—either male or female. At this same time, a small groove on the genital tubercle represents the earliest sign of the urethra. Two folds, one on each side of the body of the fetus, represent what will be either labia or scrotum, and two depressions in the center of this area are the points where

the urogenital and anal openings are developing.

During the seventh and eighth weeks of life, the baby's vulva develops rapidly. The male phallus or the female clitoris forms and, at this stage and for several subsequent weeks, is large and out of proportion to the rest of the baby's body. The urogenital membrane ruptures, forming the first opening into the baby's body for development of the urethra (or, if the baby is to be female, both the urethra and the vagina). The anal membrane ruptures toward the end of the eighth week, making the first opening for the intestinal tract to the outside of the baby's body.

Growth during the next two or three weeks allows development of the distinctive female external genitalia called the vulva.

Maturing of these tissues allows the labia majora and labia minora to develop. The clitoris, which even to this point is large and out of proportion to the baby's body, does not keep pace with growth of the rest of the body and gradually assumes its correctly proportionate size.

## 26    How does the vulva look at birth?

At birth an infant girl's labia are swollen and prominent. The hymen is succulent (soft and swollen) and, because of its thickened condition, tends to protrude outward from the vagina. The swelling of the labia and the thickness of the hymen are a result of the hormones received from the mother, since these are female tissues and are sensitive to female hormones. Most of this thickness and prominence is gone after two weeks, and at six weeks all visible signs of stimulation from the mother's hormones have disappeared. In other words, although the newborn girl's clitoris is still a little large in proportion to the rest of the vulva, as the baby matures it assumes a more proportionate size.

## 27    How does the vulva develop from birth to puberty?

The infant and child's external genital tissues stay essentially in a "resting phase" until about the seventh year of life. If the labia are spread, the tissues will look thin, shiny, and somewhat red. This redness is due to the high visibility of blood vessels in the tissues because of their thinness; it is not normally due to infection.

Between seven and nine years of age the vulvar tissues begin to mature. The mons pubis (fatty pad over the pubic bone) begins thickening up. Genital hair will eventually develop over this thickening; by the time a girl starts her menstrual periods she will have a well-developed growth of pubic hair.

During this same time fat is deposited in the labia majora and, by the time monthly periods start, the labia majora are usually large enough to cover the opening to the vagina. Although the labia minora never become as thick as the labia majora, they lose their sharp edges during this time and become somewhat rounded and full. In addition, the clitoris loses its baby size and begins thickening and elongating.

During puberty, the vulvar tissues lose their redness and become pink in color. There is a great deal more moisture present, largely a result of the growth of the Bartholin's glands which provide lubrication for the vaginal opening.

## 28    What does the vulva look like during the reproductive years?

During the reproductive years, the vulvar tissues maintain the "mature" state developed at puberty. The description of the vulva at the beginning of this chapter characterizes the vulvar makeup of a mature woman during her reproductive life.

## 29    How do the vulvar tissues change at menopause?

The cause of any change in the vulvar tissues—from those of the young child to those of the mature woman—is the secretion of estrogen from the ovaries. When menopause occurs, or when the ovaries are removed by surgery, estrogen is no longer produced by the body in adequate amounts. When this estrogen deprivation occurs, the changes to a woman's vulva simulate in reverse those changes that occurred from childhood to maturity.

After the menopause, the vulvar tissues gradually become thinner; the labia majora and the mons pubis both lose a good deal of their fatty tissue; and the labia minora become thinner, sharper, and less prominent. As a result of this atrophy, the entrance to the vagina may become smaller and tighter and cause pain with intercourse.

The urethral opening can "turn out" and become very red. This change is called urethral caruncle. Doctors who are unaware of its significance may think it is a growth of some type, when it merely indicates a lack of estrogen. Application of estrogen cream will cause the urethral opening to build up, turn back in, and lose its redness.

The changes mentioned above can be reversed, or even prevented, if a physician prescribes that a woman take estrogen regularly from menopause on. Occasionally, however, estrogen taken by mouth is not adequate to keep the vulvar tissues strong and healthy; in this situation, vaginal estrogen cream can be used. It can be applied in the vagina and also on the vulva to ease any discomfort that might have resulted from menopause. (See chapter 5 on menopause for more information, especially Q. 279).

## 30  How does the vagina develop before birth?

The vagina in an unborn female baby is formed primarily from a group of cells called the paramesonephric (mullerian) ducts. Although called ducts, they are primarily solid strands of tissue. Appearing during the sixth week of life, these ducts tunnel into the tissues of this tiny female person until they lie where the fallopian tubes, uterus, and vagina will be. These ducts will become the lining of those three organs. The ducts must fuse together in the middle to form one vagina and one uterus. If they do not, various abnormalities can develop, such as two vaginas and two uteri, or various combinations of those abnormalities.

Duct fusion for development of both the

vagina and uterus is complete by the time the fetus is ten weeks old. During the fifth month of the pregnancy, the fetal "vaginal cord" begins degenerating in the central portion, and the vagina begins to develop a lumen (cavity). The last portion to open up is the hymen—the last barrier to the vagina's opening onto the surface of the vulva.

Please remember that this is a greatly simplified description of a process that as yet is poorly understood. For example, authorities now believe the vagina forms from more than one source of tissue, but they disagree as to which tissues.

## 31  How does the vagina appear at birth?

When the infant girl is born, the hymen and vaginal tissues are thick, moist, and luxuriant. This is a result of estrogen from the mother's body that stimulated the baby's tissues during pregnancy. Six weeks after birth this effect on the baby's female organs is gone. From that point the tissues stay thin, slightly reddish, and dry-looking.

## 32  How does the vagina develop from childhood to menopause?

Between the ages of seven and nine the girl's ovaries begin producing estrogen, causing her hymen and vagina to thicken again and the tissues to become softer and more moist. The tissues maintain that change as the female goes through her reproductive years.

When the ovaries cease functioning at menopause, the female again has only small amounts of estrogen in her body. This lack of estrogen allows the process to reverse, and the hymen and vaginal tissues become very thin (atrophic). Because of this thinness, they are a little more susceptible to certain infections. The thinness can also result in relaxation of the tissues, which may cause a woman to develop weakness of her bladder so that she loses urine when she coughs or sneezes. Additionally, thin vaginal tissue can cause pain with intercourse.

Many of these changes can be prevented or cured by the use of estrogen. This estrogen treatment can be given as a pill. If the tissues do not respond well to oral medication, vaginal estrogen cream can be put directly into the vagina three times a week (See Q. 29, 273, 279).

---

## 33 How does the uterus develop in the fetus?

The uterus develops primarily from the paramesonephric (mullerian) ducts. These ducts, one on each side of the body, come together and fuse in the middle part of the baby's body by the ninth or tenth week of fetal life. The lower part of these fused paramesonephric ducts becomes the vagina; the upper part becomes the uterus.

Just as the vagina begins as a solid cord of cells, so does the uterus; just as the vagina begins developing a cavity (lumen) during the fifth month, so does the uterus. During the fifth month the cavity formed inside the uterus develops a primitive form of lining that will mature further during the latter part of the pregnancy.

If the ducts do not come together and fuse in the middle of the baby's body, the uterus can end up as two separate half uteri or, if the lower part of the paramesonephric ducts do not fuse, two vaginas can develop. Although any combination of this type of abnormality is possible, why it occurs is unclear.

The cervix of the uterus itself does not open up until the twenty-second to the twenty-fourth week of intrauterine life.

---

## 34 How does the uterus develop from birth through menopause?

The uterus of a newborn is quite large in proportion to the rest of the baby girl's body.

This is due to the presence of the mother's hormones in the infant's body at birth. The uterus becomes smaller during the next five or six weeks as the mother's hormones leave the baby's body. No active change takes place in the young girl's uterus until she is seven to nine years of age. When she begins to secrete female hormones from her ovaries, the uterus starts enlarging.

During the reproductive period of life, a woman's uterus is about the size of her fist. Prior to seven to nine years of age, the uterus is about one-third that size and, after a woman goes through the menopause, the uterus becomes much smaller again. To a doctor, the uterus of a menopausal woman feels about half the size of a reproductive-age female. This uterine atrophy does not seem to affect the way a woman feels, or her sexual responsiveness.

---

## 35 How do the fetal fallopian tubes develop?

The fallopian tubes are formed from the paramesonephric (mullerian) ducts. They arise, one on either side of the body, from the portions of the paramesonephric ducts that do not fuse to form the vagina and uterus. The open upper end of the fallopian tubes forms as early as the ninth week of intrauterine life.

By twenty-four weeks (six months) of fetal life, each tube is a thin string of tissue, approximately one-half inch long. By the time of delivery, each tube is about twice that long.

Congenital abnormalities of the fallopian tubes are uncommon except for the open end not being quite as large as it should be. It is extremely rare for a baby to be born without fallopian tubes.

---

## 36 How do the fallopian tubes develop from birth through menopause?

The fallopian tubes of a newborn girl are stringlike, very thin, and about one-half inch long. During childhood they grow proportionately to the growth of the rest of the body but maintain their thin, stringlike appearance. It is the estrogen produced at puberty that stimulates the tubes to assume their adult size. This stimulation causes the inner lining of the tube to grow and thicken and to form the hair cells, or cilia, that are responsible for the current of fluid that flows through the tubes.

The fallopian tubes attain a length of about four and a half inches at maturity. Following menopause the fallopian tubes lose much of their bulk and seem to shorten a little. Just as the vaginal lining and the other genital organs become thinner and smaller, so do the fallopian tubes. This change in size of the fallopian tubes after menopause does not affect a woman's body in any way.

## 37 How do the breasts develop in the fetus?

A female's breasts develop from the skin, just as sweat glands and hair do. The breasts represent the most significant form of development of the human skin.

When the unborn baby is ten or twelve weeks old, there is an inward budding of the skin at about fifteen different spots around the nipple area on either side of the fetal chest wall. Then there is a branching of these buds. This branching stops quickly, and these early breast structures have no further development until about the age of nine to eleven.

## 38 How do the breasts appear at birth?

As with other estrogen-sensitive tissues in the female body, the newborn's breasts may show signs of stimulation by the mother's estrogen. One or both of the baby's breasts may be slightly enlarged, and there may be some thickened breast tissue under the nip-

ples. The baby's breasts may even secrete a little milk (a further result of the hormone stimulation from the mother), and there may be slight nipple pigmentation (a result of that same stimulation). All these hormone changes will normally be completely gone after a few weeks of life.

## 39 What changes in the breasts occur from childhood to menopause?

After the mother's hormones have been excreted from the baby's body and any breast stimulation that was present at birth has disappeared, no tissue is palpable under the small, infantile nipples. When a girl is between the ages of nine and eleven, estrogen from her ovaries stimulates the primitive breast tissue that was laid down before birth. This estrogen does the same thing to her breasts that it does to the rest of her body—it causes growth and change.

In this phase of maturation, the small breast glands show further growth of the ducts of the breasts. This will often appear as a small, round mound of flesh that is a flat, button-like nubbin of tissue located just under the nipple. This firm mound of tissue soon softens, and the girl will then experience further breast development. The amount of breast development by the time a female starts her periods varies a great deal. Some girls develop only small breasts by that time, while others have almost adult-sized breasts.

As the breasts reach their adult form, they undergo further development of the duct system. The ducts become longer and branch out in order to be prepared for pregnancy.

The estrogen causes not only breast tissue enlargement, but also causes a change in color of the areola and the nipples. The first change visible will be enlargement of the nipples. They become elevated above the areola, the darker area that surrounds the

# Development of Pelvic Organs from Birth to Menopause

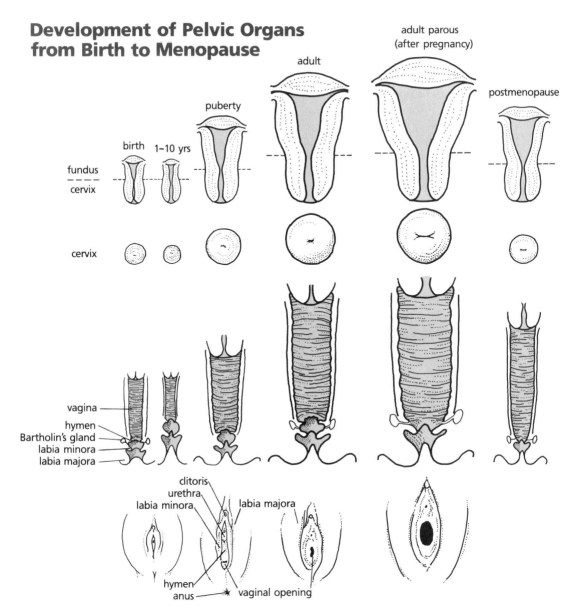

nipple. Soon after nipple enlargement, the second-stage branching of the ducts under the nipple causes thickening of that tissue, with further elevation of the nipple. The areola becomes a little darker and larger.

Because women have been trained to worry about any breast lump, and since girls occasionally form a small, flat, buttonlike disk of firm tissue under one or both of their nipples at this stage, many mothers panic. This small nubbin of tissue is normal, how-

ever, and is a sign that your daughter is developing normal, healthy breasts. Of course, it is just as "normal" for a girl not to have this nodule.

The areola thickens next. In 25 to 50 percent of girls entering puberty it almost seems to be swollen, with the appearance of a cap sitting on top of the developing breast. From this point on the breasts develop to their mature size. As previously mentioned, some girls' breasts have attained almost a mature size by the time they start their periods; others' breasts do not attain their adult size until much later.

Breasts in mammals develop along a milk line which exists on either side of the body from the underarm (axilla) the mons pubis. "Extra" nipples—and even extra breast tissue with nipples—can develop anywhere along this line. These accessory nipples exist in about 1 percent of all women.

Further changes in the breasts occur during pregnancy. The gland structure matures, enabling milk production.

After menopause the breasts become thin and atrophic and lose much of their size and shape. As the years go by breast tissue is often replaced with fat. Most older women still have visible breasts, though they may contain more fat than breast tissue.

## An Afterword

After considering the intricate development of a human being in the womb, we are reminded of Eve's words following the birth of Cain: "With the help of the Lord, I have brought forth a man." Eve obviously understood that bringing forth a child was not merely the result of sexual union—it also reflected the imprint of God's hand on that pregnancy. It seems to me that no other conclusion concerning the miracle of birth can be drawn by intelligent people than that drawn by the first mother at the birth of the first child.

Lesley Brown, the mother of the first test-tube baby sensed this too. She said, "I realize this is a scientific miracle, but, in a way, science has made us turn to God. We are not religious people, but when we discovered that all was working well and I was pregnant, we just had to pray to God to give our thanks. It seemed right and natural."

# 2

## Infant and Early Childhood Years

Healthy baby girls glow! They are pink and beautiful—and almost always normal. When they are not, they tug at our hearts even more since in some strange way, their femininity seems enhanced.

When something is wrong with a child, parents are shocked and worried. They envision entire futures ruined as they can see no way for a normal life for their child or themselves. They see a lifetime in a moment, and it overwhelms them. There is rarely a parent, in anguish and distress over a child's illness or pain, who has not cried, "Oh, that it were me instead of my child!"

It is wise for us as parents to remember that as a little girl grows, her problems are diluted by the thousands of days of her existence, making them easier for her to bear than we parents could have anticipated.

Sometimes we forget that God can teach both us and our children a great deal through problems and pain. Our family learned something about this a few years ago. Our oldest daughter, Lynne, developed pain in one foot and leg that persisted from ages fourteen through nineteen. The medical name of the problem was "reflex neurovascular dystrophy." At times the pain was so severe that she could not stand even the bedsheets touching her foot. Marion and I would often go into her room at night after she had gone to sleep and find that lonely foot sticking out from under the covers. Lynne was on crutches or in a wheelchair almost an entire year in junior high school. Finally, during her freshman year in college, an operation on some nerves stopped the pain.

None of us is bitter about those years. Lynne has told Marion and me that God used that problem in her life to bring her closer to him and to teach her lessons that she would not have learned otherwise. The rest of our family also learned a number of lessons during that time. We would not have chosen that particular way of learning, but since that is what came, we accepted it—and learned from our experience.

If you have a little girl who was born with, or has developed, a health problem, you can learn too. If you become bitter and succumb to angry despair, you increase the stress on your child and make the burden of her problems harder for her to bear. Bitterness on your part can also neutralize any lessons she and you might learn from the situation, and stunts any growth you might otherwise attain.

Fortunately, most little girls are completely normal. If you look around a hospital nursery, you will notice that almost all the babies are perfectly fine, in spite of all the things that *could* have gone wrong.

## Early Genital Health Care

**40** How do I know that my baby's female organs are normal?

There are several ways to ease your mind about this.

One way is to listen to the people who know. After her delivery, men and women who know all about newborn girls will examine your daughter carefully. The obstetrician checks her at birth; the pediatrician examines her thoroughly; and during her hospital stay her diaper is changed by professionals in the nursery who know how baby girls' bottoms are supposed to look! If all these people do not see anything wrong with your baby on the outside, she is probably normal on the inside too.

The second way to assure yourself concerning her normality is to examine her yourself. It will not hurt your baby one bit to roll her around and look her over. You can examine her closely. It is perfectly okay for you to put a thumb on either side of her perineum (the area between the vagina and the anus) and press downward and outward, spreading her labia apart slightly. Remember that for the first few weeks after delivery the hymen is thickened and enlarged and will protrude a bit from the vagina. If you see anything that you think is not quite right, check with your pediatrician.

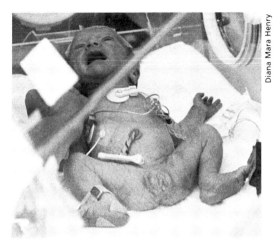
Newborn with normal genitalia.

## 41 What will happen if something does seem to be wrong?

If you or the doctor feels that something about the baby's body is not quite normal, the doctor will want to do further tests. It is important that proper studies be done promptly, since some problems can affect a girl's future health and fertility if not corrected when she is young.

## 42 What kind of examination would a doctor do if either of us suspect a female organ problem?

A doctor would want to do a complete exam of your child, including careful examination of the genitalia. If a child has an abnormality in one area, she may also have an abnormality in another part of her body.

If your daughter is an infant or small child, she will feel most secure and the doctor can best examine her if you sit on the edge of the examining table with her in your lap. In this way, you can hold your daughter's legs apart while the doctor gently examines her vulvar area. The doctor usually cannot do a vaginal exam in the office but he or she can pass a small catheter into the vagina to make sure that the hymen and vagina are normal. A rectal exam can be done to be sure there are no growths in the child's pubic area.

If you have a child between the ages of three and eight, she can lie on the examining table with her bent legs pulled back to her abdomen. The doctor may ask her to hold her own labia apart and then put his or her fingers on your daughter's to expedite seeing the area.

An eight- or nine-year-old child is usually big enough to lie on an examination table with her feet in the stirrups like an adult. Also, her vagina is large enough to allow a viewing instrument called a vaginoscope to be inserted into it. This little instrument allows the doctor to view the entire vagina and cervix in the office, with little pain to the child.

If a girl has begun having menstrual periods, she can be examined with a small speculum similar to—but smaller than—the instrument used for an adult.

Occasionally a girl must have a vaginal and pelvic exam and, because she is too young or too afraid, an office exam is impossible. A brief general anesthetic at the hospital or outpatient surgical facility can make such an exam not only possible but much less traumatic for everyone. Such an anesthetic in competent hands is quite safe. If your doctor feels it is necessary, I would recommend that you have it done.

## 43 Will a vaginal exam cause my daughter to "lose her virginity"?

No. Exams of this type done by gentle, caring doctors do no more than stretch the hymen a little. There may be a minute tearing of the edges of the hymen, which could result in a slight amount of bright red bleeding, but this is no more than might happen when a girl starts using tampons.

In any event, "loss of virginity" results from intercourse, not from a vaginal exam.

**44** **Will an examination of my daughter's vulva affect her emotionally?**

Yes, but most likely only in a positive way. A doctor should examine a girl's vulva just as he or she examines the other parts of her body during a general exam. Your daughter will accept this as routine when she is a young child because infants and young children seem not to have much sexual awareness. Having a vulvar exam established as a routine before she is sexually aware will help a girl grow into adulthood accepting her genitalia as a healthy part of herself. These exams can also establish a pattern of routine genital exams for your daughter. Not only will this help insure healthier adulthood, but it will help her accept future genital function and related activities such as periods, tampons, intercourse, and having babies.

**45** **How likely is it that problems of the female organs will develop in an infant or child before the age of fertility?**

Infants and children rarely have problems of the genital tract, but they can occur. When they do, they are minor problems about 90 percent of the time. Many problems that a child can have will be discussed in the following questions, but most of the disorders that occur in young girls have to do with vulvar or vaginal irritations or infections.

## Vulvar/Vaginal Problems in Young Girls

**46** **What vulvar or vaginal irritations or vaginal infections can occur in young girls?**

The four most common are:

infections from lack of good hygiene

venereal warts

herpes

impetigo

**47** **What is "good hygiene"? Why is it so important?**

"Hygiene" refers to practices and conditions conducive to sound health. "Good hygiene" means taking steps to maintain good health and to prevent disease.

Good hygiene, particularly of the genital area, is important for everyone, but it is especially important for females. Daily washing of the vulva with warm water and a mild soap (which contains no perfumes or other chemicals) is essential. If a girl or woman has a large amount of nonirritating, nonodorous vaginal secretions—a condition that can be totally normal—washing twice a day may be necessary. Careful drying is also important, and an application of plain (unscented) talcum powder is helpful in keeping the area from becoming irritated.

Careful washing between the folds of skin in the vulvar area is especially important if the baby or older girl is overweight. Gently spreading the labia and washing between them is also helpful.

## 48 What causes diaper rash?

Newborns have sensitive skin and need extra care. After a child is six months old, a diaper rash may be caused by ammonia. Diaper rash is usually alleviated by changing diapers more frequently, temporarily avoiding rubber or plastic pants that hold moisture against the baby's bottom, and cleansing the area thoroughly.

If the baby's bottom seems particularly inflamed and does not respond to careful hygiene, antibiotic ointments may be helpful. It may be necessary to change from detergent to soap for washing diapers or underwear, to stop using medicated or perfumed soaps, and to eliminate any medication that might be touching the baby's or young child's bottom. The baby may be sensitive or allergic to any of these things.

## 49 Is it normal for a girl to have some discharge from her vagina?

As a girl's ovaries begin producing hormones, vaginal tissues begin to grow and produce moist secretions. These secretions can collect on the vulva, and they are normal as long as they do not cause itching or odor. Of course, if a girl does not keep herself clean and dry, any type of moisture (normal secretions, swimming pool water, and so on) can cause her vulva to become irritated.

## 50 What infections might cause "abnormal" discharge?

Vaginal discharges can be caused by infection; itching, burning, and/or odor are the symptoms. Infections that can cause an adult woman to have a discharge can also cause a discharge in a child. These infections include fungus (monilia or yeast), trichomonas, gonorrhea, and gardnerella vaginitis.

(See section on diseases of the vagina in chapter 10.)

The germs that give a girl an upper respiratory tract infection may also at the same time give her a vaginal infection. Drs. Huffman, Dewhurst, and Capraro, in their book, *The Gynecology of Childhood and Adolescence* (Boston: Saunders, 1981), state that they frequently see vaginal infections develop from a week to ten days after the girl has developed a sore throat and cough.

Young girls often have pinworms, and these can cause vaginal discharge and vulvar irritation. In addition, germs that cause skin infections can sometimes cause vaginal infections with discharge.

Girls will occasionally put foreign objects into their vaginas. These can cause irritations and vaginal discharge and are usually discovered when the doctor checks for the cause of the discharge. Sometimes, but not always, they can be seen on an X-ray. (Plastic, for instance, will not show up on an X-ray.) When an X-ray does not reveal a foreign object, and there is strong suspicion that something is present, the doctor will need to look up into the girl's vagina. When the object is removed, the girl will usually stop having a discharge.

## 51 Can a child develop a vaginal fungus infection?

Fungus infections (yeast or monilia) can begin with poor hygiene, or they may start after a child has been given antibiotics. These infections cause irritation of the baby's bottom, producing a red rash, with isolated spots of red infection around the edges. A fungal infection can usually be stopped with applications of Monistat or Gyne-Lotrimin, which your doctor may prescribe.

If a child is receiving antibiotics frequently, these can cause the infections. It may be necessary to treat her bottom with fungus medication every time she takes the antibiotic treatments. If a girl is old enough, application of this medication into her vagina every night for a week may help keep fungus irritation from occurring again.

If a child is not getting well with proper medication, she should be checked for diabetes, since this can cause a persistent fungus infection.

## 52 What will the doctor do if my little girl develops a vaginal discharge or infection?

First the doctor will ask you how long the discharge has been present and what it is like. Next the child will be examined. If the doctor feels the secretions are not normal, he or she will try to determine what is causing them by testing for one of several problems.

*Pinworms.* The doctor will want you to press a piece of sticky, transparent tape against your daughter's anus with a tongue depressor and transfer the tape to a microscope slide. By looking at this preparation under the microscope, the doctor can see pinworm eggs if they are present. The entire family will need treating with Povan or Vermox if pinworms are found. If you are pregnant, do not use Vermox.

*Fungus infections.* The doctor can take a smear of the secretions, put potassium hydroxide on the smear, and see if fungus organisms are present. If they are not present, and the doctor still suspects fungus, a culture may be done.

*Trichomonas.* The doctor can look at the secretions under the microscope and see this organism moving. If so, treatment with Flagyl is necessary.

*Other germs.* To find these, the doctor will need to culture some of the secretions. Antibiotics by mouth will usually clear up these infections.

If after examination and treatment your daughter still has an infection (this is assuming good hygiene), the doctor will probably want to examine her vagina visually to see if she has put a foreign object in it. Such an exam would be done as described in Q. 42.

## 53 What are venereal warts? Can a little girl get them? How are they treated?

Venereal warts (condyloma acuminata) look like ordinary warts (somewhat firm protuberances). They are called "venereal" because they occur in the venereal (genital) area. Venereal warts are becoming quite common in our population. They are caused by a virus, and little girls can get them.

These warts are almost always caused by sexual contact. They can rarely occur without any sexual contact. You can generally assume that your child has been sexually active or molested if she develops condyloma. At least, investigate the possibility.

The best treatment for condyloma in young girls is the laser. There is a chance that the warts will return, no matter which treatment is used, but warts reoccur less often with the laser. For a baby or a young girl, laser treatment requires general anesthesia, but all the warts can usually be removed at one session. Podophyllum or freezing can also be used to treat such warts. (See Q. 1138–1145.)

It is important to have the warts treated because they can grow much larger if left alone and can cause irritation and discomfort. Surprisingly, though, such warts occasionally clear up spontaneously.

## 54 Can a baby or child get herpes?

Simple fever blisters (herpes virus type I) and true genital herpes (herpes virus II) can occur in a baby or child. Herpes I infections are not normally passed sexually. Herpes II infections generally are. Herpes II can be spread without sexual contact, however. If a child develops herpes II infections, she should be evaluated to make sure she is not the victim of sexual molestation.

If you have had herpes of your own vulvar tissues, you do not need to be terribly concerned about passing it on to your little girl. Using normal hygienic measures, such as washing your hands after touching your own vulvar area, should prevent passing the virus. It is probably best that you not bathe with your daughter if you have a herpes sore. Although unlikely, it may be possible to spread the virus in this way. Herpes virus has been cultured from hot tubs, and if it can remain alive there, it can remain active in a bathtub.

A small number of people do have the herpes virus in their mouths. If you have had mouth contact with someone who has herpes, and you develop a sore in your mouth, it would probably be wise for you to have your mouth and throat cultured to make sure you are not passing the herpes virus to your child when you kiss her.

Although herpes infections may cause burning and discomfort, they will not permanently damage a little girl's body. Like an adult, however, she may have secondary herpes episodes or recurrent outbreaks for many months or even years.

## 55 Can a young girl have impetigo of the vulvar area?

Yes. Impetigo, a contagious infection that affects the skin, is characterized by small blisters that break open and release pus. This can occur on any area of skin, including the vulvar area of a baby or young girl.

If your daughter develops an infection of her vulvar area, with several fluid- or pus-filled blisters that develop crusty scabs after maturing, she probably has impetigo. You should promptly see a physician for an accurate diagnosis and get some antibiotic oint-

ment and suggestions for care of this infection.

## 56 What other disorders might affect the vulvar skin of my baby or child?

Several conditions can affect the skin of the vulva. Unfortunately, some of them are difficult to diagnose. If your child has a condition of the vulva which your family practitioner or gynecologist is unable to definitely diagnose, it might be good to get an opinion from a dermatologist.

Conditions of this sort include psoriasis (rarely occurring before five years of age); seborrheic dermatitis (the same problem that causes dandruff); vitaligo (normal skin without its pigmentation, which appears almost pure white); lichen sclerosus; and molluscum contagiosum. (For the latter two problems, see Q. 660, 666.)

Although these problems sound serious, none of them are dangerous. Perhaps the greatest hazard would be for a doctor to overtreat the problems. In earlier days, for instance, lichen sclerosus was thought to predispose a person to cancer. We know now that it does not. It would be tragic if a well-meaning but uninformed doctor erroneously operated to remove your daughter's vulvar skin because of this problem!

## 57 Is it normal for a baby girl to have vaginal bleeding?

During the first week or ten days after birth, as her mother's hormones leave her body, a baby girl can have some "withdrawal" bleeding. This is normal and needs no evaluation unless bleeding begins again after the baby is two or more weeks old. If bleeding from the vagina occurs at any other time before puberty, she needs to see a doctor for an evaluation. She may have put a foreign object into her vagina or she could have a vaginal tumor, though such tumors are exceedingly rare. If she has other signs of sexual development plus vaginal bleeding, she may be having premature puberty.

### 58 My baby's labia seem stuck together. Is this dangerous?

No. This condition is called "labial agglutination" (labial adhesions); in this condition the edges of the labia minora have simply become stuck to each other because they have become inflamed. This situation is not dangerous, nor does anything need to be done unless the urethral opening is obstructed. This could cause a bladder infection.

Treatment, if necessary, is very simple. The doctor will probably give you a prescription for some Premarin vaginal cream or a similar estrogen preparation, to be applied to the vulva each night for a couple of weeks. This results in a thickening of the labia minora, allowing them to separate. Generally after separation the labia will not stick together again. If they do, the cream can be used again as needed.

## Vulvar or Vaginal Injury in Children

### 59 What can cause damage to my daughter's vulva or vagina? What should be done about such damage?

One of the things that can cause the vulva of a newborn baby to appear damaged is a breech delivery. When a little girl is born bottom first, her labia can be bruised. Although this looks serious, it is not dangerous. It should be left alone, as it will heal on its own.

Other causes of vaginal or vulvar injury are falls onto sharp objects, a beating or kicking or other physical abuse, and intercourse or rape.

### 60 What should be done if a young girl's vulva is injured by a beating or kicking?

Sadly, babies and young girls do get beaten. Physical abuse that involves a girl's vulva will not normally cause any significant lasting damage; a large bruise is usually all that occurs.

When a doctor examines a girl who has been abused in this way, he or she may want to admit the child to a hospital and give her anesthesia so that she can be examined and have any torn areas repaired. This is rarely necessary. The doctor will more likely merely advise the child's mother to put ice on the area for the first twenty-four hours and, after that, have the child sit in a tub of warm water for twenty or thirty minutes, two times a day. Additionally, if a great deal of tissue has been damaged, the doctor may want her to receive antibiotics. (For more information on vulvar or vaginal injury, see Q. 680, 718.)

### 61 Can a young girl be badly damaged by intercourse or rape?

A girl cannot ordinarily allow "voluntary" intercourse until she is at least eight years of age. From this age on, a girl's vulva and vagina by their own natural hormones, have been prepared to some extent for intercourse. So when a child in this age group has intercourse, the hymen is usually the only vulvar part that is torn. However, I once treated a patient who, though she was old enough to have normal menstrual periods, had the upper wall of her vagina torn the first time she had intercourse.

Even if a girl is raped, she rarely has significant tears of her vagina. These can occur, however, especially if intercourse takes place when she is younger than about eight years of age. If rape, incest, or other sexual abuse is suspected, the girl should be examined by a physician who can evaluate her in a caring and sensitive way. If forcible intercourse has torn the external area of a girl younger than eight or nine, the doctor may want the girl admitted to the hospital for an internal examination, fearing that she might have internal tears. Antibiotics may be prescribed to prevent her acquiring syphilis or gonorrhea from her attacker.

Adequate initial and follow-up counseling are needed to help overcome the emotional trauma of rape or other sexual abuse. Emotional support and help from her parents are vital for a girl who has been raped. Such parents should read extensively on the subject and obtain counseling for themselves and their daughter. Everything possible must be done to help the child overcome the trauma of the event and enable her to grow up with a healthy attitude toward sex. (See Q. 232–248 for a complete discussion of rape and sexual assault.)

## Female-Organ Abnormalities in Children

**62** **Can my daughter be born with her hymen closed?**

Yes. This abnormality is called an "imperforate hymen." It is usually detected immediately after birth when the doctor examines the baby girl's vulvar area. A bulging hymen just inside the labia minora is an indication that the hymen is closed. Secretions in her vagina are filling it, causing the bulging. These secretions indicate the effect of her mother's hormones on the little girl's vaginal tissues.

If the imperforate hymen is not detected at birth, it may not be discovered until the girl starts her menstrual periods. When this happens, abdominal pain, with no bleeding, will most likely occur. The pain is caused by the backing up of blood into the uterus, a condition which can affect her future fertility. It is best, obviously, that this problem be discovered early, when a girl is still a baby. A simple surgical procedure is required to open the hymen.

**63** **What other abnormalities of the female organs can be present at birth?**

The abnormalities of the female organs that a baby girl can have at birth are multiple and varied, and virtually no two persons are born with the same abnormality. Because of these two facts, an in-depth discussion of congenital birth abnormalities is not necessary here. Examples, however, are given below.

*Labia that are larger or smaller than normal.* This is a minor problem and is significant only if the labia are so oversized that they cause discomfort or embarrassment. In this case, a simple operation can be done to trim excessive tissue.

*Failure of the vaginal, urethral, and anal openings to form properly.* Occasionally openings for these important body parts may not develop properly. There may be no opening at all or they may open in an abnormal way. For example, the rectum may open into the vagina, or not at all; the urethra may open into the vagina; the bladder may open to the outside of the body. Many of these abnormalities are of major consequence and require specialized care.

*Other abnormalities.* Some of the other

abnormalities gynecologists see in patients are discussed in Q. 64–78.

## 64 What should generally be done if my daughter is born with an abnormality of her female organs?

If your doctor seems unsure of what to do and is not a specialist in this field, you should obtain a consultation as soon as you suspect that your child has such an abnormality. Don't delay proper treatment! A doctor should be able to lay out a plan of treatment that seems logical. In any event, delay out of ignorance should not be tolerated.

Further, I suggest that you get a copy of *The Gynecology of Childhood and Adolescence* by Drs. Huffman, Dewhurst, and Capraro (Saunders). Though this book was written primarily for physicians, reading it will give you much helpful information and advice concerning your child's abnormality. If you are unsure of your own physician's expertise in this area, you might write or phone one of the authors of that book for possible referral to a doctor in your area who is experienced in treating this type of abnormality.

## 65 Can a girl be born with two vaginas?

It is not extremely rare for a girl to be born with two vaginas (septate vagina). I have several patients with this abnormality.

The problem is not normally found until a woman is examined as an adult. The two vaginas generally cause no trouble, because one side or the other is usually large enough, not only for normal intercourse, but also for labor and delivery. Surgery is almost never necessary for this particular problem.

## 66 Can a girl be born with *no* vagina?

Occasionally a female infant is born with no vagina. Although a girl with this problem usually has normal labia, clitoris, and urethral opening, most of the time she has no uterus, and perhaps no fallopian tubes.

It is important to discover this problem early, so that the girl can be prepared for the fact that she will need to have surgery before she can have intercourse—and for the obvious conclusion that she will not be able to have children.

Another reason for finding this problem early is that if a girl does not have a vagina, but does have a uterus, menstrual blood will form in her uterus when she begins her monthly cycles. With no vaginal passage, the menstrual flow will be retained in the uterus, causing both pain and damage to the uterus and fallopian tubes. In this situation, a vagina must be surgically formed if possible, in order to allow drainage of menstrual material.

Occasionally, even if there is a uterus present, it will not be normal. The cervix may be without a normal opening, also preventing the release of menstrual products from the uterus. A hysterectomy would be necessary in this situation.

Since the ovaries originate from fetal cells that are different from those that form the vagina and uterus, the ovaries are usually normal in this situation. If a hysterectomy is done, therefore, the ovaries are usually not removed and they continue to function normally.

## 67 What can be done to allow intercourse when a girl has no vagina?

There are several surgical treatments for developing a vagina for a girl who was born without one. There is also a simple technique used to form a vagina. The girl uses a plastic test tube and daily presses the rounded end against the "dimple" where her vagina should have opened. By doing this daily and for many months, it is possible in some cases to develop a vagina that allows totally normal intercourse.

The same thing can occur with "attempted" intercourse! I saw a woman recently who, unknown to her, was born with no vagina. She had been married several years and had formed a very adequate, "normal" vagina from the pressure of her husband's penis against the "dimple" where her vagina should have been! She consulted me because she had never had a period and had not been able to get pregnant. Previous doctors had not detected the fact that she was born with neither a vagina nor a uterus.

## 68 If a vagina is present, is it always normal?

The vagina can develop with narrow places along its length. Such constrictions of the vagina can cause pain during intercourse. This problem is almost never found during childhood. A gynecologist may discover the problem on a woman's first visit for a routine checkup or because she comes to the office complaining of pain during intercourse. Repair can usually be accomplished with simple surgery, although such surgery is not necessary unless the woman is having this pain with intercourse.

## 69 What abnormalities of the uterus can be present at birth?

The formation of the uterus and vagina occur in much the same way. The mullerian ducts come together in the midline, fusing and forming one organ. If the ducts do not meet and fuse normally, variations occur in the organs they form. If they do not come together in the midline to form a normal uterus, two uteri can develop. If one mul-

lerian duct forms properly, but the other one does not, a woman may have a normal half-uterus on one side (which will usually function normally even in pregnancy), with a small, poorly developed half-uterus on the other.

Occasionally when there is incomplete fusion of the mullerian duct in the middle, a uterus may look normal but have a septum inside. This is a partition down the middle of the uterus, dividing it into two compartments. Treatment of these problems is unnecessary unless a woman cannot become pregnant or has repeated miscarriages.

## 70 Can a baby be born part girl and part boy?

A baby may be born with external genitalia that are not completely one sex or the other. This condition is called ambiguous genitalia. Unfortunately, these babies are often incorrectly called hermaphrodites. (See Q. 76.)

A couple of years ago, an acquaintance slipped up to me at church and whispered that he had a friend who had a baby with abnormal genitals. He said that this father was told by the doctors that they could not tell whether the baby was a boy or a girl, implying to the parents that the baby was some sort of "freak." My friend wanted to know if I had ever heard of such a thing. Of course, I had. Although this sort of problem is unusual, it is by no means unheard of. When it does occur, it is very upsetting to the baby's family.

Abnormalities of this kind must be handled properly. It is a tragedy if a baby is born with this problem and, because of embarrassment, parents do not allow physicians to diagnose and treat the problem properly. If such a problem is managed wisely, the child can become a totally normal person emotionally and frequently can experience normal fertility and childbearing.

If your baby is born with abnormal-appearing external genitals, make sure that your doctor can outline a plan for evaluation and treatment. If the physician seems confused or unsure of what he or she is doing or is delaying the evaluation, it is vital that you have a consultant see your baby.

One way to evaluate whether or not your doctor is handling your baby's problem correctly is to know that a competent physician should be able to tell you by the time the baby is two or three weeks old that the baby should be raised either as a boy or as a girl. The doctor will form this opinion based on both the medical evaluation and on the appearance of the genitalia. It is important that the child will eventually be able to look like and function sexually as an adult male or female.

For instance, if the child's chromosome makeup is male, but the external genitalia are inadequate for male sexual function, the genitalia may have to be surgically altered—perhaps to form female genitalia that will allow normal sexual function. Hormone therapy, adequate family counseling, and careful follow-up help complete the "change."

Obviously there are some situations in which it will be impossible for the child to produce offspring when he or she is older. This makes it even more important that the child be enabled to function sexually as either a normal male or female, except for procreation.

Remember, a person's sexuality is partially formed by the attitudes of the parents toward the child as he or she grows. In spite of "opposite" chromosomes and genitalia, a child can learn to "be" what he or she is reared to become.

## 71 How might "ambiguous genitalia" look?

When a baby is born with ambiguous genitalia, three abnormalities usually exist: first,
an enlarged phallus (too small to be a normal penis but larger than a normal clitoris); second, folds of skin that are too large to be normal labia but too small to be a scrotum (there is usually a cleft down the middle that keeps the skin from looking like a scrotum); and finally, a urethra that empties neither at the end of the phallus like a male nor at the proper location for a female.

## 72 What causes ambiguous genitalia?

There are several causes of ambiguous genital abnormalities. These include congenital adrenal hyperplasia and drugs taken during pregnancy. (See the next two questions.) Occasionally abnormal genitalia are present along with other congenital abnormalities.

If your baby is born with ambiguous genitalia, you will need a physician who can evaluate your baby, clearly tell you exactly what the problem is, and explain to you the proper treatment for your child's problem.

## 73 What is congenital adrenal hyperplasia?

The most common cause of ambiguous genitalia is congenital adrenal hyperplasia. This is a condition in which the female embryo inside her mother's uterus produces an excess of a male hormone. This hormone causes her external genitalia to become malelike, but leaves her uterus, tubes, and ovaries normal.

When I was in medical school, I reviewed all the charts on babies who had been admitted to Texas Children's Hospital in the Texas Medical Center in Houston for problems of their female organs. Most of the babies with ambiguous genitalia were there because of congenital adrenal hyperplasia.

Surgery can usually correct the genital abnormalities caused by this problem and allow the girl to look normal, have normal sex as an adult, and be able to bear children.

## 74  What drugs can cause ambiguous genitalia?

Certain drugs given during pregnancy can cause a baby girl to have ambiguous external genitalia, although these drugs may not prevent the development of a normal vagina, uterus, tubes, or ovaries. The drug most likely to cause this change is Provera, but some birth-control pills have this potential. In addition, if a woman received testosterone (the primary male hormone) during her pregnancy, a baby girl would very likely be similarly affected.

Again, this problem can usually be corrected with surgery, enabling a normal sex life and normal pregnancies as an adult.

## 75  What happens when male babies develop female genitalia?

Babies can be born with a totally male chromosome makeup, but their bodies look and function like females. Every cell in their bodies is male, and they have XY chromosomes throughout. (See Q. 294, 295 for further information on chromosomes.) Three situations can cause this.

*Males who do not develop testicles.* In this situation, because of the lack of male hormones and the effect of their mother's hormones on their bodies, these male babies develop fetally as females and are born looking like girls. They have vaginas, uteri, and fallopian tubes, but neither ovaries nor testicles. Although they cannot become pregnant, they can live otherwise normal lives as females if they are given estrogen at the time puberty would normally take place.

*Males whose testicles do not produce normal amounts of male hormones.* Children can be born as males—with testicles—but still have ambiguous genitalia because the testicles do not produce normal amounts of male hormones during development. Whether these children are reared as males or females depends on how "abnormal" the external genitalia are.

If there is enough of a penis to function, it may be best to let the child grow as a male. If the penis is too small, it may be advisable to correct the problem surgically and allow the child to be reared as a female. When this is properly done, the child, though infertile, can grow up to have normal sexual intercourse.

*Males whose bodies cannot sense the presence of the male hormones they are producing (testicular feminization syndrome).* Sometimes a child has cells that are male, and undescended testicles that produce normal male hormones, yet the child's developing body is incapable of sensing the presence of these hormones. Such a child is born with a normal vulva and a short vagina, but there is no cervix or uterus. In adolescence the child develops normal breasts. This child will be sterile but will be able to function sexually as a normal female.

There are two things different about this particular problem. First, it often will not be discovered until the "girl" does not start her menstrual periods at the time puberty should occur. Second, there is some chance of such testicles developing a malignancy. There is also the chance that the internal testicles will increase their production of the male hormone testosterone at the time puberty would occur and cause this female-appearing child to develop some male body characteristics. Because of these potential problems, such testicles should be surgically removed when the diagnosis is confirmed, after secondary sex characteristics have formed.

## 76  What is true hermaphroditism?

A hermaphrodite is a person who has both testicular and ovarian tissue present in the body. It is very rare for a child to be born a true hermaphrodite. When this does happen, the external genitals are ambiguous, and there may be variations in the development of the phallus and the vagina. There can be a great deal of variation not only in the anatomy of a hermaphrodite, but also in the chromosome makeup of the body's cells. The situation is handled just as it would be with any of the other problems of ambiguous genitalia that we have mentioned. If the child is externally male and could be expected to be able to have intercourse with the existing phallus, "he" should usually be reared as a male. If intercourse as a male would not be possible and the child might function better as a female, then "she" can be reared as a female. Although she could not become pregnant, with proper surgical treatment and psychological counseling, she would grow and function as a normal person.

---

## 77  What abnormalities of her ovaries can a baby girl have?

It is rare for a girl who has an otherwise normal female body to be born without ovaries, but the ovaries can be underdeveloped. When a female child has ovarian development abnormalities (gonadal dysgenesis), her ovaries cannot produce eggs or estrogen. At the time that puberty should occur, such girls must be given estrogen by mouth.

There are three types of gonadal dysgenesis, and none of them would normally be detected before the age of puberty.

*Normal female chromosomes but poorly developed ovaries (pure gonadal dysgenesis).* In this situation, the girl would appear normal at birth and would grow normally until the onset of puberty. Then, because her ovaries cannot produce hormones or eggs, she would not start menstrual periods and not develop sexual hair or breasts. A laparoscopy (see Q. 908), would

show only streaks of white tissue where the ovaries should be. Estrogen would be given to help her develop breasts and normal adult sexual characteristics. The girl would function sexually in a normal way as an adult, but she would not be able to conceive.

*Abnormal chromosomes and undeveloped ovaries.* This is the most common cause of gonadal dysgenesis. This girl is missing an X chromosome (see Q. 294, 295). She has only forty-five chromosomes instead of the usual forty-six and her ovaries do not develop. Her chromosome makeup is written as 45X (normal girls are 46XX). This adolescent's development would be like that described above for "pure gonadal dysgenesis" but, because of the chromosomal abnormality, there would be abnormalities in other parts of her body. The most characteristic abnormality in this situation is webbing of the neck. The second most characteristic abnormality is shortness—the girl would probably grow to no more than five feet. Other less major abnormalities, such as color blindness, can accompany this chromosomal problem.

With proper care, this girl can function sexually in a normal way, but because her ovaries do not produce eggs or female hormones, she will be unable to conceive. She will need to be given estrogen at the time puberty would normally start.

*Mixed abnormalities of the chromosomes with ovaries almost totally undeveloped.* In this situation, "mixed gonadal dysgenesis," various combinations of chromosomes may be present in a girl's body. Occasionally there will be a Y-chromosome present, and in this case a girl may have external genitalia with some masculine changes at puberty. Most of these individuals would not be fertile but could be expected to function sexually as normal adults.

If a child has mixed gonadal dysgenesis with a Y-chromosome, the ovaries, which *are* present but almost totally undeveloped, have a 30-percent chance of developing a malignancy. Such ovaries should be removed early in the child's life. This is a complicated situation and requires expert care.

## 78 Do inguinal hernias occur in girls?

Although more common in boys, these hernias do occasionally occur in girls.

An inguinal hernia is a weakness in the wall of the lower abdomen, allowing a protrusion of the internal lining of the abdominal cavity—and sometimes containing portions of abdominal organs. It can be noticed when a child cries or is pushing down with a bowel movement. Such a hernia is seen as a bulge on either side of the body just above the pubic bone.

Occasionally a girl's ovary will drop down into the hernia sac. On examination of the hernia sac, a doctor would find this as a small, solid lump. About 3 percent of the time when such a mass is felt, it is present because the child is actually a male with pseudo-hermaphroditism, even though the external genitalia look totally female. Because of this possibility, chromosome studies may be indicated. Except for this problem, such protrusion of the ovary is not in any way dangerous.

A child of either sex who has an inguinal hernia needs to have it surgically repaired.

## The "Facts of Life"

## 79 When should I tell my daughter "the facts of life"?

Sex education for your daughter begins the day she is born and continues for the rest of her life—whether or not you say a word to her about sex. The quality of her sexual understanding will be greatly affected by you and your spouse. Your attitudes, opinions, and reactions to sexual matters will be noted by your child, and your views will become a part of her attitudes, opinions, and reactions concerning sex.

In this, as well as in so many areas of life, your actions will speak at least as loudly as your words. Without doubt, your words on this subject are vitally important—so it is best that your transmission of sexual information to your daughter be done only in conjunction with your own "right attitude." This sound approach, to be ultimately effective, must be evident from infancy.

## 80 How can I be sure that I have the "right attitude" about sex?

There is only one source to which mankind can go for the answer to this question—the Bible. The wisdom of generations is held between its covers. It integrates its discussion of sex into its discussion of all phases of life, giving sex its proper place.

Where else can we look for a proper understanding of the role of sex in the human experience? We cannot take Sweden as an example—the illegitimacy rate there increased when sex-education courses, which included contraceptive advice, were made compulsory. We cannot listen to Planned Parenthood, an organization willing to sacrifice the relationship of parent and child (an obviously necessary relationship for society's health) for the less important goal of providing contraceptives or an abortion. Homosexuality does not have the answer—a lifestyle which often involves multiple sexual partners and is such abnormal activity for the male human that the body responded with an entirely new disease, AIDS. Nor can we advocate "free sex," which teaches that a person cannot be fulfilled without total sex-

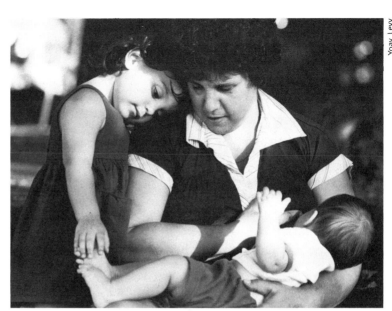

Take advantage of naturally occurring events around you to explain sexual development to your child.

ual freedom and ignores the growing prevalence of sexually transmitted disease.

In contrast to these sources, the Bible speaks with both authority and common sense about an entirely different approach for the role of sex in a person's life. Drawing from the Bible's wisdom on the subject of sex, I believe we can develop an effective plan for proper moral education of our children.

## 81 What guidelines do you suggest for the sexual and moral development of my daughter?

There are fourteen points that I advocate.

1. Beginning in infancy, treat your daughter's vulvar area as you would any other part of her body. Do not give the impression it is a "forbidden zone."
2. Don't make a big deal of it if your daughter touches or manipulates her vulva or clitoris. Children are curious and smart. They soon discover that touching their genitals brings pleasure, and it is natural that they will want to do it again. If your attitude is right and your explanations frank and open, it is unlikely that this will develop into something that will be an embarrassment in public or a problem of habitual masturbation. It is certainly appropriate to teach your child that some things are best reserved for "private occasions."
3. Don't entertain false and obsessive modesty around the house. If your child sees you or your spouse nude, accept it as a normal turn of events. I don't see any advantage, though, in family members habitually going about the house nude.
4. Use correct terms for sexual organs and do not hesitate about saying them aloud. This will show your child that her sexual organs are a normal part of her body—not something about which she needs to be ashamed.

5. Don't be embarrassed by her questions. Since sexual organs and sexual functions are a normal part of life, you should not be uncomfortable when asked questions about them. However, neither do you need to make your answers too complicated. If a five-year-old asks what a vagina is, she does not want to hear about the whole process of intercourse and childbirth. Gear your explanation to her level of understanding. Merely answer all questions in a straightforward, simple way. If you don't know the answer to a particular question, tell your child you will find it and tell her later.

6. Explain to your daughter the body changes that will occur and the normal functions she can expect. Your eight-year-old girl should know that she will start breast development, pubic hair growth, and menstruation so that she will not be frightened when these things come about. As she grows older, you should explain to her how intercourse is achieved, how pregnancy takes place, and how deliveries are accomplished.

7. Take advantage of naturally occurring events around you. The five-year-old daughter of a neighbor of ours asked her mother if there was any connection between the fact that her stomach had been large before the new baby came and now was smaller. This mother blew a great chance to explain some basic facts to the girl when she told her that there was *no* relationship between those two things! Actually, she blew a great chance much earlier. The little girl could have been encouraged to participate in the excitement of expecting a new baby by being allowed to feel the new baby kicking and mov-

ing in her mother's tummy before it was born.

8. Show your love for your spouse. When children see their parents exhibiting love toward each other and having physical contact (kissing, caressing, hugging), they will learn to associate the two in a positive way. This helps develop the attitude that physical contact between a man and a woman is associated with love.

9. Take your daughter with you for your annual physical exam. This can be a very positive aid in helping a young girl learn more about her own body. In doing this, she finds that the experience is not threatening, but is something that responsible adult women do. She can meet a physician who "takes care of Mommy," and she will learn that both doctors and the idea are "good." When my patients bring their daughters with them for their pelvic exams, the daughters accept the visit and the examining room without undue bewilderment and certainly without any fright.

10. Speak of having a baby as a miracle shared by a mother and father. This will emphasize the fact that conception and the growth of a fetus in a mother's uterus is a special thing and that the mother and father have an important role in its development. It is good to speak of "a mother and father" and not just of "a man and woman." This will help a child understand that the proper place for a baby's conception and birth is in marriage.

11. Continue with the pattern of discussing normal bodily events in a natural way as the girl grows older. For instance, when your daughter has learned that babies come from sexual intercourse, it is perfectly natural for you to explain to her that intercourse

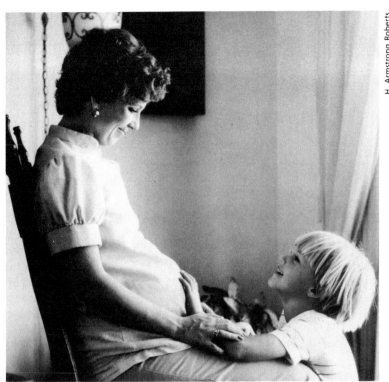
Allow young children to participate in the excitement of expecting a new baby.

does not always result in pregnancy—nor should it. A natural outgrowth of that conversation would be another conversation about contraception.

12. Teach healthy modesty concerning the body and its functions. Most girls become modest about the time they begin developing sexual hair and breasts. They begin closing the door when they dress or use the bathroom. Consideration of this sense of privacy will help your daughter understand that this is acceptable. At this point she will begin to understand why parents close the door when they dress or go to the bathroom. The right attitude in the home can help the girl develop proper modesty not only in her attitude to nudity but also in her approach to acceptable dress and behavior in society at large.

13. Use appropriate aids. There are a number of excellent books, and at least one good series of tapes that can help you with the sex education program for your child. (See Q. 86.) In addition, urge your church or any other organization that has moral values similar to yours, to conduct sex-education classes for the children from fifth grade through high school. This allows someone other than a parent to talk to your child about sex, and it is good for the entire group to receive similar sex information and therefore have a common level of knowledge.

14. Have good rules about television! A recent study of 450 sixth graders showed that 66 percent of them viewed sexually explicit shows at least once a month. Roughly 70 per-

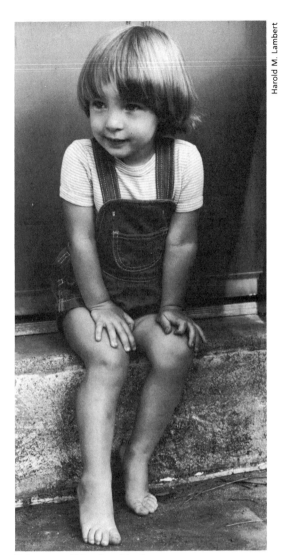

Enjoy your little daughter!

plete understanding of sexual anatomy and function and how sex is integrated into the rest of a healthy life, she will be able to make choices for herself rather than blindly follow the crowd. You will probably want your daughter to make her own decisions about how she handles her sexuality rather than doing things just because her peers do.

You want your daughter to be happy. Sex cannot be the sole source of happiness in a person's life. When a young person has been taught the facts of life from a purely physical perspective, that child may perceive sex as the ultimate source of happiness and may, therefore, continually be chasing an illusion.

Having sex fixed in a child's mind as being separate from the other parts of the human makeup—physical, emotional, and spiritual—denies what we know to be the true composition and total character of the human being. Out-of-context sex becomes intolerant, exploitative, and in the final analysis resembles nothing more than animal coitus. This approach to a person's sexuality can hinder a young person's development and may even destroy the possibility of a solid, permanent relationship in the future.

For a woman to be happy, she must integrate sexuality into her life as an important, but not the most important, factor. It is best to learn about sex from loving parents. And when sex is taught, it must be taught in the context of morality and love for it to assume its proper perspective. If this important subject is approached in that way, a child can become a mature, well-balanced person, proud of her body and prepared for the excitement and fulfillment of committed, loving sex with her spouse.

cent of these children said that their parents did not monitor the shows they watched. Common sense says that parental monitoring of television is absolutely necessary if we want to keep our children's perspective on sex appropriate.

## 82 Why is sex education so important?

Sex education for children is important for several reasons. If a child has a fairly com-

## 83 Why can't I leave my child's formal sex education to the "experts" in the classroom?

The main reason I believe parents should be responsible for their child's sex education is that their goals are likely to be different from persons who are teaching sex education in the classroom.

Parents should determine why they want to provide sex education for their child, because clarifying those goals determines what the child is taught. As an example, if my goal for my child is simply that she not get pregnant, all I need to teach her is where the sex organs are, what they do, and how to use contraception to prevent pregnancy.

If, however, my goals for my child are that she understand that her entire body is a special gift from God, something to be carefully maintained, and of which she need not be ashamed or have false modesty—and if I want her to know that sexual intercourse will be the most intimate form of communication between herself and her husband and one of the most wonderful things they do together—then the sex education I give her will have to be far more than just anatomy and contraceptive information.

---

## 84 Can sex education in a classroom setting accommodate the various goals of different parents and children?

It is my opinion that it cannot. There is much confusion and animosity surrounding the idea of sex education in a classroom, and I believe this arises from the efforts of individuals and groups with widely different goals, all trying to provide a uniform type of sex education for all children.

There are individuals and groups, for instance, who feel that no one should have any significant restrictions placed on their sexual activity, whether they are adolescent or adult. Sex-education courses designed by these people have the goal of teaching that all sex is "good" and no sexual activity is "bad," including premarital and extramarital relations, homosexual acts, masturbation, and adult-child sex. Although these goals may not be specifically announced,

they are nevertheless implied in the teaching.

When this type of so-called morality is subtly forced into my child's classroom, it draws a strongly negative reaction from me because my goal in sex education is that my children learn how precious and important sex is in the proper context, and that its expression in sexual intercourse is only for "at home, in a heterosexual marriage."

However, if I try to force my set of values into schools where the children of parents of another moral persuasion are attending class, they will react just as negatively as I do to theirs.

Because of this, I believe that formal sex education—except for a straightforward discussion of the *facts* of anatomy, the reproductive process, and sexually transmitted disease should take place only in an environment where the goals are clearly understood and where parents approve of the goals and voluntarily expose their children to the teaching.

---

## 85 What kind of sex education is most often taught in schools?

Unfortunately proponents of what I call "free sex" (for lack of a better term) hold sway in most school sex education programs. To quote Hans H. Neumann, M.D., from his article in *Medical Economics*, vol. 59, May 24, 1982, p. 35ff.:

> When I was on the medical advisory board of Planned Parenthood in the Long Island area of New York, two mothers fought strongly for the inclusion of sex education in their town's school curriculum. I supported them in their long struggle. Finally the course was offered. Barely two years later the same mothers urged even more strongly that it be withdrawn. They hadn't anticipated what its content would be or who would teach it.

I'm not opposed to providing students with basic information about anatomy, reproduction, venereal disease, hygiene, and contraception. But what we have now in many of our schools is far-reaching human-sexuality programs exploring such areas as masturbation, sexual techniques, homosexuality, and rape. The goal of reducing teen-age pregnancy has been all but lost in favor of "educating" students to achieve sexual adjustment. Instead of teaching young people how to avoid an unwanted pregnancy and its consequences, we're teaching them that the joy of sex is their human birthright.

To my knowledge, no scientific evidence exists that such courses have a positive impact on teen-age pregnancy rates. In fact, my own observation and research indicate just the opposite. When sex education became compulsory in Sweden, the illegitimacy rate, which had been declining, rose for every age except the older groups that had not received sex education. One of the three high schools here in New Haven instituted a comprehensive sex education course 11 years ago, and it's still being taught today by teachers with high academic qualifications. During this period, the other two schools offered little or no sex education. Statistics for the past seven years show that the high school with the broad-based program had a disturbingly high pregnancy rate, higher than those of the other schools.

Are there any logical explanations for this apparent failure? I believe there are quite a few.

First, coeducation classroom discussion about the joys of sex and sexual adjustment can easily become titillating. Sexual techniques, contraception, and self-gratification aren't usually discussed in social situations. Yet that's exactly what a high-school classroom is. These adolescents know each other well.

Dr. Mary Calderone, founder of the Sex Information and Education Council of U.S. (SIECUS), is an ardent advocate of sex education. In a recently published book, even she notes that masturbation is a private matter, not appropriate for living room discussion. Doesn't it follow that frank discussion of the topic is out of place in the typical high-school classroom?

One argument for comprehensive sex education courses is that "all the kids have sex anyway." Well, one recent study found that, despite a remarkable increase in sexual activity in the high-school age-group, half of all students in the U.S. are still virgins at the age of 16. By providing detailed information on human sexuality instead of limiting the instruction to basics, we may be encouraging rather than deterring earlier sexual activity. . . .

Teachers are human. They have their own beliefs. One sex educator may be an advocate of sexual freedom, while another may be an apostle of abstention. Still others may have personal leanings that they want to communicate to the class. It's a pretty big risk to take with our children. . . .

If we're going to continue to provide some degree of sex education in our schools, we should return to offering basic instruction in anatomy, reproduction, VD prevention, and hygiene. We should make our goal the reduction of the teen-age pregnancy rate, not the creation of a generation of sexually sophisticated adolescents. . . .

It's difficult to swim against the tide of education fashion. However, because parents and teachers are reluctant to appear out of touch with the latest practices, common sense is losing ground in many places.

Though I do not totally agree with Dr. Neumann's personal goals for sex education, I agree with the points he makes in his article.

---

## 86 What books and tapes do you think would be helpful to me in the sexual education of my child?

I recommend these tapes, study courses, and books:

**Cassette tapes.** Dr. James Dobson has an excellent series of tapes titled, "Preparation for Adolescence." He recommends that parents listen to these tapes with their children before those offspring enter puberty. Families that have used the tapes have found them helpful. The tapes may be obtained from most Christian bookstores.

**Study courses.** The Institute in Basic Youth Conflicts is a course taught all over the country on a regular schedule by Bill Gothard (Box 1, Oak Brook, Illinois 60521). Thousands of people have attended this course and found it extremely helpful. While it does not give specific lessons about sex, it does set the stage for young people who are in the mid-teenage years to understand the proper place of sex in their lives. Gothard's perspective on life is from the Christian viewpoint, but even those who do not accept his faith will find his insights extremely helpful for them and their children.

**Books.** The Concordia Sex Education Series is an excellent aid for sex education for children of all ages. The first book in the series, *I Wonder, I Wonder,* is for kindergarten through third-grade children; the last book, *Life Can Be Sexual,* is for high schoolers. The other books span the ages between

these two. I believe parents should make these books available to their children (Concordia Publishing House, St. Louis).

Another helpful book is *A Beautiful Gift: Your Awakening Sexuality* by Joanne De Jonge, intended to be used by ten- to twelve-year-olds in either a Christian-school classroom or home setting (Baker Book House).

*A Parent's Guide to Christian Conversation About Sex* by Irwin J. Kalb (Concordia Publishing House), is the fifth of the six-book Concordia sex education series mentioned above. Kalb has included an extremely thorough annotated book list.

*Sex Is a Parent Affair* by Letha Scanzoni (Regal Books, Glendale, Calif.) is an excellent source book.

*A Doctor Talks to Nine to Twelve Year Olds* by Marion Lerrigo and Michael Cassidy, is published by Budlong Press Company. It is available from many physicians, and has an accompanying booklet for parents.

*The Joy of Being a Woman—And What a Man Can Do* by Ingrid Trobisch (Harper & Row) is an exquisite book about a woman's sexuality for any woman from mid-teenage through menopause.

## An Afterword

In concluding the discussion on the female as a baby and child, I wish to stress again that most children are born completely normal. My purpose in mentioning some of the abnormalities that can occur is not to frighten parents but to enlighten them. Parents need to know that there is much that can be done for a child with birth defects.

Even as parents should not be fear-stricken over the possibility of having a child with abnormalities, neither should they be terrified of failing to provide "perfect" sex education for their child. As with any other aspect of childrearing, all parents can do is their best. If they do that they cannot be "failures" as parents.

Enjoy your little daughter! Her infancy and childhood will soon be a memory, and the innocence and charm of those special early years should be treasured. True, there is great responsibility—awesome, in fact!—in parenting a child. But the rewards are equally great, and there is nothing more precious than the trust and love of a little girl!

# 3
# The Adolescent Years

One of the most exciting experiences for my wife and myself has been living with our adolescent daughters during their preteen and teenage years. We have enjoyed (not always, but usually!) watching them grow from the cute little girls they were to the confident, emotionally healthy young women they are now. Those years have not been without a measure of the pain that accompanies any change, but with God's help we made the passage successfully—and the results are well worth all the effort!

An adolescent is a person in the process of growing from childhood to maturity. Obviously this involves many changes, and change is almost always a mixed blessing, bringing pleasure and pain, elation and depression, joy and sorrow. The metamorphosis of a child into an adult is not accomplished in isolation, however, since the process dramatically involves those closest to the adolescent.

Many parents live in fear of both the adolescent years and the adolescents themselves. For most parents this anxiety is unwarranted. First, fear of the teenage years is not usually necessary, since a significant parent-child communication gap does not have to exist. Neither is fear of the adolescent herself usually reasonable, because most adolescents respect their parents if those parents have earned such respect and trust. Further, the physical changes and dilemmas of adolescence that often perplex and dismay both parent and child can usually be handled smoothly with factual knowledge, proper guidance, sound medical care, and a commitment on the part of parents to be good parents.

This chapter includes medical information and guidance covering many of the major problems that may confront an adolescent female.

## The Changes and Timing of Puberty

### 87  What exactly *is* adolescence?

One dictionary defines adolescence as "growing from childhood to maturity." This growth involves every aspect of the child making that passage. For a young girl it includes:

*Emotional growth.* This is the time during which a child changes from a dependent person to an independent and mature adult.

*Physical growth.* During this period a child's physical structure becomes an adult body, the most obvious sign being the changes in contour and size.

*Sexual growth.* The changing of a girl's body into that of an adult woman includes and involves the vital change from being incapable of pregnancy to, in most cases, being fertile and able to bear children of her own.

### 88  What is puberty?

Puberty refers to the period during which a girl's body changes from being unable to bear children to the state of being fertile. The physical changes in her body during this transition involve two things—the growth of the sexual organs of the body (such as the vagina, uterus, and breasts) and the start-up

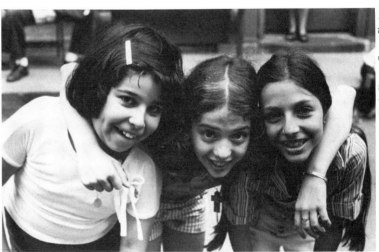

Adolescence: growing from childhood to maturity.

of the sexual hormonal cycle that precipitates the release of eggs (ova) and prepares the uterus to receive fertilized eggs for the pregnancy process.

Physicians divide puberty into different growth stages. These processes, with their medical names, are shown in the accompanying chart.

Puberty is considered complete when a girl has developed regular menstrual cycles with regular ovulation—and is, therefore, normally fertile.

---

## 89  When does puberty usually begin?

For as long as records have been kept, physicians have been noting that girls are beginning their menstrual periods earlier and earlier. It is estimated that the average beginning age for menstrual cycles, for girls in industrialized countries, has been four months earlier for every ten years that passes. This has been true for about the past twenty-five years, the time period during which accurate records have been kept. This decrease in the age of the onset of periods is only in developed countries, probably because of better nutrition.

Studies indicate that when a girl's body composition shifts into one containing a higher proportion of fat, she is more likely to start her menstrual periods. This shift occurs earlier in well-nourished children than

in children whose overall nutrition has been poor. It has been noted by researchers that children on the whole have grown significantly larger during the past eighty years, just as the age at which girls start their menstrual cycles has been decreasing.

If puberty in a female begins before the age of eight, it is considered to be early or precocious. On the other hand, if a girl has not begun breast budding by the age of thirteen, she probably is experiencing abnormal sexual development. If she has not begun menstruating by the age of eighteen, she may also have some abnormality of sexual growth. Although these ages are not absolute and a girl who is outside them may be totally normal, chances are that there is a problem.

It normally takes about four and one-half years for a girl to develop from the earliest signs of puberty (usually budding of breasts) to having regular menstrual periods. This time span may range from one-and-one-half to six years, so a mother or her child should not get upset if the development is progressing slowly. It is important that the mother and child realize that not only the age at which these things occur, but also the pattern may be different from the stated "norm." For example, it is not uncommon for a girl to develop pubic hair before breast budding, and axillary hair may not develop until after a girl has started her menstrual periods. If an adolescent understands that

### The Puberty Period

| Pubertal Change | Medical Name | Median Developmental Age |
|---|---|---|
| Breast budding | Adrenarche | 9.8 years |
| Pubic hair | Adrenarche or Pubarche | 10.5 years |
| Growth spurt | Somatic growth | 11.8 years |
| Axillary hair growth | Thelarche or Pubarche | 12.5 years |
| Uterine bleeding | Menarche | 12.8 years |

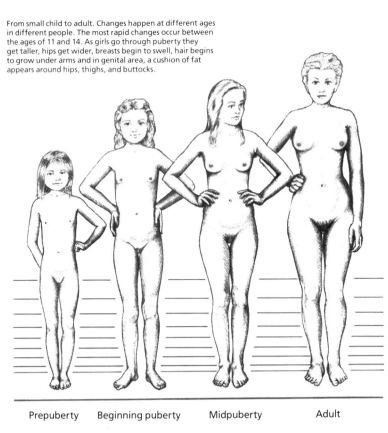

From small child to adult. Changes happen at different ages in different people. The most rapid changes occur between the ages of 11 and 14. As girls go through puberty they get taller, hips get wider, breasts begin to swell, hair begins to grow under arms and in genital area, a cushion of fat appears around hips, thighs, and buttocks.

Prepuberty    Beginning puberty    Midpuberty    Adult

## Puberty in Girls

these variations are normal, she may not worry so much if she does not develop at the same rate and in the same way that her friends do.

### 90 What causes all the changes of puberty to occur in a girl's body?

Although the statement that the "factors controlling the onset of puberty and triggering the menarche have not been identified" is true (Drs. Huffman, Dewhurst, and Capraro, *The Gynecology of Childhood and Adolescence*, Boston: Saunders, 1981.), researchers feel that the hypothalamus, located at the base of the brain and the master control unit for the female hormone cycle (and for other body hormones), has some

type of mechanism which restrains the production of the hormones necessary for initiating the female cycle prior to puberty. Other mechanisms may be operative, but no one has defined exactly why the female hormone cycle does not operate during early childhood, or specifically what causes it to begin operating at the time of puberty.

Studies have shown that the hypothalamus does "wake up" at the time of puberty (between the years of eight and eighteen). This awakening of the hypothalamus, with the resulting presence of hormones in the girl's body, produces the changes occurring in puberty. At first the hormones are responsible only for physical changes in the body, but as the hormone cycle develops to maturity, the girl begins not only menstruating but also regularly releasing eggs (ova). It is with the completion and maturing of this process that the girl becomes a fertile, mature woman.

---

## 91 Describe the female sexual hormone cycle, or the menstrual cycle.

Drs. Speroff, Glass, and Kase make this statement in their book, *Clinical Gynecological Endocrinology and Infertility* (Baltimore: Williams & Wilkins, 1978): "These hormonal changes are correlated with orthologic [physical] changes in the ovary, making coordination of this system one of the most remarkable events in biology." I certainly agree with that observation!

The first sign of this hormone function begins in the hypothalamus with the release of a hormone (GnRH—gonadotrophin-releasing hormone), which goes to the pituitary gland and stimulates it to release one of its hormones called LH (luteinizing hormone). This LH is released into the blood stream, and then it goes to the ovaries and stimulates them to begin producing estrogen, in the form of estradiol. The estrogen released by the ovaries into the blood stream is responsible for the changes of puberty.

Although the pattern for all this is incomplete at first, it is effective in initiating the physical changes that occur in puberty. As the function of the glands matures, the complete menstrual cycle is established, and the girl begins having regular menstrual periods and monthly ovulation.

The normal menstrual cycle is depicted in the accompanying diagram.

Each of these phases is discussed in the following questions.

---

## 92 What occurs during the follicular phase?

The goal of the follicular phase is to develop one mature cyst (follicle) with one mature

egg, so that this ovum can be released from the follicle at the proper time. The process begins immediately following the menstrual period and takes ten to fourteen days.

If you read or review chapter 6, Conception, now, that will help you to understand the paragraphs that follow.

Each ovary contains thousands of eggs, and almost all of these eggs are present in the ovary in individual, tiny cystic areas called primordial follicles. At the onset of puberty there are approximately 300,000 eggs in a girl's ovaries, each in its own primordial follicle. During a woman's reproductive life, for every egg she releases (usually one monthly), a thousand eggs will not grow to maturity and will die that month.

The pattern the body establishes to produce menstruation (or pregnancy) is as follows.

Because estrogen levels in the woman's body drop during the menstrual period, the production of hormones from the hypothalamus starts increasing. The primary hormone it produces at this time is called GnRH, or gonadotrophin-releasing hormone. This hormone travels in the blood only a short distance to the pituitary gland, which is hanging from the underside of the hypothalamus. This GnRH causes the pituitary to release follicle-stimulating hormone (FSH) which travels in the woman's blood stream to her ovaries where it stimulates maturation of some of the ovarian follicles. This hormone is, therefore, responsible for stimulating the development of the primordial follicles around several eggs.

Remember, follicles are the spaces or small cystic structures within each ovary where eggs are nurtured and allowed to grow

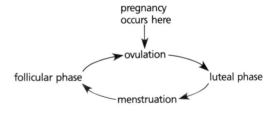

until one egg each month is mature enough to be released. During the week or two after a menstrual period, several primordial follicles are stimulated to grow and ready their eggs to be released. Except in the case of fraternal twins (or triplets, and so on), only one follicle and egg grow to maturity by the day of ovulation. This one follicle is called the dominant follicle. The other follicles and eggs grow to various stages during the two weeks, but all the follicles except one will shrivel up before maturity, resulting in the "death" of both the follicles and their eggs.

During the two weeks of its development, the dominant follicle produces increasing amounts of estrogen and releases it into the woman's body. This estrogen circulates in her blood stream, flowing back around into her uterus, stimulating the uterine lining to develop in anticipation of a pregnancy. At the same time the dominant follicle is producing estrogen, it is growing as it fills with more and more fluid. During this time the egg is maturing and being prepared to be set free from the ovary at ovulation.

At ovulation the dominant follicle ruptures, releases the egg, and then collapses. It does not die, however. This follicle now becomes the corpus luteum, which serves a vital part in the reproductive process. It produces progesterone, the hormone that completes the process of preparing the lining of the uterus for pregnancy. Just as was the estrogen, the progesterone also is secreted by the ovary into the body's circulation and is returned by the blood to the uterus to do its preparatory work. The corpus luteum is unusual in that it makes not only progesterone, but estrogen and androgens (male-type hormones), which are produced in small amounts by ovaries of all normal women.

The dominant follicle (with its egg) that forms on an ovary is normally about three-quarters of an inch in diameter and can get even larger. A doctor can often feel these ovarian enlargements when doing a pelvic exam and will often use the term *cyst* in referring to them. A competent, honest doctor does not mean that there is anything wrong when telling a woman that she has such a cyst present—because a doctor knows it as a normal part of the reproductive process. Such cysts are not to be confused with the growths and tumors that most women associate with the word. Occasionally an unscrupulous or incompetent doctor will tell a woman that she has an ovarian cyst and will insist that she have surgery to have it removed, implying that it might be cancer—when it is usually nothing more than a normal development of the ovary. If you have any reason to question your doctor's intent or ability, you should get a second opinion before you have such surgery. Most ovarian cysts do not require surgery unless they are at least two to three inches in diameter, are causing pain, or have been present for several months.

## 93 What occurs during ovulation?

The goal of ovulation is to get the mature egg out of the follicle (cyst) so that it can be picked up by the fallopian tube. At the end of the follicular phase, just before ovulation, there is a great deal of estrogen being secreted by the follicle. This high level of estrogen stimulates the pituitary to release a large amount of luteinizing hormone (LH) over a period of a few hours. Ovulation (release of the egg) occurs thirty-eight hours after this surge of LH reaches its peak.

The process of ovulation begins as the outer wall of the follicle becomes thin and stretched and the amount of fluid in the follicle increases. Hormones called prostaglandins increase in quantity in the follicle fluid and in some way seem to cause the follicle to rupture; additionally, contractions of muscle cells in the ovary apparently cause the fluid in the follicle and the egg to be squeezed out of the ovary. The rupture of the

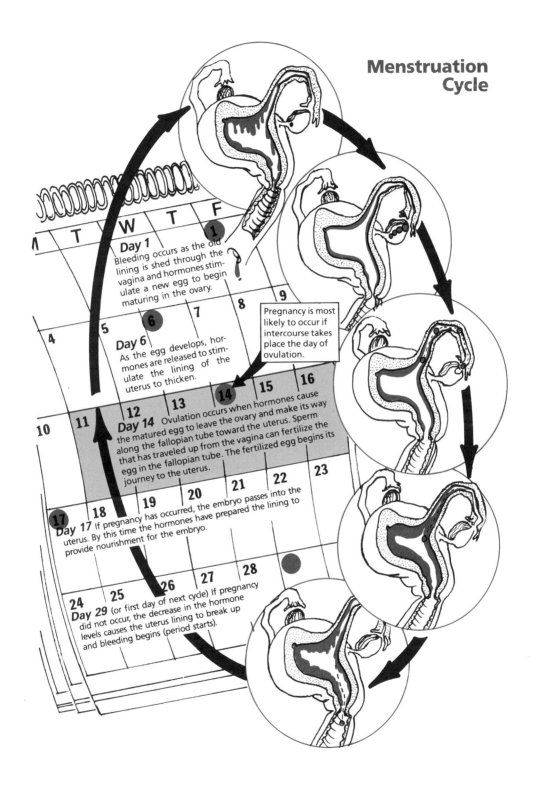

# Menstruation Cycle

**Day 1** Bleeding occurs as the old lining is shed through the vagina and hormones stimulate a new egg to begin maturing in the ovary.

**Day 6** As the egg develops, hormones are released to stimulate the lining of the uterus to thicken.

Pregnancy is most likely to occur if intercourse takes place the day of ovulation.

**Day 14** Ovulation occurs when hormones cause the matured egg to leave the ovary and make its way along the fallopian tube toward the uterus. Sperm that has traveled up from the vagina can fertilize the egg in the fallopian tube. The fertilized egg begins its journey to the uterus.

**Day 17** If pregnancy has occurred, the embryo passes into the uterus. By this time the hormones have prepared the lining to provide nourishment for the embryo.

**Day 29** (or first day of next cycle) If pregnancy did not occur, the decrease in the hormone levels causes the uterus lining to break up and bleeding begins (period starts).

follicle and release of the egg from the ovary take only a few minutes.

When follicle rupture occurs, the cystic fluid and the mature egg pass out of the ovary and are picked up by the fallopian tube. Women frequently have slight bleeding from the ovary upon ovulation. This may cause abdominal pain for a day or two *(mittelschmerz)*. It is this slight pain which signals to some women the occurrence of ovulation. Rarely does a woman have enough internal bleeding to require surgery, but it can happen. If a woman is having significant pain and seems to be bleeding inside her abdomen, the problem could be from ovulation, but it could also be from a tubal (ectopic) pregnancy or from some other dangerous problem. Because of this, severe pain with signs of internal bleeding requires an operation. A laparoscopy can be done, but occasionally a large incision is required to take care of the problem.

---

## 94 What happens in the luteal phase?

The goal of the luteal phase is to prepare the lining of the uterus for reception of an impending pregnancy. To accomplish this, the ovary secretes large amounts of progesterone, as well as estrogen. Not only does progesterone participate in preparing the uterine lining for implantation of the embryo, but it also does other things—such as suppressing the ovaries to prevent other follicles from developing until after the next period, and decreasing the irritability of the uterus so that it will hold a pregnancy and not squeeze it out.

As the luteal phase begins, the cells which line the inside of the follicle remain after the egg passes out of the follicle. These cells are called granulosa cells. Other cells, called theca-lutein cells, may participate in the formation of the corpus luteum, whose cells are responsible for production of both progesterone and estrogen.

After ovulation the granulosa cells change their appearance, developing a yellowish color. The theca-lutein cells become part of the corpus luteum and begin production of estrogen and progesterone. This production peaks eight days after ovulation and begins declining during the next two or three days.

If pregnancy occurs, HCG hormones (human chorionic gonadotrophin hormones) are released from the pregnancy tissues, supporting the corpus luteum to prevent its degeneration. The corpus luteum will then go on serving the body by producing hormones until the ninth or tenth week of pregnancy, when the placenta takes over all the production of hormones for maintaining the pregnancy, and the corpus luteum dies.

If pregnancy does not occur, the corpus luteum begins to degenerate, with a subsequent marked decrease in the production of progesterone and estrogen. The corpus luteum will continue to degenerate, and when the degeneration is complete, a menstrual period will start. The luteal phase normally lasts fourteen days from the day of ovulation.

---

## 95 What is menstruation and its function?

The goal of menstruation is to rid the uterus of the lining that has been built up during the previous month. This allows the development of a new lining that will be receptive to pregnancy the following month. Usually a menstrual period occurs from every twenty-seven to thirty days during a woman's reproductive life. Since 95 percent of all women menstruate from every twenty-one to every forty-five days, women who are within this range can consider their cycles normal. Menstrual periods occurring outside these boundary ranges may be abnormal and need evaluation.

When the corpus luteum dies, it no longer produces estrogen and progesterone, and this is what initiates menstruation. When the amounts of these hormones in the blood stream drop below a certain level, the vessels of the inside lining of the uterus go into spasm, stopping the flow of blood to the lining. The lining dies and begins sloughing out, characterized by menstrual "bleeding." Menstrual flow is made up of both dead tissue, formerly the lining of the inside of the uterus, and blood from blood vessels that have relaxed. Some of the menstrual flow is also fluid that has oozed through the raw surface of the uterine wall when its overlying surface broke down.

When menstrual flow ends, the lining (epithelium) grows once more, in response to the increasing levels of estrogen that are a result of the next follicular phase of the menstrual cycle. It is at this point, therefore, that the cycle begins all over again, developing another egg, another lining to the uterus, and the hormonal changes necessary for pregnancy.

Menstruation usually continues for three to six days, but it is also normal for a woman's menstrual flow to last only one day or as long as seven or eight days. There is a great deal of individual variation in the amount of blood that is lost during a menstrual period. It is usually from one ounce to three ounces, but it can be more or less than that. If a woman is otherwise normal and is not becoming anemic because of blood lost during menstruation, having a heavy menstrual flow is not alarming.

## Precocious Puberty

### 96 What if puberty occurs earlier than is considered normal?

If your daughter develops breasts or pubic hair before the age of eight, or if she begins menstrual bleeding before she is nine, she is starting puberty prematurely. If this happens, you should take her to a physician who specializes in problems of female adolescence. This would normally be a gynecologist, but some pediatricians are both interested and capable in this area of medicine. If a family practitioner or endocrinologist has taken a special interest in this area, he or she too might be appropriate for your daughter to see.

Girls who have precocious puberty not only require adequate medical care, but they and their families need emotional support. We must remember that they are children of only eight or nine who have developed breasts, pubic hair, and menstrual periods. They must use deodorants and sanitary napkins and have to wear brassieres. Such young girls develop some of the emotional characteristics of teenagers, such as irritability, strained relations with parents, and poor self-image. Proper counsel can help parents understand that all children with precocious puberty do not necessarily experience such teenage-type emotional upheavals. Wise counseling can help prevent the deterioration of the parent/child relationship, a situation which makes the problem even worse for both the child and parents.

### 97 How would a physician evaluate a child with precocious puberty?

If the only sign of premature puberty has been some vaginal bleeding, the vagina needs to be examined to be sure the girl has not inserted an object of some kind into it, causing a vaginal infection or tear. A vaginal exam will also rule out the presence of a tumor. This exam may or may not need to be done under anesthesia, and may be conducted in a hospital, an outpatient surgical unit, or the doctor's office.

If there are signs of puberty other than just vaginal bleeding present, an evaluation needs to be done to insure that the girl has no major disease, such as thyroid disease or a tumor growing in her brain, ovary, or adrenal gland, that requires treatment.

The doctor will want to talk to you and your daughter to see if there is any possibility of her having taken drugs that might have caused the problem. There are many reports in medical literature of children developing vaginal bleeding because they took their mother's hormones or birth-control pills.

A physical examination of the girl is very important. This includes the measurement of her height to see if hormones have caused an abnormal growth spurt, an examination of her reflexes and other aspects of her nervous system, to make sure there are no signs of brain disease; and an evaluation of changes in her sexual organs, including her breasts, vagina, and pelvic organs. For instance, if there is an ovarian tumor, it will be found during a pelvic examination.

Laboratory tests might include X-rays of your daughter's bone structure. If her bone growth is slower than it should be, she may have a thyroid problem. If it is faster than normal, this knowledge can help guide the doctor to the causative problem. X-rays of the bones may need to be taken over a period of time to see what type of development is occurring. Other studies might include X-rays of the brain, a CT brain scan, a brain-wave test, and/or hormone studies. In addition, thyroid tests will probably need to be done, as well as an evaluation of her visual fields.

The goal of all these tests is to make sure there is no life-threatening disease present, and to see if the process going on in your daughter's body is progressing or whether it was only a brief surge of hormone production that has already stopped and does not need to be treated. Testing is necessary to see what is wrong, so that appropriate treatment can be given.

## 98 What is the usual cause of precocious puberty?

In 75 percent of the cases of precocious puberty, the girl's internal time clock simply started the maturing process early. The process is begun in the hypothalamus (the tissue at the base of the brain that is responsible for starting puberty).

For some unknown reason, the hypothalamus will occasionally begin too-early production of the hormones that lead to full-blown sexual development. This process can start as early as birth and can occur at any age up to the time that normal puberty would start. There have even been rare cases of babies born with breasts who, during their first year of life, began developing pubic hair and menstruation.

## 99 What treatment should be instituted for precocious puberty, when it is caused by the normal maturing process having begun too early?

The primary physical problem with this type of precocious puberty is that the girl will be short when fully grown. Treatment is aimed at delaying the girl's maturity so that she can grow normally and attain the height she would otherwise have reached. This can be accomplished by prescribing a synthetic progesterone (Depo-Provera), given by injection every three months.

A newer and better treatment is a series of injections of LHRH analog. This is luteinizing hormone-releasing hormone. LHRH is a normal body hormone, usually released only in small, intermittent bursts from the hypothalamus. Scientists have been able to make a synthetic LHRH compound. When it is given by injection, there seems to be a flooding effect on the body that stops the premature puberty and allows breast and hair development to regress. Florence Comite, M.D., at the National Institute of Child

Health and Development, Bethesda, Maryland, is the chief investigator of this new technique. It would certainly be acceptable for you to contact her for further information if you have a child with this problem.

## 100 What disease processes can cause precocious puberty?

Early puberty caused by diseases occurs in only about 25 percent of such situations. A thorough evaluation should be done any time there is premature puberty, however, because of the possibility of such a disease. Several medical problems can cause early puberty:

*Disorders in the brain.* These disorders include brain tumors, inflammation, congenital abnormalities, and damage from accidents.

*McCune-Albright syndrome.* Although this condition is rare, it can cause premature onset of menstruation. A girl with this problem has cysts in her bones that allow easy fracturing, and she will often have light brown patches of skin (*café au lait* spots).

*Tumors of the ovaries.* These tumors produce estrogen, which causes sexual development. They may or may not be malignant.

*Disorders of the adrenal glands.* The adrenal glands may cause premature puberty by developing tumors or by overactive production of hormones (Cushing's syndrome).

*Other causes.* Occasionally an underactive thyroid can cause premature sexual development, but this is an unusual way for this problem to present itself. Other medical disorders can occur but are extremely rare.

## 101 What treatment can be given for precocious puberty caused by a disease process?

It is important, first, that the underlying medical problem be adequately evaluated and treated. Once that is under treatment, then the precocious puberty itself can be treated.

This type of precocious puberty responds to the treatment described in Q. 99.

## 102 How often does precocious puberty occur?

It is fairly common for a young girl to have slight breast development or some hair growth months or years before the age of eight, but have no other signs of puberty until after she is eight years old. This is known as *partial* premature sexual maturation. However, it is quite uncommon for a girl to have true precocious puberty (development of puberty before the age of eight). True precocious puberty—progressive sexual maturation with development of breasts, pubic hair, and menstrual periods prior to the age of eight—occurs in only about one in five thousand to one in ten thousand girls.

## 103 What might cause partial sexual maturation prior to the age of eight?

It is fairly common for a girl to experience sudden growth in one or both breasts, to develop some pubic hair, or to have a few episodes of bleeding from the uterus. When this occurs, and it is not followed by continued maturation of the sexual organs, the girl does not have true precocious puberty. She has experienced only a brief, temporary outpouring of sexual hormones, and such a situation happens frequently enough that it can almost be considered normal. Girls who have this temporary sexual development usually do start their true puberty earlier than other girls of their age.

Why this brief surge of hormones occurs is a mystery. It could be that the girls who experience this do not have mature enough hormone systems at the time to progress to normal function. It is also possible that the girl has gotten into some estrogen tablets or birth-control pills and this estrogen has caused her symptoms. Such drug intake can be suspected if the girl's nipples and areolae have developed dark pigmentation. If this is what has happened, the girl would not need medical evaluation or treatment, since taking hormones for a short time would not hurt her or make her body start puberty early.

## 104 What treatment should be administered for partial premature puberty?

No treatment is necessary for partial sexual maturation prior to the age of eight if testing has proven that only a brief production of hormones has caused the isolated or transient precocious development, and the girl has not shown an abnormal spurt of growth, the latter proven by X-rays of bone growth.

## Delayed Puberty

## 105 What should be done if my daughter's puberty seems to be abnormally delayed?

If your daughter has had absolutely no breast development, even breast budding, by the age of thirteen, or if she has not started her menstrual periods by the time she is fifteen, she may have a developmental problem. She probably needs to be examined by a physician. Since the variation in the onset of puberty is so great, however, your daughter's apparently delayed puberty may be totally normal.

Only 1 percent of all girls will not have started their periods by the age of eighteen. Any adolescent who reaches that age without starting her periods probably has a medical problem and definitely needs to be evaluated by a physician.

If your daughter does have delayed puberty and your doctor continues to tell you that she is normal and does not need an examination, he or she is obviously not familiar with this type of problem. You should find another physician who can be more helpful. I would suggest that you see an endocrinologist or a gynecologist, one interested in adolescent gynecology.

## 106 What is involved in a medical evaluation for delayed puberty?

An evaluation for a girl who has delayed puberty (no breast development by thirteen, no menstrual periods by fifteen) includes the following.

The physician will want to know about things such as when menstrual periods began among other female family members, since mother and daughters tend to start their periods around the same age. He or she will also ask about how much stress the girl is under, what kind of diet she has, whether she might be abusing drugs, and so on.

Next will probably be a complete examination, including the breasts and pelvic area. For an adequate exam of her pelvis, a laparoscopy may be necessary. (See Q. 908 for a description of this procedure.) The doctor will want to examine your daughter neurologically, which includes checking her reflexes and visual fields, and may also want to order an EKG and skull X-ray.

The examining physician will want to test your daughter's hormones to see if she is producing normal amounts from her pituitary, thyroid, adrenal, and ovarian glands. He or she may want to prescribe some progesterone to see if it will cause her to bleed from the uterus. This would prove that her ovaries are producing estrogen and that she has a normal uterus.

Normally in an evaluation of this type, the doctor does not need to do all the possible tests that are available. While working through the problem with you and your daughter, a specific test may give a hint of what is wrong and will lead to other pertinent diagnostic tools, eliminating the necessity for excess testing.

## 107 What causes delayed puberty?

The basic problem in this situation is that the girl's ovaries are not producing the estrogen necessary for the development of breasts and initiating menstrual periods in her body. The lack of estrogen may be due to defective ovaries or to some other abnormal body function.

*Hormone "time clock" set late.* In this case the girl is normal in every way except that her hormonal functioning has not started as early as that of most of her friends. If all her tests are normal, including a pelvic examination, she can be assured that she is normal. She will begin puberty and her periods later on, and she will be able to have children.

*Abnormal ovaries.* If a girl's ovaries are so abnormal that they cannot produce estrogen, she will not develop puberty. The most common cause of this is a condition called Turner's syndrome, in which the girl has abnormal chromosomes. This condition results in problems other than just a lack of normal ovaries. There are other, less-common reasons for abnormal ovarian function. She may have no ovaries at all, for

example. Most of these problems would not only keep a girl from experiencing puberty, but would also prevent her being able to become pregnant.

*Disease or health problems not located in the sex organs.* Nutrition problems and disease in the rest of the body can affect the physiology so traumatically that the female organs are affected and will not begin functioning properly. An example of this is the poor nutrition produced by anorexia nervosa (see Q. 149) or by some intestinal diseases that prevent absorption of nutrients from the intestinal tract. In this situation a girl will probably not develop the onset of menses until these nutritional problems have been eliminated.

Diseases of the base of the brain (hypothalamus) or of the pituitary gland can prevent the production of hormones necessary for initiating puberty.

*Congenital abnormalities.* Female babies can be born normal in every way except without a vagina or uterus, or with a uterus that has no opening, and so on. These girls will develop normal secondary sexual characteristics (breast development, pubic hair, hair under the arms) but will not start menstrual bleeding at the time that they normally should.

*Other problems.* Polycystic ovarian disease (see Q. 932–934), thyroid disease, adrenal gland disease, and failure of the ovaries can prevent the onset of puberty in a girl. Although these situations occur rarely, in evaluating your daughter, a doctor would have these things in mind.

## 108 What treatment is advised for delayed puberty?

First, it is important that a girl have an adequate evaluation so that the cause of the delayed puberty can be diagnosed. The treatment is dependent on the problem. If she does not have a normally developed vagina and uterus, some surgery may be necessary. (Q. 62–69 discuss this problem.)

If a girl has a medical problem, such as thyroid or adrenal gland disease, this would need to be treated.

If the problem is ovarian failure or ovaries that will not produce enough estrogen to initiate periods, she will need to be given estrogen. This should be discussed with a doctor who is competent in such treatment.

Finally, if a girl merely has a "time clock" that is set late, which means that all her other tests are normal, she can await the onset of her menstrual period for another two or three years. If, by the time she is twenty or twenty-one, she still has not started periods, and she has not already been back to a physician for an interim evaluation, she needs to return for further studies and diagnosis.

## Breast Development in the Adolescent

### 109 My daughter's breasts are developing, but one is much larger than the other. Is this normal?

No woman's breasts are totally symmetrical. In fact, you may have noticed that your own breasts are somewhat different in size and shape. This normal asymmetry between breasts is much exaggerated during the time that breasts are growing. (See Q. 37–39.)

If, after a girl has otherwise grown to maturity, her breasts are different enough in size to bother her, she can have augmentation of the smaller breast done to bring it up to the size of the larger breast. Few young women ever feel this is necessary, but, if one

does, the operation can allow her to no longer feel abnormal.

### 110 My daughter's nipples are inverted. Is this a problem?

*Inverted nipples* is a term that is used to refer to nipples that do not protrude above the level of the skin of the breasts but seem to be sunken in. They are as normal as nipples that are not inverted, and will not keep your daughter from breast-feeding a baby. They are not indicative of disease or tumor.

If a woman's (or girl's) nipples have always protruded, however, and one starts retracting (inverting), this change might indicate breast cancer. When they change, cause for concern exists. Inverted nipples that have been that way from puberty are totally normal.

### 111 Is it necessary that my daughter wear a brassiere?

There are two considerations about wearing brassieres.

As a girl's breasts are developing, she may or may not want to wear a brassiere. She will ordinarily do what her friends are doing. If her friends are wearing brassieres, it is probably best to let her wear one even before she really needs it. Some girls are embarrassed if their developing nipples show through their T-shirts, and they want to wear brassieres to cover them. Other girls couldn't care less about these little protrusions. If your daughter's nipples are quite noticeable, and you feel it is appropriate, mention this to your daughter and see if she wants to wear a bra.

Second, when a woman's breasts develop to a fairly large size, gravity starts pulling them down. Through the years this pull stretches the supporting ligaments and causes breasts to sag. Because of this physicians encourage women to wear brassieres

# Stages of Breast Development

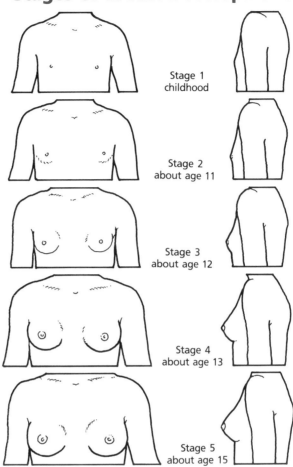

Stage 1
childhood

Stage 2
about age 11

Stage 3
about age 12

Stage 4
about age 13

Stage 5
about age 15

# Breast Changes of Puberty

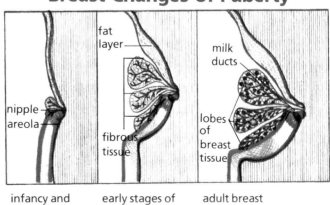

fat
layer

milk
ducts

nipple
areola

lobes
of
breast
tissue

fibrous
tissue

infancy and
childhood

early stages of
puberty

adult breast

for support. There is no real medical reason, however, for a girl or woman to wear a brassiere. It is purely a matter of cosmetics and strictly a personal decision, except that some women will have less breast tenderness if they wear a brassiere.

## Menstrual Irregularities in Adolescence

**112** **My daughter has begun her periods, but they are irregular. Should anything be done?**

One of the most common problems with girls going through puberty is irregular bleeding, and about half of all girls will have irregular periods during the first twelve months after starting their menses. In fact, it may take eight or ten years before a girl's menstrual regularity is fully established.

Obviously if a girl's menstrual periods are heavy, overly long, infrequent, or irregular the first few years, there is probably nothing to worry about. If, however, you or your daughter feel that her menstrual irregularity is too abnormal, you should call your doctor and ask if an office visit is warranted.

**113** **Which patterns of menstrual bleeding are in the normal range? Which are not?**

Patterns of menstrual bleeding that are considered normal, and about which you do not need to worry, are the following:

Periods that come as often as twenty-one days, or periods that come as infrequently as six to eight weeks.

Periods that last only one or two days, or periods that last up to six or eight days.

Bleeding that is very light, or bleeding that is fairly heavy (six or eight soaked pads a day).

Bleeding patterns about which you would probably need consultation include the following:

Bleeding or spotting which occurs on a daily or almost-daily basis, or periods that come only once or twice a year after the girl has been menstruating a year or more.

Bleeding that lasts more than six or eight days with every period.

Heavy bleeding (more than six or eight well-soaked pads a day), especially if the child seems to be getting unusually weak or tired.

**114** **What can cause irregular periods?**

The usual cause of adolescent menstrual irregularities during the first few years is irregular ovulation. The probable reason for this is the immaturity of the hormone system. Just as the rest of the body takes a while to mature, so does the hormone system. When it matures and the girl begins ovulating regularly, her periods will become regular.

There are other conditions of the teenage body that can increase the chance of a girl's having irregular periods. Some of these are:

*Dieting.* A young girl can delay the establishment of regular ovulation by starting and maintaining a rigid reducing diet. Anorexia or bulimia can cause irregular menses.

*Obesity.* It is fairly common for a teenager to gain a good deal of weight around the time of puberty. This extra fat generates extra estrogen in her body, which causes excessive build-up of the uterine lining, producing irregular spotting and bleeding.

*Exercise.* Vigorous exercise can affect a young woman's ovulation. If she has not yet developed regular ovulatory patterns and she begins exercising vigorously, she may have irregular bleeding and spotting.

*Stress.* It is fairly common for young women to skip periods in times of stress. I have had several patients, students at the University of Texas, who would have three normal periods during the summer and no periods during the nine months they were in school! The only explanation found was that the stress of school was preventing them from having periods.

*Medical problems.* There are some medical disorders that can cause a girl to have abnormal or irregular vaginal bleeding. These include problems of the hormonal system, which can cause excessive production of hormones from the pituitary, the thyroid, or the adrenal gland; blood-clotting abnormalities, which might be suspected if the girl's first period is frighteningly heavy; bleeding from an unsuspected pregnancy; growths in the uterus or vagina; and other, more unusual medical problems, such as TB or nephritis.

## 115  Should I take my daughter to a doctor for menstrual irregularities?

If there is any question about the irregularity's being abnormal, or if the irregularity is bothering her in any way, she should see a doctor.

Young women should have a gynecologic exam when they or their mothers think something might be wrong, when they become sexually active, before marriage, or when they are in their late teens or early twenties. Irregular bleeding that seems abnormal should be checked.

## 116  What can be done about irregular or abnormal bleeding?

After the doctor has discussed the girl's bleeding pattern, he or she will examine her. This exam can discover or rule out some things that can cause abnormal bleeding, such as tumors and growths.

The doctor will probably want a blood count to make certain the girl is not anemic, especially if she has a pattern of excessive bleeding. Other blood tests may be required if the doctor suspects hormonal abnormalities or other medical problems. If they are ordered at the same time, blood for all required tests can usually be drawn at once.

The problem is usually that ovulation is not taking place regularly. In spite of irregular ovulation, the ovaries can continue to put out estrogen every day, and this estrogen can stimulate the lining of the uterus to thicken. If ovulation does not take place, the lining of the uterus gets thicker and thicker. Areas of it finally outgrow their blood supply and start sloughing out, producing irregular bleeding patterns. In a woman who ovulates regularly, the ovary starts releasing progesterone into the body at the moment of ovulation. This progesterone changes the lining of the uterus so that two weeks after ovulation the entire lining will shed at one time—a normal period.

Theoretically, all an otherwise normal girl needs in order to have regular periods is production of estrogen from her ovaries most of the month and the presence of adequate progesterone in her body ten to fourteen days each month. Whether this progesterone comes from her own ovulation or from progesterone pills does not matter.

If your daughter's bleeding is caused by irregular ovulation, a common symptom in young women, the doctor may prescribe progesterone, given in the form of a pill called Provera, to establish regular bleeding. This is fine in theory but often ineffective in practice. Birth-control pills may be required to establish regular periods. (See Q. 138–144 regarding the use of birth-control pills by young women.)

## 117 What can be done about heavy menstrual bleeding?

If a girl is having a very heavy menstrual flow, she may need large doses of hormones by mouth. Birth-control pills or substances such as Norlutate, a potent, progesterone-type drug, are sometimes prescribed. If the girl has an extremely heavy bleeding episode, she may need estrogen injections every four hours several times. These injections will usually stop heavy bleeding within twelve to twenty-four hours.

If very heavy bleeding persists, Amicar, a drug not often used in the United States, might be used. This drug can occasionally be effective in stopping life-threatening uterine bleeding that might otherwise require a hysterectomy.

A dilatation and curettage (D&C) may be tried to stop bleeding, although doctors ordinarily do not like to do this procedure on young women. It is usually not particularly effective in stopping menstrual bleeding, and it is certainly better if drugs can be used for such bleeding in a young woman. (See the discussion about bleeding and D&Cs in Q. 764, 788, 789, 792–794.)

If a girl is having heavy periods, or if she has had an episode of heavy bleeding that needs treatment as suggested above, it is important that she take an iron supplement. Most teenagers do not get enough iron in their diets, and taking a supplement will help prevent anemia. An inexpensive, one-a-day iron pill is all that is necessary.

## Special Health Considerations During Adolescence

## 118 Are tampons safe, especially for young women?

Most doctors feel that tampons are the best technique for handling menstrual flow for both adolescents and older women. This is especially true in hot, humid climates, since external pads can cause the retention of moisture and heat around the vulva, increasing the chance of vulvar irritation.

Tampons have the following advantages over external protection (see Q. 682):

*Better vulvar hygiene.* As mentioned above, they keep the vulva from retaining moisture and warmth.

*Greater freedom.* A woman can swim, exercise, and so on, more conveniently and confidently when using tampons.

*Better body knowledge.* A girl who uses tampons is quite familiar with the location of her vaginal opening, and she knows how deep her vagina is and what direction in her body it takes. This knowledge and familiarity makes a young woman's first pelvic exam easier and initial intercourse less frightening.

*Detection of hymenal abnormalities.* If a girl cannot insert a tampon, she knows that something may be wrong. By trying to use tampons, she could, therefore, detect an abnormality of the hymen and have it treated before it would become a problem with marriage and attempted intercourse.

Tampons have the following disadvantages:

*Vaginal ulceration.* Occasionally vaginal ulcers can result from improper tampon insertion. Women are not normally aware that this has occurred and learn of it only during a routine examination by a doctor. This problem is easily resolved by not using tampons for a while until the ulcer heals and then, when resuming tampon use, changing the method of insertion.

*Toxic shock.* Although associated with the use of tampons, toxic shock also occurs in women who have never used tampons, and has even occurred in men. Most gynecologists feel that it is safe for a girl or woman to use tampons. If she is particularly worried about toxic shock, but wants to use tampons occasionally, she may use them during the day and use pads at night, or use pads and tampons alternately. Toxic shock is infrequent, and most doctors feel that the possibility of toxic shock does not warrant discontinuing tampon use. (See Q. 713–717 for more on toxic shock.)

## 119 Should my daughter see a female physician rather than a male physician if she must be examined for gynecologic problems as a child or teenager?

The most important characteristic of the doctor who sees your daughter, other than that of being excellently qualified, should be a warm, caring personality. Whether that professional is a man or woman is not really important as long as your daughter trusts him or her and knows that the doctor is truly concerned about her.

A physician from a major children's hospital in the United States addressed this subject recently. An evaluation was made of the relationship between girls with female-organ problems and their doctors, with the goal of determining whether it made a difference, in any way, whether the doctor was a man or a woman. No difference was detected, as long as the physician was a caring, sensitive person.

## 120 My daughter has grown an excessive amount of body hair. Why has this happened, and what can be done about it?

Most girls who have more hair growth than they think they should have, or who have hair on parts of their bodies where they do not want it, are still "normal." Because such hair growth is often embarrassing to a teenage girl, she is often convinced that it is abnormal. Roughly 90 percent of patients who consider their hair growth excessive have that heavy hair growth either because it is a family characteristic or because it is their own personal body pattern.

One fairly reliable guide is that if a girl has heavier-than-average hair growth but normal menstrual periods, her hair growth is probably a "normal" thing for her and is not due to an abnormality or disease. In spite of this, if you or your daughter think that she has an abnormal amount of hair, or that she has excessive hair growth in areas where she should not have it, you should take her to a physician for evaluation.

## 121 What hair growth is considered normal?

Hair growth on the upper lip, the sides of the face, around the nipples, and from the pubic hair up to the umbilicus (navel) is normal as long as it is not excessive. A girl can compare her hair growth with that of other members of her family. If her mother or father or other members of the family have heavy hair growth, her hair growth pattern is probably inherited.

## 122 What abnormalities can cause excessive hair growth?

There are at least five abnormalities that may cause excessive hair growth, (hirsutism).

*Ovarian abnormalities.* The most common hormonal abnormality causing excessive hair growth is the "polycystic ovarian syndrome." (See Q. 930–932.) This condition is not dangerous, but in addition to producing hair-growth problems and irregular periods, it can cause some fertility difficulties. Tumors of the ovary can cause production of increased amounts of male-type hormones, but this is rare.

*Adrenal gland abnormalities.* Excessive production of hormones by the adrenal glands can cause hirsutism. This is caused by overactivity of the adrenal glands or by a tumor in these glands.

*Thyroid abnormalities.* Hypothyroidism, or low thyroid, can cause excessive hair growth. This growth is usually on the upper lips and on the back.

*Drugs.* Male hormones, anabolic drugs unwisely taken for body building, some synthetic female hormones, and Dilantin can cause increased hair growth on a woman's body.

*Anorexia nervosa.* This condition has various effects on a young woman's body, one of which is excessive hair growth. (See Q. 149.)

## 123 What type of studies are done if bodily hair growth seems excessive?

There are several things a doctor will want to do in his or her evaluation:

The doctor will want to talk to both the girl and her mother to determine when the hair growth started and how fast it has progressed.

A complete physical exam would involve careful inspection of a girl's skin to determine the extent of the hair growth. It would include a pelvic examination to make sure there are no tumors growing on the ovaries.

Hormone testing might be done to determine whether or not there is an abnormal hormone production from the ovaries, the adrenal glands, the thyroid, or the pituitary.

X-rays, CT, or MRI scans of the abdomen might be done to determine whether or not there is a tumor growing on the adrenal glands or the ovaries.

## 124 If it is determined that excessive hair growth is problem-related, how is it treated?

Treatment of this type of hair growth is complicated by the fact that once it has occurred, the hair growth will probably continue. Rarely does the treatment of the disease that caused it result in lessening of the hair growth already developed. Treatment can prevent the growth from becoming worse, however, and this is the main reason for seeing a doctor as quickly as possible if a problem is suspected.

If the girl is dissatisfied with the hair that she has already grown, the only truly effective techniques for removing it are electrolysis and shaving or dissolving away the hair with a cream. Some physicians and patients feel that shaving and/or removing hair with hair-dissolving or depilatory creams causes the hair to become gradually more dark and coarse. If this happens, it can set up a vicious and frustrating cycle: the more treatment, the more obvious the hair becomes.

The best treatment, therefore, seems to be electrolysis. Many people dismiss the use of electrolysis because of what they have heard about its expense and discomfort. However, over a period of time electrolysis can be quite effective, and it is not very uncomfortable. Its expense and discomfort are almost always worth the good results that are usually produced.

Certain drugs have been found to be somewhat helpful with this problem— spironolactone, cimetidine, and cyproterone acetate. However, cyproterone acetate was not available in the United States at the time of this writing because of significant side effects.

Other forms of treatment depend upon what is causing the hair-growth problem:

*Abnormal ovarian function.* Use of birth-control pills will suppress the ovaries' production of male-type hormones (androgens), and other drugs may also be useful. Progesterone, one of the primary female hormones, may help suppress hair growth.

If the ovarian problem is due to a tumor, that tumor will need to be removed by major surgery. (See Q. 814–850 for a complete discussion of ovarian problems.)

*Adrenal disease.* If the adrenal glands are overactive, they must be treated with medication to suppress their activity. If the adrenal problem is caused by a tumor, that tumor will need to be surgically removed.

*Thyroid disease.* If the thyroid is underactive, thyroid medication should be administered.

*Drugs.* If the young woman is developing excessive hair growth because of Dilantin, her doctor may be able to find a substitute anticonvulsant for her. Other drugs that can cause hirsutism, such as male-hormone medications and anabolics, should not be taken by young women unless there is some unusual medical problem that makes such drugs necessary.

**125** **My husband and I are tall and our daughter is afraid she is going to be "too tall." Is there anything we can do to prevent this?**

It is possible to predict fairly accurately a person's height as an adult. If your doctor predicts that your daughter will be more than six feet tall at maturity, and this seems a real problem to you or her, you may want to consider treatment. If your doctor is unfamiliar with Bayley-Pinneau tables for height prediction, he can find them in the book, *Clinical Gynecological Endocrinology and Infertility,* Third edition, by Leon Speroff, Robert H. Glass, and Nathan G. Kase (Baltimore: Williams and Wilkins, 1978).

Whether or not to treat a girl for this predicted height attainment is primarily up to the parents, because treatment must be started *before* she begins her menstrual periods for it to be successful. At this young age, most girls would not be able to participate knowledgeably in the decision. "Late" treatment, begun after the menses have started, may be able to eliminate up to one inch of growth, however.

The treatment is safe. It consists of the use of estrogen tablets taken by mouth. This hormone treatment will cause regular periods but will stimulate the bones to complete their growth and the bones' growth centers to close, preventing the girl's height from becoming excessive.

**126** **Can tumors of the female organs develop in children and teenagers?**

Although they are rare, tumors do develop in young people, and both parents and physicians should be alert to this.

As almost half of the tumors discovered in children have the possibility of being malignant, it is important that such a tumor be discovered early. It is unfortunate that parents and doctors often discount the probability of a pelvic tumor in an adolescent. Any time a girl develops any of the warning symptoms listed by the American Cancer Society, it is important that she be taken to a doctor for examination.

In addition, if a girl develops abdominal swelling or pain, or even abdominal fullness or discomfort, she should be taken to a doctor for evaluation. The same advice applies if a girl has vaginal discharge or passes blood erratically from her vagina, or if she has an ulcer or a sore around the opening of her vagina or on her labia. As previously mentioned, if your daughter shows signs of sexual maturation before the age of eight she should also see a physician. (See Q. 96–104.)

Tumors of the female organs are rare in children, especially those below the age of sixteen, but almost any type of tumor seen in adults can also occur in children. Tumors, benign and malignant, can develop in the vagina, on the cervix, in the uterus, and in the tubes and ovaries. Ovarian tumors are the most common tumors to develop in a girl sixteen years or younger. For more information on these tumors, see chapter 10.

## 127 What type of female-organ infections can an adolescent develop?

From puberty on, a girl may have the same genital infections as an adult woman. These infections are diagnosed and treated in the same way as they are in an adult.

If an adolescent girl has vaginal discharge and itching, she needs to see a gynecologist or a knowledgeable physician to have the problem diagnosed and treated. If she has had intercourse and has developed symptoms that might be due to a sexually transmitted disease, she will also need to consult a physician for the same reason. A young girl can contract sexually transmitted disease as easily as an adult. If an adolescent is sexually active, she should also have an annual Pap smear.

Because a young woman can develop pelvic infections that may cause permanent fallopian tube damage, with resulting sterility, it is important that adolescents realize that they must weigh carefully the possible consequences of sexual activity. The best thing, of course, is for them to choose not to have intercourse until marriage, a choice which almost totally eliminates any risk of infection in the female organs that might make them infertile in later life. For a complete discussion of sexually transmitted diseases, see chapter 13.

## 128 Is it harmful for my daughter to masturbate? Should I encourage her to masturbate as a means of releasing sexual tension?

Masturbation does not produce any physical damage to a person's body. It does not cause warts, insanity, loss of hair, or infertility.

Masturbation can cause anxiety on the part of both children and parents. If you know that your daughter is masturbating, reassure her that it will not damage her body physically and also that she is not perverted or evil for having done so. I would not suggest masturbation to my child as a means of relieving sexual tension, but I would certainly discuss it with her and answer her questions if she brings up the subject.

One of the best statements that I have read concerning teenage masturbation was written by Dr. James Dobson in his book *Preparing for Adolescence* (Ventura, Calif.: Vision House, 1978). He states (pp. 86–87).

Unfortunately, I can't speak directly for God on this subject, since His Holy Word, the Bible, is silent at this point. I will tell you what I *believe*, although I certainly do not want to contradict what your parents or your pastor believe. It is my *opinion* that masturbation is not much of an issue with God. It is a normal part of adolescence which involves no one else. It does not cause disease, it does not produce babies, and Jesus did not mention it in the Bible. I am not telling you to masturbate, and I hope you won't feel the need for it. But if you do, it is my opinion that you should not struggle with guilt over it.

## 129 I think my daughter is homosexual. What should I do about that?

If you have reason to believe your daughter is homosexual, I suggest that you first go to a counselor alone. Choose that counselor with extreme care. If the counselor seems helpful to you, has good suggestions, and seems to agree with your moral values, you, your husband, and your daughter may want to visit with the counselor together. Counseling of this type, before a child's emotional makeup has jelled, can spare her tremendous unhappiness in the future. It can also help develop a healthy relationship between you and your child.

## Sexual Molestation and Abuse

## 130 What should I tell my daughter about rape and sexual molestation?

The discussion you have with your daughter depends on the child's age. It is best to bring up this subject when the child is small and continue to add to her knowledge in this area as she matures. As you talk to your daughter, remember that 85 percent of episodes of child sexual abuse are committed by someone whom the child knows and trusts. Such persons include relatives, baby sitters, or family friends. It is uncommon for

the sexual abuse to be forceable and violent and it often does not even include vaginal or oral penetration. It is much more likely to be subtle, with no physical force, partly because child sexual abuse usually develops gradually over a long period of time.

The following suggestions may help with your discussion of this topic with your child:

1. Teach your child a sexual vocabulary, so that she will know what area of her body you are referring to when you talk about sexual contact.
2. Reassure her that her body is her own and that no one has a right to touch it or handle it.
3. Teach your child that her feelings count. If someone talks to her or touches her in a way that makes her uncomfortable, she should realize that her discomfort is legitimate.
4. Teach your child that she has a right to say no. Often children feel that they must do what adults tell them to do. Children should be taught that they should not allow adults to take advantage of them.
5. Explain to your child what to do if someone will not leave her alone. Tell her that if someone tries to touch her genitalia or wants her to look at or touch their genitalia, she should say no and run away as fast as she can.
6. Teach your child to tell someone about any unsettling experience. A most important part of a child's avoiding a problem of sexual abuse is to know that it is okay to talk to a trusted adult. She should know that she can talk to you, a relative, a teacher at school, or her minister or Sunday school teacher and be believed. Help your child to develop sound relationships with people that she can trust so that she can feel free to talk to them as well as you about personal matters.
7. Be sure she knows that you will pro-

tect her from such undesired and uncomfortable episodes.

By forewarning your child about such things, she will be reassured that you are not afraid or ashamed to talk about these matters and that she should not be either. This type of discussion also allows the child to have a ready answer to someone who tries to fondle or otherwise abuse her sexually. Remember that indecent exposure is also sexual abuse. Your child should be warned about this form of harassment.

The most important aspect of the situation is that your child be reassured that if someone has already abused her sexually, or is currently abusing her, she is free to talk to you about it and you will believe her and be supportive. Children are unlikely to lie about being sexually abused. If your child tells you that this is going on, believe her and contact someone to help you decide what to do, even if a loved one or close friend is implicated.

## 131  How widespread is the problem of sexual victimization of children and adolescents?

Sexual abuse can involve rape, sodomy, oral sex, exhibitionism, fondling, masturbation, intercourse, or physical injury. Often the activity involved is "dry intercourse" in which there is no penetration of anus or vagina but rather a rubbing of the attacker's penis between the thighs and against the anus of the victim who of course cannot tell whether or not penetration was involved. No physical mark is left and the victim is therefore thought to be lying about being abused. About 10 percent of sexual abuse is continual.

According to the Texas Department of Human Resources, one person out of four experiences some degree of sexual abuse in his or her lifetime. Girls are victims 90 per-

cent of the time. Other studies show that at least one in seven women has been approached sexually by an older male at some point during their childhood or adolescent years, and that only one in ten girls who are sexually abused ever report it to authorities.

To a significant extent sexual child abuse is a middle-class problem. It is quite common for the adults involved to be highly respected citizens, even church members.

## 132  What effect does sexual abuse have on its victims?

The effect of sexual victimization on the physical and emotional health of its victims is inestimable. Of course, girls who have started their menstrual periods may become pregnant as a result, and they are subject to

### Indications of Possible Sexual Abuse

#### Younger Children

Excessive masturbation
Bed-wetting or fecal soiling
Severe nightmares
Regression in developmental milestones
Explicit knowledge of sexual acts

#### Older Children and Adolescents

Depression
Withdrawal
Isolation from peers
Drug/alcohol abuse
Chronic runaway
Increase in physical complaints
Attention-getting behavior
Suicide attempts
Physical abuse
Poor self-image
Truancy
Drop in academic performance
Limited participation in organized social activities
Overly seductive behavior
Bisexual/homosexual experimentation
Promiscuous sexual behavior

contracting sexually transmitted diseases that can leave them permanently sterile. The emotional effects of sexual abuse, however, can be even more devastating. A woman's memory of sexual abuse as a child can make it extremely difficult for her to adjust sexually in marriage. In addition, since it is so often a person whom the child trusts who inflicts the abuse, the victim may feel that there will never be anyone in the world she can ever trust again. This belief not only colors her relationships with other people, but may affect her relationship with God, the one whom she should be able to trust above all.

It is appropriate here to point out to any person who is abusing a child or who is contemplating initiating such abuse that harming a child is dealt with quite strongly in Scripture: "But whoso shall offend one of these little ones which believe in me, it were better for him that a millstone were hanged about his neck, and that he were drowned in the depth of the sea. Woe unto the world because of offenses!" (spoken by Jesus, as recorded in Matt. 18:6–7 KJV).

Another effect of sexual victimization is that as the victims grow older, they may experience unwarranted guilt, thinking that they were responsible in some way for having been molested. This creates self-doubt, which, combined with the bitter hatred they may feel, intensifies other destructive emotions that have resulted from their past experiences.

A major effect of such abuse, however, is one that is almost impossible to believe: women who were abused often become abusers of their own children. This abuse is usually physical rather than sexual, leading to beatings and emotional abuse.

## 133 Why don't little girls report sexual abuse more often?

Because sexual abuse is often a middle-class problem, when children do get the courage to tell someone that their father, a close friend, or a family acquaintance has abused them, they are often not believed. Many times a child is accused of lying because the accused is so often a "nice person," known as being moral, modest, and upright. This rejection may reinforce the child's opinion that no one can be trusted, and it can cause the child's feelings of worthlessness to grow.

When a girl's father is the one who abuses her, the problem is especially difficult. A little girl may not only fear that her mother will not believe her if she tells what is going on, but she may also be worried that if she reports her father's abuse, he will be taken to jail or will leave home, thereby hurting the entire family.

One of the major reasons more child abuse and sexual victimization is not reported, however, is the fear of retaliation. Children are often threatened by their abusers so that they will not tell anyone what is going on.

## 134 Why is sexual victimization becoming so widespread?

Why such deviant behavior is becoming so common in our society is difficult to understand, but a text from the Bible may give some insight: "Since they did not think it worthwhile to retain the knowledge of God, he gave them over to a depraved mind, to do what ought not to be done. They have become filled with every kind of wickedness, evil, greed and depravity" (Rom. 1:28).

It appears that a progression of belief, or rather disbelief, leads to immorality in our society. Each point of this progression builds on itself, leading to ultimate depravity. I see the thought sequence in our society as taking the following path:

1. God does not exist, or, if he does exist, he has no practical association with our world. . . .

2. Therefore, we are here purely as biological accidents of a universe, without a soul. . . .
3. Since we are merely accidents of nature, there is little value or importance to anything except what we want to do or what makes us feel good. . . .
4. Since everything outside of ourselves is relatively meaningless, and since there is no higher morality than pleasing ourselves, we can therefore do anything that comes to our minds.

The net effect of this thought process is the cheapening of human values; allowing us, for instance, to take the life of an unborn child when having it is an "inconvenience," or causing a man to believe that he can sexually abuse his daughter just because he "feels like doing it."

The dehumanizing influences in our society, including child abuse, incest, child pornography, abortion, and euthanasia, certainly seem to indicate a major change in the moral and ethical foundation of our entire society.

---

## 135 What can be done to prevent the tragedy of sexual molestation in my family?

There are a number of actions that you can take to avoid this tragedy in your family.

Marry a man with strong moral and emotional health. For example, if you marry a man who is continuously rebelling against authority, including his parents, he may be more susceptible to the temptations of incest, especially if he has a poor moral base for interaction with the world.

Choose healthy contacts for your child. Use the same guidelines in selecting baby sitters, including nurseries and preschools, that you use to choose a husband. If you have any question at all about the morality and

emotional stability of any of these people, including relatives, do not allow them to stay alone with your child, no matter at what age or how convenient it might be. Do not allow such persons to hold your daughter in their laps or to caress her excessively, even in your presence.

Talk openly to your child. All children should be taught about the possibility of sexual assault. They should be given rules to make the probability of sexual assault less likely. Do not wait until your children ask to give them the necessary information, since they may never ask such questions!

---

## 136 Where can I get further information on child abuse?

Several organizations can give you help:

Your local police department.

Your local county sheriff's department.

Your county health or social-welfare department.

V.O.I.C.E., Inc. (Victims of Incest Can Emerge), Grand Junction, Colorado 81501. Telephone: (303) 241-2746.

Child Sexual Abuse Treatment Program, 467 South Third Street, San Jose, California 95110. Telephone: (408) 299-2511.

Parents United, Daughters and Sons United. Counseling telephone: (408) 280-5055.

Child Help, USA, Woodland Hills, California 91370. Telephone: (800) 4 A-CHILD.

National Center for the Prevention of Child Abuse and Neglect, P.O. Box 1182, Washington, D.C. 20013. Telephone: (202) 245-2856. They offer a packet of four brochures, tips for parents, Spiderman comic book with stories about sexual abuse written especially for children, and other helpful items.

In addition, there are several books that might be helpful.

*Carol's Story* by Chip Ricks (Tyndale House, 1981).

*A House Divided* by Katherine Edwards (Zondervan, 1984).

*My Very Own Book About Me* by Jo Stowell and Mary Dietzel (available from the Lutheran Social Services, 1226 Howard, Spokane, Washington 99201). This book distinguishes between "good" and "bad" touching and does an excellent job of explaining the right not to be touched in any way a child does not like (including tickling and wrestling). This is for young children through third grade.

*Top Secret, Sexual Assault Information for Teenagers* by King County Rape Relief, 305 South 43rd, Renton, Washington 98055.

*Sexual Abuse Prevention* edited by Barbara A. Withers and Karen West (1984, United Church Press, 132 West 31st Street, New York, 10001).

*Sex Talk for a Safe Child* by Domenna C. Renshaw (American Medical Association, P.O. Box 10946, Chicago, 60610) helps parents find a way to talk comfortably and accurately about normal and abnormal sex practices.

## 137 What should I do if I was once sexually abused and have never worked through that experience?

It is normal for the human mind and emotions to respond to the trauma of sexual abuse with major emotional and psychological problems. This is just as normal as it is for the body to respond with scars as a result of severe injury in an automobile accident. If you have been the victim of sexual abuse and feel you have problems resulting from the experience, it is important that you seek counseling. Just as you would want your daughter to confide in someone if she has been abused, so it is important that you tell someone if you have been sexually victimized in the past.

Call one of the organizations mentioned in the previous question, or talk to a counselor. Life is too short for you to spend it with the pain and hurt of sexual abuse.

## Sexual Activity in Adolescence

## 138 What should I do if my adolescent daughter has started having intercourse or if I believe she may be contemplating sexual activity?

Whether or not you approve of this situation, it must be dealt with openly. Your child's future is at stake, and unpleasant as it may be for both of you, you should have a frank and honest conversation with your daughter about sexual activity. A few warnings are in order concerning the following matters.

*Sexually Transmitted Diseases (STD).* Warn your child that she can catch a sexually transmitted disease from an infected male. The disease can damage her tubes and make her incapable of bearing children in the future. (Suggest that she read chapter 13 on STD.)

*Pregnancy.* Discuss with her the fact that pregnancy is a definite possibility if she is sexually active. The pregnancy rate among teenagers is very high even when they use birth-control techniques. Remind her that pregnancy will entail major changes in her lifestyle.

*Abortion.* Even if one's moral code accepts the concept of abortion, not only is abortion expensive, but it can cause infertility problems later. Teenagers often seem to feel that abortion is no bigger "deal" than brushing their teeth. They need to understand that the consequences of abortion are not only financial and physical, but that they may also include serious long-term emotional problems. (See Q. 223–236.)

## 139 I disapprove of my daughter's having sexual relations. How should I handle this?

The majority of American parents do not want their daughters to have intercourse prior to marriage and are saddened when they learn that it is occurring. If you disapprove of your daughter's sexual activity, handling the situation well is extremely important for her well-being and your parent/child relationship.

This is a critical time in a young girl's life, and if the matter is not handled properly, it can drive her away from you to a lifestyle that she might not have chosen had you reacted more appropriately and wisely. These suggestions might help you:

1. Don't "cut your daughter off" if you discover that she has been sexually active. You must communicate to her that although you do not approve of what she is doing, you still love her and will continue to love her.
2. Continue to remind her that no matter what her friends may say about modern sexual morals, there is one right place for sexual activity: marriage. Explain how sex outside marriage only

leads to problems now and can threaten her happiness later.
3. Take her to a physician for an examination. Be sure the doctor knows that she is having intercourse and that she is checked for sexually transmitted disease.
4. If she continues to flaunt the moral codes of your home it may be necessary for you to apply some principles of "tough love." Talk with an informed psychologist or psychiatrist about this concept.

## 140 I feel such pain over my daughter's choices. What did I do wrong?

When parents have done their best to raise a child the way they feel is right and that child then seems to turn against all that she has been taught, they may feel great despair. This is one of the most difficult times for parents and their children.

Hopefully, your daughter is merely going through a period of rebellion in an attempt to establish her own independence and maturity. On the other hand, she may be starting down a path that will lead her away from you and your moral values for many years. She may never return to the beliefs that you hold and have taught her as she was growing up. But if you have provided her with a caring, nurturing, loving home—and you have not been overly legalistic in your approach—the situation is probably only temporary.

It is a good idea to counsel with your pastor or with a psychologist or psychiatrist who can help you handle the situation. In addition, there are some excellent books that you could read. Some of these are:

*Parents in Pain* by John White (Intervarsity Press).

*The Wounded Parent* by Guy Greenfield (Baker Book House).

*No Time for Fairy Tales* by Fred Grimm, (Impact Books).

*Hold Me While You Let Me Go* by Rich Wilkerson (Harvest House).

*What's the Matter with Christy?* by Ruth Allen (Bethany House Publishers).

*Easing the Pain of Parenthood* by Mary Rae Deatrick (Harvest House).

**141** **What is the safest contraception measure for a teenager?**

First, birth-control pills, or oral contraceptives, have the lowest pregnancy risk rate of any contraceptive available today. Since the whole purpose of contraception is to avoid pregnancy, it seems wise to use the one that works the best. Second, birth-control pills are medically safe. Their use is associated with an extremely small chance of medical complications, especially in young people. Birth-control pills do not offer protection against sexually transmitted diseases. (See Q.1016, 1020.)

**142** **Will birth-control pills "mess up" my teenager's hormones?**

Studies have conclusively shown that if a girl has matured enough to have regular menstrual cycles, the birth-control pills will not harm her. Even for a young teenager, oral contraceptives will not affect future fertility or her hormones. Nor will taking the pills affect her ultimate height, since if a girl has developed regular menstrual periods, she has already had her major growth.

**143** **Is the use of an IUD (intrauterine device) a good idea for a teenager?**

Most gynecologists now do not recommend the IUD for a woman who has not completed her family. An IUD significantly increases the chance of infection developing in the uterus, tubes, and/or ovaries. Since a teenager has all her childbearing years ahead of her, avoid even a small chance of becoming sterile because of an IUD-caused infection.

**144** **What about the use of condoms, or rubbers, and contraceptive foams or diaphragms for a teenager?**

The primary disadvantage of these forms of birth control is the high failure rate. Using birth-control pills, teenagers become pregnant only about 5 percent of the time. With condoms, foams, or diaphragms, the pregnancy rates vary from 20 to 33 percent. If a teenager is going to depend on one of these methods for birth control, she must use it consistently and correctly or she will probably become pregnant. The problem is, of course, that people in their teenage years are usually the least disciplined that they will ever be in their entire lives and, therefore, the least likely to use foam, condoms, or diaphragms when they need them. Most teen pregnancies occur because these methods were not used at the appropriate time.

However, there are advantages to a young person's using one of these methods of birth control as opposed to the pill or IUD. It has been shown that women who use one of these methods have less chance of contracting a sexually transmitted disease or of developing an abnormal Pap smear as a result of sexual intercourse. Using both a condom and a sponge or foam provides the best physical barriers not only to sperm but to bacteria and viruses as well.

If a girl is going to use any of these methods, she must be counseled carefully as to how to use it and motivated to use it all the time. (See chapter 12, Birth Control, and the section on abortion in chapter 4).

## Teenage Pregnancy

### 145 What are the statistics on teenage pregnancy in the United States?

The statistics are startling. In the average high-school classroom, four out of every ten girls will be pregnant before their twentieth birthday. Approximately 1.2 million teenage girls become pregnant each year, and nearly half of these pregnancies occur outside of marriage. About 40 percent of teenage pregnancies are terminated by abortion, although nine out of ten teenage mothers who deliver their babies keep them. Finally, six in ten teen mothers who deliver before they are seventeen become pregnant again before they are nineteen.

The most common reason for hospitalization of a teenage girl in the United States is for childbirth. These pregnancies represent a tremendous cost to both society and to the individuals involved. There is a high risk of birth complications for the young mothers and frequent health problems for their babies. These girls are more likely to have medical complications during pregnancy, partly because they do not have the wisdom, discipline, or money to get good medical care. The children of teenage mothers statistically have a greater chance of dying or of having serious illnesses during their developmental years. Babies born to teen mothers often have low birth weight, and this correlates closely with the incidence of neurological defects, retardation, epilepsy, and cerebral palsy.

The economic drain is tremendous, frequently resulting in poverty and the need for public support, for both health and social reasons. These young mothers drop out of school and frequently do not return. If they have jobs, they often lose them as the result of a pregnancy.

### 146 What should my attitude be if my teenager gets pregnant?

To deal with her problem, you must also deal with yours. You will feel violated, as if your teenager has defiled your trust and all that you have taught her. To dwell on those feelings, however, can ruin your relationship with your daughter both now and in the future.

It certainly is appropriate for you to let her know that you are disappointed in her actions, but you must also communicate to her that you love and accept her as a person. I have often seen parents continue to berate their children for their misconduct, even after clearly expressing their disapproval. This produces an excessive amount of guilt and self-condemnation in the girl at a sensitive age.

The relationship between parent and child is far more important than whether or not the daughter has committed an act that is repulsive and disappointing to the parent. Most girls learn their lesson adequately from the pregnancy itself, without having their parents inflict more harsh lessons on them by misdirected and unloving attitudes.

Your daughter will go through a great deal of trauma, no matter how lovingly you care for her. It seems prudent, therefore, that you treat her with as much love and acceptance as you can to help her through this time. In this way you should be able to maintain a loving and caring relationship with her, allowing the trust between you to grow and mature from her experience, instead of having it permanently damage or destroy her.

## 147 Should I suggest—or insist—that my daughter have an abortion?

In your distress and anxiety, do not hastily advise abortion. I do not believe abortion is a good choice for an adolescent. (See Q. 228–236.)

The risks of both emotional trauma and physical damage from an abortion do exist, especially for a teenager. In addition, there is the possibility of developing a pattern of activity for the future. Without wise counseling, a girl may believe that she can misuse contraception and sex, become pregnant again, and repeat the pregnancy/abortion process with no adverse effects. That is not the case.

I have seen many teenage girls in my practice who had several pregnancies aborted by other physicians before they finally reached some level of adult maturity and either stopped having extramarital intercourse or started using contraception. I see many older patients who have had repeated abortions when they were young and who are now unable to get pregnant. There is definitely a higher chance of infertility in patients who have had abortions in the past.

## 148 How should my unmarried daughter's pregnancy be handled? What if she chooses to keep the child?

It is vital that your daughter have good medical care during her pregnancy, to enable her to stay healthy and to make delivery of a healthy baby more likely.

The importance of good medical care for a teenager during pregnancy is shown by the fact that a teenager who is pregnant is about three times more likely to have toxemia of pregnancy than a mature woman. An adolescent is twice as likely to have a premature baby than a mature woman and is more likely to produce a baby with congenital abnormalities. Her baby will have a greater

chance of dying before or right after delivery and a higher risk of developmental problems in the future, including cerebral palsy, mental retardation, or epilepsy. In addition, a teenager is more likely to have trouble delivering a baby. There is a greater chance that she will need a cesarean section and have a long labor than would an older woman.

It may be best for your family that your daughter contact an adoption agency that has domiciliary care. Such an agency provides a place for her to live during part or all of her pregnancy. If you are not familiar with this type of agency in your area, you might write to an organization such as the Edna Gladney Home in Fort Worth, Texas. They can help you make contact with a similar home in your area. You might also contact the National Committee for Adoption in Washington, D.C. (202-463-7563).

Loving and Caring, Inc., P.O. Box 146, Millersville, Pa. 17551, has some excellent material on decision making, relationships, and options for unwed mothers. A counselor's manual and a series of workbooks handle the situation with insight and sensitivity.

I do have a strong bias that causes me to feel that adoption is usually the best answer for the teenage mother and her baby. My opinion stems from the fact that a great deal of my practice time is spent helping infertile women.

About 10 or 15 percent of married couples are unable to have children. If unmarried women carried their pregnancies to term and offered their babies for adoption, those couples who were unable to have children would be able to adopt them into a stable, two-parent home.

Another fact to consider is that there is more child abuse and neglect among the children of teenage mothers than occurs in the general population. Due to her immaturity, a teenage mother initially may want to keep a child because of the excitement and fun of having a baby of her own. She cannot fully comprehend the challenge and responsibility of motherhood. Later, when the child causes problems, a teenager is more likely to mistreat her child than would a more mature mother.

There are other factors. If a teenage girl decides to keep a child, her relationship with her parents is permanently changed now that she has a child to care for. Furthermore, the child can create problems in a later marriage or can end the girl's attempt to gain a higher education.

## Bulimia and Anorexia

**149** My daughter seems to be overly concerned about her weight. She is very thin and yet constantly talks about how fat she is. Her eating habits are strange. Could she be developing an eating disorder?

If your child is becoming excessively thin, or seems to be gorging food and not gaining weight, you may correctly suspect that something is wrong. She may have anorexia if she is exercising excessively and compulsively, withdrawing from friendships, becoming irritable, and has developed unusual attitudes toward food.

If a person is not gaining any significant amount of weight but is obviously overeating, she may have bulimia. This is especially true if she is storing empty food containers in hidden places, confiscating and eating food belonging to associates, missing chores, spending a lot of money (food is expensive), and spending excessive amounts of time in the bathroom after meals.

Both anorexia nervosa and bulimia often include the compulsive use of laxatives, diuretics, diet pills, and caffeine (as pills or in coffee, etc.).

Bulimia and anorexia nervosa are two diseases of a group of problems called "eating disorders," and some experts feel these disorders should be included in a group of diseases called "addictive disorders," which includes alcoholism and drug addiction. Girls with a certain personal psychological framework (similar to people who become drug addicts or alcoholics) seem to be susceptible to an eating disorder and may become bulimic or anorexic without meaning to when they "flirt" with distorted eating habits.

Bulimia (binging and purging) and anorexia (starving) may be due in part to our society's abnormal preoccupation with food, dieting, and weight, especially among high school, college, and young professional females. Experts estimate that half of the coeds at a large number of colleges in the United States regularly use self-induced vomiting to control their weight, and it is not unusual for young women to go several days without eating in order to keep themselves thin.

These young women do not realize that they are dancing on the thin crust of an abyss of quicksand that at any moment can crack open to engulf them—and, quite literally, kill them.

Bulimia and anorexia nervosa usually originate from what seems to be an innocent and well-intended attempt to control weight. Unfortunately both disorders are now epidemic among young women in our society. It is estimated that 13 percent of college coeds are true bulimics. One in 150 white females between ages twelve and eighteen have anorexia nervosa. The great majority of people with this problem are female, but for every twenty girls with one of these problems, there is one boy with the same problem.

***Characteristic family traits.*** The victims of anorexia and bulimia do not generally come from troubled, distorted homes, but rather usually have confident parents who feel that they have done a better-than-average job of raising their children. They may be described as good, directed, and ambitious parents.

The families of victims of anorexia and bulimia have few sons, with two-thirds of them having only daughters. Girls with this problem often come from upper-middle-class or upper-class families where financial achievement and social position are often high. The relatively few homes of lower-middle-class or lower-class families that produce children with eating disorders are usually upwardly mobile and success oriented.

These families are usually small, averaging about three children per family, and the age of the parents at the birth of their children is often rather high.

The mothers of these girls have frequently been career women who gave up their careers when they married. They are often submissive to their husbands in many details but do not truly respect them. The fathers, despite evident and often considerable social and financial success, feel in some sense "second-best."

These mothers are usually preoccupied with physical appearance, admire fitness and beauty, and expect proper behavior and achievement from their children. These mothers tend to be weight conscious and preoccupied with dieting. Some are obsessively preoccupied with a flaw in the perfection of their bodies.

Not only do the parents often feel that they have done a good job as parents, but the children themselves often feel that their parents have been good parents and that their home has been happy. This perception of their homes may sometimes be an outright denial of facts. These girls are often afraid of being put in a position of having to say something critical. It can also be an expression of over-conformity—what the parents say is always right—and the patients blame themselves for not being "good enough" for such "perfect" mothers and fathers.

Generally these families expect too much in the areas of appearance, good behavior (politeness is emphasized), and academic achievement. Teachers often have commented throughout the school years that the anorexic child was a joy to have in class—cooperative, reliable, and a hard worker. (From *The Golden Cage* by Hilde Bruch, M.D., New York: Random House, 1979.)

Although no one knows what actually causes these diseases to develop, children with the following characteristics seem to have the emotional framework on which to hang bulimia or anorexia nervosa:

> They are judgmental of others, feeling that they are too immature and not serious enough.
>
> They are especially hardworking and markedly helpful to less advantaged friends.
>
> They are *very* responsible, always desiring to please, and compliant at home and at school.

### Bulimia

Bulimia, the more common of the two eating disorders, is also known as the "binge-purge syndrome." The Diagnostic and Statistical Manual of Mental Disorders (p. 44) gives this definition of bulimia:

> Recurrent episodes of binge eating (rapid consumption of a large amount of food in a short period of time, usually less than two hours).
>
> At least three of the following behaviors: consumption of high-caloric, easily ingested food during a binge; inconspicuous eating during a binge; termination of such eating episodes by abdominal pain, sleep, social interruptions, or self-induced vomiting; repeated attempts to lose weight by

severely restrictive diets, self-induced vomiting, or use of cathartics and/or diuretics; frequent weight fluctuations greater than ten pounds due to alternating binges and fasts.

Awareness that the eating pattern is abnormal and fear of not being able to stop eating voluntarily.

Depressed mood and self-deprecating thoughts following eating binges.

Bulimic episodes not due to anorexia nervosa or any known physical disorder.

Victims of bulimia feel dominated by the disease and become desperate for help. They are occasionally even suicidal.

Bulimics can develop physical problems. Menstruation can be erratic or absent even though weight is normal. This does not permanently damage one's body, but pregnancy is impossible during this time. The poor nutrition that results from such abnormal eating habits can result in hair that is of poor texture, or even in partial hair loss. The complexion, too, can deteriorate.

Bulimics who have abnormally low weight can develop electrolyte (the body's salts) disturbances which can result in weakness, muscle spasm, kidney problems, and death. In addition, stomach acid which washes across the teeth during repeated vomiting episodes can dissolve the enamel of the teeth and can, if prolonged, cause the teeth to literally rot out of the mouth.

### Anorexia Nervosa

Although anorexia nervosa occurs less often than bulimia in our society, it is more widely known because the skinny bodies that are the result of the disease are so publicly obvious and because it more commonly results in death than does bulimia. Even with treatment, various studies show that from 0 to 21 percent of people die from anorexia nervosa.

The Diagnostic and Statistical Manual of Mental Disorders (American Psychiatric As-

sociation Quick Reference to Diagnostic Criteria from DSM—III, 1980, p. 67) gives the following definition of anorexia nervosa:

Intense fear of becoming obese, which does not diminish as weight loss progresses.

Disturbance of body image; for example, claiming to "feel fat" even when emaciated.

Weight loss of at least 25 percent of original body weight; or, if under 18 years of age, weight loss from original body weight plus projected weight gain expected from growth charts may be combined to make 25 percent.

Refusal to maintain body weight over a minimal weight for age and height.

No known physical illness that would account for the weight loss.

Victims of anorexia nervosa starve themselves, and this starvation results in noticeable and excessive weight loss. People with this disease often exercise compulsively, in spite of their inadequate diet, accelerating their weight loss. In addition, they will frequently use laxatives, diet pills, diuretics, and excessive coffee to help them lose weight.

It is because victims of this disease lose control, as though their exaggerated desire to lose weight is forcing them to starve, that they usually require medical care in order to regain their health.

Family or friends tend to either ignore or praise the victim's weight loss until the scarecrow-like body forces them to admit that something is dreadfully wrong. Then, typically, they respond with too simplistic advice, such as, "Just *eat*. You know you're too thin," or, more destructively, by trying to force their loved one to gain weight.

The medical problems that result from anorexia nervosa are numerous. Menstruation stops even before the person's weight is low enough to have caused such absence. The complexion and hair suffer, and there is occasional head hair loss but abnormal growth of hair on other body areas. Electrolyte disturbances can develop, and these imbalances in the amount of fluids and "salts" in the body can be life-threatening.

Anorexia nervosa is considered a form of suicide by most specialists. Although many victims threaten suicide, few patients actually commit violent suicide in the midst of their anorexic process. Studies differ, showing suicide rates up to 5.3 percent.

### Treating Anorexia and Bulimia

First of all, before there is any indication of an eating disorder parents should be knowledgeable. If yours is a family with some of the characteristics mentioned earlier, or if you have a child with some of the character traits mentioned, I encourage you to read the following books:

*The Golden Cage* by Dr. Hilde Bruch, Random House, 1979.

*Starving for Attention* by Cherry Boone O'Neill, Dell Books, 1982.

*The Monster Within* by Cynthia Joye Rowland, Baker Book House, 1984.

These books may give you the insight into your own family that will enable you to change some things for the future well being of your children.

If you suspect that a child or a friend may have bulimia or anorexia nervosa, one approach would be to set up a confrontation session with that person and those who are close to her. Observations and concerns should be communicated, along with love and support. If parents of the victim are unaware of their child's condition, they should be contacted because their involvement is vital to the healing of the disease.

The victim should immediately contact a psychologist or psychiatrist. The longer the disease is allowed to exist without treatment, the more entrenched it becomes and the more difficult to cure.

If a person refuses to admit she has a problem, and she refuses to get help, you should contact a psychologist or psychiatrist familiar with these problems to determine the appropriate next step.

Proper therapy for these patients is absolutely vital. It is the unfortunate experience of many bulimics and anorexic patients to find that many physicians, psychologists, and psychiatrists do not understand or know how to treat these diseases. Professional care for these problems should be similar to that which is discussed in the books by Bruch, O'Neill, and Rowland.

Generally, hospitalization is best at the beginning of treatment if any of the following criteria exist:

Rapid loss of more than 25 percent of body weight in less than four months

Fatigue (If a person had been strenuously exercising but has now stopped and is constantly fatigued, she is very sick.)

Fainting and/or irregularity of the pulse; abnormally low blood pressure, pulse, or temperature; abnormality of the electrolytes (the body's salts)

Failure to get well with previous therapy

Suicidal

Family situation is bad

Admission being the only way to get the patient into treatment

Other significant medical or psychiatric problem complicates bulimic condition

If the care of the patient seems to differ from the approach described above, you may want to contact one of the organizations mentioned at the end of this section or one of the specialists mentioned in one of the books to get a second opinion on the type of care being offered. Remember, care must be aggressive and good; do not be reassured when your child says that her anorexia or bulimia is not much of a problem. These patients are experts at deception and denial.

Even with proper treatment, success is not guaranteed. For example, good treatment of anorexia nervosa results in a 50 percent-cure rate and 30 percent-improvement rate. Approximately 20 percent of these patients remain chronically ill and chronically troubled by their disease.

In summary, these diseases are dangerous and indicate serious psychological problems. They can result in dangerous physical problems, and even death.

### Organizations You Can Contact for Help

American Anorexia/Bulimia Association
133 Cedar Lane
Teaneck, New Jersey 07666
Phone: 201-836-1806

Dr. Gene Ann Rubel
ANRED
(Anorexia Nervosa and Related Eating Disorders)
P.O. Box 5102
Eugene, Oregon 97404

Bulimia Foundation of America
917 Dover
Edmond, Oklahoma 73034

NAANAD
(National Association of Anorexia Nervosa and Associated Disorders, Inc.)
P.O. Box 271
Highland Park, Illinois 60035
Phone: 312-831-3438

Pat Tilton
National Anoretic Aid Society
P.O. Box 29461
Columbus, Ohio 43229

Overeaters Anonymous
Box 92870
Los Angeles, California 90009

Consult your telephone directory for information regarding local chapters. This organization offers help for all types of eating disorders.)

The following self-evaluation form, designed by K. Kim Lampson, Ph.D., 550—16th Ave., Suite 301, Seattle, Washington 98122, © 1982, can help a person decide if she needs help.

## Are You Dying to Be Thin?

The following questionnaire will give you an indication of whether or not you are living a lifestyle that indicates anorexic and/or bulimic tendencies. Anorexia nervosa (key symptom: extreme weight loss due to self-starvation) and bulimia (key symptom: binging followed by purging) are becoming more and more openly acknowledged as publicity increases public awareness and understanding.

Answer the following questions honestly. Write the number of your answer in the space at the left.

____1. I have eating habits that are different from those of my family and friends.
1) Often    2) Sometimes    3) Rarely    4) Never

____2. I find myself panicking if I cannot exercise as I planned for fear of gaining weight.
1) Almost always    2) Sometimes    3) Rarely    4) Never

_____3. My friends tell me I am thin but I don't believe them because I feel fat.
1) Often      2) Sometimes      3) Rarely      4) Never

_____4. (Females only) My menstrual period has ceased or become irregular due to no known medical reasons.
1) True      2) False

_____5. I have become obsessed with food to the point that I cannot go through a day without worrying about what I will or will not eat.
1) Almost always      2) Sometimes      3) Rarely      4) Never

_____6. I have lost more than 25% of the normal weight for my height (eg 30 lbs. from 120 lbs.)
1) True      2) False

_____7. I would panic if I got on the scale tomorrow and found out I had gained two pounds.
1) Almost always      2) Sometimes      3) Rarely      4) Never

_____8. I find that I prefer to eat alone or when I am sure no one will see me, thus am making excuses so I can eat less and less with friends and family.
1) Often      2) Sometimes      3) Rarely      4) Never

_____9. I find myself going on uncontrollable eating binges during which I consume large amounts of food to the point that I feel sick and make myself vomit.
1) 3 or more times per day      2) 1-2 times per day      3) 1-2 times per week      4) Rarely      5) Never

_____10. I use laxatives as a means of weight control.
1) On a regular basis      2) Sometimes      3) Rarely      4) Never

_____11. I find myself playing games with food (eg cutting it up into tiny pieces, hiding food so people will think I ate it, chewing it and spitting it out without swallowing) telling myself certain foods are bad.
1) Often      2) Sometimes      3) Rarely      4) Never

_____12. People around me have become very interested in what I eat and I find myself getting angry at them for pushing food on me.
1) Often      2) Sometimes      3) Rarely      4) Never

_____13. I have felt more depressed and irritable recently than I used to and/or have been spending increasing amounts of time alone.
1) True      2) False

_____14. I keep a lot of my fears about food and eating to myself because I am afraid no one would understand.
1) Often      2) Sometimes      3) Rarely      4) Never

_____15. I enjoy making gourmet, high-calorie meals or treats for others as long as I don't have to eat any myself.
1) Often      2) Sometimes      3) Rarely      4) Never

_____16. The most powerful fear in my life is the fear of gaining weight or becoming fat.
1) Often      2) Sometimes      3) Rarely      4) Never

_____17. I find myself totally absorbed when reading books about dieting, exercising and calorie counting to the point that I spend hours studying them.
1) Often      2) Sometimes      3) Rarely      4) Never

_____18. I tend to be a perfectionist and am not satisfied with myself unless I do things perfectly.
1) Almost always      2) Sometimes      3) Rarely      4) Never

_____19. I go through long periods of time without eating anything (fasting) as a means of weight control.
1) Often      2) Sometimes      3) Rarely      4) Never

_____20.  It is important to me to try to be thinner than all of my friends.
1) Almost always    2) Sometimes    3) Rarely    4) Never

Add your scores together and compare with the table below:

Under 30    Strong tendencies toward anorexia nervosa

30 - 45     Strong tendencies toward bulimia

45 - 55     Weight conscious, not necessarily with anorexic or bulimic tendencies

Over 55     No need for concern

If you scored below 45, it would be wise for you to (1) seek more information about anorexia and bulimia and (2) contact a counselor, pastor or physician, to determine what kind of assistance would be most helpful for you. Anorexia nervosa and bulimia are potential life-threatening disorders which can be overcome with the proper support and counsel. The earlier you seek help, the better, although it is never too late to start on the road to recovery.

## An Afterword

We have discussed some difficult and heartbreaking situations in this chapter, but these things are not the norm. Most females have absolutely no major health problems during childhood and adolescence. Those young girls who do develop problems can benefit from the wealth of medical knowledge and treatment available today.

If you should have problems with your child—medical or emotional—don't hesitate to seek help. Contact a physician, see a psychologist or psychiatrist, or get counsel from your pastor.

Pray a lot, whether or not you are having problems! If your child does well, you should realize that you have a great deal for which to be thankful. There is no way that you were totally responsible for the good results, or the bad. The only way loving parents can end up with mature, self-confident, well-directed, and loving children is with the help of God!

# 4

# The Reproductive Years

The reproductive years are those years in a woman's life from the time she starts having her menstrual periods until the time they stop. These are the years when her reproductive organs work the hardest, are the busiest, and are the most subject to disease. They are the years when the female hormones surge, producing characteristic ups and downs in a woman's physical and emotional self.

Because the time span of the reproductive years extends from adolescence to middle age, it occupies center stage in a woman's life. The changes that occur between the beginning and the end of this period are enormous and multiple.

The excitement, joys, opportunities, and challenges of this period of life can be overwhelming. So, too, can be the disappointments, heartaches, and pain. It is so often in this period of life that a woman goes from one extreme to another. Her body both blossoms and begins to fade. Having sex may go from being uppermost on her mind to being the least of her concerns. She both welcomes children into her life and watches them leave. She may both find her mate and lose him—all in this period of transition from little girl to mature woman!

Because the major portion of this book is devoted to the reproductive period of a woman's life (conception, pregnancy, labor and delivery, contraception, and sexually transmitted disease) this is basically a catch-all chapter. It includes these topics:

Annual routine examination

Female surgery

Endometriosis

Low abdominal and pelvic pain

Bladder infections

Premenstrual syndrome (PMS)

Diethylstilbestrol (DES)

Tuberculosis of the pelvic organs

Abortion

Rape and Sexual Assault

Many of the subjects discussed in this chapter are included because they involve more than just one of the female organs and therefore would not properly fit into the chapter on diseases of the reproductive organs; some subjects are included because it is during this reproductive phase of life that these situations are most likely to be bothersome, even though they may also occur before or after this age span. Other topics, such as rape and abortion, are included in this chapter because it is during the reproductive years that they are most likely a consideration.

Routine examinations are discussed in this chapter because it is during this time that you establish the habit of going to a physician. Often the doctor you go to early in your reproductive years is the one you still consult when you reach menopause! Hopefully you have already chosen a doctor, as outlined in the introduction.

Although I am not a urologist, I am including a brief discussion of bladder infections in this book. The reason for this is that women usually call their gynecologist, or the doctor who does their annual exams and Pap smear, for treatment of their bladder infections. Also, since bladder infections can be so intimately involved with a woman's genital function, it seems appropriate to answer here some questions you might have about this medical problem.

## Routine Medical Tests Often Included in an Annual Physical Examination

| Test | Purpose |
|------|---------|
| Blood pressure measurement | Detect high blood pressure |
| Neck and thyroid exam | Detect infection or primary tumors |
| Breast exam | Detect any lumps or other abnormalities |
| Pelvic exam | Visual and manual examination of vagina, cervix, and other female reproductive organs |
| Pap smear | Microscopic examination of cells shed from cervix |
| Digital rectal | Manual examination of rectum |
| Fecal blood | Detect microscopic blood in stool samples |
| Urinalysis | Detect sugar, albumin, or germs in urine |
| Mammography | X-ray exam of breast, occasionally between ages 35-50; regularly after age 50 |

## The Annual Routine Examination

### 150 Is it necessary to have an annual examination?

I believe that it is. In 1980 the American Cancer Society made a highly publicized recommendation that Pap smears be done every three years instead of annually. Since that time it has been found that at least 5 percent of abnormal Pap smears will worsen so rapidly that, in one or two years time, the cervix will have developed dangerous invasive cancer. Pap smears done every three years would not catch this problem until it was too late.

Further, the American Cancer Society ignored the fact that the annual examination serves other purposes than just taking Pap smears, as you will see in the next question.

Some doctors encourage patients to have examinations every six months, especially at menopausal age. This seems unnecessary unless a woman has a health problem that needs to be watched closely. True, there is a greater possibility of breast cancer as one grows older, but seeing a doctor twice a year instead of annually will not significantly increase the chance of finding a breast cancer early. Breast cancers are usually detected by mammograms or by breast self-examination, not by seeing the doctor two times a year.

### 151 What purpose does an annual examination serve?

Three primary considerations make the annual examination very important:

*Forum for questions.* The annual visit to the doctor gives you a chance to ask the questions that you have thought of during the preceding year and to discuss any problems that may have developed during that year, physical or otherwise.

*Abnormalities can be found.* Diseases and other problems can exist in your body without your being aware of them, such as abnormal Pap smears or high blood pressure. These can be found during the annual examination.

*Encouragement for good health.* At the annual examination your doctor should encourage you to keep your weight under control and to practice good health habits, similar to those suggested in chapter 15. There is new information every year about maintaining sound health, and I have something new to tell my patients almost every time they come in for a routine examination.

## 152 When should a woman start having pelvic examinations?

A young woman should start having annual examinations when any of the following occur:

There is a problem with, or question about, her female organs

She becomes sexually active

She is going to be married

She is in her late teens or early twenties, even if none of the other situations apply

## 153 What is included in an annual gynecological examination?

The routine examination varies from gynecologist to gynecologist, but the following guide provides minimum requirements for the usual checkup.

*Every year.* From the time the routine exam is started, it should include an examination of the neck, breasts, abdomen, and

pelvis, including a digital rectal examination; a blood pressure check; urine testing for albumin (for nephritis), sugar (for diabetes), and germs (for infection of the kidneys or bladder); a Pap smear; and a weight check.

*Beginning at age thirty-five.* In addition to the usual checks, the exams after age thirty-five should include an occasional mammogram. (Every other year until menopause is my recommendation.)

*After menopause.* In addition to the above, a woman should have a mammogram every year from the age of fifty on. (See Q. 851–883 for further information on breast care.)

## 154 How is the cost of an annual examination distributed?

There is a great deal of variation in the cost of an annual exam and in the way the charges might be presented to you. The following are the separate fees you might be responsible for:

Physician's fee, which will usually include a finger stick blood test for anemia, a urine test, a blood pressure check, the exam, and the question-answering time

Pathologist's fee, for the Pap smear

Mammogram

Blood tests, depending on a doctor's routine and on any signs of disease

If other than routine tests are done, there is an extra charge. If a patient has a vaginal infection, for instance, there would be charges for a smear of the vaginal secretions and for a culture, if that was necessary.

Some doctors have an arrangement with the laboratory whereby you pay only the doctor, and your doctor will be billed by the laboratory at the end of each month for all the work it has done for his or her office. The

# Bimanual Pelvic Examination

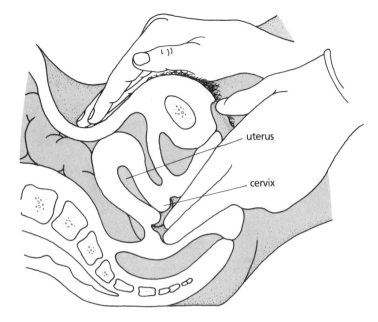

uterus

cervix

The cervix, uterus, and ovaries are palpated. The pelvis is checked for a tumor, unusual tenderness or other abnormality.

doctor normally receives a percentage of what you pay for this type of arrangement, but you pay the same amount as with other arrangements because the pathology lab charges less, in order to get the doctor's referrals.

---

**155** **What should I do if my doctor finds a problem during my annual examination?**

If your doctor finds an abnormality and recommends that you come back to the office for any reason, be sure to comply with this recommendation. Take any medication prescribed, in exactly the way the doctor tells you, and take all of it. If you have any questions about how to take your medicine, call your doctor back or ask your pharmacist.

In addition, reading is a good way to find out all you can about a problem. I hope this book serves you well in that respect. If something your doctor says does not make sense to you, consult with another physician before complying with the original suggestion. Remember, a doctor can almost always say

what has to be said in terms you can understand. If you cannot understand what he or she is trying to tell you, your doctor may be confused or unsure and may be "putting up a smoke screen" so you will not know about this confusion. If what your doctor has to say does not "add up" in your mind, or if you cannot get an adequate explanation, get a second opinion.

If your doctor suspects some type of cancer, and you cannot find another source of good information, call the National Cancer Institute's Cancer Information Service for information and confidential answers to your questions about cancer.

The main number is (800) 4-CANCER
In Washington, D.C.: (202) 636-5700
In Alaska: (800) 638-6070
In Hawaii: (808) 524-1234

---

**156** **Is it wise to have an examination by an internal-medicine specialist in addition to my annual gynecological exam?**

If you are feeling fine and your regular doctor does the exams and studies listed in Q. 153,

## Pap Smear

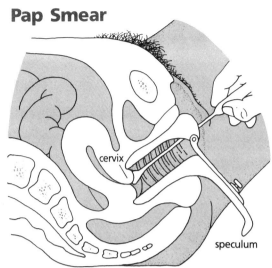

cervix

speculum

The cervix is examined and cells are scraped from the surface, smeared on a glass slide and sent to a lab for microscopic examination.

you do not need to see an internal-medicine specialist in addition to your gynecologist's annual exam. If your gynecologist finds a medical problem that is outside his or her field of expertise, you will be referred to another physician. For instance, if you have pneumonia or high blood pressure, you will be referred to a family practitioner or to an internal-medicine specialist. If a significant breast lump is found, you will usually be referred to a general surgeon. (See Q. 851–883.)

But even when your gynecologist has found nothing wrong, if you want to see an internist or family practitioner for a more complete examination, you certainly should do so. If your own doctor's exam has been thorough, however, and if you feel normal, it is unlikely that an internist would find any disease during a more detailed exam.

## Female Surgery

### 157 What types of surgery do gynecologists do?

Gynecologists perform numerous opera-

tions, and I will not try to outline them all here. However, most do the following procedures (consult Index for description).

> D&C (dilatation and curettage of the uterus for women having miscarriages or abnormal uterine bleeding)
>
> Vaginal and abdominal hysterectomies
>
> Vaginal repairs
>
> Endometriosis surgery
>
> Infertility surgery
>
> Operations for complications of pregnancy, including cesarean sections and operations for ectopic pregnancies
>
> Sterilization procedures on women. (Urologists and general surgeons do vasectomies on men.)

No one likes to have surgery. It is expensive; interrupts schedules; creates fear of dying, cancer, and complications; and is usually painful. These are all legitimate concerns, but the surgery is not done except for beneficial reasons. I encourage my patients to concentrate on what might happen to them without the surgery rather than what might happen to them during the short time it takes to get it done.

### 158 Can doctors other than gynecologists do surgery on the female organs?

Since most surgery on the female organs is generally considered "fairly easy," general practitioners, family practitioners, general surgeons, and gynecologists all do female-organ surgery. However, because of their training and expertise, gynecologists are the only group of physicians whom you should allow to perform surgery on your female organs unless you have no other choice.

I am obviously biased, but my biases are a result of the problems I have seen produced by ill-thought-out, poorly timed, or poorly done "easy" operations performed by non-gynecologists.

Here are some examples:

D&Cs done on patients who had supposedly miscarried, but who were actually still carrying normal pregnancies. Such procedures terminated pregnancies that these women wanted to continue.

Hysterectomies done for fibroid tumors on women who had not had all the children they wanted. Most of these hysterectomies could have been avoided by any gynecologist who would simply remove the fibroids from the uterus, leaving the uterus intact and the woman able to bear children.

Both ovaries removed from young women who had ovarian tumors, leaving them permanently sterile and having to take hormones every day for years to come. Any gynecologist will at least attempt to "shell" tumors out of the ovaries in this situation. Leaving some ovarian tissue present in such a patient can probably enable her to get pregnant in the future. It can also keep her from having to take hormones every day for many years.

Sterilization procedures done by making large, four- or five-inch incisions in the abdomen, when the same thing could have been accomplished by simple laparoscopy or mini-laparotomy, with very small incisions.

While the surgical procedures of gynecology seem fairly simple and straightforward, the judgment involved in deciding when to do the surgery, and what to do during the operation, is why gynecologists spend four years in specialty training following the completion of medical school. This training makes a difference for patients, and patients should avail themselves of a gynecologist's expertise.

The one exception to this is when a C-section is necessary during pregnancy. If a general practitioner or family practitioner is well trained in obstetric care, I have no qualms about such a doctor doing a cesarean section. The operation is a fairly easy procedure. The difficult part is the decision about when to do it.

## 159  What is a hysterectomy?

Hysterectomy refers to removal of the uterus. The cervix is part of the uterus; the fallopian tubes and the ovaries are not. Removal of the uterus can be accomplished through an incision in the abdomen or through the vagina. The decision of which method to use is not based on the surgeon's personal preference or a flip of the coin. There are definite reasons for doing either procedure.

In addition, it may be necessary to remove the tubes and ovaries along with the uterus. Most women think of this as a "complete hysterectomy," but that is not the correct term. A complete hysterectomy involves removal of the uterus only. When the tubes and ovaries are also removed, the procedure is called a "complete (or total) hysterectomy *and* bilateral salpingo-oophorectomy." It is no wonder the term *total hysterectomy* has been adopted by lay people to mean "they got it all!"

Briefly, the different operations and their impact on the body are:

*Hysterectomy.* This is removal of only the uterus, but including both parts of the uterus—the body of the uterus and the cervix. The tubes and ovaries are left in place. The term *total abdominal hysterectomy* means the same thing: removal of the uterus with its cervix. A hysterectomy means that there will be no more periods, no more pregnancies, no possibility of ever having cancer of the uterus or of the cervix, and no hormone change. The ovaries will continue functioning as they always have until menopause. Sexuality is unaffected.

***Supracervical hysterectomy.*** This term means a hysterectomy in which only the upper part of the uterus is removed, leaving the cervix in place. This operation is much simpler to do than a regular hysterectomy, and even doctors who are not well trained in gynecologic surgery can do it quite easily. It was used a great deal many years ago, but there are only two situations that call for a supracervical hysterectomy these days: first, if a patient is having massive uterine bleeding and the doctor must remove the uterus in a hurry; second, if a woman has ovarian cancer in her pelvis that would make it unwise for the doctor to remove the cervix at the time of the hysterectomy. If there is massive ovarian cancer in a woman's pelvis and the cervix is removed at a hysterectomy, the ovarian cancer can sometimes more easily grow down into the vagina, causing bothersome bleeding and discharge. I have done only a few supracervical hysterectomies on patients with

# Types of Hysterectomies

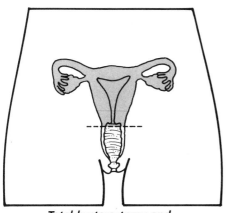

**Total hysterectomy and salpingo-oophorectomy**
Uterus, ovaries, and tubes removed.

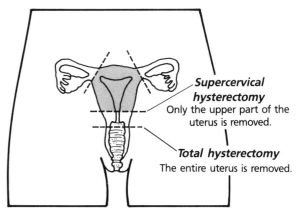

***Supercervical hysterectomy***
Only the upper part of the uterus is removed.

***Total hysterectomy***
The entire uterus is removed.

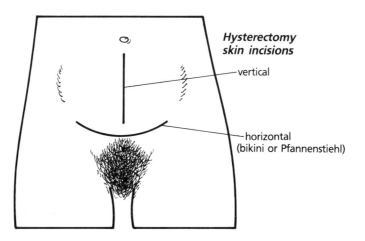

***Hysterectomy skin incisions***
vertical

horizontal (bikini or Pfannenstiehl)

ovarian cancer, but have never had to do one as an emergency, and such a situation is rare. A supracervical hysterectomy will mean no menstrual periods, no pregnancies, no hormone change, no change in sexuality, and no possibility of uterine cancer in the future. It is still necessary to have a Pap smear once a year, however, because there is still a possibility of cervical cancer, since the cervix is still in its original position.

*Hysterectomy with removal of tubes and ovaries.* Physicians call this "total abdominal hysterectomy and bilateral salpingo-oophorectomy" (or "panhysterectomy"). This surgery means no more periods, no pregnancies, and no possibility of cancer of *any* of the female organs except the vagina or vulva. Because the ovaries have been removed, there will be no female hormones being produced in the body. This necessitates taking supplemental hormones if the woman has not already gone through menopause at the time of the hysterectomy.

---

## 160 Is it true that many unnecessary hysterectomies are done?

It is true that more hysterectomies than any other major operations are done in America, and that 25 percent of all women will eventually have their uterus removed. This is not an indication that doctors are doing "too many" hysterectomies, however. If you question this, take a poll of your friends who have had hysterectomies and ask them if they regret having had the procedure done. I expect that you will find that they are almost unanimously glad that they had a hysterectomy and are thrilled at the beneficial changes in their bodies.

The few patients who are unhappy with having had a hysterectomy are usually those who had some medical problem that made their hysterectomy necessary before they had a chance to complete their family. These women, though, would not be counted in the number that some experts say represent "unnecessary hysterectomies."

The truth of the matter is that many of the doctors who write articles about so-called unnecessary hysterectomies are in academic environments and do not have to deal with patients on an everyday basis. They would probably even say that many of the situations that most doctors agree definitely warrant hysterectomies (see Q. 162) would be unnecessary indications. If their guidelines were followed, women would have to live with female organ problems that cause their quality of life to be worse than it needs to be.

Furthermore, hysterectomy is perhaps the safest major operation done today. Patients rarely have any complications during the operation or during recovery. It is for this reason that a hysterectomy can be done for problems that are not life-threatening and that some doctors might label "unnecessary."

---

## 161 In general, when should a hysterectomy be done?

A hysterectomy should be performed when a woman, regardless of age, is having enough "female trouble" or disease associated with her uterus that it needs to be removed or that she wants it removed. Fortunately most of the uterine problems that occur in younger women are not ones that demand a hysterectomy. Women can normally delay a hysterectomy until they have had all the children they want.

Many women delay a hysterectomy unnecessarily, however. I had a patient who finally had the needed surgery, after delaying it for years. She came back to my office feeling significantly better and questioning why she had put it off so long. She made an interesting statement: "I felt that since I was so young, I ought to have a uterus, even if it was diseased!"

Doctors occasionally tell patients they

should have a hysterectomy to avoid ever developing cancer of the cervix or uterus. Fear of having cancer in the future should have little influence on your decision to have a hysterectomy now. A hysterectomy should be done for specific problems, not for what might develop in the future. Besides, cervical and uterine cancer can almost always be discovered by your doctor before they become dangerous.

I tell my patients that there are hysterectomies that (a) *must* be done and those that (b) *can* be done if a woman feels her problems are serious enough. Examples of both situations are discussed in the next two questions.

---

## 162 What situations definitely require a hysterectomy?

Hysterectomies must be done in the following situations. A complete discussion of these disorders is found in chapter 10.

Cancer of the uterus

Severe precancerous changes in the uterus

Severe endometriosis with large pelvic masses made up of endometriosis tissue

Severe bleeding that produces anemia and is not corrected by other treatment

Severe pelvic infections that do not respond to antibiotics. Such infections, if allowed to progress, can result in death.

Fibroid tumors the size of a three-month pregnant uterus or larger

If a hysterectomy is not done in these situations, major health problems or even death may result.

---

## 163 What are the situations in which a hysterectomy can legitimately be done if the woman chooses so?

Hysterectomies can be done, if a woman is bothered enough by a problem, in the following situations:

Prolapsed uterus (or prolapsed uterus with looseness of the vaginal walls)

Pain when deep penetration occurs during intercourse

Looseness with intercourse

Enough difficulty having a bowel movement to necessitate a woman using her fingers to press on her tissues (either in the vagina or just above the anus) in order to have a bowel movement

Excessive loss of urine with coughing, sneezing, or laughing

Fibroids

Pelvic pain

Heavy bleeding with periods

Certain low-grade infections

Severe premenstrual or menstrual problems

Some physicians might argue with my suggesting a hysterectomy for severe PMS, severe cramps, or severe headaches that may occur just at the time of menstruation. There are some women, however, who have had all the children they intend to have and whose lives are wrecked by these symptoms. If such a woman is having debilitating problems and has been unable to get relief from her symptoms any other way, a hysterectomy will sometimes help. She would want to proceed with such a major step only after consultation with a competent gynecologist, so that she can know that her chances of cure from such a procedure are good. In order to assure a good response to such surgery, it is sometimes necessary to remove the ovaries too. This, of course, would not be advisable for younger women.

A woman can tolerate any of these problems and not have a hysterectomy, and many women prefer to do just that. The choice is an individual one in most cases.

I suggest that you check the Index for a complete discussion if you are bothered by any of the problems listed above. The majority of this information is in chapter 10.

## 164  What are the advantages of having a hysterectomy?

Having a hysterectomy can result in these advantages:

It can be life-saving in certain situations.

It can improve your enjoyment of life by removing a nagging and troublesome problem.

It means no more menstrual periods; not a reason to have a hysterectomy, but a pleasant side benefit.

It usually means no more premenstrual tension and the end of symptoms caused by the rise and fall in hormones. Most women stop having these symptoms even if they do not have their ovaries removed.

It means no more pregnancies and no need for contraception.

Furthermore, if you ask, your doctor can remove your appendix during a hysterectomy, which means you will never have appendicitis. If you have already gone through the menopause or are older than forty at the time of hysterectomy, the doctor can also remove your ovaries, permanently eliminating the risk of ovarian cancer. (See Q. 166.)

## 165  What are the disadvantages of a hysterectomy?

The drawbacks of a hysterectomy are:

No more pregnancies. A woman may have to undergo a hysterectomy before she completes her family. Since this obviously would be unfortunate, in this situation a woman should not have a hysterectomy unless it is mandatory for life and health.

There is some discomfort the first three or four days after a hysterectomy, although pain medication generally makes this problem tolerable. Patients should ask for pain medicine as often as it is allowed, which is normally every three hours. This not only keeps them from feeling tense during the first few days after surgery, but will actually allow them to feel better sooner than if they let themselves hurt.

Although complications from hysterectomies are extremely rare, all surgery carries some risk, and this is no exception. For example, complications and even death can occur from the anesthetic. Bleeding during or after surgery that would require transfusions from which one *might* get AIDS or hepatitis is a risk from all types of surgery. Other possible complications from a hysterectomy are a hole between the bladder and vagina, ureteral damage (involving the tube carrying urine from the kidney to the bladder) a bowel obstruction, or an infection in an ovary.

## 166  Does a hysterectomy make a woman "different"?

There are many myths that surround hysterectomy. Such myths include:

*"The vagina becomes 'just like a sack' for the man during intercourse."* I have not had a single patient whose husband could tell that she had had a hysterectomy by the way her vagina felt to him during intercourse. Actually the upper vagina is somewhat more snug after a hysterectomy because of the way the top of the vagina is sewn together and heals.

It is normal for a husband to be afraid of having intercourse for many weeks after his wife has had a hysterectomy. He can picture his penis pushing right out through the top of his wife's vagina. However, once a woman's vagina is healed and the doctor says it is okay for intercourse, intercourse is okay, no matter how deep or vigorous the vaginal penetration. Common sense says for a couple to take it easy at first.

Many women ask what happens to the space in the body where the uterus was after the uterus is removed. To understand the amount of space involved, remember that the uterus is about the size of a small orange, approximately three to four ounces in weight. When it is removed the intestines merely fall into the space where the uterus was. This repositions the intestines so that the abdomen flattens out just enough to take up the place where the intestines were. Even if the uterus is fairly large, this repositioning of the abdominal contents is not enough to make much difference in the flattening of a woman's abdomen.

*"Menopause will come sooner if a woman has had a hysterectomy."* This is not true if the ovaries are still intact. The ovaries are independent of the uterus and feed their hormones to the body through the blood stream. The uterus seems to have no effect on the way the ovaries function.

*"Women who have their ovaries removed have to take hormones the rest of their life."* Women who are forty years old or older but still not past menopause can choose to have their ovaries removed at the time of a hysterectomy to eliminate the future possibility of having ovarian cancer. They should then start taking estrogen as described in Q. 275, 276 because young women who are without estrogen in their bodies are more likely to develop osteoporosis. When they reach the average age for menopause, fifty-one, they will be no different from other postmenopausal women and can then decide if they wish to continue taking estrogen. I recommend that all such women take estrogen and progesterone.

*"A woman's sexual interest will decrease after a hysterectomy."* Studies have shown quite clearly that a woman's sexual interest and responsiveness are not related to her uterus, tubes, and ovaries, once her sexual responsiveness has been established. There is no change in a woman's sexuality after a hysterectomy unless she develops a psychological hang-up about it. If a woman expects that she might have some emotional problem about this, she should see a counselor before she has the hysterectomy.

*"There is less sexual feeling with intercourse."* A woman's sexual feelings are primarily located in the undisturbed portion of her vagina and vulvar tissues, not in the uterus. Her feelings during intercourse and orgasm, therefore, will not be disturbed by a hysterectomy.

*"Women get fat after a hysterectomy."* There is no relationship between the female organs and the body's metabolism. Therefore, women do not get fat after hysterectomies *because* of the surgery. It just so happens that women often gain weight in their forties and fifties, and this is when they most often have hysterectomies.

*"There is no lubrication with intercourse."* Some women seem to have a little less vaginal moisture than before a hysterectomy. This may occur because the cervix does produce some secretions into the vagina which can increase the moisture around the opening of the vagina. The cervix, however, does not contribute to sexual lubrication. Therefore, there should be little or no change in sexual lubrication after hysterectomy.

---

**167**  **I am afraid I will feel "castrated" if I have a hysterectomy. Is this feeling unusual?**

This is not an unusual thought for a woman to have, in spite of all the reassuring information she might read. It would be best for you to see a psychologist, psychiatrist, or other counselor if you need a hysterectomy and feel this way. If you have had a hysterectomy and you now feel a sense of loss, regret, or castration, don't let it build up in your mind or try to sweep it under the rug. Talking to a counselor, or a friend who has gone through the same experience, will usually help a great deal.

## 168 Which is best, a vaginal hysterectomy or an abdominal hysterectomy?

Medical conditions usually dictate whether your hysterectomy should be done through an incision in the abdomen or through the vagina. Both are sound procedures. A vaginal hysterectomy is not done blind, as the doctor can see the area quite well while he or she performs the surgery. Believe it or not, there is almost always plenty of room for good visualization during vaginal surgery if there are no significant adhesions or growths.

Generally you should agree to the technique your doctor recommends. If you question his or her recommendations based on the information in the next two questions, you might want to get a second opinion.

Some gynecologists are not comfortable with nor good at doing vaginal surgery, and the advantages of the vaginal over the abdominal procedure are not important enough to warrant changing doctors if yours does not want to do the hysterectomy vaginally. The advantages of vaginal surgery include less pain, shorter hospitalization, quicker recovery, no abdominal scar, and no chance of infection or hernia of an abdominal wound.

Occasionally the supporting ligaments of a woman's uterus hold the uterus so high that a doctor cannot remove it through the vagina. Of course, if the surgeon doing a vaginal hysterectomy finds blood vessels he or she cannot get to through the vagina, or adhesions are fusing the pelvic organs together, the surgery may have to be finished by doing an abdominal incision. This is not a "complication," but rather a turn of events that is always possible when a doctor is doing vaginal surgery.

## 169 What medical situations would best be handled by an abdominal hysterectomy?

An abdominal hysterectomy is best in these cases:

*Uterine growths are too large to be removed through the vagina.* Once a uterus is the size of a two-month pregnancy or larger, it is best that it be removed through an abdominal incision because of difficulty in getting it out through the vagina.

*Ovarian growths are present.* If you are having surgery for ovarian growths, and you are going to have a hysterectomy at the same time, it must be done through an abdominal incision. It is often difficult or impossible to remove the ovaries through the vagina, and

## Vaginal/Abdominal Hysterectomy

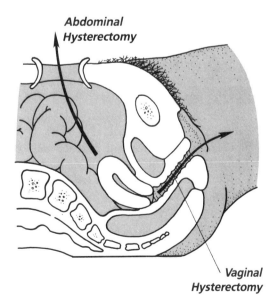

Abdominal Hysterectomy

Vaginal Hysterectomy

if cancer is present, more extensive evaluation and surgery must be done.

*Pain is the indication for a hysterectomy.* When surgery is being done because of pelvic pain, it is usually best that it be performed with an abdominal incision, so that the doctor can evaluate the entire pelvic area and the upper abdomen. Occasionally the pain is coming from some part of the body other than the uterus. It is best, therefore, to have the entire abdomen explored at the time surgery is performed for pain, because the doctor cannot see much of the abdomen above the level of the uterus, tubes, and ovaries when operating vaginally.

*The uterus is infected.* If you are having a hysterectomy because of infection, it must be performed through an abdominal incision. When infection is or was present, it can cause the organs inside the body to stick together as though glue had been poured on them. The bands of scar tissue that hold the internal organs together in this situation are called adhesions. A doctor operating through the vagina would not be able safely to cut adhesions and remove the uterus. In trying to cut adhesions, the surgeon might cut into the bladder or bowel.

## 170 What problems are best handled by a vaginal hysterectomy?

A vaginal hysterectomy can usually be done when the following situations exist.

*Bleeding.* If you are having a hysterectomy because of bleeding problems, and your uterus is normal size, it can most easily be done through the vagina.

*Pelvic relaxation.* If you are having a hysterectomy because your uterus is prolapsed, or because your vaginal walls are relaxed and a hysterectomy is necessary to repair the problem, this is best accomplished through the vagina. (Both the hysterectomy and vaginal repairs can be done in the same surgery.)

*Uterine growths that have not enlarged*

*the uterus too much.* A uterus with fibroids that have not enlarged to the size of a two-month pregnancy can often be removed through the vagina. If your vagina is too tight, the doctor might have to finish the operation with an abdominal incision.

*Precancerous changes in the lining of the uterus or of the cervix.* Generally this condition can be successfully taken care of by a vaginal hysterectomy.

## 171 Does surgery for vaginal relaxation involve a hysterectomy?

Surgery for vaginal relaxation (see Q. 699–702 for more information) normally includes removal of the uterus, because if the vagina is loose, the uterus is also probably inadequately supported by its ligaments. Even if the uterus is not prolapsed, a better bladder repair can be done after the uterus is removed.

Once the uterus has been removed, vaginally or abdominally, and the top of the vagina closed, the doctor reinforces the vaginal walls, "taking up the slack" by pulling in and tying normal supporting tissues under the bladder to give it good support. If necessary, the same can be done on the back wall of the vagina, giving the rectal wall better support too.

When the surgery is completed, the rectal and bladder walls are both well supported and, in the process, the vagina is made more snug, an advantage for intercourse.

Vaginal repairs must be done with skill and care to avoid recurrence of the same vaginal problems in the future.

## 172 Will you describe normal hospitalization procedure for a hysterectomy?

The hospital procedure for a hysterectomy is basically the same as with other major surgery.

Before surgery the following things are routine:

Blood tests are taken.

Urine is collected for a urinalysis.

Your medical history will be taken. You will sign a permission form for the surgery.

The anesthesiologist will talk to you.

You will often be given an enema and a vaginal douche.

You will be given nothing to eat or drink after midnight the night before surgery because any food in your stomach might be vomited up into your lungs during the administration of the anesthetic, an extremely dangerous situation. If you cheat on this rule, be sure to tell your anesthesiologist or your doctor so they can delay your surgery for a day. This can be a life-or-death matter.

About an hour before surgery you will often receive an injection to relax you. The shot will not usually put you to sleep. An antibiotic is often included in the injection. Given before surgery, this helps prevent infection.

Following surgery the standard procedure is:

You will receive fluids in your veins for one or two days. If you start eating immediately after surgery, before your intestines start working, the fluid and food can back up in your intestines and cause severe bloating and gas pain. (Blood transfusions are not usually necessary following a hysterectomy.)

You will have a catheter in place when you wake up from surgery. If you have not had a vaginal repair, this catheter will usually be removed the day after surgery.

You will normally stay in the hospital about five to seven days after surgery,

and you will receive pain medication, which you should not hesitate to take if you are uncomfortable. You will not feel any different if you have had uterus, ovaries, and tubes removed or only the uterus removed.

If you have had a vaginal hysterectomy with no vaginal repairs, you will probably have less discomfort than with an abdominal operation. You should be able to go home a day or two earlier than if you had had an abdominal operation.

If you have had vaginal repairs done, you will have either a regular Foley catheter or a suprapubic catheter in your bladder. The suprapubic catheter is inserted through the skin above your pubic bone into your bladder. This is more convenient for you, because you will not have a catheter in your urethra. When you begin voiding urine again, the suprapubic tube measures how much urine is left in your bladder. When you are emptying your bladder completely, the tube can be painlessly removed. If you have a Foley catheter, you will normally have it removed five days after surgery to see if you can void. If you cannot, the catheter will be reinserted and taken out again the next day or two. This procedure will be repeated until you are able to empty your bladder.

I warn my patients who are having bladder repairs done that they may not be able to urinate normally for two months after surgery, although this is not generally the case. About half my patients are able to empty their bladders and have the suprapubic tube or Foley catheter removed before they leave the hospital. The other half usually can have these devices out within one or two weeks of leaving the hospital. Remember, though, being unable to void normally for two or three months after vaginal surgery is *not* a complication. It merely means that a good, tight bladder repair was done.

---

## 173 What will my recovery at home be like after a hysterectomy?

I give my patients the following suggestions as they leave the hospital to go home after a hysterectomy.

*The first two weeks.* Let someone else do the cooking and housekeeping. If patients go home and assume the responsibilities of running the household, it often takes them months to recover from the resultant tiredness and fatigue. If they go home and take it easy for two weeks, they feel much better more quickly, with less lingering tiredness. As soon as they get home patients can climb stairs slowly, take leisurely walks, and ride in a car. They can drive a car as soon as they know they will be able to hit the brake in an emergency.

*Resuming normal activities.* I tell my patients not to plan on resuming normal activities, including going back to work, for six weeks after the day of surgery. However, after three weeks they can resume many normal activities if they feel like it. If they don't feel like it (and many do not), they should wait for three more weeks, or until they feel up to it. Occasionally patients do not feel truly normal for up to six months. I encourage such slowly recovering patients to start an exercise program of walking, six weeks from the day of surgery. This will usually make them feel better.

*Exercise.* I encourage my patients not to begin exercising for six weeks after surgery, and then to start back slowly with an exercise program. The patient who starts immediately doing sit-ups, jogging, and other vigorous exercise will strain ligaments and muscles that have gotten weak from inactivity. However, after six weeks a gradually accelerating exercise program will help a patient feel better than if she does not exercise.

*Bleeding from the vagina.* Two or three weeks after a hysterectomy or vaginal repairs, as the sutures absorb out of the vagina, a woman may have some bright red vaginal bleeding. This is nothing to worry about unless it becomes heavier than a normal menstrual period. If that happens she should call her doctor. It is also just as normal for this *not* to occur.

Two or three weeks after surgery, a patient may notice a few dark strings falling out of her vagina. These are sutures that have completed their job, and does not mean that the tissues are separating.

*Intercourse.* Before resuming intercourse after a hysterectomy, a patient should be checked by her doctor to be sure she is healed. Patients are normally healed well enough to have intercourse five or six weeks after the day of surgery, but this is not always the case. Intercourse may be mildly uncomfortable for up to a year following vaginal repair. Scar tissue is hard and takes a while to soften up. Until it does there may be discomfort with intercourse. The eventual improved sexual enjoyment, good urine control, absence of bowel problems, and elimination of pressure and pain in the pelvis more than make up for the temporary discomfort.

*Granulation tissue.* Granulation tissue, often called "proud flesh," is commonly found in the vagina along the incision lines after a hysterectomy. It is comparable to the bright red tissue that is visible when a scab is knocked off a sore.

The vagina heals by forming granulation tissue with no scab. This can cause bleeding, spotting or discharge, and pain with intercourse. If this happens, the doctor will have you come back every week or two to have silver nitrate applied to the granulation tissue to burn it off until you have total healing. This may require from one to ten or more treatments. This type of treatment causes essentially no pain and is quite effective.

*Follow-up exams.* After your granulation tissue is gone and you are healed and feeling well, your doctor will want you to come back for annual exams as usual.

## Endometriosis

## 174 What is endometriosis?

Endometriosis is the presence of normal tissue in the wrong place. When the lining of the uterus, the endometrium, is found anywhere else in the body, it is called endometriosis. Female hormones circulate all through the body, stimulating endometrial tissue, no matter where it is, building it up during the month. When the hormone levels drop to produce menstrual bleeding, the endometrial tissue, wherever it is, will bleed too. Endometrial tissue in the uterus will bleed out into the vagina, but in other parts of the body the blood cannot escape and pockets of blood will form in the tissue containing it. These pockets are irritating and will cause the tissues around them to develop scarring. Endometriosis is often found on the outside surface of a woman's uterus or on her tubes, ovaries, bladder, or intestines. It can occasionally be found in other areas of her body, and it has even been found in otherwise normal men.

## 175 Why is endometriosis such a major problem?

Endometriosis can cause a great deal of pain in the pelvis, and the scarring along with other changes that result from endometriosis can cause infertility. Endometriosis can collect to such an extent that it forms large accumulations of bloody fluid, surrounded by scars and adhesions. These are called endometriomas, commonly referred to as "chocolate cysts."

Endometriomas can become so large that they can be felt by your doctor during a pelvic examination. When the condition becomes this extensive, a woman will normally have a great deal of pain with her periods and also pain in her pelvis. This is not always the case, however. A woman who had been feeling almost totally normal came to me because her general practitioner found an ovarian enlargement during a routine exam. A laparoscopy revealed large endometriomas of both ovaries. They were so large that they were touching each other behind the uterus and were "scarred down" and immovable, but the woman had had only minimal pelvic discomfort!

There are several ways to treat endometriosis, depending on the extensiveness of the problem, whether or not a woman wants to have more children, and so on. These situations are discussed in the following questions. An extensive discussion of endometriosis and its symptoms is also found in Q. 953–960.

## 176 If I have endometriosis, and I do not want to have any more children, what should be done?

If your endometriosis is causing significant discomfort, you probably should have a hysterectomy. There are some facts to consider in this situation, however.

Your doctor could be wrong about your having endometriosis. A doctor cannot definitely diagnose endometriosis without seeing it at surgery or laparoscopy. Therefore, you should not have a hysterectomy because of the "possibility" of endometriosis. Have a hysterectomy only if your discomfort is bad enough for surgery, or if growths in your pelvis are large enough to warrant surgery, whether or not endometriosis is present.

If you have pain that is bothersome enough to require investigation, but not bad enough for a hysterectomy, or if your doctor insists that your pelvic exam suggests a problem that must be looked into, the best procedure is a laparoscopy. With laparoscopy, endometriosis can be confirmed, if present. Then, if you are not too uncomfortable, you can choose to leave it alone, take birth-control pills to keep it from progressing, or use Danocrine (as discussed in Q. 956) to suppress it so that the symptoms will stop. If endometriosis is present but not too extensive, the laser can be attached to the laparoscope to get rid of the endometriosis without making a larger incision.

If your doctor feels enlargements or growths in your pelvis that are as large as two inches across, exploratory surgery is necessary, because the growths could be ovarian cancer.

## 177 If I have endometriosis and want to have more children, what should be done?

There are two methods of treatment. The first is the use of the drug danazol. The second is surgery. The surgery can sometimes be done with laparoscopy but often a major incision is necessary. Endometriosis can recur after either one of these procedures. (See Q. 957, 958.)

Surgery to remove your endometriosis, which leaves your female organs capable of reproduction, can be performed. There is a recurrence rate of 15 percent even if most of the endometriosis was removed during the first surgery. (See Q. 957, 958.)

## 178 If I have not had all the children I want, but my doctor says my endometriosis is too extensive for fertility surgery, what should I do?

First, be certain that you are in the hands of a doctor who is enthusiastic about fertility surgery. It is far easier for a doctor to do a hysterectomy than it is to do surgery for removal of only the endometriosis. If your doctor is enthusiastic about working with patients who have fertility problems and still recommends a hysterectomy, it is likely that your female organs have been damaged so extensively that a fertility-type operation would be useless, merely leaving you with a great deal of scarring, no chance of pregnancy, and the possibility of another operation in the future.

If it is worth it to you to take the risk of repeat surgery, you can ask your doctor to do fertility surgery anyway, with the understanding that you will not allow a hysterectomy. I do recommend, though, that you give your permission to go ahead with removal of the uterus, tubes, and ovaries if the surgeon finds that he or she is unable to leave you with any normal ovarian tissue. In this situation you would need to accept the fact that you have done your best, as has your doctor, and neither of you should have any regrets in the future. A second opinion might be helpful in this situation.

## 179 If I have *significant* endometriosis in my pelvis and do not want to have more children, what should be done?

A hysterectomy is the solution in this case, because endometriosis is almost always attached to the uterus or to its supporting ligaments in some way. Even if only the ovaries are involved, a woman would not want to have her ovaries removed and have her uterus left intact. This would cause her to bleed vaginally every time she took a course of hormone pills. In addition to having your uterus removed for endometriosis, it is also necessary to have your ovaries removed. If they remain, the estrogen they produce can cause endometriosis to again develop in your pelvis, making another operation necessary later.

If your uterus, tubes, and ovaries are removed for endometriosis, you should take estrogen tablets. Your doctor will normally have you take something like Premarin (1.25 mg a day, on days one through twenty-five of the calendar month), and Provera (10 mg a day with the last fourteen of your estrogen tablets).

While it is true that these estrogen pills can cause the endometriosis to grow back (as can estrogen produced by your ovaries), the estrogen tablets can be stopped if symptoms of endometriosis recur. The only alternative, if the doctor does not take out the ovaries and the endometriosis started growing back, would be another operation to remove the source of the estrogen—the ovaries.

It is important to prevent endometriosis from growing back after a hysterectomy. For example, if endometriosis is not controlled, it can eventually obstruct the colon or can rupture into the vagina and cause pain and vaginal bleeding. Although it is extremely unusual for endometriosis to grow back after the uterus, tubes, and ovaries have been removed, it is not unusual for this to happen if only the uterus has been removed.

## Low Abdominal and Pelvic Pain

## 180 What is meant by "low abdominal and pelvic pain"?

The type of pelvic pain we will be discussing in this section is not a sudden, acute, severe pain. That type of pain is usually easier to diagnose and does not require the observation and testing that the persistent, long-term pain involves.

Low abdominal and pelvic pain varies from mild to moderately severe. It is rarely disabling, but it may include pain with intercourse, severe or unusual pain related to menstrual periods, or severe and abnormal pain at the time of ovulation.

Patients occasionally experience pain of the skin surfaces, either of the low abdominal area or the vulva. This discomfort is usually due to herpes if on the vulva or to shingles if on the low abdomen or vulva. (Herpes zoster is the medical term for shingles.) Pain from these two problems is usually not too difficult to diagnose and is not usually confused with the pelvic pain we will discuss in the next few questions.

## 181 What causes low abdominal and pelvic pain?

Low abdominal and pelvic pain is a problem for both patients and their doctors. It is not only difficult to diagnose, but it can also be just as difficult to treat. Many articles written by well-qualified physicians state that 50 percent of the pelvic pain that women experience is not due to physical abnormalities, the implication being that the pain is often psychological in origin. Although I do not doubt that some pelvic pain is due to emotions, my experience has been that this is uncommon. I believe that if a patient and her doctor pursue evaluation of the pain, the cause can almost always be found and treated. Some of the physical causes of this type of pain are discussed in the following eight questions.

## 182 What symptoms might indicate a pain problem that is related to my female organs?

If the pain you have gets worse at the time of your menstrual periods or during the time of ovulation, and it goes away at other times during the month, its origin is probably your female organs. If your pain is not affected by the regular monthly menstrual cycle, or if it is affected only very little by it, you probably do not have a problem of your female organs. Your problem is more likely related to your urologic or intestinal system. (See Q. 185, 186.)

One standard action I take in the event of pelvic pain is to remove an IUD if one is being used. Even if a woman does not think her problem is caused by the IUD, it must be removed because it could be the cause of the pain. An IUD can cause pain in the back, side, upper abdomen, and upper legs. The only way to know for sure that a pain is IUD-caused is to remove it. (See Q. 1022–1041.)

## 183 What problems of the female organs might cause low abdominal and pelvic pain?

There are several gynecologic problems that can cause low-grade but persistent pelvic pain.

Endometriosis (See Q. 174–179.)

Adenomyosis (See Q. 782–783.)

Pelvic-congestion syndrome (See Q. 784–785.)

Pelvic relaxation. If the vaginal tissues are relaxed and the uterus is prolapsed, a woman can experience pelvic discomfort, usually felt as a "bearing down" or "bottom falling out" feeling.

Pelvic inflammatory disease with adhesions. Women occasionally have low-grade infections with no fever. Although the pain may be present some months and not present other months, typically this PID pain will be present with menstrual periods.

Ovarian growths. Occasionally an ovary will twist on its supporting ligaments, cutting off its own blood supply, causing pelvic pain. This can be difficult to diagnose because the ovary and tube can untwist and look totally normal at laparoscopy, and then twist back again a few days later. Also, a growth on an ovary will sometimes hurt.

## 184 If my pelvic pain is not related to my menstrual cycle, what is the procedure for diagnosis?

If your pain is not related to the menstrual cycle at all, there will not usually be anything wrong with your female organs. For that reason, with this type of pain I usually do no testing at the time of the first visit. If there is no abnormality found during a thorough pelvic exam, I refer the woman to a gastroenterologist (intestinal specialist) and, if he or she finds nothing, I refer her to a urologist (bladder and kidney specialist).

I will definitely refer a patient to a gastroenterologist (GI specialist) if she has any of the following symptoms and a normal pelvic examination.

Abdominal bloating

Nausea

Diarrhea

Constipation

Pain that increases upon eating or drinking

A history of intestinal disease, such as an irritable or spastic colon.

I definitely send a patient to a urologist if she has a normal pelvic exam and has symptoms related to the urologic tract, such as:

Burning with urination

Unusual frequency of urination

Inability to hold urine when the bladder is the least bit full

Blood or pus in the urine

History of urologic problems, such as stones or infection

## 185 What would the GI doctor do, and what might be found wrong?

The gastroenterologist would take a medical history in an attempt to find the nature of your problem and will often do a proctoscopy. This involves insertion of a tube through your anus into your colon to look for colon polyps or tumors. X-rays of your intestines may be ordered to check for intestinal growths or kinking of the intestines. In patients with low abdominal pain, the doctor often discovers an irritable (spastic) colon, an extremely common problem. Such a patient is usually put on a high-fiber, low-

sugar diet. If a woman follows these suggestions, her pain will almost always go away.

An occasional patient will have chronic appendicitis that flares up periodically. The pain from this is normally more severe and occurs less often than the pain of an irritable or spastic colon. The gastroenterologist would be the doctor to diagnose this but would then refer such a patient to a general surgeon for an appendectomy.

## 186 What would a urologist do, and what might he or she find wrong?

A urologist would usually want a urinalysis and a urine culture and would also look into a woman's bladder with a cystoscope to check for signs of inflammation of the urethra or of the bladder, if this was felt necessary. The urologist may also take a kidney X-ray, called an IVP (intravenous pyelogram), in which a special X-ray dye is injected into a vein. X-rays of the kidneys are taken as the dye collects in them.

An irritated bladder, urethritis (irritation of the urethra), or cystitis (infection of the bladder) can cause persistent pelvic pain. If you have cystitis, antibiotics will be used. If the urologist believes that your bladder is merely spastic, you might be put on Ditropan, or some other drug, to relieve the spasms. If you have urethritis, the doctor will often dilate your urethra. This compresses the small glands of the urethra, squeezing out the pus so that the infection will go away. Antibiotics may also be prescribed. Urethral irritation is a fairly common cause of pelvic discomfort in women, but it is often hard to diagnose. Be sure to see a good urologist if you have persistent pelvic pain that can be caused by this problem.

## 187 What other problems might produce low abdominal or pelvic pain?

A few of the problems that can cause pelvic pain are:

**Hernias.** If you notice a bulge in the groin when you strain or have bowel movements, you probably have a hernia. Hernias in women are sometimes difficult to find. If you have persistent pain in the groin, and the doctor does not find any abnormality, including no enlarged lymph nodes, he or she may order a CT scan (see glossary) to see if there is a bulge, a telltale sign of a hernia. If the CT scan is negative, your pain is almost certainly not a hernia but is probably a problem with the ligaments in the pelvic area. In this case you should see an orthopedist for evaluation of those ligaments and bones.

**Hematomas of the abdominal wall.** In both young, athletic women and in older women, tears of the rectus muscles, the muscles of the central part of the abdominal wall, can cause bleeding into these muscles. This causes pain and a thickening that can feel like a growth in the pelvis. If your pain increases when you lift your head and goes away when you put your head down, you probably have a hematoma of the abdominal wall. Occasionally, in a relaxed position, you can actually "pick up" part of the muscle in your fingers and feel the knot in it where the blood has accumulated. This accumulation of blood is a clot, but it is not the dangerous kind that can break loose and go into your lungs or heart, nor does it require surgery. The blood will absorb out of the area. A heating pad to the area and aspirin are usually all the treatment needed.

**Enlarged lymph nodes.** Lymph nodes can become enlarged in the groin area and cause pain. If these nodes remain for several weeks, you need to have them evaluated.

I want them to come back to me so that we can continue trying to find the problem. Those who do come back need a more thorough gynecologic evaluation. Only a few patients return for this purpose, because on their first visit to me I would have diagnosed most of the typical gynecologic problems. The urologist and gastroenterologist would have done the same with patients having problems in those particular areas. This usually leaves very few patients who are still having pain without a diagnosis.

The first thing I would do after doing another pelvic examination would be a laparoscopy. For a description of this procedure, see Q. 907. The laparoscopy will occasionally show some adhesions, some mild inflammation of the tubes, or some other abnormality that the physicians did not suspect from the history and examination in their offices.

If a laparoscopy is normal, a hysterosalpingogram might be the next step. This procedure is an X-ray of the uterus (see Q. 905) which would show whether or not there are abnormalities in the uterus that might be causing pelvic pain.

If these two procedures have identified no abnormality, the process of elimination has narrowed the possibilities of physical problems down to two probable choices: pelvic congestion syndrome and adenomyosis. (See Q. 781–785.) These problems will normally get worse at the time of the menstrual period and get better afterward, but this is not necessarily so. When diagnostic procedures have been exhausted and no physical cause of the pain has been discovered, the possibility that the pain is of emotional origin must be considered.

## 188 If no one is able to find the cause, but my pain persists, what should I do?

I tell my patients that if their pelvic pain persists after evaluation by other specialists,

## 189 If the gynecologic and related evaluations fail to find a cause for my pain, what else can be done?

If you have gone through the complete evaluation process and are still having pain, you can be sure that there is nothing seriously or dangerously wrong and that you have nothing to worry about, even though you may still have discomfort. Empiric treatment can now be tried. This is treatment with a technique that might stop the problem, although there is no specific indication. Empiric treatments for pelvic pain may include:

*Birth-control pills.* If a patient has pain in her female organs, birth-control pills are sometimes useful in eliminating it. They essentially put the female organs to sleep and can cause endometriosis and adenomyosis to become inactive. Unfortunately, if a woman has pelvic-congestion syndrome, birth-control pills can occasionally make that worse.

*Danocrine.* If a doctor suspects adenomyosis, Danocrine can be tried. (See Q. 956.) Danocrine can cause adenomyosis to clear up, and if that has been the problem the patient's pain will lessen. A patient can stay on Danocrine for only six months. However, if her pain recurs after one round of treatments, Danocrine can be tried again. But if pain persists after a second round, most physicians recommend that a woman discontinue using Danocrine because it obviously is not going to be a permanent cure.

*Psychiatric consultation.* Women do occasionally have pain in their pelvic organs that stems from an emotional disturbance. If you have been physically evaluated to no avail, and you know that you are under significant emotional stress, have your doctor refer you to a good psychologist or psychiatrist. Such a specialist can often help you rid yourself of not only the burden of pain but also of the underlying problem that produced it.

*Surgery.* Presacral neurectomy (see Q. 957–58), cutting the nerves that go by the cervix (paracervical uterine denervation), and D&C are procedures that can occasionally help a woman with pelvic pain. If these procedures do not seem wise, a hysterectomy might be useful.

Doctors who write research papers and talk about unnecessary hysterectomies would frown at this approach, but my feeling is that if a woman's quality of life is being affected by her pain, and she has been unsuccessfully and thoroughly evaluated for every other cause—and the pain seems to be from the female organs—then hysterectomy is useful. My experience, and the experience of many other gynecologists, has been that this procedure does stop patients' pain if thorough evaluation has preceded such surgery.

Doctors opposed to this approach to pelvic pain will say that the patient's pain was "emotional" to start with and that she will, a few months after the hysterectomy, begin feeling pain in some other part of her body. This may occasionally be true, but in the patients I have treated, there have been only a few recurrences.

## Bladder Infections

**190** **What causes bladder infections, and why do they occur more often in women than in men?**

Bladder infections or cystitis are caused by germs that invade and infect the bladder. These germs cause the lining inside the bladder to become red and inflamed, just as your throat does when it gets infected. Since pus cells and germs from the infection are passed in the urine, it is often easy to diagnose a bladder infection by urine tests.

Bladder infections occur frequently in women because the urethra, the tube through which the urine leaves the bladder and empties to the outside, is so short (one and one-half to two inches long). This makes it easy for germs from the vulva to get up through the urethra to the bladder.

Germs can be worked into the bladder with intercourse, and most women do not have bladder infections until they start having intercourse. Poor toilet habits can also introduce germs into the bladder. For this reason a woman should wipe her vulva from front to back after urinating or having a bowel movement.

## 191 What are the symptoms of cystitis or bladder infection?

A bladder infection usually comes on suddenly. A burning sensation when urinating and the need to urinate frequently are common symptoms. Other symptoms are blood in the urine and pain in the lower abdomen, behind the pubic bone. When she first notices these symptoms, a woman should immediately call her doctor and get medication, whether it is night or day. If she does not, she can quickly get extremely uncomfortable.

## 192 What is "honeymoon cystitis"?

Honeymoon cystitis is a term applied to a bladder infection that develops after a woman first starts having intercourse. This type of cystitis is often merely an irritation in the urethra, but sometimes it is an irritation of the bladder caused by the penis thrusting against it. Many times this is not a true infection of these tissues, and all that is required is a drug to soothe the bladder and urethra.

Honeymoon cystitis can also occur when a woman resumes intercourse after several months of abstinence. It does not necessarily occur immediately, but sometimes develops several weeks or months after resuming or starting sexual activity.

## 193 Are there other things related to sexual practices that might encourage cystitis?

There are two sexual practices that might contribute to bladder infections: oral sex and anal sex. If your husband stimulates your clitoris and vulvar areas with his mouth and tongue, he may be contaminating the area with germs. For most women, oral stimulation by their husbands is not a factor in their cystitis and is generally a normal, healthy sexual activity. If you have a frustrating problem with recurrent bladder infections, you might try stopping this practice for a few months to see if it makes any difference.

The same applies to anal, or rectal, intercourse. If you do have anal intercourse, gynecologists recommend that you not allow your husband to insert his penis into your vagina after it has been in your rectum because this puts large numbers of germs from your rectum into your vagina. If you practice anal intercourse and are having a major problem with bladder infections, you should stop this practice completely even if your husband does not go back into your vagina after rectal intercourse. If you notice that this helps clear up your bladder infections, you should discontinue anal intercourse.

One other sexual practice that may contribute to cystitis is the penis entering the vagina from the rear. If you feel that you get a great deal of poking on your bladder from your husband's penis with this or any sexual technique you normally use, change that technique if you continue to have problems with cystitis and see if it makes any difference.

## 194 How is cystitis treated?

Treatment for cystitis is classified into three categories.

***First cystitis episode.*** You should call

your doctor immediately when you have symptoms of cystitis. If it is inconvenient for you to take a urine speciment to a laboratory—for instance, if the problem develops at night or while you are out of town—the doctor will probably prescribe medications anyway. The medications might be Pyridium to soothe the bladder, and an antibiotic such as Septra, Macrodantin, or Ampicillin to kill the germs. Pyridium will color your urine orange. Since this can stain your clothing, you need to be careful about getting this colored urine on clothes that you value.

With this type of medication, the burning will usually stop within twelve hours. It was once thought that women needed to be treated with antibiotics for ten or twelve days, but it has recently been found that treatment with an appropriate antibiotic for five days, or even for one day, will get rid of most bladder infections. However, it is vitally important that you take all the medication your doctor prescribes.

***Repeat episodes of cystitis.*** It is common for cystitis to return, even though it has been treated properly. Most doctors want a urine culture done if a woman calls back with another infection within a month or two of the first infection. This is done to determine which germ is causing the infection and to find out which drug is most likely to cure it. (If the germs responded to the drug previously used, the same drug may be given again.)

This time, though, the doctor may encourage you to drink cranberry juice and take vitamin C. This promotes an acidic urine in which germs grow poorly. He may want you to drink more water to promote flushing of the bladder. He may also suggest that you urinate after each act of intercourse to wash any germs from your bladder and urethra, and to keep stagnant urine from staying in your bladder.

***Recurrent cystitis infection.*** If you continue to have bladder infections, you should see a urologist because the infection may actually be coming from germs that have infected the kidney and are coming down in the urine to infect the bladder. Of course, the reverse could happen: continued presence of germs in your bladder could eventually result in your kidneys becoming infected.

Recurrent bladder infections may be caused by a stricture of the urethra, a condition in which the opening of the urethra is so tight that it prevents complete emptying of the bladder. Stagnant urine can provide excellent culture media for the growth of germs.

A urologist will normally check to be sure your urethra is not too small. The doctor will look inside your bladder by cystoscopy to make sure you do not have a growth that might be causing the infection, and will normally order a kidney X-ray (IVP) to make sure your kidneys do not show signs of chronic infection. You will then be treated and kept under the urologist's care for the treatment of your bladder or kidney problems. You should call the urologist (rather than your gynecologist) when symptoms reoccur.

There are many patients on kidney machines today because their kidneys were destroyed by neglected kidney disease. There is no need for you to take any risk of this happening to you.

## Premenstrual Syndrome (PMS)

### 195 What is PMS or premenstrual syndrome?

Premenstrual syndrome is a term used to describe the symptoms a woman may experience prior to her menstrual period. These symptoms may begin at the time of ovulation and last until the period begins. Since ovulation generally occurs fourteen days before the start of the period, premenstrual symptoms may exist for up to fourteen days.

If a woman has symptoms that are present the entire month, she does not have PMS and should be evaluated by a physician for other medical problems.

The body changes that cause PMS begin with the production of progesterone from the ovary at the time of ovulation. They cannot start before that. It is for this reason that some researchers think that PMS is caused by an abnormal production of progesterone. (See Q. 200.)

## 196 What are the symptoms of PMS?

The accompanying chart describes the several common PMS symptoms.

### Symptoms of Premenstrual Syndrome

| Pain Group | Psychological Group | Edema/Water Retention |
|---|---|---|
| Abdominal cramps | Tension | Breast tenderness |
| | Irritability | Weight gain |
| Headache | Depression | Swelling of joints |
| Backache | Anxiety | of extremities (fingers, ankles) |
| Muscle spasms | Mood swings | Bloating |
| | | Abdominal heaviness Pelvic pressure |

Other symptoms that are reported with some frequency but which do not fall into one of these groups include food cravings, clumsiness, acne, dizziness, nausea, fatigue, insomnia, and difficulty in concentrating. There are other symptoms. Some physicians have listed as many as a hundred different PMS symptoms their patients have had.

## 197 Is PMS "real" or is it only "in a woman's head"?

Prior to the 1950s women were often told by their physicians that emotional changes associated with their menstrual periods were "all in their heads" and not due to any physical change at all. We know now that is not true. These problems are due to actual physical changes in a woman's body.

These changes can produce traumatic problems. Since 1945, studies have shown that 70 to 80 percent of the violent crimes committed by women occur during the premenstrual time. Certain medical problems, such as epilepsy, asthma, migraine headaches, breast soreness, acne, clumsiness, irritability, bloating, and depression, are all associated with the woman's premenstrual period more often than with other times during the month.

This is not to say that premenstrual changes make a woman a murderer or a child abuser. Premenstrual syndrome merely aggravates any already established predisposition to antisocial behavior. However, because of the physical aspect of PMS, it has been successfully used as a defense by several women in England at their murder trials. In recent trials in the United States, PMS has not been allowed as a defense for a woman's criminal behavior.

## 198 If I have PMS, does it mean that there is something wrong with my body, that I am just "emotional," or that I am spiritually out of touch with God?

On the contrary. It is important that you realize that PMS is not a sign that your body is abnormal but evidence that the hormones in your body are working just the way they are supposed to work. (See Q. 200 for a further discussion of this.) If you have PMS, you do not need to worry that you have a disease in your body that is going to be dangerous for you. Rather, you can concentrate your efforts on doing things to make yourself feel better and not spend time trying to determine why you feel the way you do.

The irritability, anger, depression, and other psychological changes associated with PMS do not mean that a woman is weak or unstable, or that she has lost touch with God. These changes are a result of physical changes, not a sign of emotional or spiritual weakness. While it is certainly appropriate to pray about these feelings, if they affect a woman's relationship with her husband, her children, or her friends, she should also seek medical help.

## 199 Do all women experience PMS?

Almost all women experience premenstrual syndrome to some extent. Doctors divide women into two groups. The first group includes those women who, in relation to PMS, are considered "normal." Their symptoms of PMS are limited to "premenstrual awareness." They are differentiated from the women who are diagnosed as having true PMS by the severity of the symptoms that they have.

As many as 30 to 50 percent of all women are in the second group. These women experience severe symptoms during the premenstrual time span. They need medication during that period and are, to some extent, incapacitated by their symptoms.

## 200 What causes PMS?

Premenstrual syndrome is related to the production of progesterone by the ovary. When ovulation occurs, the follicle on the ovary from which the egg is released collapses and turns into a corpus luteum. (See Q. 91–95.) This corpus luteum produces progesterone. Ovulation occurs fourteen days before the menstrual period in almost all women. Since prior to ovulation the only hormone produced by the ovary is estrogen, PMS cannot exist more than fourteen days prior to the start of a period.

Deficiency of progesterone, abnormal production of progesterone, or production of an abnormal-type progesterone is thought by some researchers to be the cause of premenstrual syndrome. Therefore advocates of the abnormal progesterone theory as the cause of PMS propose that the ovary's corpus luteum is producing progesterone in an abnormal way. This has not been proven, and blood tests to measure progesterone in women with PMS do not reliably show abnormalities.

Many other theories have been proposed, such as the imbalance between progesterone and estrogen in a woman's body, too much estrogen, vitamin deficiency, stress, hypoglycemia, hormone allergy (the body rejects the progesterone that is produced), and abnormal amounts of endorphins in the brain. Endorphins are the body's own opiate-like hormone. They are often discussed in connection with long-distance runners whose supposed increase in endorphins explains the "high" they receive when they run.

## 201 How can I know if I have PMS?

Make a calendar like the one below and keep a record for three months. If, according to the calendar, your symptoms always occur after ovulation and tend to go away at the time your menstrual flow starts, you probably have PMS. If you seem to have PMS by your calendar, you may be able to control your PMS symptoms by using some of the suggestions offered in the answer to Question 203. If you cannot, you may want to take your calendar to your physician and talk about further therapy.

If your calendar does not show that you are free of PMS symptoms for at least a week

# A PMS Calendar

Use this type of calendar to record your *three worst symptoms.* Two sample months are shown at right.

***A—Anxiety***
***AB—Abdominal Bloating***
***BT—Breast Tenderness***
***H—Headache***
(M)***—Menstruation***

In Chart "A" the woman is diagnosed as having PMS. In Chart "B" the timing of symptoms does not have a clear relationship to the menstrual cycle; this woman's symptoms may have another cause that should be investigated.

| | Month 1 | Month 2 | Month 3 | Chart A | Chart B |
|----|---------|---------|---------|---------|---------|
| 1 | | | | | |
| 2 | | | | | *A* |
| 3 | | | | *H* | *A* |
| 4 | | | | | |
| 5 | | | | | *A* |
| 6 | | | | | |
| 7 | | | | | |
| 8 | | | | | *H* |
| 9 | | | | | |
| 10 | | | | | |
| 11 | | | | | |
| 12 | | | | | |
| 13 | | | | | |
| 14 | | | | *A* | |
| 15 | | | | *HA* | *H* |
| 16 | | | | *a* | *A* |
| 17 | | | | *a* | |
| 18 | | | | *A* | *A* |
| 19 | | | | *A* | |
| 20 | | | | *HA* | |
| 21 | | | | *H* | |
| 22 | | | | *H* (M) | *H* |
| 23 | | | | (M) | |
| 24 | | | | (M) | (M) |
| 25 | | | | (M) | (M) |
| 26 | | | | (M) | (M) |
| 27 | | | | | (M) |
| 28 | | | | | (M) |
| 29 | | | | | *H* |
| 30 | | | | | |
| 31 | | | | *H* | *A* |

after your menstrual period, you do not have PMS. Or, at least all your symptoms are not due to the premenstrual syndrome.

When you keep a PMS calendar, *record only your three worst symptoms*. Otherwise such a chart will be almost unreadable.

## 202  What is the treatment for PMS?

Even though doctors are not sure exactly what causes PMS, they have found some ways to control it. These methods can be divided into two groups. The first includes common sense, nonmedical changes in your life which may alleviate your problem if you do not have severe PMS. The second group includes medical treatments.

## 203  Which nonmedical changes might help control PMS?

There are several nonmedical measures you can adopt to control your PMS:

*Adjust your life to your cycle.* Live with your menstrual cycle; don't fight it. In her book, *The Joy of Being a Woman*, (Harper & Row), Ingrid Trobisch suggests that women should be aware of when they will have their premenstrual symptoms and reserve that time for the quiet activities of life, such as reading and doing things that do not require much interaction with other people. If a woman works, she can concentrate on work-related duties that require less intensity. A woman should not plan big dinner parties or a household move at the time of her premenstrual symptoms if she can avoid it. Obviously no woman can control these things completely, but it does help to re-

member to schedule the events in your life around your cycle.

*Talk about PMS.* Discuss your PMS with your family and, if appropriate, with close friends. This will help them be aware of what is going on. It would certainly be appropriate for you to warn those you are closest to as soon as you sense the onset of PMS symptoms.

I suggest that husbands keep up with where their wives are in their cycle so that her PMS symptoms may be anticipated. A husband will usually find that doing "something nice" for his wife during that time will be greatly appreciated. It is helpful if the husband dispenses hugs and kisses and shows his wife tenderness during the time of her PMS. This should be the type of physical closeness that does not demand intercourse as a reward. Many women do not hug their husbands as often as they want to at this time because they "know what will happen" if they do!

*Cut calories and eat more frequently.* Decrease your intake of calories, not just at premenstrual time but all month long. This helps control body weight, decreasing the swelling during the premenstrual days. Cutting calories might also lessen the symptoms of hypoglycemia during this time.

Eating more frequently can also help decrease hypoglycemia, resulting in help with PMS. Try eating some cheese or a small meal every three hours during the time of your PMS, whether or not you have the disease of hypoglycemia. Such meals should include a minimum of sugar.

*Increase physical activity.* This too should be done all month long. It will not only decrease body fat but will also improve your health and general sense of well-being.

*Cut salt intake.* Follow a low-salt diet, especially during the premenstrual time. This helps decrease swelling.

*Discontinue use of caffeine.* Avoid the intake of caffeine during PMS time because caffeine may increase your level of agitation. This means drinking caffeine-free coffee, tea, and colas and not eating chocolate.

---

## 204 What medical treatments can help alleviate PMS symptoms?

Vitamin B6 and progesterone are two treatments that may prove helpful in the treatment of PMS.

*Vitamin B6 (Pyridoxine).* I start my patients on 150 mg of vitamin B6 a day. I have them begin taking this medication a day or two before their PMS symptoms usually appear. They continue taking the pills until the time that their symptoms are usually gone, whether it is at the beginning or end of their menstruation. If this treatment causes nausea, I cut them back to the highest dose they can take without being nauseated at all.

A recently-published, highly advertised study showing neurological damage from high doses of vitamin B6 made many patients afraid to use it. The patients involved in this study, however, were taking a minimum of 4,000 mg a day. Taking 150 mg or less of vitamin B6 daily has never been shown to be harmful.

Although no one really knows why B6 helps, some patients have had a beneficial and dramatic response to its use.

*Progesterone.* Natural progesterone, used from the time that the PMS symptoms start until the onset of the period, has been found to help many patients. This can be taken in the form of intramuscular injections, as vaginal suppositories, or as rectal fluid or suppositories.

Most doctors suggest starting with 200 mg a day, and it seems safe to increase it to as much as 1,200 mg a day, if necessary. The disadvantages of using progesterone are the expense, the messiness, and the inconvenience, but if your symptoms are bad enough, it may be worth it.

Since some patients will find that their symptoms get worse when they use pro-

gesterone, you should be aware of that possibility.

The progesterone may cause menstrual flow to become irregular. This may be seen as a delay of the onset of the menstrual period or bleeding during the days you are using the progesterone. This can become so bothersome to some women that they stop progesterone therapy.

Progesterone is not a contraceptive. Reliable contraception should be used while taking it, because of the possibility of its effect on a baby you might conceive. Actually, the type of progesterone used for PMS is the "natural" kind that is often given pregnant women to help keep them from miscarrying. However, during pregnancy the dose is usually lower.

---

## 205 Are there other prescription drugs that are sometimes used to treat PMS?

Other prescription medications have been suggested for the symptoms of premenstrual syndrome, but none has been suggested as often or as widely used as B6 and progesterone. Here is a list of such medications.

- *Oral contraceptives.* These stop ovulation and are, for some women, a good solution.
- *Prostaglandin inhibitors.* Motrin and similar drugs are excellent for menstrual cramps, and many patients find them helpful for relief of PMS symptoms.
- *Tranquilizers.* Some patients find that taking a 2 or 5 mg Valium tablet two or three times a day for a few days before the period is all they need to handle their symptoms. This is a simple, safe therapy, and I recommend it. A woman can almost not get addicted to tran-

quilizers if she uses them only on this cyclic-type basis.

*Diuretics.* If a woman's primary problem is fluid retention, all she needs to do is take a diuretic (Aldactone, 25 mg three times a day) each day she has swelling until her period starts. Spironolactone is useful if there is a major problem with water retention. Occasionally a woman will respond dramatically to this drug, which is usually used for hypertension.

*Bromocriptine (Parlodel).* If breast discomfort is a major problem, this drug is useful. If a woman wants to try this, she can take 2.5 mg twice a day for ten to fourteen days prior to the menstrual period.

*Danocrine (danazol).* Recent reports indicate that women with PMS symptoms have responded positively to the use of this drug.

## 206 What about over-the-counter drugs for PMS?

Over-the-counter drugs are available to help with some of the symptoms of PMS. An example is Premensyn—PMS. Such drugs contain a mild diuretic for the swelling, an antihistamine for the tension and cramps, and acetaminophen (such as in Tylenol) for the pain associated with the premenstrual time. These drugs, and others of similar makeup, may be moderately useful.

## 207 What about PMS clinics?

If you have a major problem with PMS that is not being helped in any other way, a PMS clinic may be helpful. If your problem is not major, however, I recommend that you counsel first with your own physician. PMS clinics are usually quite expensive, and their specialized care is not necessary for the majority of patients with PMS symptoms.

## Diethylstilbestrol (DES)

## 208 What is diethylstilbestrol (DES)?

DES is a synthetic compound which produces the same effect in a woman's body as estrogen. DES can be used interchangeably with estrogen compounds in numerous situations, such as for women who need estrogen after menopause and for women with a fertility problem who need extra estrogen to make their cervical mucus receptive to sperm. (See Q. 916, 917, 939.)

*Except for use during pregnancy,* DES is in no way more dangerous or unhealthy than any other estrogen-type compound.

The dangers of taking DES while pregnant were exposed in 1971, at which time doctors stopped prescribing it for pregnant women. Eight to ten million people were exposed to DES in their mothers' wombs between the years of 1941 and 1971, but since the drug is no longer being used during pregnancy, we can expect no more people to join this group. Because many women's lives have been affected by DES, we should discuss this topic.

The youngest girls born after exposure to DES were born in 1971. Therefore, the only women in our society who have been exposed to DES before birth are, at the time of this publication, in their late teens up to their late forties.

The problems connected with DES are generally much less severe than was first feared when the dangers of DES were exposed. Knowing this should help those who are concerned about it to relax and not worry so much about their DES exposure. It should also help those women who took DES while pregnant to feel less guilty about having taken a drug that might have affected their offspring.

## 209 Why was DES ever used in pregnancy?

Starting in 1941, studies indicated that DES helped decrease the chance of miscarriage. Subsequent studies showed that DES was also useful if a pregnant woman had diabetes or toxemia of pregnancy. Because of these findings, doctors felt that a woman who had a previous miscarriage, who had diabetes, or who had toxemia with a previous pregnancy would benefit by taking DES during a subsequent pregnancy. Since 20 percent of all pregnancies end as miscarriages, and since any patient who had previously had a miscarriage was supposed to be helped by DES, one can easily see why such a large number of women received DES while pregnant.

## 210 Did DES use in pregnancy always cause abnormalities?

If women used less than 1.5 mg of DES a day during pregnancy, their babies were not affected. Likewise, if a woman did not take DES until after the twenty-second week (fifth month) of her pregnancy, her child was not affected.

## 211 What abnormalities are seen in women who were DES-exposed while in their mothers' wombs?

All of the DES-caused abnormalities in women are seen in their female organs: the vagina, the cervix, the uterus, and the breasts. While the abnormalities may have been present at birth, because of the nature of the abnormalities, most were not discovered until much later in life.

It is not known exactly how DES caused its damage, but the most logical theory is that it went through the placenta and into the baby's body during its early developmental stages. Once in the fetus, DES competed with the mother's and the baby's natural estrogen, effectively blocking the normal growth stimulation of the baby's vagina, cervix, and uterus at a critical time in their development. There is no other time in a person's life when that particular set-up exists again. Consequently, outside of the early few months of fetal life, DES cannot in any way be more dangerous than any other estrogenlike drug. Recent studies have shown that DES-exposed women have a greater chance of developing breast cancer in later life. Therefore they should carefully examine their breasts monthly and have them checked by a physician regularly.

## 212 What vaginal abnormalities are seen in DES-exposed women?

Vaginal changes, which are seen in about 30 percent of women who were DES exposed in the womb, include the following:

*Adenosis.* The vaginal lining may develop adenosis, a condition in which the vaginal lining (squamous epithelium) is replaced in spots by the type of lining that covers the inside of the cervix (columnar epithelium). This "substitute lining" is a type of glandular epithelium that is normal for some parts of the body but, in this situation, was caused to be in the wrong place. This tissue is not dangerous, and it should not be treated unless it is causing a great deal of mucus secretion. The laser is the best instrument for eliminating adenosis if it is causing enough trouble to be treated. (See Q. 708 for more information about laser treatment of vaginal abnormalities.)

*Cancer.* Doctors were tipped off to the effect of DES by a rare cancer of the vagina called "clear-cell adenocarcinoma." Prior to the use of DES in pregnancy, this type of cancer was almost unknown. In the patients who were exposed to DES while in their mothers' wombs, more than three hundred cases of clear-cell adenocarcinoma have now been found. The encouraging thing for those who have been exposed to DES is that almost every one of the patients who have had clear-cell adenocarcinoma already had it the first time they were examined by a doctor. This means that patients who have been exposed to DES do not seem to be developing clear-cell adenocarcinoma of the vagina as the years go by. It is unknown whether this means that the condition existed from the time of birth, but the chance of developing this cancer later in life seems to be almost zero. In other words, if you did not have it when you were first seen by your doctor, you will probably not ever get it.

***Cervical intraepithelial neoplasia and vaginal squamous cell cancer.*** Precancerous and cancerous growths of the cervix develop more often in DES-exposed women. The adenosis that is found in the vagina is a type of lining usually found in the cervix. This seems to increase the chance of developing a cervical-type precancerous or cancerous growth. (For a complete understanding of this type of growth, see Q. 742–756.)

An annual examination, including Pap smears and colposcopic visualization of both the cervix and of areas of adenosis in the vagina, is the ideal method of watchcare for most DES-exposed women. If a woman has a large area of adenosis in her vagina, however, it is probably best that she be seen every six months instead of once a year.

A colposcopy is useful in making sure that a patient is not developing abnormal cells of the vagina or cervix, and in finding such changes early if they are developing. For the patient who has normal Pap smears of her adenosis and of her cervix, and whose annual examination does not show any change in her tissues, colposcopy annually may not be absolutely necessary for routine care, but it is best that it be done if available. (For a discussion of colposcopy, see Q. 421, 751.)

## 213 What cervical changes are seen in DES-exposed women?

About 30 percent of women who were exposed to DES while in their mothers' wombs will have structural abnormalities of their cervix. These changes do not damage a woman's body or affect pregnancy, but they can be a tip-off to an alert doctor that the patient's mother may have taken DES while she was pregnant. The changes vary from one woman to another but may consist of any of the following:

Smaller-than-normal cervix

Ridges of tissue, sometimes called "cervical collar"

Irregularities that make it appear that polyps are present, although true polyps are not actually present

A protrusion of the upper part of the cervix, sometimes called a "cockscomb"

## 214 What uterine changes are seen in DES-exposed women?

Almost half the women who have had DES exposure in the womb have an abnormal shape to the inside or the outside of their uterus. The most common abnormality is found by an X-ray of the uterus, a hysterosalpingogram, (HSG see Q. 905). Instead of the normal triangular-shape, about one-third of the women who have been DES-exposed will have a T-shape to the inside cavity of their uterus.

Other abnormalities that may be found, either by HSG or laparoscopy, may vary from a uterus that is smaller than normal, an irregular-shaped inner cavity, or a too-wide lower uterine cavity.

If a woman has a DES-type uterine abnormality, it may be best for her to have a purse-string suture put around her cervix (called a cerclage) in early pregnancy to keep the abnormal uterus from aborting her pregnancy or to keep it from causing a premature delivery. (See Q. 420.)

## 215 Can DES exposure in her mother's uterus affect a woman's fertility?

Half of the women who were exposed to DES have no abnormalities and their fertility is unaffected, so far as researchers know now.

If a woman is found to have an abnormality of her uterus as a result of DES exposure, the probability of her having a premature baby increases. One study showed that if a woman had an abnormal uterus from DES, she had only a 51 percent chance of carrying a pregnancy to term and giving birth to a live infant. A more recent study has shown that 82 percent of DES-exposed women will eventually have a normal, full-term pregnancy.

Tubal ectopic pregnancies occur more often in DES-exposed women who have an abnormal uterus. Approximately 13 percent of the pregnancies in this group end up as tubal ectopic pregnancies, whereas only 1 percent of the DES-exposed women with a normal uterus will have tubal ectopic pregnancies.

Women with an abnormal uterus also seem to have more miscarriages than women with a normal uterus, but the difference is not significant.

The important thing for a DES-exposed woman with uterine abnormalities to realize is that although childbearing for her may be more difficult than for most women, she still has an almost normal chance of eventually having healthy, normal children.

## 216 Were the sons of women who took DES while pregnant affected?

One study showed that about 30 percent of the DES-exposed sons had some abnor-

mality of their genital tract. In spite of these abnormalities, however, DES seems to have no effect on a man's fertility or sexual function, nor on his age of puberty, first ejaculation, first intercourse, hormone levels, sperm count, or sperm quality.

Abnormalities that have been seen are mild abnormalities of the penis, the testes, and the epididymis. The most common abnormality is epididymal cysts (an insignificant finding) present in 20 percent of the males who were exposed to DES while in the womb.

No cancer has been found to be more common in men who were DES-exposed than in other men.

## 217 Where can I get more information about DES exposure?

The best source of information about DES is the National Cancer Institute. This organization has an ongoing study, The DESAD Project (Diethylstilbestrol and Adenosis Project). Institutions participating in this study, and the principal investigators, are:

Massachusetts General Hospital
Harvard Medical School
Boston, Massachusetts
Dr. Ann Barnes and Dr. Stanley J. Robboy

University of Southern California
Los Angeles, California
Dr. Duane E. Townsend

Baylor College of Medicine
Houston, Texas
Dr. Raymond H. Kaufman

Mayo Clinic
Rochester, Minnesota
Dr. David G. Decker

Your own physician may have information about DES, and there is a lay group, DES Action National, which is publishing information for DES-exposed men and women.

Their address is 1638-B Haight Street, San Francisco, California 94117.

## 218 If I was exposed to DES before birth, what examinations or treatment should I have?

If you have been exposed to DES, it is important that you have an annual examination, but this is no different from what other women should do, since all women need an annual examination and Pap smear. The one addition to your examination that your doctor might feel is necessary would be an annual colposcopy, a magnified view, of your cervix and vagina.

I also recommend that you do not let doctors perform unnecessary procedures on you. There is much greater understanding of DES exposure now than there was when the problem was first recognized. Many women had areas of adenosis of their vagina surgically removed, and others had their cervix frozen, cauterized, or lasered. We now know that most of those procedures were not necessary.

One encouraging note is that studies are showing that at least 50 percent of the DES-caused abnormalities in women's vaginas and on their cervixes disappear over the years. A cervix cannot get bigger, of course, but the collars, ridges, and cockscombs seem to flatten out with time and areas of adenosis seem to get smaller. Because of this trend, it is unlikely that DES-exposed women in the future will develop unusual malignancies more often than other women.

## Tuberculosis of the Pelvic Organs

## 219 What is tuberculosis of the pelvis?

This is a tuberculosis infection that develops in the pelvis, usually from TB infection in the lungs. It causes scarring and adhesions that can block the fallopian tubes and cause infertility. About 10 percent of the women who have tuberculosis of the lungs develop it in their pelvic structures.

Women are generally unaware that they have tuberculosis of the pelvis. They do not usually discover it until they try unsuccessfully to get pregnant.

Because tuberculosis itself is uncommon in the United States, tuberculosis of the pelvis is also uncommon. In my private practice I have never treated a patient with this disease.

Most women with tuberculosis of the pelvis are in the reproductive age. Physicians believe that the fallopian tube is the first structure in the pelvis that becomes infected and that the disease spreads into the uterus and ovaries from there.

## 220 How would tuberculosis of the pelvis be found?

The diagnosis depends on the severity of the disease:

*Mild tuberculosis of the pelvis.* If you are unable to become pregnant, you will probably see a doctor for an evaluation. The pelvic examination might reveal no abnormalities, but a complete fertility evaluation would show the presence of pelvic TB. In other words, the discovery of only mild pelvic tuberculosis would probably be a finding of a fertility evaluation. You would be completely unaware that you had TB. A complete infertility evaluation would include a uterine scraping. If you had pelvic TB the pathologist would usually see the changes of TB on those tissues. Also, a hysterosalpingogram might show that your tubes were blocked. When laparoscopy was done to find the reason for that, the tissues of the fallopian tube would be seen to be thickened and have small, elevated nodules (tubercles) over their surface from pelvic TB infection.

*Advanced pelvic tuberculosis.* A patient may not feel any symptoms of the presence of even advanced tuberculosis of the pelvis. The doctor might find, on examination of the abdomen, that there is a "doughiness," caused by the tissues of both the pelvis and the intestines being "stuck together" by the scarring and adhesions of advanced pelvic TB.

---

## 221 What diagnostic procedures would the doctor perform if tuberculosis of the pelvis is suspected?

There are several techniques for diagnosing tuberculosis of the pelvis:

*TB skin test.* Because tuberculosis of the pelvis is one cause of infertility, I now do a TB skin test on each of my infertility patients. Your doctor would do a TB skin test if TB of the pelvis is suspected.

*Chest X-ray.* If tuberculosis of the pelvis is suspected, a chest X-ray would be ordered. TB of the pelvis does not generally develop for several years after the person has had TB of the lungs, but it is possible for a woman to have active tuberculosis of the lungs and also to have pelvic tuberculosis. Remember, pelvic TB essentially always comes from a primary infection of the lungs.

*D&C.* If TB of the pelvis is suspected, your doctor would want to do a thorough curettage or scraping of your uterus to see if you have changes that confirm tuberculosis. However, 50 percent of the time a D&C will not show the disease, even when it is present. The doctor may prescribe birth-control pills for you to use for two or three months without a break, so that a D&C done at the end of the three months will show the TB. This is because the monthly shedding of the uterine lining with the menstrual flow can prevent TB from showing up on a D&C. If a woman takes birth-control pills every day without stopping, she will usually not have any uterine bleeding until she stops the pills.

If she has TB in the uterus, this will allow the germs and infection to build up on the uterine lining and be found by a D&C at the end of three months.

*Culture of the menstrual flow.* The doctor may want you to collect some of your menstrual flow so that it can be cultured. It has been reported that as many as 90 percent of the patients with TB of the pelvis will show positive cultures in this way. A collection of menstrual fluid can be done with a plastic cup that is inserted in the vagina much like a diaphragm.

---

## 222 How is TB of the pelvis treated?

If a woman has TB of the pelvis and plans to become pregnant either now or in the future, she would be treated with antibiotics. Several different antibiotics are effective against TB. Your doctor would choose the right ones for you. These drugs enable some women to achieve pregnancy after treatment, but, unfortunately, most women who develop tuberculosis of the fallopian tubes will be permanently sterile.

If a woman's tuberculosis has become so bad that the doctor can feel masses, and the masses do not get smaller after three or four months of treatment, surgery is usually necessary. Or if the masses disappear and then return, surgery is also necessary. Likewise, if a woman's tuberculosis produces abdominal pain that does not get better with treatment, or if the tuberculosis causes excessive bleeding from the uterus, an operation is required.

Surgery for tuberculosis consists of removal of the uterus, tubes, and ovaries. Before surgery, a patient should receive antibiotics for up to two months. After the surgery, she should receive the antibiotics for a period of from several weeks to several months.

## Abortion

### 223    What does the word *abortion* mean?

Abortion is a medical term that refers to the ending of a pregnancy, for whatever reason, before the baby is mature enough to survive outside the mother's uterus. Physicians usually use the term when a pregnancy ends before the twentieth week. After that time, or if the baby weighs more than about one pound, the loss of the pregnancy is considered to be a premature delivery. A birth is considered premature until delivery within two weeks of the due date for the birth.

Most people call the spontaneous loss of a pregnancy a miscarriage rather than an abortion. When abortions were legalized in our country in January 1972, even doctors began using the term *abortion* for the pregnancy that a woman terminated and the term *miscarriage* for a pregnancy that she lost spontaneously. Although this helps avoid confusion, technically any loss of pregnancy before the twentieth week is termed an abortion, no matter what causes the loss.

Doctors use these terms to define abortion.

*Spontaneous abortion.* This term describes the spontaneous loss of a pregnancy before the twentieth week.

*Missed abortion.* This refers to a loss of pregnancy before the twentieth week of growth but—because the contracting mechanism of the uterus did not start working when the baby stopped growing—the dead tissue inside the uterus was not delivered. Once doctors are certain that a woman has had a missed abortion, a D&C or a suction curettage is done to remove the dead or remaining material from the uterus.

*Miscarriage.* This is the spontaneous loss of a pregnancy before the twentieth week. It is a lay term and is not actually a part of the medical vocabulary.

*Elective (voluntary) abortion.* This refers to the termination of a normal pregnancy at the decision of the mother or a guardian.

*Therapeutic (medical) abortion.* A therapeutic abortion is one done because of medical problems of the mother that might make pregnancy dangerous for her, or because of problems that might cause grave physical abnormalities or mental retardation of the baby. Pregnancies that result from rape or incest are also considered by most physicians to be an indication for therapeutic abortions.

Although these abortions are called "therapeutic," they are still elective for the mother. The decision about having a therapeutic abortion is hers alone. There is no law that says a woman must have an abortion because the child might be born with abnormalities or because the mother's health would suffer if she does not have an abortion. A woman whose doctor tells her this in an attempt to convince her to have an abortion should consider changing doctors if she does not want to have an abortion.

### 224    When does a baby become a human being?

Life clearly begins at the moment of conception. It does not matter at what stage of development from that point on that a pregnancy is terminated; a life is destroyed and a person no longer exists.

From conception on, a baby's growth and development are continuous. The birth itself does not change a person from one type of organism into another. Birth is merely one of many significant events that occur in a person's life. Some oriental cultures seem to understand this better than our own: when a baby is born, it is considered to be one year old.

A baby's total dependence on its mother

before birth does not make it less a person than it is after birth, nor does it mean the baby is merely an appendage to the mother's body. There is a change in the form of dependence that a baby has on its mother, but there is no less dependence of that baby after birth than there was before birth. An astronaut, for example, is no less a person when he or she is confined to a space suit and dependent on it for all life functions than when walking on the ground, free of the restrictions of the space suit.

Studies have shown normal human functions are detectable in a baby's body very early in pregnancy.

*EEG studies.* Electroencephalograms have shown brain activity in the baby after six or eight weeks of development. The brain activity shown is much like that of a sleeping adult. This brain activity does not change abruptly at the time of birth.

*Heartbeat.* After only two weeks from the day of conception, the tiny baby's heart contracts occasionally. Thirty-one days after conception the heart has begun the normal, rhythmic contractions it will have for the rest of its life.

*Hormones.* By the sixth week of life in the uterus, the baby's adrenal and thyroid glands are functioning. These glands continue to function for the rest of that person's life.

*Physical identity.* By the twelfth week of intrauterine life, the baby's fingerprints have developed. He or she can be identified as an individual from that point until death by those same fingerprints.

*Activity.* By the marvel of ultrasound viewing, the baby can be seen moving its arms and legs, sucking its thumb, and turning somersaults. Fetal movements have been recorded on film as early as the thirty-sixth day (fifth week) of development inside the uterus. By the sixth or seventh week of intrauterine life, the baby is developed enough to respond to touch. Later the unborn baby can be seen to be urinating, holding on to the umbilical cord, and doing all the things you would expect a baby to do. Ultrasound allows us to appreciate the fact that "a baby is a baby," whether inside or outside the uterus. This emphasizes the fact that birth is only an event in the baby's life, not an act that turns a baby from a nonhuman to a human.

---

**225** **Do doctors believe that a fetus is a human being?**

Make no mistake, most of the doctors who perform abortions know that they are killing babies. Doctors have enough scientific orientation to know that the signs of the humanity of the fetus cannot be ignored.

A few years ago doctors did not have the evidence we have today that shows the humanity of a fetus. There were no instruments accurate enough to measure the signs of life in a young fetus. Consideration of the many facets of this complicated problem led Bernard N. Nathanson, M.D.—former director of what was the largest abortion clinic in the world at that time—to state in *The New England Journal of Medicine* (Nov. 28, 1984): "I am deeply troubled by my own increasing certainty that I have, in fact, presided in over sixty thousand deaths. There is no longer serious doubt in my mind that human life exists within the womb from the very onset of pregnancy, despite the fact that the nature of the intrauterine life has been the subject of considerable dispute in the past."

---

**226** **Does the Bible speak about the baby inside the uterus as a human being?**

Yes, in many places and from many perspectives:

*Psalm 51:5,* NIV. Surely I have been a

sinner from birth, sinful from the time my mother conceived me.

This is not the place for a theological discussion about sin. The point is made here that the baby in the uterus is considered to be more than just living tissue.

Psalm 139:13–16, NIV.
For you created my inmost being;
You knit me together in my mother's womb.
I praise you because I am fearfully and wonderfully made;
Your works are wonderful,
I know that full well.
My frame was not hidden from you
When I was made in the secret place.
When I was woven together in the depths of the earth,
Your eyes saw my unformed body.
All the days ordained for me
Were written in your book
Before one of them came to be.

Genesis 25:22, NIV. The babies jostled each other within her and she said, "Why is this happening to me?" So she went to inquire of the Lord.

This verse speaks of the conflict between Jacob and Esau. They were twins who began their conflict with each other *even before they were born,* causing their mother, Rebekah, to inquire of God before she delivered them why they were fighting each other inside her uterus.

Luke 1:41, NIV. When Elizabeth heard Mary's greeting, the baby leaped in her womb, and Elizabeth was filled with the Holy Spirit.

John the Baptist, *while in his mother's uterus* leaped for joy when his mother was in the presence of Mary, the mother of Jesus, while she was pregnant with Jesus.

Jeremiah 1:5, NIV. Before I formed you in the womb I knew you, before you were born I set you apart. I appointed you as a prophet to the nations.

These words were spoken by God to Jeremiah. God had a plan for Jeremiah from before the time he was born.

Based on these and other similar passages, I believe that God created every person and that he knows every person from conception to death. (See also chapter 6, especially the introductory paragraphs.)

---

## 227  How are abortions performed?

The method of abortion is determined by how far along a woman is in her pregnancy.

***Suction curettage (dilation and evacuation or D&E).*** If a woman is in her first three months of pregnancy, a suction technique is normally used. The suction is applied through the end of a thin tube, called a cannula. If an abortion is done very early in pregnancy, a straw-sized cannula can be used. If the pregnancy is more advanced, a larger cannula is necessary and the cervix must be dilated slightly to allow the cannula in.

Suction curettage is normally used through the twelfth week of pregnancy. It cannot be used from the twelfth to the fifteenth weeks because the developing baby's body is so large that it will clog even the largest cannula that might be used to suck out the baby.

Once the cannula is pushed up into the uterus, powerful suction is applied and the baby, with its placenta and membranes, is pulled apart and sucked through the cannula into the collecting bottle.

A paracervical block is usually used for pain relief and is moderately effective.

***Dilatation and curettage (D&C).*** This procedure is the same one that is done when a woman has bleeding problems or has a miscarriage, but in this case the pro-

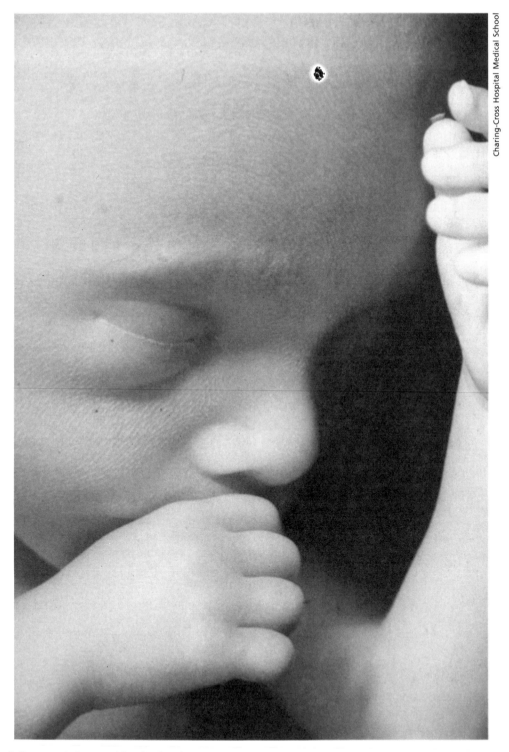

A five-month fetus sucking its thumb.

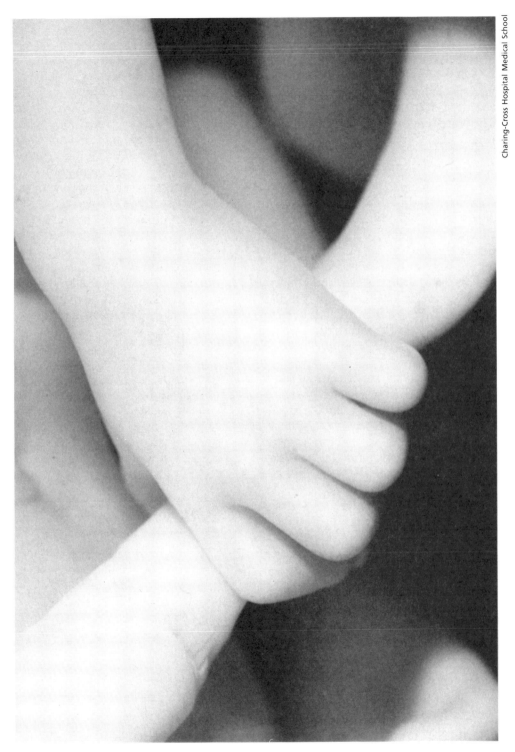

A five-month fetus gently holding its umbilical cord.

cedure is used to end a pregnancy. The baby, the placenta, and membranes, are scraped or pulled out of the uterus.

A D&C is normally done with a paracervical block, but it may be done with general anesthesia if the pregnancy is very far along. The procedure can be used through the fifteenth week of pregnancy.

To do the D&C, the doctor dilates the cervix, breaks the bag of waters, and if it is a very early pregnancy merely scrapes the tissue out. If the body parts are large, the doctor may use instruments to reach up inside the uterus, grasp the parts of the baby that can be reached, and pull them out, tearing them away from whatever part of the baby is still inside the uterus. If the pregnancy is past the fifteenth week, the baby's head is so large that it is difficult to remove, although all the other parts of the body may have been pulled out. It is for this reason that a D&C is not used past the fifteenth week. By the end of the fifteenth week, the baby is about eight inches long, has reached half of its height at birth, and could weigh as much as one-half pound. By this time the mother will usually have felt movement.

***Saline or prostaglandin abortion.*** These techniques are used when the pregnancy has progressed to sixteen weeks or more. They are not effective prior to this because: (1) it is difficult to put a needle into the bag of waters because it is so small prior to the sixteenth week, and (2) the uterus does not contract well earlier than sixteen weeks.

With this procedure, either salt water or prostaglandins (hormones that make the uterus contract) are injected into the amniotic fluid. After a few minutes or up to twelve hours, the uterus begins contractions, stimulated by the drugs that have been injected. These contractions cause the expulsion of the baby and the placenta (afterbirth). Occasionally the placenta does not come out when the baby is expelled. A D&C is necessary in that event.

Normally the saline solution kills the baby before delivery, because the salt solution is more concentrated than that in which human tissue can live. If prostaglandins are used, they do not kill the baby; the baby dies because of the pressures of labor on its delicate body. With prostaglandin abortions babies are occasionally born alive.

***Hysterotomy and hysterectomy.*** The uterus can be opened up and emptied of its contents, or it can be removed with its contents still in place. Either one of these procedures ends the pregnancy.

Hysterotomies are normally done only when a pregnancy is more than sixteen weeks along, and then only when other methods have failed or there is some reason that they cannot be used. Hysterectomies can be used at any stage in pregnancy. They are normally done as an abortion procedure only when a woman is planning to have a hysterectomy anyway. The abortion only serves as a reason for her to go ahead with the surgery.

For both hysterectomy and hysterotomy, a major incision in the abdomen is necessary. This requires a general anesthesia, a spinal, or an epidural, and the usual five or six days of recovery in the hospital.

---

**228** **What complications can result from abortions?**

There are numerous complications of abortions, and the further along a woman is in her pregnancy, the more likely they are to occur. Many physicians who perform abortions do not discuss the possible complications with their patients. I feel strongly that they should, especially with young women. I have found that women below the age of twenty often are not aware of the medical complications that can result from abortion.

In an article from the Center for Disease Control, printed in *Obstetrical and Gynecological Survey,* 1979, physicians wrote that although abortion is basically a safe surgical procedure, the further along the pregnancy is when the abortion is done, the more likely a woman is to have complications. These complications may include:

*Uterine hemorrhage.* A patient may bleed heavily after any D&C, but if she is pregnant when the procedure is done, there is even more chance of heavy bleeding. If a woman is more than thirteen weeks pregnant at the time of abortion, there is a truly significant risk of bleeding heavily.

*Perforation of the uterus.* The instruments used for doing an abortion can make a hole in the wall of the uterus. It is difficult for a doctor to feel the difference between the fetal tissue and the tissue that makes up the wall of the uterus. In trying to get out all of the tissue of pregnancy, the doctor may push the instruments through the wall of the uterus. When this perforation occurs, bleeding into the abdominal cavity and/or infection may result. Occasionally a major operation may be necessary to take care of this complication.

*Injury to the cervix.* No matter what type of abortion is done, the cervix can be damaged. Cervical trauma is a common and potentially serious complication of abortion. The damage includes tears, scars, and stenosis, scarring so extensive that the opening of the cervix is made too small for fertility or, if future pregnancy does occur, for normal delivery.

*Risk from anesthesia.* Any time a patient is given a general anesthesia, there is a slight risk of major problems or even death. Even with a paracervical block there is some risk to a patient's health.

*Embolism.* Amniotic fluid or air can be forced into the mother's blood vessels during the abortion procedure. If these pass to the brain, they can cause brain damage or death.

*Infection.* After an abortion, the inside of the uterus is raw. Since the instruments that were inserted inside the uterus can carry germs, infections can occur. This happens often enough that some doctors recommend that all women having abortions be given antibiotics.

*Other problems.* Other problems have been known to develop following abortion. These include menstrual irregularities, infertility, future spontaneous abortion, tubal pregnancies, prematurity of later pregnancies, and death of the mother.

---

**229** **Why do I read in newspapers and magazines that abortion is a "safe operation" if all these things can occur?**

Those who favor abortion usually refer to the fact that it is safer, physically speaking, for a woman to have an abortion than it is for her to carry a pregnancy to term and deliver the baby. They also mention the fact that few women are made infertile or sterile by an abortion. Percentagewise this may be true, but the number of women in our country who have been made sterile by an abortion runs in the thousands.

The unifying facts in this puzzling maze of information have to do with numbers. If physicians perform an operation that has a low percentage chance of complications, they consider it a low-risk procedure, and abortion definitely has a low chance of problems. But abortions are done in such huge numbers in the United States that physicians and even medical organizations have lost sight of how many individual people have been hurt or killed by abortion. The chart on p. 164 describes potential risks of these abortion procedures.

It is not until we realize how many such operations are done in our country and understand how many women are being made sterile, or have loss of later desired pregnancies, that we comprehend the extent of damage that is being done. The sad thing is that one-fourth of those who are being hurt are teenagers who usually have not yet had their families and who do not realize the

## Complications from Legal Abortions
## Performed Annually in the United States[1]

1,300,700 women, one-third of whom
were teenagers

| Complication | Number of Women Damaged | Percentage of Women Who Had Abortions |
|---|---|---|
| Death | 7 | |
| Pelvic Inflammatory Disease (PID)[2] | 50,730 | 3.9 |
| Damage to cervix from suction curettage (can cause spontaneous abortions or premature babies) Risk increases to 16–24% in repeat abortions[3] | 104,061 | 8 |
| Risk rate doubles for teenagers below 17 (15% of all aborted women)[4] | 3,317 | 1.7 |
| Hysterectomy[5] (1 in 20,000 abortions) | 65 | |
| Major complications in teens having suction curettage[4] | 52-156 | .1–.3 |
| Major complications in teens having saline abortion (4 or more months pregnant, 6–12% of teenage abortions)[4] | 338-676 | 1.3 |
| Loss of later pregnancy due to 2 or more abortions[3,6] | | 2–3 times greater than normal |

1. Based on statistics gathered by Center for Disease Control—admittedly under-reported.
2. From E. Quistad et al, "Pelvic Inflammatory Disease Associated with Chlamydia Trachomatis Infections After Therapeutic Abortions: A Prospective Study," *British Journal of Venereal Diseases*, 59:189-192, 1983.
3. 23% of women having abortions are having their second or more abortion.
4. Figures on teenage abortions are from W. Cates, Jr., et al, "The Risks Associated with Teenage Abortion," *The New England Journal of Medicine*, 309:621–627, 1983.
5. From J. E. Hodgson, "Major Complications of 20,248 Consecutive First Trimester Abortions: Problems of Fragmented Care," *Planned Parenthood*, 9:52, 1975.
6. From A. Levin, et al, "Association of Induced Abortion with Subsequent Pregnancy Loss," *Journal of the American Medical Association*, 243:2495-2497, 1980.

implications of being made infertile by the abortion of the only pregnancy they might ever have.

## 230 How significant is the emotional trauma of abortion to the women and men involved?

A book called *Men and Abortion: Lessons, Losses and Love*, by Arthur Shostak, Gary McLouth, and Lynn Sing (Praeger, 1984), states that most of the men whose wives or girl friends had abortions felt isolated, angry at themselves and their partners, and fearful of the physical and emotional damage done to the women. One of the many men surveyed stated, "It is a wound you cannot see or feel, but it exists." This is from the man's perspective and he is not the one whose body is pregnant and undergoes the abortion.

Women do have an emotional response. The psychological reaction varies from individual to individual, but almost all patients who have had an abortion remember the experience as being unpleasant, both physically and emotionally. Many women seem to have no regret, others seem to have a lingering sadness. Patients who have had abortions, even those who have no guilt associated with it, often fail to mention an aborted pregnancy when they list all previous pregnancies for their physician. It seems that they are trying to forget the event. Patients who subsequently have problems with their fertility, especially if damage to pelvic organs resulted from the abortion, often experience regret for having had the abortion.

I advise my patients not to have abortions. Although they may think they will not feel guilt or regret if they have an abortion done, they can definitely carry around in their minds, emotions, and bodies for the rest of their lives the memory of a most unpleasant experience.

complicated situation. If the doctors involved are convinced that your life is in danger, however, I feel you should follow their advice and have an abortion.

*Abnormalities of the fetus, incompatible with life.* There are certain abnormalities of the fetus that are totally incompatible with life. In these cases I feel that the wisest choice is an abortion. One example of this type of problem is a baby who has no brain development (anencephaly). Since this condition is totally incompatible with life, terminating the pregnancy is not killing a baby which could have survived outside the uterus. With this pregnancy over, the couple can go on with their lives and, if they desire, another pregnancy.

## 231 When are abortions considered necessary?

There are several problems for which most physicians recommend medical, or therapeutic, abortions, but less than 5 percent of abortions in the United States are done for those reasons.

*Medical problems of the mothers.* Medical problems can exist that endanger the life of the mother if the pregnancy continues. These include severe heart disease, disseminated lupus erythematosis, severe hypertension (including severe toxemia), and cervical cancer. An abortion or induction of premature delivery may be necessary in these situations to save the life of the mother.

Contrary to what many people think, this is not a choice between the life of the mother and the life of the child. If the mother is so gravely ill that an abortion is necessary, both she *and* the baby would probably die if she did not have an abortion. If you have been advised to have an abortion because of a health problem, and you do not want one or feel it is necessary, I recommend that you get a second opinion, and even a third. Some doctors use abortion as an easy way out of a

## 232 Are there other medical reasons for abortion?

Other reasons for abortion are not absolute indications for abortion, although many physicians and lay people may recommend them. Whether you have or recommend an abortion for one of these reasons depends on your own morality as it relates to abortion.

*Genetic/chromosome problems.* Often a woman will decide to abort if she knows she is carrying a child with a disorder such as Downs syndrome. There is much help now available for children suffering from this disorder. No longer does the presence of this and other syndromes necessarily provide justifiable reasons for an abortion. (See Q. 495–516 for more information on genetic/chromosomal problems.)

*Incest.* Generally, if a girl is old enough to become pregnant, she is old enough to deliver a child. Delivering a child is a normal, sexual function, and even a young woman can accept that as a natural part of the function of her body. Abortion, however, is *not* natural, and it can leave adolescents and young women with tremendous emotional and physical scars.

*Rape.* Rape almost never results in pregnancy. Studies in Pennsylvania and Minnesota have shown that as many as five thousand rapes have occurred without a single pregnancy resulting. Even though a pregnancy begins as a result of rape, however, a mother must realize two things: half of that baby is from *her,* and no matter how it was conceived, the baby is still a baby. If an abortion is done for this reason, there is always the danger that a mother's emotional and psychological make-up may be even further damaged. Two wrongs cannot make a right or correct the first wrong.

*German measles (rubella).* If a mother develops German measles during the first three months of pregnancy, there is a 15-to-50–percent chance of having a baby with a major abnormality. However, this means that if an abortion is done because of German measles, there is a 50-to-85–percent chance that a *healthy, normal* child has been aborted. (See Q. 520–523.)

There are obviously a few valid reasons for which doctors and lay people advocate abortion. Unfortunately, however, it is often recommended because it is an easy solution to a problem or worry. Every woman who becomes pregnant must realize that there is an "automatic" 3-percent chance of having a baby with a major abnormality. There is no absolute way that a woman can be totally sure that she will have a healthy baby. Any good thing that comes into our lives involves some element of risk.

---

**233**  **Is an abortion necessary because drugs were taken or after radiation exposure just before or early in pregnancy?**

There is almost no drug in common use, either prescription or over-the-counter, that routinely causes abnormalities in fetuses. Even the drugs that *can* cause problems rarely do so, especially if taken only for a

brief time. Because of this, an abortion is not usually necessary because a woman has taken medications or drugs while pregnant.

The same is true for radiation exposure. There is no reason a woman should ever have an abortion just because she has had X-ray examinations. Careful research has shown that there is no diagnostic X-ray that can add up to enough exposure to cause any danger to a fetus.

Radiation treatment such as that done for cancer in the pelvis *is* dangerous to the fetus. In fact, this type of X-ray therapy would usually kill the baby. Unfortunately this therapy is sometimes necessary for cervical cancer if a pregnant woman is found to have such a cancer.

---

**234**  **Are babies still alive when they are aborted?**

Sometimes a baby is delivered alive after an abortion. This is because doctors in most states are not legally bound to perform abortions only in early pregnancy. Consequently, there are babies being aborted today who are the same size and maturity as many premature babies being successfully cared for in intensive-care nurseries all over the nation.

Abortions during the second three months of pregnancy are commonly done. Because of this, we occasionally see headlines such as appeared in the *Dallas Times Herald* (AP) on March 23, 1983:

Six Live Births After Abortions
Cause Furor

Madison, Wisconsin—The live births of six babies whose mothers had abortions at Madison hospitals in the past ten months have shocked residents and become a rallying point for abortion foes.

The births also have prompted one hospital to drastically curtail the surgical procedure.

All six babies died within twenty-seven

hours of birth, four at Madison General Hospital and two at the University of Wisconsin Hospital.

## 235 What advice do you have for women considering abortion?

There may be several factors to be considered if a woman is thinking about having an abortion, but one thing is certain: she should not let anyone push her into having the abortion. The relationship a pregnant woman has with the baby she carries is too personal for her to let the baby's father, whether or not he is her husband, her parents, or anyone else convince her to kill her baby.

My advice is:

*Don't take the easy way out.* There are many examples in life that show us that the easiest way is not necessarily the best way. In chapter 15, for example, we point out the importance of exercise in maintaining a body that will do what we want it to do. It is not easy to exercise, but the "hard" way is best.

Since most abortions are performed because of the inconvenience of the pregnancy and not because of medical reasons, abortion can be considered in this same light. Though an abortion may be the easiest way out of a difficult situation, it may not be the best solution.

I received the following letter from a patient who came to me in early pregnancy, planning to have an abortion. After we talked for a while, she decided not to have the abortion.

Dear Dr. McIlhaney,

If you have a woman come in and wants to abort or her husband wants her to, as mine did . . . please show her this picture and tell her I almost made the biggest mistake of my life and had it done to this beautiful boy. Maybe it might save a life . . . it is a life . . . anything that can make

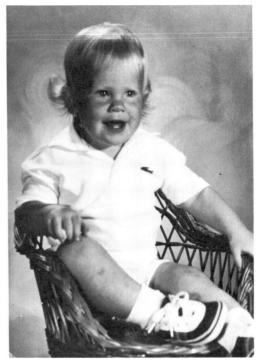

"...I almost aborted this beautiful baby."

you that sick (when pregnant) has got to be a life.

Thank you for bringing two of the most precious children in the world into this world and into my life.

Name Withheld

*Be realistic.* A woman should not be naive when she considers an abortion. The people who perform abortions often picture it as a simple, straightforward procedure. Most women who have an abortion report that it was a very traumatic experience. Many women complain of being handled "like cattle" in abortion clinics and compare an abortion with rape—as a procedure that leaves a woman feeling violated.

*Be prepared for guilt.* For many women, guilt following abortion is inescapable. This procedure is one that a woman will never forget, and one that she may regret for the rest of her life.

*Expect possible infertility.* Doctors who treat women with infertility problems re-

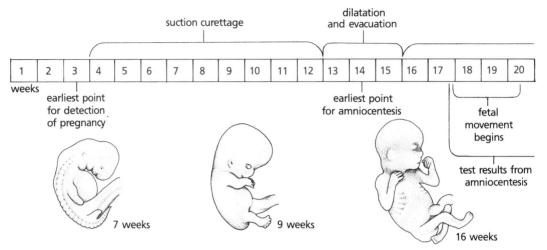

suction curettage

dilatation and evacuation

| 1 | 2 | 3 | 4 | 5 | 6 | 7 | 8 | 9 | 10 | 11 | 12 | 13 | 14 | 15 | 16 | 17 | 18 | 19 | 20 |

weeks

earliest point for detection of pregnancy

earliest point for amniocentesis

fetal movement begins

test results from amniocentesis

7 weeks

9 weeks

16 weeks

port that often the difficulty is somehow related to a previous abortion.

*Don't base an abortion on finances.* Do not overplay your own poor economic situation. There is never a good time, financially, to have a baby. Almost no one feels that she can really afford adding a baby to her family. However, just like millions of other parents in America, you will, somehow, be able to provide for your child. It is your *love* the baby needs primarily, not the material things you can provide for the child.

There is a great deal of rhetoric about abortion from both sides of the issue. I encourage you to read and give honest consideration to the information in this chapter. I urge you to consider the consequences of a decision to end a human life.

## 236 What advice do you have for a woman who has had an abortion?

It is possible that you will never regret having had an abortion, but many women do. If you are one who does have such regrets, it is important that you not let these regrets dominate your life. There are several things that a woman can do to help keep a past mistake from weighing on her for the rest of her life.

If you are having a major problem with guilt and self-blame, see a counselor (pastor, psychologist, or psychiatrist). Be sure you choose a counselor whose viewpoint is compatible with your own. Otherwise he or she can cause you more frustration than you are now experiencing.

If you find yourself blaming your husband, boyfriend, or parents, you must realize that blaming others will not accomplish anything and that the ultimate decision to have an abortion was yours. If you cannot overcome the anger toward the people that may have influenced you in your decision, talk to a counselor.

Ask for God's forgiveness, accept it, and then forgive yourself. It is helpful to remember examples of God's forgiveness. King David, for example, got Bathsheba pregnant and then, to cover his tracks, had her husband killed. When Nathan, God's prophet, confronted David with his sins, David thought God would not forgive him. His response was not a mere statement, "I have sinned." He was truly sorry and expressed his repentance to God, whose response was complete forgiveness. God will do the same for you. When God forgives you, you must forgive yourself so that guilt does not ruin the rest of your life.

# Method Selection

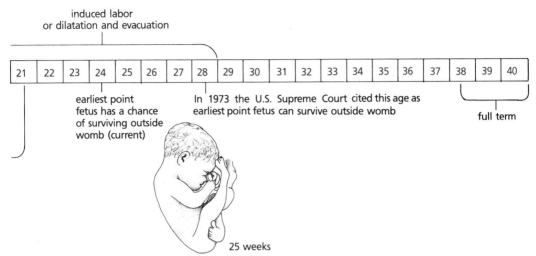

induced labor
or dilatation and evacuation

| 21 | 22 | 23 | 24 | 25 | 26 | 27 | 28 | 29 | 30 | 31 | 32 | 33 | 34 | 35 | 36 | 37 | 38 | 39 | 40 |

earliest point
fetus has a chance
of surviving outside
womb (current)

In 1973 the U.S. Supreme Court cited this age as
earliest point fetus can survive outside womb

full term

25 weeks

Become a "counselor" for those who are considering abortion. Those who have the best insight into the abortion problem are those who have had one. If you have decided, since your abortion, that abortion is not the best solution to a problem pregnancy, you could very well serve as a helpful counselor for someone who finds herself pregnant and is considering abortion as a solution.

## Rape and Sexual Assault

**237** **What is the definition of rape?**

According to the dictionary, rape is the crime of forcing a woman to submit to sexual intercourse. The technical definition, however, does not do the word justice, because the word *rape* evokes such horror, fear, and dread in a woman that mere words cannot express it. The powerful emotions that even the thought of rape evokes are due, no doubt, to the fact that rape is not just an act against a woman's body, but an act against the very essence of her womanhood.

Even the most powerful emotions must sometimes be reduced to legalities, however, and rape and other sexual crimes are no exception. There has recently been a change in the legal terminology used in reference to sex crimes. Most states and most police departments now use these new terms. Old terms such as *rape, statutory rape,* and *aggravated rape* have been replaced by:

*Sexual Assault.* Forced sexual activity which includes rape and intercourse with someone incapable of giving knowledgeable consent. This term does not apply to a child under fourteen years of age. Sexual assault is a second-degree felony offense.

*Aggravated sexual assault.* Forced sexual activity that includes: the involvement of a weapon; or serious bodily injury; or intercourse with a girl under the age of fourteen, even if she consents to such activity. Aggravated sexual assault is a first-degree felony offense.

*Attempted sexual assault.* Activity which indicates by words, acts, or deeds that a person intends sexual assault but who does not, for some reason, have the opportunity to carry through with his or her intent. This is a third-degree felony offense.

*Indecent exposure.* This term refers to an act in which a person exposes himself (or herself) to another person. An example would be a man exposing himself to a woman while masturbating. This is a Class B criminal offense.

*Indecency with a child.* If a man or woman exposes himself or herself to a child under seventeen years of age, it is referred to as "indecency with a child." Other acts are included under this heading: putting the mouth on a girl's breast, or touching a child's genitalia (both of these are second-degree felony offenses); indecent exposure to a child. This is a third-degree felony offense.

## 238 What do statistics reveal about the act of rape?

Rape is the fastest-growing violent crime in the United States. Some facts concerning this horrible crime are:

Ten times as many rapes occur as are ever reported to authorities.

Fewer than 50 percent of the rapists who are caught are ever brought to trial, and very few of those are convicted.

One woman in ten will be the victim of rape or attempted rape during her lifetime.

About 85 percent of women who are the victims of rape are also beaten or threatened with physical force.

Roughly half of all rapes occur in the homes of the victims.

Rapists do not choose their victims according to their appearance or age. Every woman is a potential victim.

The incidence of rape in women over sixty has increased by 800 percent during the past fifteen years.

About 50 percent of rapists have committed prior crimes.

Students constitute 11 percent of rapists.

Over half the victims who report rapes know their attacker.

Over half of convicted rapists are married and have "normal" sex lives.

Almost three-fourths of arrested rapists will repeat the crime at some time in the future.

Rape is not usually spontaneous. Over 70 percent of all rapes are planned and victims and place are picked out ahead of time.

Rape is a crime of violence, not "passion."

## 239 What can I do to protect myself and my daughters from rape?

First, you must learn all you can about rape and teach what you learn to your daughters. Next, you must practice precautions against rape and teach your daughters to do the same. The often-used saying, "It's better to be safe than sorry," is extremely applicable in this case.

If at all possible, take a self-defense course. Being able to react quickly and effectively may give you the advantage you need to repel an attacker and get away from him.

Further suggestions include:

Secure your home so that visitors can enter only when you admit them. When you are alone at home, never allow any man inside unless you know that you can trust him completely. Insist on identification even from "authorized" service personnel.

Never walk in an unsafe or secluded area. Avoid eye contact with strangers. If you must be in areas where you will be alone, carry a loud whistle or take a dog with you.

Travel only in a well-maintained automobile on major roads or highways. Do not travel alone if you can avoid it, especially at night. Keep your car doors locked and never give rides to hitchhikers or stranded motorists. You can always offer to call for help for them. If you are stranded, do not accept a ride with a stranger.

## 240 What should I do if I am attacked by a rapist?

If you are attacked, you may be able to avoid rape by the right reactions. Rapists often say that they are more likely to rape a woman if she shows no emotion and stays quiet. Therefore do the following:

React strongly and physically. Kick the man in the genitals; poke at his eyes with a comb or pen; scratch, tear, and bite.

Make all the noise you can, scream as loud as you can.

If you can throw the attacker off guard, run. The idea of using self-defense is to get him off guard so that you can get away without being hurt.

Fighting, screaming, and running are not always possible nor the best tactic. When your life is threatened if you do not submit to an attacker's demands, you must decide whether to endure the sexual demands of the rapist or risk serious injury or lose your life.

There is no cut-and-dried answer that fits all situations or all women. Some women, for instance, would rather die than submit. Others are able to deal with the horror of rape by realizing that, they at least preserved their life.

## 241 What should I do if I am raped?

If your attempts at preventing an attack fail, and you become the victim of rape, the following suggestions may help.

Do not alter your surroundings, your appearance, or your body in any way. The best evidence of what has happened to you is the physical changes of your surroundings and your body. For example, do not straighten up the room or the area; leave any torn clothes where they were thrown by your attacker; do not wipe off any secretions; do not change clothes; do not urinate or have a bowel movement; do not douche; do not shower or bathe.

If you are physically injured, phone for help. Call the 911 emergency number if available in your area; call your local emergency medical service; or call an ambulance, a hospital, or a doctor.

Also call the police, the sheriff, or some other law enforcement official immediately.

Have a medical examination as soon as possible.

## 242 What doctor should I use following rape?

Whether or not you plan to bring charges against your assailant, it is important that you go immediately to a doctor. If possible, call your own physician. If he or she is able and available to do the examination, you will be in the hands of someone who you know will be caring and comforting. If your doctor is not familiar with the process of examining a rape victim, however, you may be advised to go to a local emergency room.

Emergency-room doctors try to be understanding with a rape patient, but their main job is to care for gravely ill people. Because of this, rape victims often feel neglected and poorly treated by emergency room personnel. For this reason it is best, if possible, that a woman get her own physician to examine her.

A local Rape Crisis Center may also be able to give you advice, encouragement, and help during this time. They will usually have someone come to the emergency room to be with you.

### 243 What does the medical examination following rape consist of?

The doctor and nurse will talk to you and record in great detail what has happened to you. In addition, they will ask what contraceptive technique you have been using and when your most recent episode of intercourse prior to the rape took place. The physician will also want to know if you have bathed or douched or changed clothes since the assault.

A complete physical examination will be done. The physician will record your emotional state, note any bruises or cuts or broken bones, and look for bruising, cuts, and swelling of your female organs.

The doctor will attempt to get specimens from your body to confirm the rape. This evidence will require:

Combing your pubic hair to remove any hair or thread that might be from the assailant.

Obtaining small specimens of your own pubic hair to differentiate it from the attacker's pubic hair.

Obtaining vaginal secretions that would be tested for the presence of sperm and acid phosphatase. There is a high concentration of this chemical in semen. If the man has had a vasectomy there would be no sperm, but the presence of

this chemical can confirm that he ejaculated.

The doctor will also obtain blood from you to check for syphilis and order a culture of your vaginal secretions to make sure the attacker did not pass gonorrhea germs to you. If there is any question of your being pregnant at the time of the attack, the doctor will obtain a serum pregnancy test to determine whether or not this is the case.

### 244 What medical treatment might be necessary because of rape?

If you have had injuries from a rape attack, these will be treated by the doctor with traditional therapy. In addition, you will probably be given a 4.8-million-unit injection of procane penicillin and one gram of probenecid by mouth to keep you from contracting gonorrhea or syphilis. If you are allergic to penicillin, the recommended drug is Trobicin (spectinomycin), 4 grams, I.M.

If you have not been using contraception, and the attack occurred at a time when you might get pregnant, your doctor may recommend that you use a high dose of estrogen by mouth in order to prevent pregnancy. This therapy is controversial because these high doses of estrogen can cause congenital abnormalities in a baby if a woman is already pregnant at the time of the rape, and sometimes this technique does not prevent a pregnancy. This is a situation you must discuss with your physician.

### 245 Is any follow-up treatment necessary?

If pregnancy as a result of the rape is a possibility, you should see a physician in two or three weeks. By that time a serum blood test for pregnancy could be positive.

You should also have a vaginal culture

and another blood test for syphilis twelve weeks after the assault, to be sure that you did not contract a sexually transmitted disease. Of patients who were raped and not treated at the time of the first medical exam, 3 percent developed gonorrhea and 0.1 percent developed syphilis.

## 246 Is counseling important for rape victims?

Counseling is very important, and I encourage you not to hesitate to get it. You should not feel abnormal if you respond to rape with deep emotional upheaval. All rape victims are left with some degree of fear, and there is often a feeling of helplessness in which a woman feels that she no longer has control over her own life and destiny.

Women who do not get counseling after rape often find that the greatest damage from the rape has been emotional rather than physical. It is important, therefore, to undergo counseling to keep these emotional problems from becoming deep seated and permanent.

In addition to formal psychological or psychiatric counseling, Rape Crisis Centers can be useful. Counseling is often free, and it will often involve not only the victim but her family as well. In addition, these centers can help a woman through the legal procedures necessary for bringing charges against her attacker. Support groups, which can be very helpful, are also available at most Rape Crisis Centers.

## 247 Is it really important to file charges against a rapist?

Although you may feel strangely guilty and/or embarrassed about being raped, you should not let this keep you from filing charges against your assailant. People who work with rape victims are often dis-

couraged by the failure of these women to press charges. It is important to remember that almost three-fourths of arrested rapists will repeat the crime. All of us should do whatever we can to keep these men from having an opportunity to commit rape again.

## 248 Where can I get further information about rape?

Because rape is the fastest-growing violent crime in the United States, it is important that we all become better informed about it. All women should learn how to protect themselves against rape, and both men and women must learn how to protect their children against it. Sources of information about rape include the following.

Your physician may or may not have information about rape for you. If he or she does not, your doctor can probably get it from the state or county medical society or from the state department of health.

Emergency-room personnel often have information about rape or will know who might have such information.

Almost all large cities in the United States have a Rape Crisis Center. You can probably find the phone number in the phone book, or call information. If you live in a town that does not have such a center, call the Rape Crisis Center in the nearest large town. They can send you information or can help you if you have been a rape victim.

Rape is a crime. Because of this, your local law enforcement agency has dealt with rape victims many times. The agency's personnel will have information not only for rape victims, but for those seeking to learn more about rape. They are vitally concerned with reducing the incidence of rape as are the thousands of other men and women around the country who are sickened by this horrible crime.

The National Center for the Prevention and Control of Rape. This organization has booklets and pamphlets available for individual use as well as sight/sound material for group use. You may want to contact them (Room 6C-12, Parklawn Bldg., 5600 Fisher's Lane, Brockville, Maryland 20857; Phone: 301-443-1910).

## An Afterword

During the reproductive years, a woman's body is working hard and it requires good care. If a woman maintains a healthy lifestyle during this important period of her life, her body will usually serve her well during the reproductive years and in the years beyond. A woman should keep herself in good condition, have regular health check-ups, and get good medical care for any problem that she may have. This chapter provides the information a woman needs to maintain and preserve her health and vitality.

Many of the topics discussed in this chapter also affect other aspects of a woman's life and are discussed in different parts of this book. Please use the index to locate related discussions so that you can be fully informed on these topics.

# 5

## Middle Age, Menopause, and Maturity

The poet Robert Browning expressed a possibility which most of us do not consider when we are younger:

> Grow old along with me!
> The best is yet to be,
> The last of life, for which the first was made.
> Our times are in his hand
> Who saith, "A whole I planned,
> Youth shows but half;
> Trust God: see all, nor be afraid!"

Youth is only half a life; the other half is lived as a middle-aged or older person and it can be the best part.

The Book of Isaiah speaks of God's care for us as we get older:

> I will be your God through all your lifetime,
> Yes, even when your hair is white with age.
> I made you and I will care for you.
> I will carry you along and be your Savior
> (Isa. 46:4, LB).

How gracious of God to assure us that he will carry us along in our old age, and to remind us that he made us and has been with us since our youth. If we are assured of God's watchcare in our later years, how can we dread the years of maturity?

There is much more going for midlife, menopause, and maturity than mere survival, but misinformation and fear of change often cause young women to look with dread on midlife years. While change is always difficult, the anticipation and dread of change are even worse. I hope this chapter will help not only those who are already in the midlife and mature years but also those who are younger. A clear understanding will enable young women to enter the best of life "for which the first was made" without fear or dread.

Young women seem to dread middle-age and the mature years, for fear that they cannot be as physically active and healthy, as mentally alert, or as physically attractive as they once were. One goal of this chapter is to introduce to younger women the idea that if they live healthy lives in their youth and carry these good health habits into their middle years, they can be much healthier and freer from disease and more mentally alert in old age than they thought was possible. And because of the glow of good health and the charisma of a sound mind and happy heart, their physical attractiveness will be maximized.

The goal is the same for those women who are already middle-aged or older. If they do not have well-established good health habits, they should understand that much of the deterioration they are experiencing is due to poor health habits, not to the inevitability of age decline. A program begun now for improving their health will pay off in their feeling better and being healthier both now and in later years.

There are older people who have apparently done nothing to

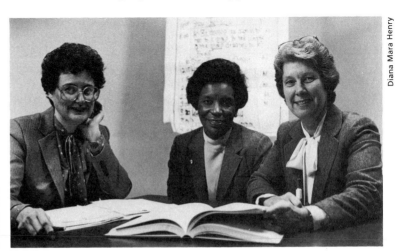

Diana Mara Henry

The glow of good health and the charisma of a sound mind and happy heart maximizes physical attractiveness.

care for their bodies or minds, yet seem to be alert, healthy, and active. A visit to a nursing home, however, will show many folk whose health has declined. Why should you take a chance? The better you care for yourself now, the more likely you are to be healthy in the future. Wouldn't it be nice to be healthy and vigorous up to the end of your life?

Good health should not become an obsessive goal or the god of your life. Doing whatever is necessary to insure and maintain your health, however, will enable you to attain your life's goal and to reach your maximum potential for serving God.

## Some Basic Definitions

### 249 What is the meaning of the various terms which are used to refer to this particular time of life?

The definitions of these various terms and the ages at which they occur tend to blend into each other and overlap. The following definitions and ages are generally accepted.

*Midlife.* The years between the ages of forty and sixty are considered the middle age of life. This term has nothing to do with menopause except that it usually occurs during the midlife years.

*Climacteric.* This term applies to the period of life that starts when the ovaries begin having decreased estrogen production. It includes the menopause, continues for several years, and ends when all the estrogen-sensitive tissues in the body have thinned out (atrophied) as much as they ever will. The entire climacteric period can last for thirty years.

*Premenopause.* This period extends from the time a woman's ovaries have begun producing less estrogen until she has her last period. This is the first phase of the climacteric.

*Menopause.* The menopause is actually a woman's last menstrual period. In our society the term *menopause* is usually used, even by medical personnel, when they are talking about the climacteric. The meno-

pause occurs in most women from the age of forty-eight to fifty-five, with the average age being fifty-one. This is the second phase of the climacteric.

*Postmenopause.* This term describes the time from the last menstrual period through the rest of life. A woman is postmenopausal when the menopause is totally over. Normally, menopause is considered complete when twelve months have elapsed without a menstrual period.

*Change of life.* This nonmedical term usually applies to the time from the first changes in a woman's body due to decreased estrogen, through the last menstrual period, or menopause. It is often used to refer to the few years after menopause, during which a woman has hot flashes or trouble sleeping that result from her climacteric. This period of time roughly corresponds to the climacteric. Most lay people use this term in reference to the symptoms of the climacteric.

*Mature years.* The years from about sixty until death encompass the years of a woman's "maturity."

## General Health Care in Midlife

### 250 Can good health habits help me feel better during the last half of my life?

Progressively worse health and increasing disease are not an inevitable part of the sec-

# Menopausal Terms

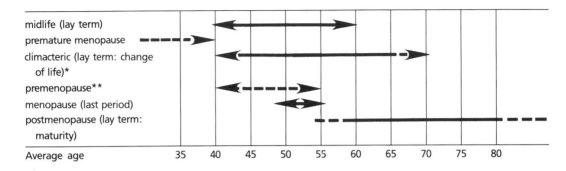

*years between first sign of decreased estrogen until all estrogen-sensitive tissues complete their process of atrophy
**years between first sign of decreased estrogen and last menstrual period (menopause)

ond half of life. Many of the health problems of older people are a result of the lifestyle they had as young adults. Obviously there are many middle-aged and older people today who are alert, active, and healthy. Others seem to be ill, inactive, and feeling poorly most of the time. It is easy to assume that their health is a result of the way their bodies were made. Actually it is likely that most of these people are reaping the results, both good and bad, of health habits they established years ago.

If you will do the things suggested in this chapter and in chapter 15, you will probably feel better now. The improvement in health from adopting sound habits is not just for the future, but for the improved sense of well-being and healthiness for today.

Although chapter 15 includes a more complete guide to good health, a summary of health habits particularly pertinent to women in midlife or maturity are discussed in Q. 251–257.

## 251 What major health hazard should be avoided by women seeking optimum health in later years?

Smoking! Studies show over and over again that smoking is the worst health hazard for Americans in general, and that it is particularly detrimental for the woman who is growing older. Besides increasing the wrinkling of skin and making a woman look older, smoking increases the incidence of lung cancer and is responsible for the fact that lung cancer is now more common than breast cancer in women. Smoking greatly increases a woman's chance of having heart disease, strokes, and poor circulation, and it limits the amount of oxygen distributed from the lungs to the rest of the body, decreasing energy and making a woman less likely to exercise. All of these effects are devastating to a woman as she grows older.

Studies are beginning to confirm that if a woman stops smoking she is more likely to remain a nonsmoker if she exercises regularly.

## 252 How is exercise related to growing older?

Many women get into a vicious cycle as they enter midlife. First, in the back of their minds they believe they are supposed to slow down as they get older. Then, at a picnic or on vacation, they perform some unusual physical activity and strain a ligament or muscle, confirming in their minds that they really do need to slow down. As a result they engage in even less activity. This downward spiral causes these women to do less and less physical activity and assume that this is normal for the human body.

This attitude and approach to physical activity from the middle-aged years on is absolutely wrong. Women should continue exercising until the day they die if they can.

They are many good books about exercise and how much exercise a woman should have. One such is Ken and Millie Cooper's book, *Aerobics for Women* (Bantam Books). If you participate in the exercises recommended in these books for your age group, you will find that you will stop having strained muscles and ligaments on vacations or family outings, and that you will generally feel a great deal better.

Studies have shown that poor vision and lack of exercise cause the majority of falls in elderly people. Ophthalmologists can usually take care of the visual problems, but the responsibility of exercising is up to you. Start this habit right now.

## 253 How will my current eating habits affect my life later?

The normal American diet—high in fat, high in sugar, low in fiber—is detrimental to the human body. It may take a long time for the effects to show up, but a poor diet produces a chain of events in the body that will probably eventually cause disease.

The diseases that poor diet cause (which include heart disease, colon cancer, hemorrhoids, hiatus hernia, and diverticulitis) have been accepted for years as being natural for older people. It seems clear now, however, that if women will eat a proper diet that is high in fiber and low in fats and concentrated sugar, they can avoid many of these problems, or at least be less likely to have them. (See chapter 15 for further information.)

## 254 Why is estrogen important for the menopausal woman?

A woman who has gone through the menopause is much safer taking estrogen (hormones) for the rest of her life than she is not taking them. The primary reason for this is that taking estrogen can help prevent the broken bones which occur so often in older women. In addition, women who have annoying symptoms from menopause will feel better if they take estrogen. They will sleep better, feel more like exercising, and will maintain better health. (See Q. 265–273.)

## 255 Are routine mammograms recommended for older women?

The American Cancer Society recommends a mammogram every other year from the age of thirty-five to fifty, and one every year from age fifty on. This one procedure would decrease the death rate from breast cancer for women over fifty by more than 40 percent! A mammogram can detect a breast cancer two years before a lump is large enough to be felt on breast self-examination. When a lump is found this early, a woman has a 95 percent chance of being cured by surgery for that cancer. Although breast self-examination (BSE) will not detect a cancer as early as a mammogram, BSE is still an important procedure for every woman to do every month. Mammograms are not perfect, and even they can miss a breast cancer.

## 256 What other special tests are important?

Colon cancer is so common in our society that routine testing is worthwhile. The American Cancer Society recommends that every person over forty years of age have a digital (with the finger) rectal exam every year. An examiner can feel a cancer growing in a patient's rectum if it is within reach of his or her finger. In addition, since a colon cancer will usually bleed into the intestines even when it is very small, a simple test for blood in the stools will often detect the presence of a colon cancer quite early. You can get a small inexpensive test packet to check your stools from your doctor, your local cancer society, or your pharmacy. The American Cancer Society recommends that you check your stools every year from the age of fifty on. Because this test is so cheap and easy to do, I feel that a person might as well do it from the age of forty on.

In addition, the American Cancer Society recommends that a person who is age fifty or over have a proctoscopy every three to five years. This is recommended after a person has first had a proctoscopy two years in a row to make certain there are no existing abnormalities.

A proctoscopy requires that your doctor insert a metal tube through your anus into your rectum, so as to see the interior of your colon and determine whether or not there are growths present. Proctoscopies are not done by gynecologists. They are usually done by gastroenterologists (intestinal specialists), internal medicine specialists, general surgeons, and family practitioners.

### 257 Is a yearly physical still important once a woman is past reproductive age?

Yes! It is important to have an annual physical examination for the rest of your life. This exam should include a blood pressure check, a blood count, a urine analysis, and a Pap smear. The doctor should, at minimum, check your thyroid, your breasts, your abdomen, and your pelvis. This basic examination will detect most abnormalities that an otherwise healthy woman might not know she has. In addition to the annual exam, if you have pain, discomfort, or other symp-

toms, you should go to the doctor for that. (See Q. 150–156 for a more complete discussion of the annual exam.)

## Menopause

### 258 What causes menopause?

Menopause comes when the ovaries no longer manufacture enough estrogen to produce menstrual periods. The ovaries stop producing estrogen when the ovarian follicles—small cysts which contain egg cells—die. When all these egg cells with their follicles are gone, the ovaries no longer produce estrogen, and a woman can no longer have periods. When this occurs the ovaries are essentially dead. Over the next few years they shrink, becoming small nubbins of fibrous tissue no more than one-half inch in diameter in the eighth and ninth decades of life.

### 259 At what age does menopause normally occur?

Menopause usually occurs between the ages of forty-eight to fifty-five, the average age being fifty-one. It is also normal for women to go through menopause as early as forty or as late as sixty. About 30 percent of women will have had menopause by the time they are forty-five and 98 percent will have had menopause by the time they are fifty-five.

There are variations.

*Premature menopause.* If a woman has menopause before the age of forty, she is said to have "premature menopause," and even adolescent girls can experience this. The medical term is "premature ovarian failure." This is a permanent condition, and there is nothing that can be done to make the ovaries begin again to produce eggs or hormones. Obviously a woman with premature menopause cannot become pregnant.

It is vitally important that a woman begin taking estrogen immediately if premature menopause occurs. Women who have early menopause are much more likely to have osteoporosis and fractures of their bones as they grow older than women who go through menopause at the usual age.

*Surgical menopause.* A woman is said to have "surgical menopause" if she has her ovaries removed by surgery. She will not go through "natural" menopause. Menopause will not result from the removal of one ovary if the other ovary is functioning normally. As a matter of fact, the remaining ovary will increase its production of estrogen and eggs to allow normal function and near normal fertility.

*Menopause after the age of sixty.* This is a fairly common occurrence among American women. If a woman continues to have periods after the age of sixty, most doctors feel that she should have an endometrial biopsy, or scraping of the inside of the uterus, to make sure that cancer is not present. If a woman's periods persist into her sixties, she is more likely to have endometrial cancer than if her menopause had occurred earlier. If you are such a woman, make sure your doctor does an endometrial biopsy, or a D&C, every year or two.

## 260 Are women having menopause later in life now than they did in the past?

The age at which a woman goes through menopause has not changed through the years. It only seems that more women today are having late menopause because women are living to an older age than they did in the past.

Menopause is apparently fixed in a woman's genes at birth and is unaffected by diet or any other factor. A woman's menopause is unrelated to when her periods started and has nothing whatsoever to do with her having taken birth-control pills or fertility drugs in the past.

## 261 How will I know that I have gone through the menopause?

When you have gone twelve months without a period—and your female organs are otherwise normal—you have probably gone through the menopause.

A blood test for FSH (follicle-stimulating hormone) will positively indicate whether or not you have gone through the menopause. If your ovaries are no longer functioning, your pituitary will increase its production of FSH in an effort to force the ovaries to produce follicles, eggs, and estrogen. An FSH blood test will detect a significantly elevated level. If your FSH level is elevated to the postmenopausal level, you cannot get pregnant and do not have to worry about contraception anymore!

## 262 How will I feel before and after menopause, in other words, during the climacteric?

There are several changes in your body that may occur during this time.

*Changes in menstrual pattern.* As the ovarian production of estrogen decreases and the ovaries stop putting out eggs regularly, your periods may change. You may have decreased menstrual flow or you may have increased menstrual flow. Your periods may be irregular and you may have spotting between them.

Unfortunately, it is impossible for you or your doctor to know whether spotting between periods and/or unusual bleeding is due to premenopausal changes or to uterine cancer. Because uterine cancer is so much more likely to occur from the age of forty on, doctors will usually recommend a D&C or endometrial biopsy if a woman in that age group has unusual bleeding.

After the menopause, a woman should not have any more vaginal bleeding unless she is taking hormones. If she is not on hormones and has bleeding, she always needs a D&C or a thorough endometrial biopsy to be sure she has no uterine cancer.

*Hot flashes and sweating.* A hot flash has been described as being "a welling up of heat inside that begins in the chest and moves up into the head." A woman may perspire and turn red in the face with a hot flash, but most of the time a woman feels much redder in the face than she really looks! These flashes may last from only a few seconds to an hour, and it is common for hot flashes to occur at night.

*Trouble sleeping.* Because hot flashes often occur at night and may wake a woman, she often does not sleep well. This insomnia leaves her continually in need of sleep and constantly tired.

*Joint aches.* Patients who are going through the climacteric often have aching of the large joints of their body or of their back. This may be because of calcium changes in the body from decreased estrogen.

*Thinning of the estrogen-sensitive tissues of the body.* This problem is primarily noted as the vagina thins out, causing dryness and discomfort with intercourse. Tissue atrophy can also affect the bladder, producing pain with urination and later a weakness of the bladder that causes a leakage of urine when a woman coughs, sneezes, or laughs. (See Q. 699–704.) In addition, a woman may notice that her breasts are becoming thinner and droopier at this time of life.

*Other problems.* Lack of estrogen can produce depression and irritability in some women. Others will have headaches and decreased interest in sex.

## 263 Do all women have symptoms of inadequate estrogen after menopause?

No. Some women go through the menopause with no symptoms at all, and they are almost surprised when they remember that it has been a year since their last menstrual period. Other women have severe symptoms. At least half of the women who go through menopause find that some type of medical treatment for their symptoms is helpful.

Three factors seem to be associated with the degree of problems that menopause can cause. Drs. Speroff, Glass, and Kase state, in their excellent book *Clinical Gynecological Endocrinology and Infertility* (Williams and Wilkins) that the three factors associated with the severity of a woman's symptoms are:

The amount of estrogen depletion and the rate at which estrogen is withdrawn.

The collected inherited and acquired propensities to succumb or withstand the impositions of the overall aging process.

The psychological impact of aging and the individual's reaction to the emotional implications of a change in life.

The woman who will probably have the most trouble with menopausal symptoms is the one whose estrogen levels drop suddenly, whose body is so made that it readily senses these changes, and who, because of her psychological makeup, reacts more emotionally to the changes in her life than other women do.

## 264 What causes hot flashes and how long do they last?

Hot flashes are a real symptom of menopause and are definitely related to physical change in a woman's body. Many other symptoms during this time may be due to the psychology of midlife.

Hot flashes are not a result of *no* estrogen; they are a result of *change* in estrogen levels. This explains why a woman can have hot flashes even though she is still having menstrual periods. In that case, she is still producing estrogen or she could not have any menstrual bleeding at all.

About 75 percent of women who undergo natural menopause will have hot flashes, and one-third of these women will experience severe hot flashes. The more severe the symptom is, the greater the change in estrogen levels. Half of the women who have hot flashes have them once a day; one-fifth of women with hot flashes will have more than one "attack" daily. Hot flashes usually last from one to two years, but rarely more than five years.

Hot flashes are a result of an increased flow of blood through certain parts of the body. This increase seems to be due to instability of the autonomic nervous system, the part of the nervous system that controls the degree of dilation of blood vessels, the amount of sweat that is put out by sweat glands, and sexual lubrication. This instability is termed "vasomotor instability" and usually produces heat, redness, and sweating of the face, neck, and upper chest. Studies show that the woman's body does not return to normal for about thirty minutes after a hot flash.

There are those who believe hot flashes are caused by hormones from the pituitary gland trying to make the ovaries work. In other words, they think the increased amount of FSH in the body causes the hot flashes. This is not the usual mechanism, however, if it is part of the cause of hot flashes at all. Women who do not have pituitary glands can have hot flashes.

Hot flashes may occur at night and may wake a woman from a normal, sound sleep. If a woman is thin, or below her ideal body weight, she is more likely to have hot flashes than if she were heavier. This is because the estrogen production in fatty tissues of a heavier woman keep her estrogen levels from changing dramatically as menopause occurs. This also explains why women who are overweight have less osteoporosis following menopause than thin women.

## Estrogen After Menopause

### 265 Should women take estrogen after menopause?

Yes! Although there has been a great deal of controversy about this in the past, there is almost no controversy now. Estrogen is so important for your health during the entire last half of your lifetime that if your doctor will not prescribe estrogen for you, when there is no medical reason for your not taking it, you should change doctors.

Taking estrogen after menopause will not make a woman ovulate or become fertile. Menopause means the ovaries stop functioning and nothing will reactivate them.

Also taking estrogen will not increase the risk of developing breast cancer.

### 266 Why should a woman take estrogen after the menopause?

There are several reasons a woman should take estrogen:

*Osteoporosis.* This thinning of the bones, which begins when the estrogen levels in some women's bodies start decreasing, makes the bones weaker. Therefore, when a woman's ovaries stop producing estrogen her bones become more susceptible to fractures. Experts estimate that 25–50 percent of white females will experience some degree of osteoporosis.

*Reduction of heart disease.* Premenopausal women have a lower risk of heart attack than men of the same age. Postmenopausal women who do not take estrogen soon begin having heart attacks at the same rate as men. Recent studies show that if a woman will start taking estrogen immediately after menopause, she can lower by two-thirds the possibility of having a heart attack. This fact probably will become the most significant reason for using estrogen after menopause.

*Symptoms of climacteric.* If a woman is having annoying symptoms of inadequate hormones, estrogen will relieve those symptoms and help her feel "normal" again.

*Symptoms after menopause.* Estrogen helps to keep the vagina from becoming dry (allowing comfortable intercourse) and prevents the vaginal tissues from weakening, thus helping to decrease the possibility of hysterectomies and vaginal repairs later in life.

*Psychological and physical symptoms.* Estrogen helps provide a sense of psychological well-being. It will usually prevent irritability, headaches, anxiety, and depression.

### 267 What effect does estrogen have on the symptoms mentioned above?

Estrogen is without question the best treatment for these pre- and postmenopausal symptoms. Excellent studies show that when women with menopausal symptoms are given estrogen, the symptoms almost always cease to be a problem.

If a woman cannot take estrogen (see next question), the use of progesterone is the next best thing. Progesterone, however, requires high doses to stop hot flashes. This is not dangerous, only expensive! Twenty mg of Provera in pill form a day will usually stop hot flashes. A less expensive, but just as effective, way to take progesterone is through an injection of 150 mg of Depo-Provera every three months.

### 268 Who should not take estrogen?

There are several groups of women who should not take estrogen.

Women who have tumors that might be stimulated by estrogen. The most common of these is breast cancer. Estrogen will not cause breast cancer but can make an already present cancer grow faster.

Women with liver disease. An internal medicine specialist can determine if liver disease is too severe for taking estrogen.

Women who have a tendency to form blood clots. Your doctor can determine if your tendency to blood clotting is severe enough to keep you from taking estrogen.

Women who are unlikely to have osteoporosis. Since extremely obese people and black women are unlikely to have osteoporosis, they probably do not need to take estrogen except for other menopausal symptoms.

Women who have problems when they take estrogen. For example, women who have had migraine headaches will sometimes start having them again when they take estrogen. Some women will bleed from the uterus excessively if they take even small doses of estrogen. Other women just do not feel well if they take it.

If you cannot take estrogen for alleviation of bothersome menopausal symptoms, you may want to ask your doctor to try one of the other drugs that has been found effective for the relief of these symptoms. Such drugs include Depo-Provera, Bellergal Symmetrel, Catapres, and Aldomet. It is possible that Depo-Provera may have some effect on delaying osteoporosis. The other drugs are not hormones and do not prevent osteoporosis.

### 269 Should I take estrogen if I have fibrocystic breast disease?

Because breast cells are sensitive to hormones and fibrocystic breast disease is thought to be caused by over-reaction of breast tissue to these substances, women who have fibrocystic breast disease with bothersome pain and increased nodularity may have more breast problems if they take estrogen. However, by taking a three-month course of Danocrine (see Q. 956), a woman's problems may be alleviated or diminished to the point where she can take estrogen. It is wise to resolve problems associated with fibrocystic breast disease so that a woman can take estrogen after menopause. Again, taking estrogen will not increase the risk of developing breast cancer.

### 270 Is osteoporosis really a serious enough problem to warrant taking estrogen for the rest of my life?

Yes, it is. The following statistics show the problems that osteoporosis produces in women in our society.

Bone loss for women begins about age thirty-five and continues at the rate of .5 percent annually until menopause. After menopause bone loss increases dramatically. Ten years after menopause women have lost from 15–20 percent of their bone mass and, at that point, can begin having fractures. Most of the time, however, a fracture indicates a loss of about half of the bone mass of a woman's body. Many women who have a fractured vertebra have lost two-thirds of the bone of their body. If you have suffered a fracture of any of your bones after menopause, you have probably been losing bone mass faster than the average woman. You should use that as a warning and consider the advice in this section even more seriously than the average woman.

By the age of sixty, 25 percent of all women have compression fractures of the vertebrae of the spine. This explains why they get shorter and have humped backs. By the age of seventy-five, 50 percent of the

women have had fractures of bones somewhere in their body.

About 40 percent of white women have had a fractured hip by the time they reach ninety, and 15 percent of these women die within six months of that hip fracture. Those who do not die are often left invalids.

In a study about hip fractures in *The Journal of The American Medical Association* (August, 1982), it was reported that of a group of 108 patients who were treated for hip fractures (all over fifty years of age) 41 percent were discharged to nursing homes. After one year, nine (8 percent) had died and the majority of these patients were still in nursing homes.

Dr. Bill Creasman of Duke University calculated that a woman has a one in sixty chance of dying of a hip fracture or of its complications if she lives past the age of seventy.

About 40 percent of women over sixty will lose their teeth because of jawbone

## The Effects of Osteoporosis

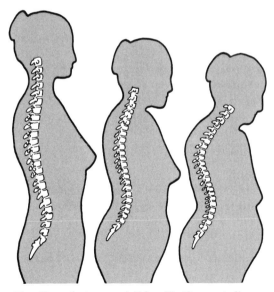

The effects of osteoporosis. When 30 - 40 percent of bone loss occurs, the vertebrae start to collapse and as much as five to eight inches in height can be lost, all from the upper part of the body. The lower spine curves inward and the abdomen protudes.

tissue loss. Women who have osteoporosis between the ages of fifty and sixty are three times as likely to need dentures as women who do not have it.

Ten years after menopause, women have ten times as many arm fractures as men of the same age.

### 271 Is estrogen really effective against osteoporosis?

If a woman starts estrogen right after the menopause, she will not lose bone mass and will not be subject to the risk of fractures that occur if she does not take estrogen. The routine that is used by most physicians includes progesterone. Recent studies have shown that the combination of estrogen and progesterone not only keeps a woman from losing bone, but actually increases existing bone mass.

In addition to these benefits, taking estrogen seems to reduce by 50 percent the risk of dying from a heart attack. One reason for this may be that women who take estrogen have a higher level of HDL cholesterol (the protective "good" cholesterol) in their blood.

It is important to know that if you use estrogen for a few years and then stop taking it, you will lose bone mass faster than is usually normal—until the weakness of your bones is, within about four years, where it would have been if you had never taken estrogen at all. If you start taking estrogen, therefore, you need to make a lifelong commitment to taking it. The only thing that would change this course of treatment would be if some better treatment were discovered before the time of your death, or if you develop a medical problem that makes it unwise for you to take estrogen.

### 272 Are there women who are more likely to develop osteoporosis and, consequently, bone fractures?

Yes, there are several groups of women who are more likely to have problems with osteoporosis. These women face great risk for future fractures if they do not take estrogen.

Women who exercise so excessively that their menstrual periods cease. Such women probably need to start taking estrogen and progesterone as though they were postmenopausal.

Women who have had their ovaries removed surgically before the menopause occurs or who start menopause early.

Smokers. Women who smoke are more likely to have early menopause and will lose bone faster.

Diabetics.

Women who have taken cortisone for a long time.

Inactive women (or women who have been immobilized longer than three weeks).

Tall women.

Women who have been exposed to minimum amounts of sunlight. Such women have inadequate Vitamin D in their bodies and have probably not been absorbing adequate calcium from their diet.

Thin women.

Heavy alcohol consumers.

Women who have never had a pregnancy. Studies show that they are at greater risk than women who have been pregnant.

### 273 If I am not in any of the categories listed above, can I wait to see if I develop osteoporosis before I start taking estrogen?

If you wait, it will be too late. Once bone loss has occurred in your body, it is impossible to do anything to make those weak bones strong again. If a woman waits until she begins having health problems of *any* kind, measures to repair damage are not nearly so effective as preventive measures would have been. Estrogen is in this category. Early use will prevent later problems.

### 274 Are there other things I can do to help prevent osteoporosis?

There are several things a woman should do to help maintain her healthy bone structure. None of these will take the place of estrogen, but each is a good health practice.

*Take calcium.* Although many women want to try to take enough calcium so that estrogen is not necessary, enough calcium to keep the bones healthy would cause kidney stones if it would work at all! Before menopause, women need to have about 1,000 mg of calcium a day; after menopause they need 1,500 mg daily. If a postmenopausal woman is taking estrogen, she should take 1,000 mg of calcium daily.

A normal diet contains about 400 to 500 mg of calcium a day. A woman, therefore, needs to take enough supplemental calcium to make up the extra calcium needed. She can take one or two 250 mg calcium pills with breakfast and one or two with the evening meal.

Vitamin D is included in many calcium preparations but is not necessary for most women. The majority of women get enough vitamin D from everyday exposure to the sun. If a woman is exposed to adequate sunlight, her body will manufacture enough vitamin D for its needs.

The intake of more than 1,000 units of vitamin D a day may actually cause bone loss, so do not overdo the intake of vitamin D. Vitamin A can also cause bone loss if taken in dosages larger than 5,000 units a day.

There are several forms of calcium available on the market. I would suggest that a woman choose the one which is least expensive. Os-Cal, Caltrate 600, and BioCal all contain calcium carbonate and are good sources of calcium. Tums Antacid is pure calcium carbonate and is just as good a source of calcium as the drugs just mentioned, and generally the least expensive. There are two sources of calcium that women should avoid: bonemeal and dolomite (tablets and powder)—both have been found to be contaminated with lead.

*Exercise.* Next to estrogen and calcium, weight-bearing exercise appears to be the most important technique for preserving bone. Exercise actually stimulates the formation of new bone in a woman's body. Some studies indicate that adequate exercise on a regular basis stops bone loss, even if a woman is postmenopausal!

Weight-bearing exercises that involve the use of the entire body are the best for this purpose: walking, jogging, bicycling, and jumping rope. Exercise done now is very beneficial in helping avoid bone loss in the future. It is good to get in the habit of exercising now, so it will be a natural part of your life as you get older. Remember, these exercises need to be started before the damage is done, not after bone loss has already developed. Once a woman has developed significant osteoporosis, she should avoid activities that involve strain to her bones, such as running or jogging, but she still needs—vitally needs—to exercise. Walking can be the ideal exercise.

I do not recommend that a woman depend on exercise for maintenance of her bone mass as an alternative to taking estrogen. Although future studies done over many years with women who have exercised to keep their bones healthy, and have not taken estrogen, may prove that exercise is just as good as estrogen in keeping the bones healthy, we do not presently know this is true.

*Other means of maintaining healthy bones.* No other treatment seems to be acceptable. Although some doctors advocate the use of fluoride to keep bones healthy, at least one-third of patients who take fluoride in adequate dosages for this purpose have side effects from it. In addition, the bone formed when a person takes this drug is not normal bone. It is less elastic and possibly more fragile than normal bone.

A drug called calcitonin, which has an effect similar to calcium, may be approved by the FDA at some time in the future and may be useful in maintaining bone integrity or in helping women with osteoporosis develop healthy bone again.

A 1982 study suggested that a combination of calcium, estrogen, and fluoride could increase the bone mass in a woman's body. This treatment regimen would be especially useful for those women who have begun developing fractures.

A long-acting preparation, Depo-Provera, in large dosage cannot only stop hot flashes and reverse vaginal atrophy, but also has positive effects on the bone if a patient takes enough calcium by mouth.

## 275 What is the best way to take estrogen?

Estrogen can be taken conveniently by using a patch that sticks to the skin. The patch must be changed twice weekly. Since studies haven't conclusively shown how effective this form of estrogen is for the bones and heart, it is probably best to take the pill form. The treatment schedule that seems best is to take one 0.625-mg tablet of conjugated estrogen or 0.05 mg of ethinyl estradiol from the first day of the calendar month until the twenty-fifth day. With the last fourteen estrogen tablets you should also take a daily progesterone pill, such as 10 mg. Provera. The schedule would then be this: take an estrogen pill each day from the first day of the month through the eleventh day. From the twelfth day until the twenty-

fifth day, take both an estrogen tablet and a Provera tablet.

From the twenty-sixth day of the month until the first day of the next month, no medication is taken. During this time it is normal for you to have a period. Some women have only light bleeding and some have no bleeding at all. If you have periods with these hormones when you first start taking them, you will probably continue to have them. Some women will have a period every month the rest of their lives; other women will gradually stop having any bleeding as the years go by. The hormones do not make it possible for you to get pregnant. When you stop taking the hormones your periods will totally stop.

If this dose of estrogen is not enough to prevent the symptoms of menopause, you can increase it so that you are taking two, three, or four times the original dose. The 0.625-mg-a-day dose is enough to maintain healthy bones.

If you have vaginal spotting or bleeding other than when expected (on days off the hormones), you should immediately see your doctor, who may want to do a D&C or an endometrial biopsy to make sure you do not have uterine cancer. In addition, before staying on the hormones indefinitely, I feel that you need to make sure that you do not have endometrial cancer. I normally let my patients try this hormone routine for two or three months. If they then decide they are going to continue the regimen, I have them come to my office for a scraping of the lining of the uterine wall. Studies done in the past few years have shown that many of the cases of uterine cancer once thought to be caused by estrogen were actually already present when the patients started taking estrogen.

A new regimen uses 0.625 mg estrogen and 2.5 mg of medroxyprogesterone (Provera) every day of the month. This eliminates menstrual periods. Taking hormones in these dosages causes the lining of the uterus to thin to the point (in a month or two) where no bleeding occurs. Any bleeding on this regimen should be reported to your doctor immediately. The dosage can be adjusted if a woman does not feel well on it.

Some women cannot tolerate conjugated estrogen. Alternatives are other types of oral estrogens, an injection of estrogen, or using a skin patch containing estrogen. The skin patch, which has not been available long enough to be totally evaluated, does produce good estrogen effect in the body and give good protection to the bones. It may not give much protection to the heart and blood vessels.

## 276 If I have had a hysterectomy, how should I take estrogen?

If you have had a hysterectomy, you can take your hormones on the schedule outlined in Q. 275. You can start on 0.625 mg of estrogen, but if you continue to have symptoms of menopause you can increase the dosage. Take enough estrogen so that you do not have menopausal symptoms, but remember that a higher dose can cause breast tenderness. You may have to choose an amount that makes you reasonably comfortable with menopausal symptoms but does not cause too much breast pain.

Once you have determined the dosage that you need, you might continue it for a few years and then try to decrease the daily dosage back down to 0.625 mg, the minimal dose necessary for keeping your bones strong.

Recent studies have not been conclusive that a woman who has had a hysterectomy should take estrogen and progesterone. A woman who has had a hysterectomy will, of course, not have bleeding when she takes the progesterone. Studies indicate that if a woman is taking estrogen and progesterone during the postmenopausal years, she has less chance of breast cancer occurring later in life than if she were on no hormones. Be-

cause of the expense and trouble of a woman having to take two hormones, if I have her take progesterone after hysterectomy, I now prescribe only estrogen. Further studies may be more conclusive about the use of progesterone and estrogen in women who have had hysterectomies.

## 277 Why should progesterone be taken with estrogen?

If a woman who still has her uterus takes estrogen without progesterone, there is an increased chance of her developing uterine cancer. If a woman takes progesterone for ten to fourteen days each month, this "balancing hormone" neutralizes any cancer-producing effect of the estrogen. As a matter of fact, if a woman is on this estrogen/progesterone program, she has less chance of developing cancer of her uterus than a woman who has gone through menopause and who takes no hormones at all! Progesterone also augments the healthy effect of estrogen on bones.

Cancer that results from estrogen is caused by the constant, uninterrupted stimulation of the uterine lining by estrogen. The unrelenting growth of the uterine lining caused by such stimulation can ultimately result in the development of abnormal cells in the uterine lining; eventually these abnormal cells become cancerous.

Some women will have such heavy, bothersome periods when they take progesterone with the estrogen that they do not want to take it. These women should do two things: (1) Take as small a dose of estrogen as possible for the first twenty-five days of every month, but not less than 0.625 mg a day; (2) Have the uterine wall scraped and the tissue studied by a pathologist every two or three years and any time there is unusual bleeding, to make sure there are no cancerous changes in the uterus.

## 278 Aren't hormones dangerous?

No. Circulating in your body are literally hundreds of different types of hormones, without which you would not even be alive. Further, if your body had not begun producing estrogen, a hormone, you would not have developed as a woman. Hormones are extremely important for your overall health.

All hormones cannot be lumped together. You should not confuse birth-control-pill hormones with those used for menopause. The dose of estrogen used for treating menopausal and postmenopausal symptoms is the same amount of hormone that you have been producing in your own body, with your own ovaries, all your reproductive life! The amount of hormones in birth-control pills is many times higher than that which you would take for menopause and is used for a different purpose.

Also, the birth-control estrogen is different from the more natural estrogen used for menopause. The chemical makeup of these hormones makes the birth-control-pill hormones much more potent than those needed for alleviation of menopausal symptoms.

A few studies over the past few years have indicated that estrogen might increase the chance of breast cancer, but other very large and adequate studies have shown that there is, in fact, no increased risk of breast cancer if a woman is taking estrogen. In addition we now have the studies we have already mentioned that show that there is less breast cancer in later years in women who take the estrogen/progesterone combination than in women who take no hormones.

In summary, studies have shown that a woman is more likely to be unhealthy and more likely to have an early death if she does not take hormone pills than if she does take them after the menopause. An excellent report (*The Journal of The American Medical Association,* April, 1983) showed that a group of women who were taking hormones generally lived longer than a similar group of women who were not taking estrogen. Exactly what produced this difference was not clarified by the study, but it may be that a woman who is on estrogen has some protection against heart attacks in addition to being less likely to die from bone fractures.

## 279 I continue to have vaginal dryness even though I take my hormones. What should I do?

Even though a woman is taking enough estrogen by mouth to stop her other menopausal symptoms, vaginal dryness and resulting discomfort with intercourse may still be a problem. In this case a woman needs to use vaginal estrogen cream in addition to the hormones taken by mouth.

An application of vaginal estrogen cream each night for seven to ten days will normally stop vaginal discomfort. Once the problem is under control, a smaller amount of cream used less frequently—such as one-half an applicator-full two or three times a week—is usually adequate.

An added benefit of the use of the vaginal cream is that if a woman has gone through the menopause and begins leaking urine when she coughs or sneezes, the vaginal cream may strengthen her tissues enough to stop such a loss. (See Q. 699–704.) Hormones may not be adequate to stop such urine leakage, and surgery might then be necessary.

Whether a woman is using estrogen only by mouth, only vaginal estrogen cream, or a combination of the two, it seems important that she take a 10 mg Provera tablet every day for ten to fourteen days every month to help prevent any chance of developing uterine or breast cancer.

It has been found that women who have intercourse after menopause have healthier vaginas with thicker vaginal linings. It is important for a woman to realize that intercourse is healthy for the vagina just as physical activity is good for her body in general.

## 280 Are some pelvic problems aggravated by taking estrogen?

Some women with endometriosis cannot take estrogen because estrogen increases that problem; other women have fibroid tumors of the uterus that become larger if they take estrogen. In these cases there are two choices. One is not to take any estrogen; the other is to have a hysterectomy so that estrogen may be taken.

Consideration of the information we have just reviewed would suggest that as a woman grows older it would be healthier for her to have a hysterectomy, so she can take estrogen, than not to take estrogen. This, of course, would be a personal decision for you to make with your doctor's professional guidance. But if you have any of the high-risk factors mentioned in Q. 272 making you more likely to have osteoporosis, you should strongly consider proceeding with a hysterectomy.

## 281 I am still having periods, but I am also having an occasional hot flash and other menopausal symptoms. What should I do?

Symptoms of this type may indicate the need for estrogen. You might start with a small dose, such as 0.625 mg once a day, beginning on the fifth day of your menstrual cycle, and stopping them on the twenty-eighth day, or when you start your period. If this seems to help, but you still do not feel as well as you would like, you can double, triple, or even quadruple this dose. If the pills do not help at all, then your symptoms are not due to menopause, but are more likely

due to the stress of the midlife time that you are in.

## Adjusting to Midlife Change

## 282 My doctor says that I am not having symptoms of the climacteric, but I am depressed, irritable, and do not have any interest in intercourse. I tried estrogen and it didn't help. Is my doctor right?

True symptoms of the climacteric are caused simply by a lack of estrogen, and estrogen intake will reverse them. Symptoms that are "left over" after you have started taking adequate amounts of hormones are not due to the menopause but to other causes, such as midlife crises.

It has been aptly stated that "menopause chooses a bad time to come!" It is difficult sometimes to decide whether midlife pressure or decreasing levels of estrogen are causing you to feel bad. The best way to determine this is by taking some hormones for a few months to see if your symptoms go away.

If your symptoms do not go away, they are probably due to your being in a stressful time of life. Sometimes your physician can help you deal with this stress. Occasionally it is helpful to get away from your daily pressures for a vacation, and sometimes it is advisable to see a counselor, such as your pastor, a psychologist, or a psychiatrist.

Many things are going on during midlife that can cause stress.

Your children are leaving home, making you feel that your primary job in life is over. Or this may be creating financial strain due to college and living expenses, and so on.

Your husband may have become more involved in his work, making you feel that he is less interested in you.

Your body is changing. Wrinkles and gray hair begin to appear. Perhaps "middle-age" spread has set in.

Your parents are getting older. There is often great stress in taking care of sick, elderly parents, and severe stress in facing their deaths.

Sexual monotony may be a reality. It is during midlife that many couples fall into predictable patterns in their sexual relationship. This can lead to boredom and dissatisfaction. Medications commonly prescribed at this time in life, especially those taken for hypertension and irregularities of the heart, can affect sex drive and orgasmic response.

### 283 What about sex during my later years?

It is normal for people to have intercourse right up until the day they die of old age! One warning, though: if you have not enjoyed a healthy and happy sexual relationship with your husband when you were young, you are less likely to have a happy sexual relationship as you get older. So, if you and your husband have some problems in this area, work them out now, so they do not become ingrained, blighting the many years you have left together.

There are advantages to sexual relations after menopause.

First of all, you do not have to worry about getting pregnant, and many women find this increases their sexual interest. Many couples also report that they become much more relaxed and comfortable with each other as time goes by. This, plus the increased mutual sexual understanding that time can produce, greatly heightens the sexual experience for many couples.

Since the children are not around any longer, you can have intercourse whenever or however you like without worrying about being seen or heard!

Sex in the later years can be a major part of "communication" between you and your spouse. You should anticipate its having great importance in your relationship in the years to come.

### 284 Are there any health problems of the female organs that are specifically related to the postmenopausal time?

There are no problems that are specifically related to this age in life, but there are many suggestions for the care of your female organs. (For a more complete discussion, see chapter 10.)

*Breasts.* Regularly do a breast self-examination (BSE), and have a mammogram every year from age fifty on. If there is any question about a breast problem, see your doctor without delay.

*Ovaries.* After menopause your ovaries shrink to about one-half inch in diameter. Unless you are extremely thin, your doctor cannot feel them. If the doctor is able to feel an ovary, it means that it is enlarged and probably has a tumor. You should allow the doctor to operate, as there is a 50-percent chance of ovarian cancer if there is such a growth after menopause.

*Uterus.* After menopause the uterus rarely causes any problems, although it can develop cancer. If you have any bleeding at all after the menopause, you should immediately see a physician, who will probably recommend a D&C. If you are taking hormones regularly, it is normal to have bleeding each month, but, even if you are taking estrogen, if bleeding occurs at an unusual time, you should notify your physician immediately and anticipate that a D&C or an endometrial biopsy will be required.

*Cervix.* An annual Pap smear is indicated, even after the menopause. There is almost no reason to have a Pap smear more often than once a year after menopause.

*Vagina.* The vagina can become loose after menopause, causing loss of urine when a woman coughs, sneezes, or laughs. The vagina can also seem very loose during intercourse.

An additional problem can be a bulging of the back wall of the vagina with bowel movements. This bulging can be so marked that a woman must push with her fingers in her vagina, or just above her anus at the opening of the vagina, to help the stool be expelled. Gynecologists call this "rectal splinting." Surgery can be performed to correct these problems.

Occasionally estrogen vaginal cream will help such problems. At times it takes both the estrogen cream and surgery to solve a problem of vaginal looseness, loss of urine with coughing, or problems with bowel movements. Gynecologists lump all these conditions together in the term *symptomatic pelvic relaxation.*

In addition, the vaginal lining can become so thin and sensitive after menopause that intercourse is uncomfortable. If a couple then limits intercourse, the vagina can shrink, causing even more pain with intercourse. A vicious cycle has developed that results in a couple no longer being able to enjoy intercourse, even though they would like to. If this happens see your doctor. A little estrogen cream can totally reverse this process and allow normal, comfortable intercourse.

*The vulva.* If an area of your vulva itches persistently, or if you have a small growth on it, you should insist that your doctor biopsy it. Such a biopsy can easily diagnose a cancer of the vulva long before it becomes dangerous.

## 285 Does psychological or emotional health play an important part in a woman's adjustment to midlife and the mature years?

Psychological and emotional health are overriding health concerns at all ages. If we do not feel good emotionally and psychologically, we tend to say, "What's the use?" about the rest of life. Many poor health habits are a subconscious statement that "life is not any fun anyway, so why should it be prolonged by staying healthy?"

Emotional and psychological health are particularly important to those women entering the middle age of life. It is common for people who allowed certain psychological excesses or weaknesses to affect their lifestyle when they were younger to see those tendencies become exaggerated and a major part of their personalities later. For instance, a woman who allows herself to have fits of anger may see this become a major part of her character as she gets older, causing her to become a lonely, isolated, angry person. Likewise, the woman who allows money, clothes, or sex to be her god when she is younger may find that the only thing that interests her when she enters middle age or beyond.

If there is an emotional or psychological problem in your life, take care of it now. Do not tolerate that excess or weakness. It can ruin happiness now and the joy of your later years.

I am absolutely convinced that a life cannot have the balance and joy it is meant to have without a woman's opening herself up to God and doing what she feels is his desire. Solomon, the writer of Ecclesiastes, has been called the wisest man who ever lived. He built houses for himself and planted vineyards; made gardens and parks and planted all kinds of fruit trees in them; amassed silver and gold and the treasures of kings and provinces. Solomon denied himself nothing his eyes desired, and he had seven hundred wives and three hundred concubines. At the end of the Book of Ecclesiastes, however, Solomon summed up his discoveries about life with this advice: "Remember your Creator in the days of your youth," adding, "Fear God and keep His commandments, for this is the whole duty of man" (Eccles. 12:1,13). Solomon's final conclusion was that life without God is utterly meaningless (v. 8).

---

## 286 What can I expect during the postmenopausal years?

The postmenopausal years can be extremely fulfilling and rewarding in many ways. In fact, you can anticipate a growing satisfaction with life. Most women in the postmenopausal age develop a serenity about life and an acceptance of situations that they cannot change. That illustrates maturity.

You can expect a lot of company! In 1982, 11.7 percent of the population of the United States was sixty-five years or older. There were over twenty-six million Americans in this age group, and elderly women outnumbered men by three to two. Today the life expectancy of women is still longer than that of men.

In this age you can look forward to having time to do things that you have never had time for before. You might be able to go back to school and earn a degree. There will be time to do things for your church or to develop some skills that you never had, such as painting, writing, or tennis.

You can also expect to have an increased influence on younger people. Paul, in the Book of Titus, tells older women that they "are to teach what is good and so train the young women to love their husbands and children." The older a woman, the more influence she can have on the people around her because of her maturity.

There will probably be a growing and maturing relationship with your husband. Of course, people do divorce, but most do not. Partners are also lost to death, but there are usually many good years before that happens. The years that follow menopause can be the golden years of life. It is in these years that you and your husband are truly companions to each other—meeting each other's needs, spending time together, and cashing in on investments that you have made in each other's lives through the earlier years of your marriage.

In these years you can also grow in your relationship to God. There is nothing in the world more beautiful to me than to visit with an older woman who has grown in her love for God and her relationship with him. Such a woman literally glows with joy, peace, and love. It almost seems as though God, in a very special way, is able to shed his love around a community through the life of one of his very special, beloved women. As Psalm 92:12–15 (NIV) says:

> The righteous will flourish like a palm
>    tree,
> they will grow like a cedar of Lebanon;
> planted in the house of the LORD,
> they will flourish in the courts of our
>    God.
> They will still bear fruit in old age,
> they will stay fresh and green,
> proclaiming, "The LORD is upright;
> he is my Rock, and there is no wickedness in him."

---

## 287 Are there any books that I can read, or organizations I can contact, that can help me during this time of life?

There are several.

Among the books are:

*The Joy of Being a Woman,* by Ingrid Trobisch (Harper & Row, 1975), has a good chapter called "Menopause—Chance for a New Beginning."

*After Forty Health and Medical Guide* (Better Homes and Gardens, Des-Moines: Meredith, 1983) contains an excellent section on the climacteric.

Some organizations to contact are:

The National Institute of Aging
Building 31, Room 5C35
Bethesda, Maryland 20205

U.S. Administration on Aging
    U.S. Department of Health, Education, and Welfare
Social and Rehabilitation Services
Washington, D.C. 20201

National Council on the Aging
1828 "L" Street, N.W.
Washington, D.C. 20036

National Council of Senior Citizens
1511 "K" Street, N.W.
Washington, D.C. 20005

American Association of Retired Persons
1909 "K" Street, N.W.
Washington, D.C. 20006

The Grey Panthers
3700 Chestnut Street
Philadelphia, Pennsylvania 19104

## An Afterword

As a closing thought for this chapter, I'd like to share this appropriate prayer:

### Seventeenth-Century Nun's Prayer

LORD, thou knowest better than I know myself that I am growing older and will someday be old. Keep me from the fatal habit of thinking I must say something on every subject and on every occasion. Release me from craving to straighten out everybody's affairs. Make me thoughtful but not moody; helpful but not bossy. With my vast store of wisdom, it seems a pity not to use it all, but thou knowest, Lord, that I want a few friends at the end.

Keep my mind free from the recital of endless details; give me wings to get to the point. Seal my lips on my aches and pains. They are increasing, and love of rehearsing them is becoming sweeter as the years go by. I dare not ask for grace enough to enjoy the tales of others' pains, but help me to endure them with patience.

I dare not ask for improved memory, but for a growing humility and a lessening cocksureness when my memory seems to clash with the memories of others. Teach me the glorious lesson that occasionally I may be mistaken.

Keep me reasonably sweet; I do not want to be a saint—some of them are so hard to live with—but a sour old person is one of the crowning works of the devil. Give me the ability to see good things in unexpected places, and talents in unexpected people. And, give me, O Lord, the grace to tell them so. *Amen.*

# Part Two

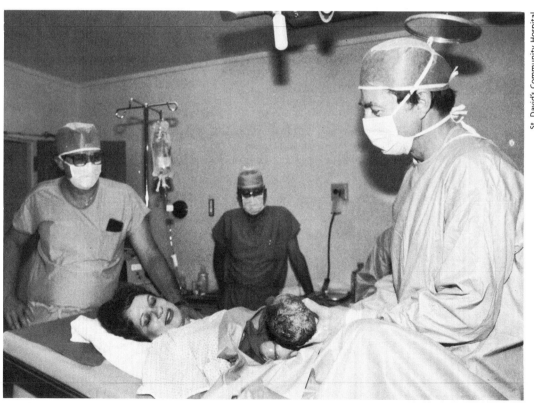

St. David's Community Hospital
Teresa White

192

# Bearing a Child

# 6
## Conception

The most exciting, mysterious, and complex event of your entire life took place in the darkened, hidden recesses of your mother's abdomen. The event occurred without applause, without recognition, without appreciation.

You were completely unaware of your debut into the human race. And even your mother was unaware of the miraculous superdrama being enacted within her body.

God, however, knew. The one who masterminded the creation of all life from the beginning was also responsible for yours.

It is my firm belief that your beginning was not merely an accumulation of matter. You were created by God with a distinct value and purpose—from the moment of conception.

Conception is not a trivial event. Although its occurrence might seem routine, it is truly a miracle of the highest order. There is no better illustration anywhere of God's handiwork than the delicate, fascinating, awe-inspiring event of conception.

One edition of Webster's dictionary describes life as "the form or quality of existence that distinguishes animals and plants from inorganic or inanimate things." The definition states further: "There are four characteristics of life that are shared by all living organisms: growth, reproduction, metabolism, and the capacity to respond to stimuli." According to that definition, there is no doubt that the miniscule collection of cells created at conception is already "life."

However, it is more than mere life itself, for the personhood of the newly created life is instantly established when egg and sperm unite. The new person has already been programmed—created with a definite pattern—for life.

At the moment of conception many things are determined, including your sex, genetic makeup, and physical appearance.

At the point of conception you are unique; the only "you" that has ever been or ever will be again.

And the entire process is absolutely fascinating.

This chapter will explain as simply as possible a truly complex, fascinating process. It begins with the first moment of your life and the steps leading up to that moment; then it looks at the reason why you developed into a female rather than a male. It showcases the most unique aspect of womanhood: the ability to conceive and carry a new life.

## The Marvel of Conception

### 288 How does life begin?

You came into existence the moment your father's sperm united with your mother's egg. This union is called fertilization, a complex procedure that will be discussed at length in the following questions. A very simple illustration can be used to introduce the subject.

For fertilization to occur, the stage must be set for the drama. A leading lady (the egg) must be waiting in the wings (the fallopian tubes) for an eager, determined leading man (the sperm) to approach her.

As she waits passively, he struggles valiantly through a labyrinth of dark, slippery passages in search of his mate.

He is strong and hardy, employing speed and endurance in his frantic, desperate race against time and competition. He is one of hundreds making the same quest but, when he is accepted by the egg, all other suitors are immediately dismissed.

The newly united pair "honeymoon" for three days at their meeting place in the tube. Here they rest and grow together to prepare for the completion of their journey.

After these three days, the united egg and sperm continue their voyage, eventually "settling down" in the uterus, their home for approximately nine months.

A new life has begun.

### 289 Where do the egg and the sperm meet, and how do they get there?

The meeting of the sperm and egg usually occurs in the outer half of the fallopian tube, the half farthest away from the uterus.

Sperm reach the meeting place via a journey from the vagina, up through the cervix and uterus, and into the tube. This is accomplished by swimming, with their progress being aided by contractions of the uterus and fallopian tubes. Tubal contractions are called peristalsis, the same activity used by the intestines to propel food. The entire trip takes only about ten to twenty minutes.

The egg cannot swim. It is expelled from the surface of the ovary where it floats passively and freely in the abdominal cavity. This freedom is short-lived, for the egg is quickly taken in by the fallopian tubes.

The fallopian tubes do not connect the ovary to the uterus, as many people imagine. This explains how an egg can be produced by one ovary, cross to the tube on the other side, pass down that tube into the uterus, and grow into a normal pregnancy. This has happened to women who have had an ovary removed on one side and a tube on the other side.

The egg is captured and brought into the tube by small tentacles called fimbriae on the end of the tube. These tentacles are vigorously active. They sweep over the surface of the ovary, and when the egg escapes, the fimbriae capture it.

This procedure has been photographed in animals. Richard Blandau, M.D., Professor Emeritus, University of Washington, has used time-lapse photography to produce some enthralling films that show fimbriae catching eggs and sweeping them toward the openings of the fallopian tubes, where the tubes suck in the eggs like miniature vacuum cleaners.

This action starts the egg on its passive journey to the womb.

The egg's trip is aided, as is the sperm's, by the muscular activity of peristalsis. It is further helped along by small hairlike structures, the cilia. These line the inside of the fallopian tubes and are also present on the fimbriae. They are beating constantly, physically sweeping the egg, which is sticky, into and through the tube.

The cilia also cause a small current of fluid to flow through the tubes and into the uterus. This current helps the cilia draw the egg into the tube.

## 290 Do the egg and the sperm unite immediately when they meet in the fallopian tube?

Neither the egg nor the sperm is capable of fertilization at that point. Both must go through a cleansing process termed "capacitation" before they can become fertile. This fact, and the parallel sequences that must take place prior to fertilization, make the act of conception just that much more fascinating.

As the egg passes into and through the fallopian tube, it is scrubbed clean of material that has clung to it from the ovary. When the sperm and the egg meet, the egg is further cleansed by "hyaluronidase," an enzyme produced by the sperm.

A sperm, however, is unable to produce the hyaluronidase until substances that prevent its production are removed during the journey through the uterus and tubes. This is accomplished by the sperm's exposure to uterine and fallopian tube secretions.

Many sperm, all now capable of producing hyaluronidase, work together to change the surface of the egg until it is finally possible for *one sperm* to penetrate the egg. Once fertilization occurs, all other sperm are immediately repelled.

## 291 What happens after fertilization of the egg?

The fertilized egg remains in the fallopian tube for about three days. If it were to get into the uterus earlier, it would be too immature to adhere to the uterine wall and would pass on out of the uterus as a very early miscarriage, even before the mother would miss a menstrual period.

The tube acts as a preincubator, allowing the fertilized egg to grow to just the right degree of maturity for its start in the uterus. Scientists think that the hormones of the normal menstrual cycle cause this tighten-

# Fertilization and Cell Division

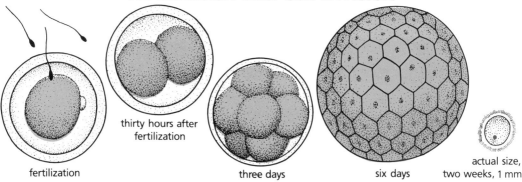

fertilization

thirty hours after fertilization

three days

six days

actual size, two weeks, 1 mm

ing and loosening of a tube's opening into the uterus.

Upon its entrance into the womb, "home" for the next nine months, the baby has grown to be about twelve cells in size. The fertilized egg can now adhere to the uterine wall because it has had time to develop a small amount of placental tissue. This tissue has the ability to stick to the wall of the uterus, thus drawing life-sustaining oxygen, fluid, and nourishment from the mother's tissues.

---

## 292   What happens to an unfertilized egg and the sperm that did not fertilize an egg?

An unfertilized egg lives about twelve to twenty-four hours. Sperm have a useful life of forty-eight hours, although they may live four or five days.

If an egg has not been fertilized, it either disintegrates or passes on out of the uterus into the vagina. In a normal, healthy female, the process will be repeated again in another month, when another egg is produced, released from the ovary, and begins its journey through the tube.

Sperm are deposited by the millions into the vagina, but only one of them will achieve fertilization. The remainder will gradually be filtered out by the woman's reproductive

tract until the few that remain alive at the end wander aimlessly until they die.

When the sperm are deposited into the vagina, they swim out of the semen, which consists mainly of mucus, into the cervical mucus. Some sperm immediately pass on through the uterus into the tubes, some swimming through one tube, some through the other. Some never make it into the cervical mucus and drain with the semen from the vagina.

Excess sperm that do make it into the tubes help cleanse the egg and prepare it for penetration, but those not accepted merely swim right on through the tubes and out into the abdominal cavity where they are absorbed by the body.

Sperm, which live much longer than an egg, have been found in the uterus and tubes up to sixty hours after intercourse. Though they may live that long, they are usually fertile only the first twenty-four to forty-eight hours of their life.

---

## 293   What are the chances for fertilization to occur?

Fertilization depends on many factors, such as the abundance and health of the sperm, the time of intercourse, and the health of the partners (see chapter 11).

Even if everything is functioning properly and the act of intercourse is timed perfectly,

# Fertilization and Conception

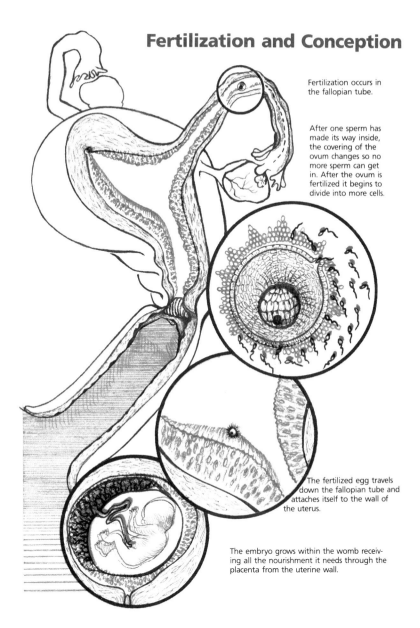

Fertilization occurs in the fallopian tube.

After one sperm has made its way inside, the covering of the ovum changes so no more sperm can get in. After the ovum is fertilized it begins to divide into more cells.

The fertilized egg travels down the fallopian tube and attaches itself to the wall of the uterus.

The embryo grows within the womb receiving all the nourishment it needs through the placenta from the uterine wall.

there is at most only a 25 percent chance of pregnancy occurring each month. Within a year's time, however, 85 percent of couples actively trying to conceive will be successful.

It has been estimated that 70 percent of human pregnancies are aborted naturally. Most of these are very early pregnancies, and most of the time the woman is not even aware that she had conceived.

Many of these spontaneous abortions occur because the conceptions are abnormal. Something has gone wrong in the fertilization process and the resulting fetus could not develop normally. This high percentage (70 percent) of miscarriage has led some people to say that human reproduction is inefficient.

Fertilization is obviously a difficult and exacting procedure. When successfully accomplished it is further proof of the miracle of conception.

## XX and XY Chromosomes

### 294   What determines the sex of a fertilized egg?

It is the chromosomes within the egg and sperm that determine both a baby's sex and many other characteristics. A chromosome is a microscopic piece of protein, several of which are present in the nucleus of every living cell. Each chromosome is made up of hundreds of smaller units called genes. These are responsible for your (and your husband's) ability to transmit to your child such characteristics as small feet, curly hair, and blue eyes.

Each cell has forty-six (twenty-three pairs) of chromosomes. Out of those twenty-three, only one pair carries the sex determinants and are thus called sex chromosomes.

The remaining twenty-two pairs are called autosomes and have little to do with determining sex, although they carry hundreds of genes that guide the growth of the rest of the body.

Geneticists (scientists specializing in the study of genes and genetic problems) are able to identify and number individual chromosomes. Sex chromosomes, however, are not numbered but are labeled XX or XY.

The male's sperm carry the sex chromosomes that determine the sex of the offspring. All eggs always carry X chromosomes, while sperm may carry either X or Y chromosomes. Whether or not the child is a boy or girl depends on which sperm—an X-chromosomed or a Y-chromosomed—fertilizes the egg.

Every normal baby is conceived with either XX (female) or XY (male) sex chromosomes. Every cell in a person's body will have one of these chromosome pairs making each of us totally male or totally female, no matter what is done to our sex organs or what kind of hormones we take.

Technically, there is a fifty-fifty chance of producing a boy or girl when the egg is fertilized. Two simple addition problems will explain what happens:

    Egg     with an X chromosome (all have this)

+ Sperm   with X chromosome (half have this)

= GIRL

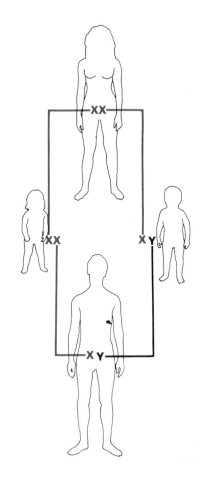

Egg     with X chromosome (all have this)
+ Sperm  with Y chromosome (half have this)
= BOY

To reiterate: it is always the man who is responsible for the sex of a child!

---

**295** **How does an XX chromosome create a woman and an XY chromosome create a man?**

XX chromosomes cause a baby to develop ovaries, whereas XY chromosomes cause a baby to develop testicles. Beyond this statement lies a combination of theory and fact. Further research may prove some of the following information wrong, but, as it is understood today, here is a brief look at this fascinating process.

### If Your Baby Is Going to Be a Boy

The sex-chromosome pair for a boy is XY and is determined at fertilization by the type of sperm that catches the egg.

After four weeks of growth, two little nubbins of tissue will have developed in the male embryo, one on each side of what will become his abdomen. These are sex organs, or gonads, which at that point look as if they could become either ovaries or testes. The baby is only about one-fourth inch long at this time.

The Y chromosome begins to stimulate the small "neutral" gonads to become testes instead of ovaries. This appears to be all the Y chromosome does, as it does not create any further detectable difference in the development of male characteristics in the child.

Researchers have wondered for years how the Y chromosome produces its effect on the testicle. Recently they found a protein substance, "hy antigen," produced by the Y chromosome. Theoretically, this substance is responsible for organizing the gonad into a testicle.

The gonads are now true male organs, and they begin their work of changing this seemingly sexless little fetus into a male being by doing three things.

The first duty of these male organs is to suppress the cells in the body of the fetus that would have developed into female organs (mullerian cells). They accomplish this by secreting a compound termed "mullerian inhibiting factor."

The secretion of this compound is the very first hormonal function of these new male hormone glands called testicles. It takes place in the seventh week of pregnancy.

With the production of the mullerian inhibiting factor in the little boy's body, most of the female cells are suppressed into inactivity. A few, however, do persist. Instead of becoming female organs as they would have done had this baby been a girl, they help form part of the connection to the testicle (the vas deferens) which will transport the sperm out of the testicle in later life. The suppression process is complete by the end of the third month of pregnancy.

The second duty of the testicles began even before the mullerian cell regression was complete. The production of the major male hormone testosterone by the testicles began during the ninth week of pregnancy. Testosterone "stabilizes" the cells of the fetus's body (wolffian duct cells) that will form the seminal vesicles, the vas deferens, and the epididymus. This allows these organs to begin their development properly and to form completely, under continued testosterone stimulation.

The third function of the fetal testicle is to produce the enzyme "five alpha-reductase." This enzyme causes some of the fetus's testosterone to change into dihydrotestosterone. The male fetal body requires this altered form of testosterone to form a penis, a scrotum, and a prostate gland.

The remainder of the pregnancy, as it relates to the boy, merely provides the important time that is necessary for his male sexual organs to grow and develop, a process which includes the descent of his testicles into the scrotum.

### If Your Baby Is Going to Be a Girl

The sex-chromosome pair for a girl is XX. This is also determined at fertilization.

After four weeks of growth, the girl's gonads, or sex organs, have developed in the area that will eventually be her abdomen. These little ovaries begin producing small amounts of estrogen, the major female hormone, when the fetus is about two months old.

Over the next seven months, estrogen is responsible for the development of the girl's female organs, which include a complete uterus by eighteen weeks of pregnancy and a complete vagina during the last three months of pregnancy.

An interesting fact to consider in the development of a female baby is that although she is producing small amounts of estrogen, her mother's body has a huge amount of estrogen constantly bathing the fetus. No one knows how much influence the baby's own estrogen has on its development and how much effect the mother's estrogen has, because a human fetus has never yet developed outside a mother's body and away from the mother's estrogen.

Since a male fetus is subjected to the same bathing of maternal estrogen, it cannot be presumed that estrogen determines the sex of the child. It has been shown, however, that if a fetus does not receive "normal" sex chromosomes at the time of fertilization and does not have a Y chromosome, it will always develop female sex characteristics.

It appears that the development of the fetus as a female may be in part a passive process, aided by the mother's hormones.

This entire process is much more complicated than indicated in this answer. For instance, although XX and XY chromosomes are the most important ones in sexual development, at least nineteen other genes are involved in the development of the sexually normal adult man and woman.

---

**296** **At what age can the sex of a baby be determined following miscarriage?**

If a pregnancy is two and a half to three months along, and the baby has continued normal growth up until the miscarriage, the doctor can probably determine the sex. At that point the baby would be about one and a quarter inches long.

---

**297** **Is it possible to choose the sex of my child?**

There do seem to be some ways to improve your chances of choosing your child's sex, but there is no technique that will give you your choice 100 percent of the time. Because of the impossibility of complete accuracy, it may not be wise to become pregnant if you are not willing to accept your child's sex and love the child without reservation.

The major consideration in any conception should be the parents' full acceptance of the baby, not that the baby fit all the preconceived ideas the parents have as to what that baby should be like.

---

**298** **What techniques might I try so that I can increase my chances of choosing my child's sex?**

The first widely read, modern book on the subject of sex determination was *Your Babies' Sex: Now You Can Choose*. This was written by David M. Rorvik and Landrum B. Shetles, M.D., and was published by Bantam

Books in the 1960s. The ideas advocated for sex selection in this book have now been generally discarded.

In a book, *Boy or Girl?* (New York: Bobbs-Merrill, 1979), Dr. Elizabeth Whelan reports that if you follow her suggestions, you will increase your chance of having a boy from about 50 percent to 60 percent, and your chances of having a girl from about 50 percent to 57 percent. Briefly, here is a summary of her suggestions, most of which require determining carefully which day you ovulate. This can be done by:

Watching for *"mittelschmerz."* This is a pain in the low abdomen that some women feel at the time of ovulation.

Watching the calendar. Most women ovulate about 14 days prior to the start of their next period.

Taking your basal body temperature. Ovulation usually occurs twenty-four to forty-eight hours prior to the sustained rise in temperature, as recorded the first thing in the morning before getting out of bed.

Observing changes in cervical mucus.

When ovulation occurs, a moderately heavy vaginal discharge may be noted.

According to Dr. Whelan, once you feel confident about predicting your ovulation date, you should then time your intercourse to improve your chance of having a child of the desired sex.

If you are attempting to have a boy, you should have intercourse on the sixth, fifth, and fourth days prior to ovulation. This is necessary because, while it is true that sperm do not have a useful life of five or six days, ovulation *may* occur earlier than expected. If you are trying to have a girl, you should have intercourse on the third and second days prior to ovulation. While Dr. Whelan points out that statistics show that this system works, no one knows exactly why it works.

Either way, avoid intercourse or use contraception during the other days of the cycle.

Dr. Whelan has gone into much more detail in her book. For further information on this subject, a study of the methods stated in the book may prove helpful.

The most recent techniques for sex selection that have been posed are filtration tech-

## Basal Body Temperature Chart

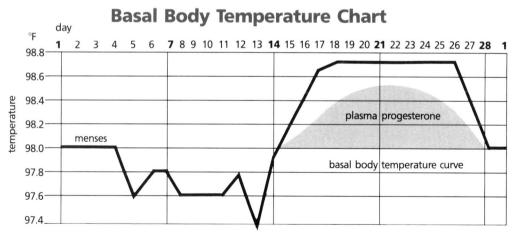

To get a basal body temperature curve, a woman's temperature is measured immediately upon awakening and charted according to the day of the menstrual cycle. The hormone progesterone, which is produced only after ovulation, makes a woman's basal temperature rise. Thus if ovulation has occurred, the basal body temperature curve will show a rise and a plateau after ovulation. The rise and fall in basal temperature somewhat parallels the rise and fall of progesterone levels.

niques. Using these methods, the man's sperm is filtered through special media to separate "female" from "male" sperm. The prospective mother is then inseminated with sperm that would be expected to produce the desired sex. A form of this procedure is being developed by Ronald Ericsson, a Ph.D. in reproductive physiology. He is president of a company in Sausalito, California, called Gametrics, Ltd., which is marketing Ericsson's technique by training individuals in the performance of the techniques, and licensing clinics around the country. His company claims a success rate of 77 percent in producing male infants. Ericsson's technique cannot be used to increase the chance of having a female child, although Gametrics and other groups are working on this too.

If you have an infertility problem or want to get pregnant as quickly as possible, any attempt at sex determination will only slow your attempt to become pregnant, and I would advise against trying such a procedure.

## An Afterword

Conception is truly a miracle. Even the brief study of conception contained in this chapter fills us with wonder and delight as we consider the incredible precision, intricacy, and mystery that surrounds the creation of a new life.

# 7
## Pregnancy

There are, perhaps, no three words in any language more pregnant with meaning than the words *You are pregnant!* These words have evoked the gamut of emotion—joy, pride, disbelief, fear, dismay, thanksgiving, wonder—for countless generations of men and women. Whatever your reaction to the confirmation of your pregnancy, you can be assured that you are neither the first nor only woman who has felt exactly that!

If you have never had a baby before, you are faced with many unknowns. Your body has never been swollen with pregnancy. Will your husband like the way you look? Will you like the way you look? What will labor be like? Will you be able to nurse the baby? What will your infant look like? Whom will he or she look like? Will your baby be normal? Will you be a good mother?

If you have already had a child, you face different problems. Your family is enlarging. Is there enough love, time, and money to go around? With a new baby you may face serious financial strain, and certainly emotional and physical pressures. Can you handle it? Will you be a good mother to more than one (or two, or three, or more) children?

As your pregnancy progresses and each new hurdle is passed, both mother and father begin to identify with the child in the uterus. Both can feel movement, hear the heartbeat, and even "see" the baby on an ultrasound machine.

One thing seems clear to me. In spite of our advanced medical and technical knowledge, infertility clinics, in vitro fertilization programs, obstetric clinics, and home deliveries, human beings can't make a baby. It is quite obvious that the psalmist was right: *"Children are a gift from God"* (Ps. 127:3,LB).

## If You Think You Are Pregnant . . .

**299** **Are there any very early symptoms of pregnancy that I might notice?**

Possibly. Some women experience early symptoms; others notice nothing out of the ordinary. In any case, the hormones of pregnancy are secreted into the body soon after fertilization takes place. Although they are produced in tiny amounts, they do begin changing the body even before a menstrual period is missed.

Occasionally, even before the first missed period, some women have been able to tell that something is different. They guess, often correctly, that they are pregnant. Most of the early suggestions that might herald a pregnancy, however, will not develop until after the missed period, and even then may not be noticed.

The earliest symptoms of pregnancy may include the following.

*Feeling that the missed period is about to start.* For most women, that a period fails to arrive on time is the first sign of pregnancy, and usually the failure of the menstrual flow to start is accompanied by the feeling that it is going to begin at any minute. The typical sensation is of pelvic fullness and low abdominal bloating. When that feeling accompanies the failure of a flow to start, you are probably pregnant. This is especially so if you have always had regular periods.

This feeling that you are going to start menstruating at any minute is a little trick your body plays on you. Many women assume that they cannot be pregnant because they have such a strong feeling that the period is about to start. Accordingly, they delay coming in for a pregnancy check until many days after they have missed their period. This is especially true for infertility patients who cannot believe they are really pregnant!

*Cramping.* Cramps are common at the time the period is missed and for a few days afterward. This is a normal sign of early stages of pregnancy—accept it as such. There is no need to limit activity or do anything different because of these cramps. Bleeding with the cramping, however, may indicate the beginning of a miscarriage. If this occurs, contact your physician immediately.

*Nausea.* Morning sickness, as this nausea is commonly called, does not come only in the morning; it can occur at any time during the day. It usually begins just after the missed period but can start even before. The

### Signs of Pregnancy

| Indication | First Appearance |
| --- | --- |
| Blood or urine contains HCG | Day 9-10 |
| Sleep patterns change | Week 3-4 |
| Cervical tissue softens | Week 3-4 |
| Breasts enlarge | Week 4 |
| Nipples darken | Week 4-5 |
| Mild constipation | Week 4-5 |
| Cramping | Week 4-5 |
| Frequent urination | Week 4-5 |
| Nausea | Months 1-3 |
| Dizziness | Months 1-3 |
| Uterus enlarged at exam | Week 9 |

nausea may be either mild or severe and may include vomiting. (See Q. 306–I.)

*Constipation.* Mild constipation is a common, early sign of pregnancy and will often occur soon after a woman misses her period.

*Breast changes.* Soon after missing a period, you may notice that your breasts are more tender and full. A doctor can almost as easily detect the early state of pregnancy by examining a woman's breasts than by examining her uterus. This is not always true, but it points out that the breasts do change quite significantly and quite early in pregnancy.

*Frequency of urination.* You may experience more frequent urination early in pregnancy, soon after the missed period.

*Tiredness and sleepiness.* These symptoms do not usually start immediately, but the feelings of tiredness and a need for more sleep can occur before you miss your second period. These feelings usually disappear toward the end of the third month. If you are experiencing nausea and vomiting, the tiredness will often go away when your nausea disappears.

*Fainting.* It is normal for a woman to have fainting spells and/or feelings of dizziness. When and if you think you are going to faint, lie down immediately so that you do not hit your head on a sharp object.

mean that you are pregnant, and a negative test that you are not. The results can be wrong in a small percentage of situations. Vibration of the fluid during the test, too much heat or sunlight during the test, high levels of protein in the urine (caused by a kidney or bladder infection), or the presence of certain drugs can affect the test result.

Office pregnancy tests are more reliable, but more difficult to do. They may be done on either blood or urine. (We no longer use frogs and rabbits for testing for pregnancy; modern tests are much more accurate.)

*Urine pregnancy tests.* These are not as reliable as blood pregnancy tests, partly because the urine may contain drugs, blood, or pus cells, or may vary in its acidity. Any of those things could distort the results. If none of these factors is present, the test can be quite reliable and can indicate pregnancy even before a period is missed.

*Blood pregnancy tests (serum pregnancy tests).* These tests, if done by a reliable laboratory, are quite accurate. They can determine pregnancy even before a missed period, as early as seven or eight days after conception. If a woman wants to know before (or at the time of) her missed period whether or not she is pregnant, because of its greater reliability she should have the blood test rather than the urine test.

## 300    What should I do if I think I may be pregnant?

The first thing to do is to get a pregnancy test. Some women will want to try a home pregnancy test; others would rather have the doctor or laboratory make the diagnosis.

Home pregnancy tests, done by testing the woman's urine, are accurate and easy to do. They are reliable from about the ninth day after a missed period. If a test shows negative and you still think you are pregnant it would be wise to repeat the test a week later. A positive test does not necessarily

## 301    What do pregnancy tests detect?

The tests detect a compound called human chorionic gonadotrophin (HCG), which is produced by the placenta. Trophoblastic cells (which contribute to the formation of the placenta through which the embryo receives nourishment from the mother) produce this hormone. These cells can hardly be called a true placenta only seven or eight days after conception, but that is basically what they are.

The HCG hormone is necessary for the pregnancy to stay in the woman's body. It is produced only in pregnancy, with the exception of abnormal conditions, such as tumors associated with abnormal placentas from a previous pregnancy and certain types of cancer. The ability to test for pregnancy is one of the modern medical miracles. It is amazing to be able to detect the presence of relatively few trophoblastic cells by the presence of their secretions of HCG in blood or urine.

## 302 Isn't a physical examination by the physician the best way to know that I am pregnant?

When frog-and-rabbit testing for pregnancy was still in use, the physician's exam was often the most accurate way to determine pregnancy. With the advent of the new urine and blood pregnancy tests, however, this exam is the less accurate way.

It is best, when you have skipped a period and think you may be pregnant, to do a pregnancy test at home or take a urine specimen to your doctor's office for testing. It may be suggested that you have a pregnancy test done at a laboratory.

When the test is positive, you can be fairly confident that you are pregnant. It may be best, however, not to tell all your friends and family until after a visit to the doctor's office confirms the accuracy of the pregnancy test.

## 303 If a pregnancy test at home or in the office is positive, when should I see my doctor for a physical examination?

Patients should come in for an examination after their second missed menstrual period. A pelvic exam at that time will usually confirm pregnancy—the uterus will be enlarged. At this time the doctor can usually tell whether or not the uterus is progressing normally in its growth, and if it is the size it

should be in relation to the date of the last menstrual period that the woman had. Occasionally the uterus will not be quite as large as would seem compatible with the last period. In this situation it is better for patients not to announce their pregnancies until the doctor examines them three weeks later to confirm that the uterus is continuing to grow.

If the uterus is not enlarged at that examination, it is fairly certain that the woman is not pregnant or has become pregnant only recently. If her pregnancy test was positive, but the uterus is not enlarged and she has had some bleeding, she can be fairly sure that she either is miscarrying, has miscarried, or has an ectopic tubal pregnancy.

An examination before the second missed period will not definitely confirm pregnancy. Although the uterus may be a little enlarged upon examination at this time, a little enlargment or a little softening of the uterus does not always indicate pregnancy. Women who skip a period, but are not pregnant, will often have a uterus that is slightly swollen, boggy, and enlarged. I have had many patients come to me after other doctors told them, incorrectly, that they were pregnant. This assessment was based on an exam that was done too early; what the doctors felt was only the swelling from a missed period.

## The Role of the Doctor Early in Your Pregnancy

## 304 What will the doctor do on my first examination?

Your physician will do a complete physical examination. This includes checking your heart and lungs, as well as doing a pelvic examination. If you have not had a Pap smear in the past year, your doctor will want to do one. This will not disturb your pregnancy. When your doctor does a Pap smear, he or she merely scrapes the surface of the cervix; any bleeding that occurs comes from that surface, not from or inside the uterus.

If this is your first pregnancy, or if it is the first time you have seen this doctor, he or she will examine your pelvic bones to check for any prominence or deformity. This is called a clinical pelvimetry. The size of your pelvis would also be measured, to see if there is any indication that you will not be able to deliver a baby normally. A clinical pelvimetry that shows an adequate pelvis, however, does not mean that you will be able to deliver without a cesarean section. Cesarean sections are done for other reasons that have nothing to do with the size of the pelvic bones.

Following the physical exam, the doctor will discuss pregnancy and delivery with you (see Q. 306), answer your questions, and probably schedule a return visit in three or four weeks.

## 305  How will the doctor determine my due date?

The formula is simple. (See the accompanying chart.) The doctor calculates from the *first* day of your *last* normal menstrual period. Conception normally occurs approximately two weeks after that day. The doctor subtracts three months from that day and then adds seven days to it to determine the day you are most likely due. I tell my patients that this due date is plus or minus two weeks.

This technique is based on a pregnancy schedule of 280 days from the first day of the last period (nine months and seven days). One recent study indicated the following figures:

48 percent of babies were delivered within seven days of calculated date,

28 percent of babies were delivered between seven and fourteen days of calculated date,

26 percent of babies were delivered more than fourteen days before or after calculated date (pre- or postmature).

The length of time from actual conception to delivery is normally about 270 days. This can be confusing. Some of the time your doctor will be talking about your pregnancy as though it began on the first day of your period and at other times as though it began at the time of the actual conception. You may need to listen carefully to the terms to know which gestation time (length of pregnancy) is being discussed.

## 306  What general advice might my doctor give me during my first visit to the office?

There is a great deal of general information that should be discussed during this visit. The program that I outline is fairly standard, although the opinions of individual doctors may vary in some particulars. Various staff members may assist in explaining some of this basic information.

The following list covers most of the information provided during the first visit.

*A. Appointments.* You will probably visit the doctor every three weeks through the seventh month of your pregnancy, every two weeks until the last month, and once a week during the last month.

*B. Fees and other expenses.* It is important that patients know what kind of expense they are facing during pregnancy and delivery. Fees vary widely from doctor to doctor, and hospital expenses will be determined by many factors, such as the hospital

# Gestation Chart

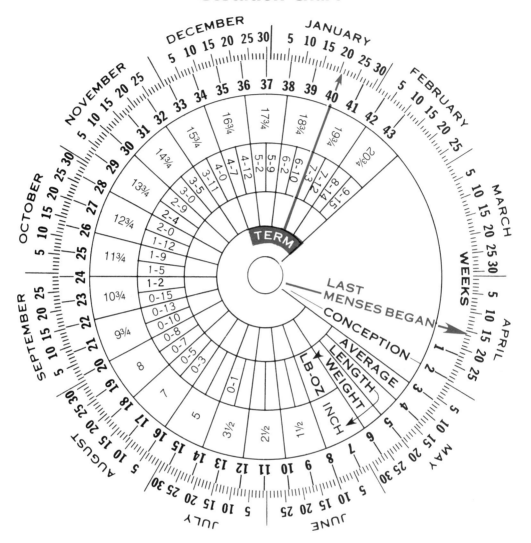

used, what kind of delivery is done, and whether there are any complications. Additional expenses throughout the pregnancy may include extra tests, such as ultrasound, or special laboratory work. Whether or not the couple has insurance is a major financial factor to be considered.

As each case is different, it is impossible to give definite figures in relation to expenses. These matters should be discussed early in the pregnancy, preferably on the first visit, so that you will know what to expect.

Incidentally, patients do have the right to change doctors during a pregnancy. If you are unhappy with your care, ask for a refund of money paid toward the delivery fee and find another doctor.

*C. Activity.* With a normal pregnancy you may engage in almost any activity that you wish. If you have not had a history of repeated miscarriages and seem to have a normal pregnancy with no bleeding, you should live a normal life.

I advise all my patients that they may

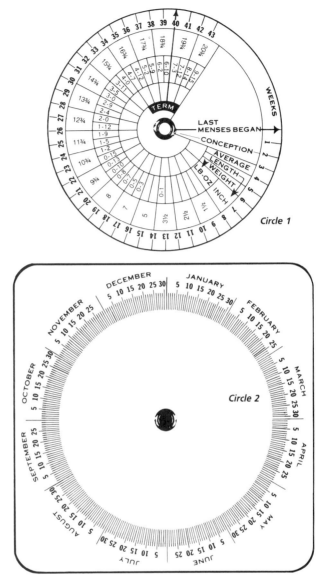

Circle 1

Circle 2

To make a gestation chart for each of your pregnancies, photocopy the two parts above, cut out circle 1 and center it over circle 2, tape the larger arrow to the beginning date of your last menstrual period, and circle the projected date of delivery at the point of the arrow in Week 40.

continue to do the things they did before pregnancy, which may include climbing mountains, water-skiing, and riding horses. I qualify this freedom with some blanket advice, however: Don't do anything you are uncomfortable doing or feel might be dangerous. Also, you should not participate in any of these vigorous activities unless you already know how. For example, a fall from a horse could interfere with your pregnancy as well as injure you.

When a patient is involved in a particular

sport or activity, I offer pertinent advice, such as suggesting that joggers not jog long distances or at a fast pace after the first half of the pregnancy. Vigorous exercise can shunt a lot of blood away from the placenta and fetus.

There is little evidence that intercourse is harmful during any stage of pregnancy. Dr. James L. Mills of the National Institute of Health did a study involving more than 10,000 women. He found no relationship between any problem they had during pregnancy or after delivery that was associated with intercourse during pregnancy. Although there have been some studies which indicate that intercourse can be associated with problems such as infections, my feeling is that Mills's studies are correct. I tell my patients that they may have intercourse at any time during pregnancy until the cervix is significantly dilated (two centimeters or more). This usually occurs during the last month.

**D.** *Exercise.* I ask my pregnant patients to walk three miles a day, or to swim or bicycle regularly, and I suggest that they start exercising as soon as their nausea and tiredness are diminished enough to allow them to be active. Exercise early in pregnancy will make you stronger and will make you feel better later in your pregnancy. Exercise also helps keep weight down.

The major benefit of exercise during pregnancy is that being in good shape physically can make labor easier. Labor is a physical activity and cannot be done as well by someone who is weak and in poor physical condition.

The American College of Obstetricians and Gynecologists has excellent pregnancy and postnatal exercise programs available in videocassette, record album, and audiocassette form. Check with your doctor before ordering from ACOG Exercise Programs, 3575 Cahuenga Blvd., W., Los Angeles, California 90068. (Phone: 1-800-443-4040, ext. 165; in California, 1-800-531-1212, ext. 165).

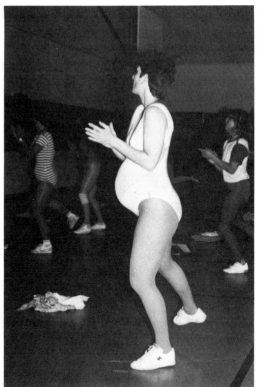

Exercise during pregnancy will keep a woman in good physical condition and can make labor easier.

These programs were designed by health officials who understand the special needs of pregnant and postnatal women.

**E.** *Diet.* A balanced diet is of great importance during pregnancy. There is some evidence that if the baby is poorly nourished during the last three months of pregnancy or during the first eighteen months of life, the brain is permanently affected and intelligence is decreased.

Studies have shown that the development of the baby's brain is most sensitive around the time of birth. During the last three months of pregnancy, when the brain cells are growing and dividing the fastest, and during the first eighteen months after birth, when the brain cells are maturing, a balanced diet for mother and infant is crucial.

**F.** *Weight gain.* A two-pound weight gain per visit (between twenty-five and thirty pounds during the pregnancy) is what I suggest to my patients. Pregnancy is not a time to diet excessively. A healthy weight gain (up to thirty pounds) provides the best nutrition for the baby. However, if you are not gaining that much weight do not consume candy and colas in order to gain. As long as you are eating a healthy, balanced diet everything is fine.

Frequently patients who are overweight when they become pregnant want to diet during pregnancy. It is better to diet after the baby is born. During pregnancy eat a healthy diet for the benefit of your baby. Eating only wholesome, healthy foods, however, can result in safe, steady weight loss throughout the pregnancy, or at least insure that no more unnecessary fat is added.

**G.** *Rest.* You should get an adequate amount of rest. During the early and late months of pregnancy you may feel tired; it is best to respond to your body's demands and get more rest at those times. Pushing yourself would only make you more tired. I recommend that my patients lie down for thirty to forty-five minutes at midday during the last two or three months of pregnancy. If you are particularly tired either early or late in the pregnancy, lie down for thirty to forty-five minutes both morning and afternoon.

**H.** *Medications.* You should take as little medication as possible during pregnancy. Prenatal vitamins, which are to be taken every day throughout the pregnancy, will likely be the only "medication" you will need. These vitamins may be taken with the evening meal, if necessary, to prevent their causing increased nausea. Their use may even be safely suspended until the nausea of pregnancy subsides, even if it persists several months.

It is imperative that you inform your obstetrician of any medication prescribed for you by another physician. For example, tetracycline or sulfa antibiotics should not be taken during pregnancy without consulting your obstetrician. Tylenol (or a sim-

## Distribution of Weight Gain During Pregnancy

| Trimester | Weight Gain of Mother |
|---|---|
| 1st (months 1-3) | 3 - 5 lbs. |
| 2nd (months 4-6) | 10 - 12 lbs. |
| 3rd (months 7-9) | 10 - 13 lbs. |
| **Total** | **23 - 30 lbs.** |

ilar medication containing no aspirin) should be used instead of aspirin during pregnancy. (See Q. 395, 468, 469, 477–492.)

**I.** *Morning sickness.* Morning sickness is real. Don't let anyone tell you it is just imagination. Though researchers do not know what causes it, they do know that morning sickness is due to the changes in the body produced by pregnancy.

More than half of pregnant women experience nausea and vomiting to some degree early in pregnancy. Morning sickness usually appears soon after the first period is missed, and usually spontaneously disappears at the end of the third month. When the nausea goes away, the accompanying tiredness usually also leaves.

The term *morning sickness* is misleading

## Causes of Weight Gain in Pregnancy

| Cause | Pounds |
|---|---|
| Baby | 7.7 |
| Placenta | 1.4 |
| Uterus | 2.0 |
| Breasts | 0.9 |
| Amniotic fluid | 1.8 |
| Blood volume increase | 4.0 |
| Body fluid | 2.7 |
| Other (fat deposits) | 3.5 |
| **Total** | **24** |

and physicians prefer to label this normal complaint "nausea and vomiting of pregnancy." It may occur at any time during the day and the severity can vary greatly. The nausea may be so mild that it does not interfere in any way with a woman's schedule or diet. She may have no vomiting. Other women will have more severe nausea with occasional, or even daily, vomiting. Then there is a small group of women who get very ill from this nausea and vomiting. They lose weight and can become dehydrated from lack of or loss of fluids. Sometimes the problem is severe enough to require hospitalization and then it is called hyperemesis gravidarum.

The treatment of the nausea and vomiting of pregnancy depends on its severity. A woman does not *need* treatment until her nutrition and body fluids are significantly affected. She may *want* it before that occurs.

These hints may help a pregnant woman experiencing nausea and vomiting:

Nibble on toast or crackers all day. Have crackers at your bedside. Start nibbling when you awaken.

Eat smaller, more frequent meals.

Do not eat spicy food unless you know it does not upset your stomach.

Avoid foods that seem to cause nausea.

Eat foods that seem soothing to your stomach.

Do not cook if that upsets your stomach. (I learned to cook during the months my wife had morning sickness accompanying her three pregnancies.)

Use medications if your problem is especially bothersome, i.e., if you do not seem to be able to keep much food down and are sick most of the time. (Check the discussion of medications that follows.)

Consult with a nutritionist. The hospital at which you will deliver probably has a nutritionist that would be happy to help you choose a diet that you could not only tolerate but also one that would be nutritious.

Do not take prenatal vitamins until the nausea is gone; they can aggravate nausea.

As long as you are not becoming dehydrated and are not losing weight, the problem is "awful" (my wife's word), but not dangerous. However, when your symptoms are severe and hyperemesis gravidarum results, your doctor will probably want to give you some medications. You may need to go to the hospital to get fluids in your veins. If you do go into the hospital, your doctor will want you to be able to rest. You will be allowed to have very few, if any, visitors. Your room may be kept cool and darkened. You will feel much better with such medical care.

Medications can be helpful. Many women have a negative attitude toward taking drugs for morning sickness. As long as this attitude is not carried to the extreme, it is a healthy position. Unfortunately, I have had patients who were so afraid of such medications that they refused to use them when they should have and as a result began to lose weight and became dehydrated. At this point poor nutrition would seem as likely to hurt a developing baby as any medication a careful obstetrician might prescribe. But a fetus is tough and probably would not be harmed by either factor.

Because of the media attention given to Bendectine, it was taken off the market. It had helped thousands of women with their nausea problem and reliable studies proved its safety to be almost absolute. However, 3 percent of all newborn babies have some type of abnormality and the parents of some of these unfortunate babies sued the manufacturing company claiming that Bendectine caused the abnormalities. The claims were unfounded but the company chose to stop making the product rather than to defend itself against unwarranted lawsuits.

I felt safest with a woman taking Bendectine for her nausea. Although this drug is not available, its component parts are sold without a prescription. One Unisom tablet and two 50-mg capsules vitamin B6 equal two Bendectine tablets. Daily dosage should not exceed the equivalent of four Bendectine tablets. It is probably best to take half of a Unisom and one vitamin B6 before arising and repeat the dosage later in the day. A full dose (equal to two Bendectine tablets) may be taken at night if necessary.

Other medications given for nausea include Combid, Phenergan, Tigan, and Thorazine. A small patch containing medication worn behind the ear is often helpful. It is called Transderm Scop. Some doctors give patients vitamin B6 shots or prescribe vitamin B6 tablets. Care must be taken not to give a patient an excessive amount of this drug. Neither a doctor nor a patient knows which drug will be helpful. Keep trying until you get relief. Remember, however, that it is possible that none of these drugs will relieve your symptoms.

**J.** *Swelling in Pregnancy*. Swelling of the body during pregnancy is a normal response to the hormones circulating throughout the body. If you experience some swelling, don't worry about it, unless it is very sudden and severe. Diuretics (medications that increase the amount of urine output, thereby relieving some of the swelling caused by excess fluid) are used much less frequently these days than in the past. If swelling is a problem, try other means of dealing with it. You could increase your water intake to three quarts a day; prop up your feet when you sit to allow fluid to drain from them; and decrease (but do not eliminate) your intake of salt. If those means do not provide relief, and the swelling causes significant discomfort, some doctors will prescribe diuretics. Obstetricians who have trained more recently will almost never prescribe diuretics,

even for this problem. This is probably the best approach, so don't argue if your doctor feels it is not healthy for you to use diuretics. (See Q. 490.)

**K.** *Prenatal classes*. If you have not already done so you should attend prenatal classes, sometimes called natural-childbirth or Lamaze classes, even if you plan to have general anesthesia during delivery. The classes are popular; you should enroll in one early in order to insure getting in. (See chapter 8.)

**L.** *Nursing*. If you plan to nurse your baby, "brushing" your nipples once or twice a day with a dry washcloth during the last month of pregnancy will help toughen them. Follow this treatment by massaging *Masse Cream* or another lubricant your doctor might suggest into the nipples. This nipple cream may also be used after each nursing to help keep the nipples from cracking or getting dry.

**M.** *Dental work*. See your dentist as necessary. If X-rays are needed, they should be taken after the third month and *the abdomen should be protected with a lead shield.* Your dental cavities may be filled as needed during the middle three months of pregnancy; it is preferable that your dentist use only a local anesthetic. However, I recommend that you have as little dental work as possible done during pregnancy, because bacteria from your gums move into your blood stream when you have dental work.

**N.** *Travel*. You may travel wherever and whenever you wish until the last month of pregnancy. At that time, you should stay within an hour's drive of home so that your baby can be delivered at your own hospital as planned. Babies can come prematurely and in inconvenient locations. A reasonable cutoff time for long-distance travel seems to be four weeks before your due date.

If you travel long distances by car, get out each hour and walk around the car a couple of times. This will keep you more comfortable and help your circulation. Air travel, either commercial or private, is permissible, except during the last month. During long flights you will want to walk in the aisle occasionally.

*O. Problems during pregnancy.* I tell my patients to call me any time, day or night, if a problem occurs. It is better and safer to call when there is a small problem, rather than to wait until there is a serious one. I assure my patients that I, or one of my partners, will be available at any time.

If you can tell from the initial visit with the obstetrician you have chosen that he or she will be difficult for you to communicate with, difficult to reach, or is one whom you would hesitate to "bother" with a problem or question, you should consider changing doctors. A good relationship with your physician makes for a happier, healthier, safer pregnancy and delivery.

---

**307** **May I continue to work while I am pregnant?**

It is fine to continue all normal activities during pregnancy; this includes working. An exception would be if you are in a job that might cause problems for your body or damage to the baby.

If you are on a job that requires a great deal of lifting, you should probably stop the lifting after the fifth or sixth month. Continuing to lift in the latter part of pregnancy could cause you to injure your back. If you work where you are exposed to strong chemical fumes, you probably should change jobs while you are pregnant.

Some reports indicate that continued exposure to high temperatures during the first part of pregnancy can damage the baby. It is therefore probably best not to be on a job that exposes you to high temperatures, although it is highly unlikely that you could tolerate working in such a situation while you are pregnant.

Radiation (X-rays, radioisotopies) can be harmful to both you and your baby and should be avoided during pregnancy.

Studies have also indicated that a large number of "questionable" work or environmental factors do not seem to be harmful to the fetus. These include video displays, TV screens, magnetic or electronic fields, noise, or ultrasound.

Other reports indicate that it is not good for a pregnant woman to be exposed to very high altitudes, or to dive in deep depths, or to experience compression or decompression more than that experienced in normal air travel. Air travel itself is allowed during pregnancy, whether or not it is in a pressurized aircraft.

If a woman has previously had a premature baby, it might be best for her to stop working during the last three months of her pregnancy and to rest both morning and afternoon. Some studies have indicated that if a mother rests more during the latter part of her pregnancy, she is more likely to carry that pregnancy to term and to have a larger, healthier baby.

---

## Changes to Expect During Pregnancy

---

**308** **What physical changes can I expect during pregnancy?**

The hormones of pregnancy are produced in huge amounts, and these hormones, coupled with the growth of the baby, produce truly amazing bodily changes. Some of the major changes are as follows.

*The abdomen.* By the time most patients see a physician (after the second missed period), their abdomens feel bloated. Since at this point the uterus is about the size of a man's fist, obviously the uterus is not causing the bloated feeling. The feeling occurs because of the swelling effect of the hormones on all the tissues of the lower abdomen and pelvis.

Toward the end of the third month, the abdomen is a little more protuberant. At about this time the doctor, and sometimes the mother herself, will be able to feel the uterus as a lump extending about two inches above the pubic bone.

Most pregnant women can still "hide" their pregnancy, if they so wish, until between the sixteenth and twentieth weeks of pregnancy. By the twentieth week, the end of the fifth month, the top of the uterus is at the level of the navel, and most women cannot conceal a pregnancy once it is that far along.

As the abdomen becomes larger and larger, women often wonder how much bigger they can get. The capacity of the uterus and the abdominal wall to expand are almost beyond belief. The uterus is not limited by the rib cage and can expand as much as it needs to, for twins, triplets, or more.

Women often ask about the use of maternity girdles. These girdles are safe during pregnancy, and some women feel more comfortable while wearing them. Most patients, though, do not seem to be helped much by maternity girdles, and if you are pregnant during a period of warm weather, you may feel too hot to wear one. The only way to know if you will benefit from a maternity girdle is to get one and see if it helps both your abdomen and your back feel more comfortable.

**Breasts.** During pregnancy the breasts change almost as much as the uterus does. Early in pregnancy the breasts may be tender and full. After the second month they increase in size and become nodular, or lumpy. The nodularity is due to the growing and thickening glands that are necessary for the production of milk after delivery.

The nipples may or may not produce a thick yellow fluid called colostrum, but its production at this point is unrelated to the ability of a woman to nurse. Don't worry if you begin having colostrum after only a few weeks of pregnancy, as it is not abnormal for this to happen.

A darkening of the nipples and areola (the skin around the nipples) is normal. This change in color is due to the effect of hormones on these tissues. Also, small elevations on the areola are the so-called glands of Montgomery, oil glands that are increasing in size during pregnancy.

Blue veins may appear beneath the skin overlying the breasts. These are normal during pregnancy. The body's blood vessels carry 40 percent more blood during the latter part of pregnancy than they normally do. It is also normal for stretch marks (see the next paragraph) to be present in the skin of the breasts.

**Skin.** Many people are not aware of the fantastic changes, caused by hormones, that the skin undergoes during pregnancy. The most obvious change involves stretch marks *(striae gravidarum)*, the pinkish lines that resemble scars and appear on the abdomen, breasts, and thighs of some women. These marks occur in about one-half of all pregnancies; remaining even when the skin returns to its normal position after pregnancy. Stretch marks will become much lighter and much less visible after the pregnancy is over.

Stretch marks are not, as commonly thought, due to stretching, but to changes caused by the hormones of pregnancy. Moisturizers and lubricants may make the skin feel better, but they will not prevent stretch marks.

In addition to the darkening of the skin of the areola and nipples, which usually occurs with the first pregnancy, a dark line *(linea nigra)* will often develop from the navel down to the pubic hair. These discolorations usually get darker with each pregnancy.

Facial discolorations develop in many

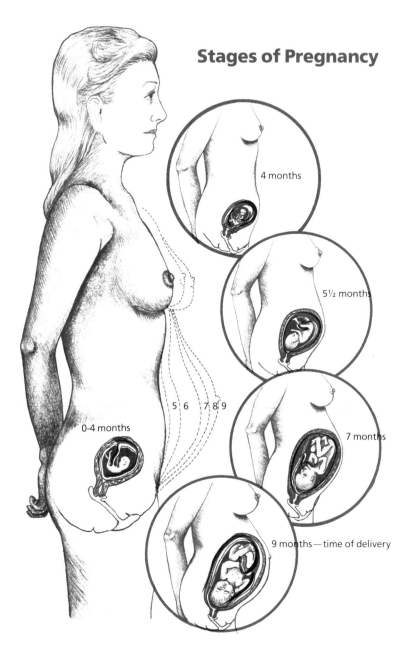

## Stages of Pregnancy

4 months

5½ months

0-4 months

5 6 7 8 9

7 months

9 months — time of delivery

pregnant women. These various-sized brown patches *(chloasma)* are often called the mask of pregnancy. Although the discoloration usually fades after delivery, the skin does not normally return to its original color. Birth-control pills can produce the same change.

Vascular spiders develop in about two-thirds of white women and approximately one-tenth of black women during pregnancy. These are small (one-quarter to one-eighth inch) red discolorations of the skin, occurring most commonly on the face, neck, upper chest, and arms. From the central spot, small red lines extend outward. The blood drains from them and they blanch when they are touched lightly. These are also known as *nevus, angioma,* or *telangiectasia.*

Redness of the palms is common in pregnancy, occurring in about two-thirds of white women and one-third of nonwhite women. This condition usually disappears after pregnancy.

Skin tags, small, flesh-colored growths of skin of about the size of a small tick, often develop during pregnancy. Changes in the color of moles also will often occur. Skin tags usually go away after pregnancy; moles usually lighten but remain. Some women are afraid that such changes mean they have skin cancer. This is highly unlikely, but if there is any question, you should have your doctor check.

**Arms and legs.** Occasionally a pregnant woman will develop numbness of her hands. This is called the *carpal tunnel syndrome.* If a patient has occasional numbness, nothing is usually done about it. However, if her hands become totally numb and this numbness lasts twenty-four hours or longer, I suggest that she see a neurosurgeon or a plastic surgeon, who can perform a simple operation that will relieve the pressure on the nerves to her hands. This can prevent permanent damage to the nerves of the hands.

The veins of the legs become prominent during pregnancy because vessels are carrying so much more blood than they normally do. In the latter part of pregnancy, small blood vessels are at least 50 percent larger than normal, making it possible to see small veins and capillaries that are not ordinarily visible. These veins are generally not varicosities. A varicose vein is normally one that is enlarged to at least the size of your little finger, large enough to make the skin bulge over it. For small collections of veins or small isolated veins, there is no treatment. Besides, most will usually go away after pregnancy. Your skin, though, will never be the way it was before your first pregnancy,

and some of these veins will continue to be visible.

Varicose veins are normally not very responsive to any particular recommendations during pregnancy. I have not found it useful to have patients wear elastic stockings. In the southern part of the country, elastic stockings are uncomfortable to wear because of the heat. Most women choose not to wear them. If a patient has such severe varicose veins that she must do something for them, she can have custom-fitted elastic stockings made. These are probably the only ones that are significantly helpful if the varicose veins are quite bad.

***Changes in the internal parts of the body.*** During pregnancy remarkable changes occur in almost every system of the body. The kidneys and the tubes from the kidneys to the bladder (ureters) change in an extraordinary way. The actual work of the kidneys also increases remarkably. The stomach and intestines change and are "displaced" by the enlarging uterus. The lungs change because the growing abdomen pushes up the diaphragm, thus reducing the volume of air in the lungs. The actual function of the lungs is not impaired by pregnancy, but certain diseases of the lungs, such as pneumonia and bronchitis, are more common in pregnancy.

One of the most dramatic changes in your body during pregnancy has to do with your heart and blood-vessel system. The heart rate increases ten or fifteen beats a minute, and the output of blood from the heart increases, especially during the first three months of pregnancy. In the past, doctors were afraid that pregnancy was hard on a woman's heart and gave stern warnings of the danger of pregnancy to women with heart disease. There certainly are some problems associated with severe heart disease in pregnancy, but these are not nearly so all-encompassing as was felt in the past.

**Gums.** Your gums may become soft and may bleed easily during pregnancy. These changes seem to be related to the hormones of pregnancy and usually disappear after delivery. The best treatment seems to be good dental hygiene, which includes flossing and brushing.

A condition called *epulis* (a swelling of the gums in a specific spot which resembles a growth) can occur during pregnancy. If that happens, your dentist should check to be sure that this is merely a swelling and not a growth.

There is no evidence that there is any truth in the old wives' tale: "The baby sucks the calcium away from its mother's teeth and causes them to decay."

Dental work should be done during the middle three months of pregnancy. During that time the placenta is at a healthy stage and is better able to filter out bacteria that may be released into the blood stream while the dentist works on your gums and teeth. If you have an abscess or any sign of infection, this must be treated. You are certainly a lot safer having that taken care of than letting it go untreated while you are pregnant.

**Muscles and bones.** Several things happen to your muscles and bones, the most obvious of which is a change in posture. As your uterus enlarges and grows forward, you must lean back to balance yourself. This is called *lordosis* and is one of the most common causes of discomfort of the low back during pregnancy. This tendency to experience pain in the lower back is one reason patients are encouraged to start exercising early in pregnancy. Exercise makes the muscles strong enough to help support the body during the latter part of pregnancy when there is more stress on it.

A patient may develop aching, numbness, and weakness in the arms. This is due to the tendency to lean back, pulling the neck forward and thereby pulling on the nerves that go down to the arms.

There is also a softening of the ligaments between your joints, not only of your arms and legs but also of the pelvic bones themselves. This relaxation seems to be what causes the bones to grate against each other, to pop, and to produce some of the discomfort that a woman feels in her arms, legs, back, and pelvis. These changes are important. X-rays reveal the amazing way that the pelvic bones separate during labor to allow the baby's head through for delivery.

---

**309** **Are there any ways to avoid or ease low back pain during pregnancy?**

Suggestions for avoiding back pain, in addition to beginning exercise early in pregnancy to keep the muscles toned up all along, include the following.

*Resting.* Lie down; don't sit. Lie on a firm surface with your knees elevated by a pillow. When you get up, roll over on your side and lower your legs to the floor without jerking your back.

*Lifting things.* When you lift, squat down directly in front of the object you are planning to lift. Do not bend over. Pregnant women usually do more injury to their backs when they already have one baby; their tendency to bend over and pick up that small child, with a back that is weakened by the present pregnancy, is a real problem. Be careful with your back if you already have a young child to care for.

*Sitting.* When you sit, avoid soft, low chairs that allow you to sink down into the upholstery. It is easy to hurt your back when you stand up. Never sit for more than fifteen minutes at a time if you can avoid it, especially late in pregnancy. Get up and move around as frequently as possible.

*Driving.* Push the car seat forward so that your knees are higher than your hips. It is vital that you always wear your seat belt. If you are in an accident and hit your uterus against the dashboard or steering wheel, you can damage your unborn baby.

*Standing and walking.* When you are pregnant, you are naturally a little more clumsy. Be careful when you are stepping over curbs or walking on rough ground. Don't stand in the same position for more than a minute; shifting from one foot to the other occasionally will help.

*Physical work.* Get on your knees to do jobs that you might be tempted to do by leaning over. When your back is really hurting, don't do any physical work that will aggravate your condition.

---

**310** **What are some of the most common complaints during pregnancy?**

Inevitably, because of the numerous and major changes being made in your body, there will be some discomfort and possibly pain. I believe these aches and pains are more easily borne if they are understood and if a woman knows why she is hurting. An explanation of some of the more common problems follows.

***Round ligament pain.*** This type of pain is probably the most common during pregnancy. It can begin after only a few weeks of pregnancy and can occur at any time during the pregnancy. The pain, which can be as severe as appendicitis, may be brief or may last for days, occurring in the lower abdomen on either side. If the pain is bad, you should see your physician to determine exactly what it is. He or she can usually confirm that it is round ligament pain by merely pressing on the areas where the round ligament inserts into the uterus and finding tenderness in that spot.

This pain is caused by shifting, coughing, or moving in such a way that it pulls one of the round ligaments, located one on each side of the uterus. These ligaments help stabilize the uterus and hold it from abnormal positions.

***Braxton-Hicks contractions.*** These contractions are commonly called false labor pains. Many people have the idea that they occur only as a warm-up for labor, but this is not true. The uterus contracts and relaxes all the time, even when a woman isn't pregnant. However, during pregnancy, as the uterus is being stretched, it does contract more and with stronger contractions than it does in the nonpregnant condition.

Braxton-Hicks contractions will normally become less frequent and less strong if a woman rests, but can be intensified by physical activity and intercourse. When a patient is having discomfort with false labor pains, the best thing is to rest and to refrain from intercourse for a short time.

***Vaginal discomfort.*** It is common, especially in the latter part of pregnancy, for a woman to feel "shooting pains" into her vagina, as though the baby were putting its foot through the cervix and out into the vagina. This is not usually a sign that the baby is about to come. These pains, which may vary from pressure to a sharp, shooting sensation, are not a danger sign and nothing needs to be done. If the pain is quite bothersome, you may need to lie down. This will allow the baby to float up out of the pelvis a little and relieve some of the discomfort.

The vagina and the vulva can both feel swollen in the second half of the pregnancy. Occasionally this is uncomfortable enough to make intercourse unpleasant. Many women, whether or not they have problems of this type, do not desire intercourse anyway, especially during the latter part of pregnancy. This situation, of course, puts a great deal of pressure on the husband; his sexual drive is unabated.

Unfortunately, some men cannot stand sexual deprivation (or think they can't). This is shown by the fact that there is a greater incidence of infidelity during pregnancy. You can alleviate some of his stress—and show your love for him—by meeting his sexual needs. If vaginal sex causes actual pain for you, you might use your hands to bring him to ejaculation occasionally.

***Feeling the baby move.*** Although many women feel occasional discomfort when the baby moves, sometimes they don't know whether the baby is moving or something is wrong. It is usually easy for the doctor to tell. When you feel really uncomfortable and are not sure whether it is the baby or your own body, see the doctor and let him or her tell you.

It is normal to have a tender place in the uterus as a result of the baby poking the uterine wall. This sensation may stay for several hours or several days before going away. It is normal, too, to feel a fairly sharp and uncomfortable pain under the ribs, and this will often happen as early as six months. It can be caused by both the stretching of your ribs and/or the baby's movement. There is nothing you can do about the baby's movement; it is a normal part of the baby's growth and indicates that the baby is healthy inside the uterus.

Some women worry about the baby moving too much. They feel it must be an indication that something is wrong, or that they will have a hyperactive child. In 1983 William F. Rayburn of the University of Michigan studied more than 900 pregnant women who kept charts of fetal movement. Forty-seven of the women recorded more than forty movements of the baby per hour, signs of excessive fetal activity. All of these babies were healthy and normal when they were delivered; none died, and studies on them since that time have shown that none of them had unusual temperaments or delayed development.

Mothers frequently complain that their babies have a repetitive "bumping" activity. This is hiccups, and when I mention this to mothers, they immediately recognize it as such. Studies have shown that all normal babies have hiccups at least once a day from the seventh month on. Don't worry, though, if you don't feel the baby's hiccups; they can occur at night when you are asleep. And it is certainly not worth losing a night's sleep to see whether or not the baby is hiccupping once a day.

On the other end of the scale is the quiet baby. This one is usually normal. You should not worry if you are not constantly aware of your baby moving around. Mothers frequently fail to feel a baby move for one or two days at a time and become worried. Normally this fear is unwarranted. If you have any questions about the baby being inactive for an entire day, you should see your doctor and have the baby's condition checked. You might also try "poking" the baby, eating something sweet, or standing by a loud radio. These things will often awaken a quiet baby.

*Leg cramps.* Women often get leg cramps during the last half of pregnancy. This is usually due to drinking too much milk. Cow's milk contains excessive phosphorous, which lowers the amount of calcium in your blood. If you experience leg cramps, you should stop drinking cow's milk altogether and start taking calcium pills. These may be obtained without a prescription at a drugstore. If the cramps stop, you can begin to drink milk again, up to the amount that causes the cramps to return.

*Insomnia.* Many patients have trouble sleeping during the last month of pregnancy, which makes them feel tired and weak. Although I do not like to prescribe sleeping pills during pregnancy, if the woman is really miserable from insomnia—and because this problem is almost exclusively a "last-month" problem—I will offer Benadryl (25–50 mg) to take when they go to bed.

*Nausea late in pregnancy.* Nausea during the last month is fairly common. For nausea of this type, I prescribe Combid. I feel that the baby at this point is almost fully developed and likely not affected by a drug such as Combid. Women often think that they have a virus or some other illness when late nausea starts. This can be true, but usually it is due to the pregnancy.

*Hemorrhoids.* Hemorrhoids are fairly common both during and after pregnancy. It has been thought that these are due to the pressure in the veins from the pregnant uterus, and that after pregnancy hemorrhoids are present because of the woman's pushing during labor. This may be true in part; however, in societies where more fiber and less sugar are eaten, women almost never have hemorrhoids, even during pregnancy. It is felt, therefore, that hemorrhoids are related more to the type of diet that we eat in the Western world than to pregnancy.

Hemorrhoids can be treated with cool, moist compresses, Nupercainal ointment, or a cortisone-containing ointment prescribed by your doctor. Because hemorrhoids protrude, it is tempting to push them back inside the anus. Don't do this. Pushing them back will often irritate them and make them more sensitive.

*Heartburn or indigestion.* This is common in pregnancy and results from the stomach slowing down its function and passing food through sluggishly. This problem can often be helped by avoiding rich, greasy, or spicy foods. One report associates the use of antacids with congenital anomalies in babies. Most physicians, though, do not feel that antacids are likely to cause any problem with the baby. I personally feel that it is permissible to use antacids in pregnancy, but, as with any medication, it is probably best to use them only if you cannot make yourself comfortable by other techniques, such as adjusting your diet.

*Ill feeling.* Some women simply do not feel well when they are pregnant. They feel uncomfortable, full, tired . . . just wretched. At the time it seems like small comfort, of course, but I often tell my patients that feeling miserable is a small price to pay for a beautiful new baby.

Other women feel great while they are pregnant. My wife has frequently remarked that she felt better while she was pregnant than she had ever felt in her life.

There really does not seem to be much you can do to make yourself feel better except to keep in good physical shape through sensible exercise and eating. After your doctor has assured you that nothing is wrong, don't worry if you feel wretched. Keep yourself in good shape and tolerate that miserable feeling until the baby comes. It will be worth it!

*Lightening.* Normally, pregnant women do not complain about lightening, or dropping, of the baby in the few weeks before the onset of labor. However, it can cause increased pelvic discomfort. Some mothers will notice a few weeks before the start of their labor that the baby seems to have dropped lower in their pelvis. They will notice a little extra room at the upper part of their abdomen. Sometimes they may be able to breathe a little easier. After this has occurred, the mother will notice that she has more pressure in the pelvic area. She will often have the feeling that the baby is poking its foot or its hand into her vagina. Occasionally it will be more difficult to walk because of the feeling of pressure in the hips. Increased frequency and urgency of urination as well as increased backache may also occur.

This dropping of the baby occurs most dramatically in mothers who are having their first baby. After the first baby, it seems that the pregnancy starts low, stays low, and does not usually have the lightening that occurs with the first baby.

---

**311** **Is it true that a husband may experience symptoms of pregnancy too?**

Yes. Not only may you experience nausea in pregnancy, but so may your husband. When this occurs, it may include not only nausea, but also other symptoms that mimic the discomfort and problems that you may feel, such as abdominal pain, vomiting, diarrhea, and even burning with urination and blood in the urine. These symptoms, called couvade syndrome, are most always psychogenic and not due to any disease in the male.

About 14 percent of expectant fathers are likely to have some symptoms of this type. Most of the time the husband's problems will go away on their own. Men with this problem are not psychiatrically abnormal; they don't need anything more than encouragement and a little insight into what is going on.

## How Your Baby Develops

### 312  What is the month-by-month development of my baby inside the uterus?

The growth of your baby is a rapid, miraculous, fascinating chain of events. The accompanying chart gives a broad overview of fetal growth.

The chart of fetal development is only a broad outline of the amazing, miraculous process of growth in the uterus. It is a process that no human engineering can make happen. There is almost no process in all creation that more clearly demonstrates God's creative genius.

### 313  How does the placenta function during pregnancy?

The placenta begins forming during the second week after fertilization, and it continues to grow, compatible with the size of the pregnancy, right on through the pregnancy. The placenta stays attached to the uterine wall until after the birth of the baby. Then it separates and is also delivered.

During the last month the baby's heart is pumping 300 gallons of blood a day through the placenta. The fluid that the baby drinks is absorbed into its blood stream, and is then carried through the blood vessels into the placenta. The placenta secretes the fluid back into the uterine cavity around the baby. The baby drinks *a gallon of fluid every day*.

By the time of delivery, the placenta normally weighs one to two pounds.

## Monitoring Your Health During Pregnancy

### 314  What are the reasons for routine office visits throughout pregnancy?

Your doctor wants to be sure that your pregnancy is progressing normally. He or she checks for indications that all is well and will watch carefully for signs of any current or potential problems.

Some of the routine procedures involved in this process are these:

*Blood pressure check*. Your blood pressure throughout pregnancy is an important indicator; it will be checked each visit. Early detection of blood-pressure elevation allows prompt treatment and a healthier pregnancy. One of the most common causes of poor fetal growth and fetal death is a mother's high blood pressure.

*Weight*. Checking your weight regularly is important for four reasons:

Gaining too much weight makes it more difficult for you to deliver the baby, because the birth canal stores fat just as the rest of the body does.

Gaining too much weight indicates that you may not be eating a healthy diet, which is extremely important for both you and the baby.

Excessive weight gain can also indicate that you are retaining too much fluid in your body. In this event, the doctor may suggest decreasing your salt and increasing your water intake.

Failure to gain weight, or extreme weight loss, might be an indication of a problem; if this happens your doctor will want to determine the cause as soon as possible.

*Urinalysis.* Your urine will be routinely tested with a dipstick. This helps detect possible kidney damage, which can be caused by toxemia of pregnancy, a metabolic disorder characterized by hypertension, edema or swelling, and protein in the urine. This condition can cause several problems. (Q. 405–414.)

Diabetes can also be detected by routine urine tests. If you are diabetic, your blood stream is carrying too much sugar; that excess sugar will spill over into the urine and can be detected by the urinalysis. (See Q. 380–389.)

A third test, usually done with the same dipstick, is a test for infection in your urinary tract.

*Abdominal exam.* During each visit the doctor will feel your abdomen to check the location of the top of the uterus. This test shows the size of the uterus and its monthly growth. The doctor will measure it with a tape measure, with his or her hands, or with a measuring instrument of some type, checking to see whether there is continued growth of the uterus from visit to visit. This tells the doctor not only if the baby is growing at the rate that it should be, but also if the uterus is getting larger than it should be, indicating the possibility of twins or triplets. Until after the fifth month the doctor cannot tell by an abdominal exam whether there is more than one baby.

*Fetal heartbeat check.* The doctor will listen for the baby's heartbeat. Using a Doppler instrument, the doctor can pick up the heartbeat when the baby is about ten weeks along or he or she can hear it with a fetoscope (a stethescopelike instrument)

about the end of the fifth month. The heartbeat cannot indicate the baby's sex. If someone tells you the sex of your baby based on its heartbeat, he or she is just guessing.

*Check for swelling.* The doctor will usually check your legs for swelling. The presence of swelling is not especially significant, as long as your blood pressure is normal and you do not have any protein (albumin) in your urine. Swelling is usually a normal part of pregnancy. (For suggestions on dealing with it, see Q. 306.)

*Pelvic exam.* Although the doctor probably did a pelvic exam on your initial visit to the office, he or she may want to do another on the next visit or two to make sure that your uterus is growing as it should.

If you are having any bleeding, a pelvic exam will be done to make sure the cervix is not dilating. Early dilation of the cervix can be forewarning of miscarriage or premature labor.

During the last month the doctor will usually do pelvic exams each time (every week) you come to the office. These exams will indicate if the baby is coming head first or bottom first (breech), or if the cervix is dilating and effacing (thinning out), a sign that you may begin labor soon. A contraction during a pelvic exam in the last month can also be an indication that you may go into labor soon.

If the baby's head or bottom is not dropping down into the pelvis during that last month, that may be the first indication that you might need a C-section. (See Q. 639–653.) There is no need to worry if your doctor tells you this, since most of the time when labor actually starts, the baby does drop down.

*Development of a relationship with your doctor.* Your obstetrician is interested in developing a good relationship with you, one that will inspire confidence on your part in your medical care. If this is your first baby, the doctor knows that you may be somewhat apprehensive. The relationship you

# Fetal Growth

| Time from Fertilization | Growth |
| --- | --- |
| 24-35 hours | The egg divides into two cells. This occurs in the fallopian tube where the egg and sperm unite. |
| 21 days | The heart begins beating and the brain begins to develop. |
| 26 days | Arm buds develop. |
| 28 days | Legs begin to develop. The baby is the size of an apple seed (about ⅙ to ¼ inch in length) and is 10,000 times larger than the fertilized egg from which it started. |
| 35 days | The eyes begin forming and by the end of this (second) month the ears, nose, lips, and tongue can be clearly identified. |
| 40 days | The baby's brain waves can be detected, recorded, and even read by a doctor. |
| 8 weeks | The fetus now looks like a little human baby. *Fetus* in the Latin means "young one" or "offspring." It now has muscles, and cartilage that will soon change into true bone. Movement begins, although the mother won't feel it for another few weeks. For several weeks now the baby has been capable of feeling pain; it can even be taught conditioned responses. |
| 3rd month | During this month the baby grows to more than two inches in length and weighs an ounce. Its movements become very graceful, and the fingerprints form. Fingernails and toenails appear, and sexual differentiation is obvious enough to tell whether the baby is a boy or a girl. The baby begins having respiratory motion that exercises the chest muscles for eventual breathing at birth; it begins drinking some of the fluid which surrounds it; and it excretes fluid from the kidneys. The baby will drink more fluid if it is sweet and less fluid if it is bitter or sour. This information was discovered by injecting these substances into the amniotic fluid. A mother cannot make the amniotic fluid more sweet or more sour by anything she eats or drinks. The vocal cords form during this time and if the baby were outside the body and could breathe adequately, it probably could make a noise. |
| 4th month | By the end of this month the baby is 8 to 10 inches long, half its height at birth. It can weigh about one-half pound or more. It is during this month that the mother begins to "show" and to feel the baby's movements. The baby begins growing hair on its head, having facial expression, and developing its own individual appearance. |
| 5th and 6th months | The baby is fully formed as far as its organs and systems are concerned. Its ears are developed enough for it to hear and recognize its mother's voice. The baby's eyes open and are able to perceive the light and shadows that penetrate the wall of the abdomen and uterus. Sounds provoke energetic reactions and repetitive signals may bore the fetus. The body becomes covered with a white, greasy material called vernix, which is composed of secretions from the oil glands of the body, hair that has fallen from the skin, and other secretions. By this time the baby weighs 1–1½ pounds. If the baby is born at this stage, it has a chance of living. |
| 7th through 9th months | During this time the baby gains weight, has further maturing of its organs, and grows to about 20 inches in length. It is in this period that the doctor can usually feel the baby's head in the low part of the mother's abdomen just above the pubic hair line. Most babies are positioned head down from the very first time that you or your doctor are able to feel its position. |

build as you see him or her on frequent visits is valuable and in your best interest.

## 315 Are there any special problems for teenage pregnancies?

Quite definitely. Teenagers are more likely to have medical complications, partly be-cause they do not often have the wisdom, discipline, or money to get good medical care. The children born to teenagers have a statistically greater chance of dying or having serious illnesses during their developmental years.

The frequent low birth weight of these babies correlates closely with the occurrence of neurological defects, retardation, epilepsy, and cerebral palsy.

To avoid serious or fatal consequences for themselves and their babies, these young girls must see a physician regularly during pregnancy and be serious in observing the guidelines that the physician gives them. (See Q. 145–147.)

## Multiple Births

**316** **What is a multiple pregnancy, and how is one detected?**

When we use the term *multiple pregnancy*, we are talking about pregnancies with two, three, or more babies. As the doctor follows you in your pregnancy, he or she will not automatically assume that you have only one baby, although that is the most likely situation. Twins are much less common than one-baby pregnancies, and pregnancies of more than two babies are unusual. The incidence of twins in pregnancy is about one per hundred and of triplets about one in eight thousand.

When monitoring the growth of your uterus, your doctor may notice that it seems larger than it should be for the length of time you have been pregnant. This is almost never obvious during the first three or four months of pregnancy. It is usually during the fifth to sixth months of pregnancy that the doctor might notice that your uterus is larger than it should be. You or your friends may start commenting that you look as though you are ready to deliver any time.

If you are carrying twins, you may feel a great deal of activity in the uterus, with lots of kicking in all directions. This, of course, is not a certain sign of twins; a very active baby can make you think you are carrying half a dozen! Some women feel that kicking in two different places might indicate twins, but this is not necessarily true, either. One baby can kick the lower uterus with its feet and butt its head up against the top of the uterus just as actively as though there were two babies.

Patients often ask me if I can hear two heartbeats. Much of the time it is impossible to tell whether there is more than one baby just by listening to the heartbeats. With great care, and with two people listening at the same time, it is possible to tell a difference, but this is a difficult way to identify a multiple pregnancy.

The most reliable method for determining a multiple pregnancy is with an ultrasound machine. Because it is important to know if a twin pregnancy exists, some doctors feel that every pregnant woman should be scanned at about the fifth month. Personally, I feel that eventually every pregnant woman will have such a scan at least once during her pregnancy. This will not only allow detection of multiple pregnancy but also of some congenital abnormalities. This, however, is not accepted practice today.

An X-ray, too, can tell whether or not you have a multiple pregnancy, but this is not reliable until the fourth to fifth month, when the baby starts depositing calcium in its bones. With the presence of ultrasound scans, however, the use of X-ray for this purpose is not needed, and certainly all unnecessary X-rays are to be avoided.

**317** **Would my pregnancy be handled differently if I were found to have twins?**

Yes. The main "treatment" might be bed rest. Many doctors recommend that a woman carrying twins rest (in bed) a great deal of the time from the sixth month on.

**318** **How does bed rest help in a multiple birth?**

Studies show fairly conclusively that if you will stay in bed a good deal of the time in the last few months of pregnancy, your babies will weigh more when they are born. This is due primarily to the fact that you would be less likely to deliver the babies as early as you would if you did not stay in bed.

As with any baby, carrying the pregnancy to full term is safer and healthier for the child, and twins are certainly no exception to this rule.

**319** **Is a normal vaginal delivery or a cesarean section the best method of delivery for twins?**

The answer to that question is determined by several factors. It is really impossible to give an absolute answer, since postbirth health studies of twins are not conclusive one way or the other.

Most physicians seem to feel that if the babies are going to be born prematurely, by four weeks or more, a cesarean section should be done. If the babies are within four weeks of being due when labor starts, it is probably best to deliver vaginally unless some complication arises during the progress of labor or delivery.

Occasionally, and rightly, a doctor delivers the first baby through the vagina, discovers at that point that the second baby might have problems, and decides to do a cesarean section for its delivery.

As a matter of interest regarding the vaginal delivery of twins, the first baby (twin A) is born head first 75 percent of the time; the second baby (twin B) is born head first 53 percent of the time.

**320** **How are twins produced? How often are they identical?**

Twins result from two types of development.

*Identical twins.* About one-third of the time twins are identical, meaning that every cell of the two babies will be the same as they grow, and the genes are the same in every cell. These twins result from the fertilization of one egg which divides into two different parts early in its development. Since one sperm fertilizes one egg, every cell of both parts of that egg are genetically the same.

*Nonidentical twins (fraternal twins).* Twins of this type are the result of two separate eggs fertilized by two different sperm. After fertilization, these eggs grow as nonidentical twins. This type of twinning is most common, occurring in about two-thirds of all twins. These babies, of course, can be just as different from each other as any two nontwin children of the same parents can be.

Multiple birth of triplets (or more) may also occur as identical or fraternal babies, or even as a combination of both!

**321** **If there are twins in our family, am I likely to have them? Do twins "skip" generations?**

If there are twins in your family or in your husband's family, there may be a slightly increased chance of your having twins. The chance is not very great, however; you should not assume that you are going to have twins. Statistically you probably will not. If there is a tendency of twinning in your family, it does not skip generations and is as likely to affect you as it is your children.

**322** **What are the chances of having more than two babies?**

The occurrence of multiple births greater than twins is so uncommon that the subject

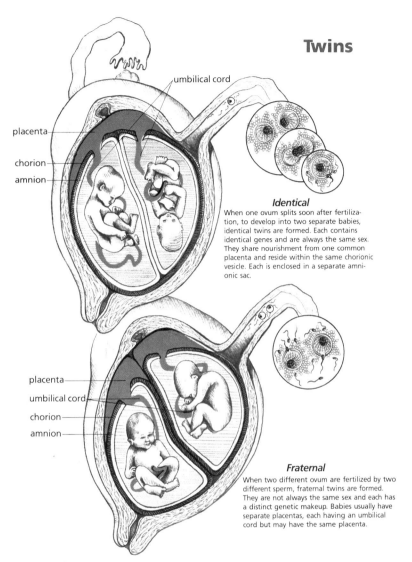

placenta
chorion
amnion
umbilical cord

**Identical**
When one ovum splits soon after fertilization, to develop into two separate babies, identical twins are formed. Each contains identical genes and are always the same sex. They share nourishment from one common placenta and reside within the same chorionic vesicle. Each is enclosed in a separate amnionic sac.

placenta
umbilical cord
chorion
amnion

**Fraternal**
When two different ovum are fertilized by two different sperm, fraternal twins are formed. They are not always the same sex and each has a distinct genetic makeup. Babies usually have separate placentas, each having an umbilical cord but may have the same placenta.

is barely mentioned in one of the major textbooks of obstetrics commonly used in this country. The chance of a woman having triplets is one in 8,000, and the chance of quadruplets is one in 700,000 pregnancies.

For infertility patients using drugs to cause ovulation, however, the statistics are quite different. Women who use clomiphene to ovulate have a 10 percent chance of conceiving twins, rather than the normal 1-percent chance. The chance of their having triplets is 0.5 percent, and there is 0.3 percent chance of conceiving four or more babies.

In the past seventeen years, with all my clomiphene patients, there has been only one set of triplets; this is in spite of the fact that I administer clomiphene quite often.

Clomiphene is not the fertility drug that causes most of the multiple births you hear about. The drug that causes three-, four-, five-, or six-baby pregnancies is usually Pergonal. Modern techniques of administering this drug are making pregnancies of more than triplets much less common than in the past.

Women who conceive by in vitro fertilization (test-tube-baby technique) also have

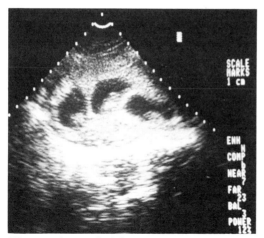

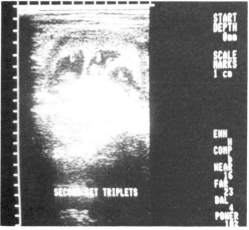

Ultrasound scan of triplets.

Ultrasound scan of triplets.

a chance of a multiple pregnancy. (For complete information on fertility drugs and techniques, see chapter 11.)

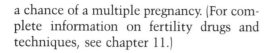

### 323 How are the pregnancy and delivery of more than two babies handled?

Very carefully! A multiple pregnancy requires more frequent visits to the doctor's office and more pelvic examinations. A woman must have more bed rest to keep her cervix from dilating too early. As in the case of a twin pregnancy, frequent bed rest decreases the chance of premature birth. The mothers must be carefully watched for toxemia, because toxemia is more prevalent with a multiple pregnancy.

The possibility of delivering by cesarean section is greater with a multiple birth, and most obstetricians would not argue with any physician who wanted to do a cesarean section for three or more babies before labor ever begins.

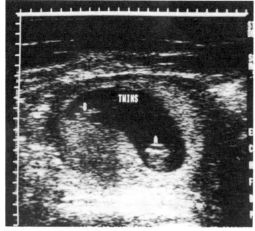

Ultrasound scan of twins.

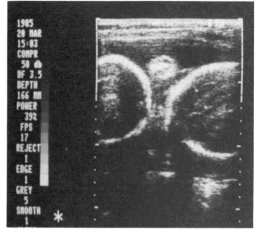

Ultrasound scan of twins in twenty-seventh week of development.

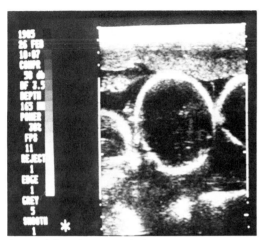
Same triplets three months later.

## Miscarriage

**324** **What is a miscarriage and how often does it occur?**

*Miscarriage* is the term used to describe the spontaneous ending of a pregnancy before the twentieth week of pregnancy. Medical persons call this a spontaneous abortion. Abortion actually means the end of a pregnancy, by an abortionist or by miscarriage, before the twentieth week of pregnancy. (See Q. 223.)

Miscarriages occur in 10–20 percent of pregnancies that are far enough along for a woman to know that she is pregnant. Now that pregnancies can be diagnosed so early by serum pregnancy tests and ultrasound scans, we know that miscarriages actually occur much more often than 20 percent of the time. A study done by Dr. D. Keith Edmonds at South Hampton General Hospital in England showed that 62 percent of all pregnancies were lost within the first twelve weeks of pregnancy! Most of these, of course, occurred before the mother was even aware that she was pregnant. These early

pregnancies, and their loss, were detected with serum pregnancy tests.

What this means is that you may "lose" many fertilized eggs, pregnancies that you will never know about. According to Nathan Kase, M.D., of Mount Sinai Medical Center in New York City, this loss of fertilized eggs is probably due to defects in either the egg or the sperm that would prevent normal development of the baby during the next few months.

Women often ask me if the heavy periods they are having each month are miscarriages. This is most unlikely. If the pregnancy is a very early pregnancy at the time you lose it, whether before or at the time of your period, you would probably not notice any unusual bleeding or change in menstrual flow.

**325** **What might cause the miscarriage of an established pregnancy, one the mother is aware of or that is several weeks along?**

The cause can be due to abnormal hormones (about 23 percent); an abnormality of the uterus that "squeezes the pregnancy out" (about 15 percent); abnormalities of the baby (25 percent); and unknown reasons (about 37 percent).

**326** **If I have had a previous miscarriage, will I ever be able to carry a pregnancy? Should further testing be done?**

The facts are quite well confirmed that usually after one miscarriage, there is nothing you need to do. Your next pregnancy will, in all probability, be a normal pregnancy with a normal delivery.

Even more surprisingly, the same good chance of eventually having a baby still holds after a second (or third or fourth) miscarriage. This is sometimes referred to as habitual abortion. The encouraging statistic is that even if you have had four miscarriages in a row, you still have a 60 percent chance of having a live baby in the next pregnancy.

These statistics, though, do not mean that studies and tests on women who are having miscarriages should not be done. They should. If a woman is thirty years or older and has one miscarriage, I will usually recommend some tests. When the woman is younger than thirty, I usually do not suggest any testing after one miscarriage. This is because women who are over thirty, and therefore have "less time to waste," need to be sure there is nothing wrong or get the problem treated as quickly as possible if one exists.

Women under thirty generally feel that they have a little bit more time to see how things turn out with the next pregnancy. Although statistically most women who have miscarriages will eventually have a normal pregnancy, some do have abnormalities which cause their miscarriages.

---

**327** **What does an evaluation for the problem of miscarriage involve?**

Such an evaluation involves several things:

- A pelvic examination is done to make sure there are no tumors, cysts, or growths in the pelvis;
- An X-ray of the uterus (hystero-salpingogram, HSG) is done to make sure that the uterus is formed properly. A uterus with a septum can abort a pregnancy, even though the baby and placenta may be healthy.
- A general evaluation for existing or potential medical problems is made. For example, thyroid disease, diabetes, and collagen-vascular diseases such as lupus erythematosus should be looked for because they can cause miscarriage.

- A D&C and diagnostic laparoscopy may be done to guarantee the absence of pelvic disease, endometriosis, or severe pelvic adhesions that might cause miscarriage.
- The presence of mycoplasma and chlamydia germs is considered since they can cause miscarriages. Although culture for these organisms is possible, laboratories frequently will not find them even when they are present. I usually treat a patient who has repeated miscarriages with a tetracycline or erythromycin antibiotic in case those germs are there.
- Testing for inadequate hormones is done, using a basal body thermometer, or a test to measure the progesterone in the blood stream or an endometrial biopsy. If a patient seems to have inadequate hormone production in the last half of her menstrual cycle (the luteal phase), progesterone vaginal suppositories can be used to try to correct the problem and prevent further miscarriages.
- Genetic testing on the mother and the father may be conducted, because if either has abnormal genes and cannot produce normal eggs or sperm, this can result in a baby that is abnormal enough to be miscarried. The testing is expensive (about $1,000 for the couple) and, if there is a genetic problem, it cannot be corrected. The only course of action would be artificial insemination with donor sperm if the husband had the problem, or adoption.

All these tests are usually not necessary for every patient. I would do part of the testing if a woman over thirty miscarries once and wants to undergo the testing. If a woman is under thirty, and has had two miscarriages or more, I would suggest some of the testing. In both situations I am referring to a woman who has never had a baby. If a woman has had a previous full-term, healthy, normal baby and later has a miscarriage or two, I would probably not suggest any testing because she has proven that she and her husband have all the ingredients necessary for producing a baby. If such a couple continue having miscarriages, then it would be wise to do some testing.

## 328 What is a midtrimester loss of pregnancy, and what might cause it?

A midtrimester pregnancy loss is a loss of the pregnancy during the middle three months; it is much more likely to be due to an abnormality of the uterus than is a miscarriage in the first three months. If a pregnancy loss occurs this far along, a medical evaluation should be done.

Some of the things this evaluation might reveal include an abnormal uterus; a fibroid tumor in the uterus; or an incompetent cervical os (cervix not strong enough to hold the pregnancy). (See Q. 420.)

If an incompetent cervical os exists, it would be wise for you to have a minor operation, a cerclage procedure, either before or during your next pregnancy. In this operation a suture is put around your cervix in purse-string fashion to keep the cervix closed.

If an abnormal uterus (tumor, structural abnormality, scarring inside) is discovered, you should have the problem corrected surgically. This usually calls for major surgery, but can possibly be accomplished by hysteroscopic surgery. (See Q. 919, 920.)

Although most miscarriages in the middle three months are due to abnormalities of the structure of the uterus, approximately 25 percent of them are due to abnormalities of the baby's chromosomes. In this situation the abnormalities are not severe enough to cause early miscarriage but may cause loss of the pregnancy before it reaches full term.

## 329 Can chromosome abnormalities cause loss of pregnancy in the last three months also?

Yes. This is much less common, causing only about 5 percent of the pregnancies lost during the last three months. Of course, if a baby who is chromosomally abnormal is not delivered so early that it dies of prematurity, it will be born with its abnormality, such as Down's syndrome or Turner's syndrome.

## 330 How is it determined that my miscarriages are genetically abnormal, or that I or my husband have abnormal genes? What can we do?

Tissue from a miscarriage can be examined by a geneticist and, if there are genetic abnormalities, they will be identified. This evaluation is not frequently done, as it is expensive and cannot usually determine conclusively that your next pregnancy will have the same problem. Therefore this type of study is not usually recommended, nor is it usually useful.

If you or your husband have been tested and have been found to have genetic abnormalities, consult a geneticist who may recommend artificial insemination if the husband has the genetic problem or adoption if the wife is genetically abnormal.

Genetic engineering is still a far-distant development. At the present time there is no way to alter genes to insure a genetically normal baby.

## 331 How will I know if I am having a miscarriage? What should I do if I think I am?

Vaginal bleeding may be the first indication of a miscarriage. Occasionally there will also be cramping. If you begin to bleed, call your doctor. He or she will probably want to examine you. If you are not bleeding heavily and are not cramping, you may be asked to wait until the next morning to come to the office for an exam.

— Less than half the pregnant women who bleed in early pregnancy actually miscarry. Pregnant women will bleed occasionally at the time they would have had a menstrual period, and sometimes each month for several months during the first part of their pregnancy. This bleeding is implantation bleeding, meaning that as the placenta is "eating its way" into the wall of your uterus to implant itself, it causes bleeding. This invasion of the uterine wall is necessary for a normal pregnancy because the placenta must implant itself in order to provide food and oxygen for the baby.

Significant bleeding in the early part of pregnancy (the first three months) is often referred to by obstetricians as a threatened abortion. Bleeding as heavy or heavier than a normal period, will often be given this name because it so often ends up as a miscarriage. If you do not miscarry, the bleeding will not have hurt your baby. This bleeding is not from inside the sac where the baby is located. It comes from the area between the placenta and the wall of the uterus. So do not worry about the baby. Just be thankful that your bleeding stopped and that you did not miscarry.

If you should begin bleeding in the middle three months or midtrimester of your pregnancy, when you have had no bleeding before, it is imperative that you let your doctor know immediately. This slight bleeding, with perhaps mild cramping, may be a sign that your cervix is dilating. If this is the case, and the pregnancy is otherwise healthy, your doctor may be able to hospitalize you and close your cervix with stitches to help hold the pregnancy. (See Q. 328, 420.)

---

**332** **What might my doctor advise if he or she thinks I may be going to miscarry?**

After examination, your doctor will proba-

bly advise you to stay in bed for two or three days and get up only to use the bathroom. He or she will also suggest that you not have intercourse until about a week after the bleeding has stopped.

Unless it is felt that you have a hormone deficiency, most doctors will not want you to take any hormones. Hormones do not help prevent miscarriage, except where there is a definite hormone inadequacy.

If you continue to bleed after resting for several days, my feeling is that you may as well get up and go on about your business. If the fetus is healthy, it will "stay" whether or not you get up and return to normal activities. If it is not a healthy fetus, losing it is inevitable; bed rest will not prevent the loss of an abnormal fetus.

— If after bed rest you still have a slight increase in bleeding (only an occasional change of your pad), and you are not cramping, there is no urgent need to go back to the doctor. Even if there is increased bleeding with slight cramping, there is nothing the doctor can do until he or she knows for sure you are miscarrying.

If you continue to have increasingly heavy bleeding, especially with significant cramping, you are probably going to miscarry soon. If your water breaks (amniotic fluid surrounds the fetus even in the first few months of pregnancy, and this small bag can break, resulting in a gush of fluid), this means you will definitely miscarry. Call your doctor immediately.

---

**333** **What will the doctor do if it is certain I am going to miscarry?**

Once it is established that you are miscarrying, your doctor will do a D&C, dilatation of the cervix and curettement (scraping) of the uterus. The material inside your uterus is already degenerating; if it is not removed it can cause heavy bleeding or infection. An infection in the uterus can cause scarring and damage to the uterus and the fallopian tubes, which could limit your ability to get pregnant later. With new and improved suction apparatus, many doctors now are doing the curettement on an outpatient basis or in their offices.

However, if your miscarriage occurs only a few days past your first missed period, your uterus is very small, you are not bleeding much, and you are not passing too much tissue, you may not need a D&C. Frequently even if it appears that you have had a "complete" miscarriage, there may be continued spotting and bleeding for many days. If this goes on for more than a few days, it is probably best for you to go ahead with a D&C of the uterus to remove any remaining tissue.

## 334 What is a "missed abortion"?

A missed abortion occurs when a fetus dies and the uterus does not expel the pregnancy tissue. This happens fairly frequently. There may be no cramping or bleeding at all.

In this situation, the woman will stop being nauseated (if she has been having nausea) and her uterus will stop growing. She will even lose a little bit of weight. If the woman feels that something is wrong or that the pregnancy is not progressing, or if the doctor determines that the uterus is not growing, an ultrasound (sonogram) will probably be ordered.

If the sonogram shows that the fetus has died, the doctor will want to use a suction machine to withdraw the pregnancy tissue from your uterus. If the material is not removed, an infection or a dangerous coagulation problem—disseminated intravascular coagulation (DIC)—can develop (See Q. 647). For your health, as in the case of a "regular" miscarriage, the doctor will want to be sure that all the material is removed.

## 335 Is it normal for me to feel so emotional about my miscarriage?

Yes, definitely, since you have experienced, in effect, the death of a child, one you loved and wanted to hold in your arms. Your sadness and sense of loss are to be expected for several months. Feeling as if you have lost a child may remain for the rest of your life.

A miscarriage is often treated by friends and medical personnel as "just one of those things"; something that is not as important as you feel that it is. Quite normally, they will forget it sooner than you do. Many women, however, have had miscarriages themselves. They know how you feel, whether or not they can express their empathy.

It is especially normal to feel sad on the day your child would have been born if you had not miscarried, especially the first time that date occurs. Knowing this can help you prepare yourself and your husband for it.

This is an especially helpful book: *When Pregnancy Fails—Families Coping with Miscarriage, Stillbirth, and Infant Death* by Borg and Lasker (Boston: Beacon Press) 1981.

There are support groups (SHARE) for couples who have suffered miscarriages or stillbirth. For more information write: Sister Jane Marie Lamb, SHARE, St. John's Hospital, 800 E. Carpenter St., Springfield, Ill. 62769.

## 336 What can I say to help a friend who has had a miscarriage?

The following excellent suggestions, written by Leslie Snodgrass were published in *Stepping Stones*, an infertility newsletter, (Wichita, Kansas: Oct. 1982).

1. Don't avoid a loved one who is hurting simply because you're afraid you won't know what to say! The Lord gives us grace and wisdom for each moment (see Exod.

4:12), and the feeling of being alone and forgotten during such a difficult time only adds insult to injury.

2. Don't assume your friend doesn't want to talk about it! Chances are, she probably does. I have found that talking about it, re-living the details, helps the person to face the reality of the loss and this is an integral part of the healing process. You can't *assume* she *does* want to talk either, so you must be sensitive to what she says (or doesn't say).

3. If she does want to talk about it, let her! Often, those with the best intentions find themselves filling in an awkward moment by recounting their own personal tragedies, blurting out suggestions or throwing out scriptural reminders without allowing the person in need to get a word in edgewise. *Listening* is the key word; in doing so, you'll be able to learn what your friend's special need is. (What is she having trouble coping with—the loss itself, why God allowed it to happen, whether she did something wrong, whether it is wrong to be angry, etc.?)

4. Don't assume you have all the answers to her questions (or feel inadequate if you don't)! You may not have the answer because the Lord wants your friend to find it in Him. Miscarriage or loss of a child often leads one to feel alone (even with a multitude of family and friends), or abandoned, or even angry. The insatiable need to know the "why" to a myriad of questions will draw her into the arms of the only Person with the answers which give relief to the pain.

5. Do remind her she's loved and being thought of often! You don't have to camp on her doorstep to show her you care. Besides being physically worn-out, she needs time alone, too. Pray for creative ways to show her you care; for example, a ready-to-heat meal is a blessing after a stay in the hospital. A flower stuck in the mailbox with a note attached is a pleasant surprise, or what about a series of unsigned postcards with comforting scriptures?

6. Don't use cliches! They may or may not be true, but more often than not they come out sounding callous and insensitive. For example:

a. "It's probably for the best." To someone whose hopes and dreams for a child have just been shattered, no matter what the reason, it's hard to believe it could be for the best. (While it may be true, it's a statement that hurts more than helps.)

b. "You're young, you'll be able to have more." Again, it probably is true, but the fact is that even if more children do come along, it doesn't mean the one lost didn't mean as much. Just because it was a life unborn, didn't mean it was any less a life already loved and cherished.

c. "Don't give up, I had a friend who lost two, but then carried a baby full term." This is meant to be hopeful, but what it says is "be glad, it could be worse." It is true, I'm sure, but it also says that the pain they just endured could very possibly happen again. Hurt isn't minimized by comparison. It's a concept that works well in theory but not in practice. Your friend is trying hard to overcome her own grief—she doesn't need to try to work through someone else's!

d. "Time will take care of it." Time may heal the wound, but the memory will probably last forever. I lost my baby three years ago, and have been blest with a beautiful daughter since, but I haven't forgotten.

7. Do continue to be sensitive to your friend's loss in the months that follow. In my own case, it took a while for the initial shock to wear off and when it did, I was left with an incredible emptiness. I needed to be constantly reminded that the Lord loved me, and that He hadn't forgotten me. My loss was more difficult because I knew how long it had taken me to get pregnant, and it took several years to get pregnant again. Special friends and family continued to pray, and I was sustained by those prayers.

If you continue to find yourself emotionally

torn by your miscarriage, see a counselor. Your intense feelings do not mean that you are abnormal. A counselor can often help you, sometimes after just one or two visits, and I suggest that you take advantage of that help if you need it.

## Molar Pregnancy

### 337 What is a molar pregnancy?

Molar pregnancies, invasive molar pregnancies, and malignant molar pregnancies are growths that result from abnormal pregnancies referred to as trophoblastic diseases. Doctors often use the term *mole* to describe some of these problems; this has nothing whatever to do with a mole on the surface of the skin. The term *trophoblastic disease* is derived from the name of the trophoblast cell, the cell that makes up the placenta.

"Molar pregnancy" is the informal term for what doctors call hydatidiform mole: an abnormal pregnancy in which there is no baby, just an abnormal placenta. As it grows, segments of the placenta (chorionic villi) swell into cloudy, grapelike structures. Often all the chorionic villi change into these cystic structures. When this happens, the uterus becomes literally filled with hundreds of these small, fluid-filled sacs. These little growths are shaped like green seedless grapes and are often about the same size.

About half the time a molar pregnancy results in an apparently normal miscarriage. When this happens, treatment would be the same as with a normal miscarriage. Unless you were told, you would not know that you had had a molar pregnancy instead of the more usual type of miscarriage.

The 50 percent of women who do not miscarry a molar pregnancy may have other problems that indicate an abnormal pregnancy. They may have bleeding; the uterus may grow faster than it should, indicating development of the multiple cysts; or it may not grow as fast as would be expected. When a pregnancy seems to be developing in an abnormal fashion, the doctor will ordinarily order an ultrasound scan. This scan can usually show that a hydatidiform mole is present.

Molar pregnancies are not extremely rare. They occur in about one out of every two thousand pregnancies in the United States. Each country, strangely, seems to have its own rate for this problem. Some countries have fewer cases and some have more cases than the United States.

### 338 How is a molar pregnancy treated?

If your molar pregnancy shows up as a miscarriage, a D&C would be done. If your molar pregnancy was discovered by ultrasound because the pregnancy was not growing properly, the doctor would probably give you general anesthesia and use a suction machine to curette the tissue from your uterus.

After the molar pregnancy has been removed from your uterus, the doctor will want to do blood tests for human chorionic gonadotrophin (HCG). See also the discussion about therapy for malignant moles, Q. 339–343. Immediately after the D&C is done, the doctor will order an HCG test. HCG is produced by the cells of a molar pregnancy. From then on, you will probably have an HCG test every week until you have had three consecutive normal tests. Following that you should have an HCG test every month for six months, and then every other month for six more months to make sure all abnormal tissue is gone from your body.

If your HCG level stops falling and stays the same for three consecutive weeks, or if it starts rising, you need to be treated with chemotherapy, just as does a woman who has a malignant mole. You should have normal HCG levels three to four months after having had the D&C, but it may take several months for the HCG levels to return to normal. The important thing is that your doctor be aware of the importance of following your HCG levels if you have had a mole and makes sure that they do go down to normal.

## 339 What is invasive molar pregnancy?

An invasive mole (chorioadenoma destruens) is a condition that is halfway between a molar pregnancy and a true malignant mole. The molar tissue grows into the wall of the uterus, but under the microscope the cells look more like molar tissue that has grown down into the wall of the uterus than they do malignant molar cells.

Remember, in order for the placenta to implant itself in the wall of the uterus to establish a normal pregnancy, it must be able to invade the mother's uterine wall. When trophoblasts start growing abnormally, however, they can become invasive, even highly invasive.

This molar growth that has become mildly invasive requires chemotherapy. Occasionally, but rarely, a hysterectomy might be necessary because the growth may perforate the uterine wall and cause bleeding.

## 340 What is a malignant molar pregnancy?

A malignant mole is called a choriocarcinoma. This is a condition in which the trophoblastic cells have become cancerous. A malignant mole starts growing only in women who are or have been pregnant, and can occur after a molar pregnancy or after a normal pregnancy. It can also occur after a miscarriage or after a tubal pregnancy. Doctors know that this type of growth always

starts with a pregnancy, but it may not be detected until many months after a pregnancy is over. I realize that this is confusing; it also confuses physicians. One of my patients was found to have a choriocarcinoma growing in her lungs months after a normal pregnancy. She had been admitted to the hospital for tiredness, and a chest X-ray showed the growth.

This malignancy of the trophoblastic cells is the most invasive type of cancer that can occur in humans. If treatment is delayed, or if a woman does not respond to proper treatment, this can be a truly devastating malignancy. Before treatment was available, almost everyone with this cancer died very quickly. On the other hand, because the cells of this tumor grow so fast (much faster than normal cells), they are more responsive to chemotherapy than most other cancer cells; the cure rate with chemotherapy is almost 100 percent, better than with any other solid tumor that can spread in the body.

## 341 How would I be treated if I had a malignant molar pregnancy?

It is essential that you be treated promptly and properly. If this type of tumor is allowed to grow for very long, it can be irreversible.

Treatment is with chemotherapeutic drugs. You would be referred to a specialist in the use of these drugs. He or she would discuss with you which drugs you need and what their side effects are.

Your doctor will want you to have blood tests done frequently to see how much tumor is left in your body during each step of the treatment. Remember that placental cells, even those of malignant molar tissue, produce the hormone human chorionic gonadotrophin (HCG). This is the hormone identified by a pregnancy test. (See Q. 301.) The production of HCG by only a few thousand placental or molar cells can be detected with the test. The doctor will want to keep treating you and testing you until all signs of HCG and, therefore, all vestiges of the choriocarcinoma have been eliminated from your body.

If your doctor does not test for HCG on a regular, organized basis during your treatment, he or she does not understand how to care for this type of tumor. In this situation you should seek further consultation. I suggest that you phone a cancer hospital, such as M. D. Anderson Cancer Hospital in Houston, Texas, and talk with one of the physicians in the department of gynecology.

### 342 What is the drug cure rate for molar pregnancies, invasive molar pregnancies, and malignant molar pregnancies?

The results are good. For a regular molar pregnancy that must, for some reason, be treated, the cure rate is 100 percent. For an invasive mole (chorioadenoma destruens), the cure rate is also 100 percent. For a malignant mole, the cure rate is 100 percent if the mole has been contained within the uterus and has not spread to any other part of the body.

With proper chemotherapy, one is almost guaranteed a complete cure. Once a cure is effected, a woman is able to stop the chemotherapy and live a normal life in the future. Chemotherapy, in this particular situation, is almost always effective and worth taking.

### 343 If I have had a molar pregnancy, should I avoid future pregnancies?

You must not become pregnant until your HCG level has become normal and stayed normal. It is best that you use birth-control pills to prevent pregnancy until such normal test results have been obtained. Birth-control pills will not affect the test result.

Once the tests have become normal and stayed normal, you should consult with your physician about the advisability of pregnancy. Generally it is safe to say that if you have had a hydatidiform mole or invasive molar pregnancy, you can become pregnant once the tests have stayed normal for more than a year. If you have had a choriocarcinoma, a pregnancy may be allowed after an extended length of time. The decision about getting pregnant again must be made after careful consultation with your physician.

## Ectopic Pregnancy

### 344 What is an ectopic pregnancy and how often does it occur?

An ectopic pregnancy is one that is developing anywhere outside of the uterus. About eight in a thousand pregnancies are ectopic, and the rate is increasing rapidly.

Ectopic pregnancies occur in the fallopian tube 95 percent of the time. The remaining 5 percent may be in an ovary, in the abdominal cavity, or in the cervix.

In an April 1983 American Medical Association journal, an editorial by David Eschenback, M.D., and Janet Daling, Ph.D., pointed out that there has been a dramatic increase in the number of ectopic pregnancies diagnosed during the past twenty years. In the past ten years there has been a twofold increase in the rate of ectopic pregnancies, and in the past five years this rate has been increasing even faster.

# Ectopic Pregnancy

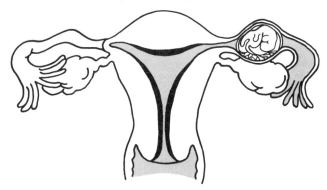

## 345 Why do ectopic pregnancies occur, and why are they increasing?

Ectopic pregnancies can be caused by abnormalities of the tube due to infection, scarring, poor development, inability to transport the egg, or tumors. Or they may result from failure of the egg to get into the tube. The egg can be fertilized outside the tube.

The increased rate of ectopic pregnancies seems to be related to things that are going on in our society. Changed sexual mores have produced more venereal disease (which includes infections in the uterus and tubes), the use of the IUD (intrauterine contraceptive device) has increased, and the number of abortions has increased. In addition, infertility treatment, such as surgery to repair damaged or blocked fallopian tubes, surgery to reverse sterilizations, and the use of fertility pills and drugs is more common. Finally, more women over thirty are having babies. All of these factors have been shown to increase the rate of tubal pregnancies.

## 346 What happens with a tubal pregnancy, and is a tubal pregnancy dangerous?

The only place where a baby can safely grow to term size is in the cavity of the uterus. There is no other place in the body where a placenta can properly implant and erode its way into the surrounding tissue to gain adequate nutrition, and enlargement can occur that is adequate to hold a baby at all stages of pregnancy.

When a pregnancy begins in the fallopian tube, rupture of that tube will occur before many days have passed. The tube can stretch only a small amount. When the tube stretches, the growing placenta pulls loose and bleeding starts. This detachment of the placenta kills the fetus, and the bleeding that occurs will often continue until the mother either dies or has surgery. Occasionally, when surgery is done for an ectopic tubal pregnancy, a fetus will be found, but usually none is seen in the tissue.

Although from 10 percent to 50 percent of ectopic pregnancies, if left alone, would be absorbed back into the body, it would be dangerous to allow the ectopic pregnancy to continue to see if this occurs. Tubal pregnancies will grow to the point where the tube ruptures, causing excessive bleeding and even death. In 1978 there were thirty-seven deaths in the United States from ectopic pregnancy, amounting to 11.5 percent of *all* deaths from pregnancy in this country.

It is most important, therefore, that as soon as an ectopic pregnancy is suspected, a definite conclusion be reached as quickly as possible as to the existence and location of the pregnancy.

Occasionally a woman will have a pregnancy develop from conception in the abdominal cavity. Also occasionally, a tubal pregnancy will be squeezed by its tube out into the abdominal cavity without the mother knowing it. Here the pregnancy can grow and the baby can develop. A pregnancy that is developing in the abdominal cavity can grow to near term size, but most abdominal pregnancies do not carry to full term because of bleeding and pain. The placenta must attach to something as it develops. That attachment can be to portions of the intestine, the outside of the uterus, the ovaries, or the lining of the abdominal cavity. There will be bleeding from these different areas as the placenta pulls and tears during the stretch and strain of the mother's normal activities. The bleeding can cause abdominal pain.

---

## 347 What are the symptoms of an ectopic pregnancy?

You should suspect an ectopic pregnancy if you miss a menstrual period or seem to have a delayed period, and then have vaginal spotting or bleeding and pain in the lower abdomen. The flow may be heavy and the pain intense, or there may be only spotting and minimal pain. If a menstrual period is missed or was much lighter than normal, and you know there is a possibility of your being pregnant, you should contact your doctor immediately when you begin bleeding from the vagina and experience low abdominal pain.

It is important that a diagnosis be made before a tubal rupture, if possible. An early diagnosis can prevent loss of blood, but, more importantly, it can prevent loss of the fallopian tube and ovary.

---

## 348 How is an ectopic pregnancy diagnosed?

Your doctor should suspect an ectopic pregnancy if you experience the symptoms just described, and a diagnosis can be made, based on his or her suspicion of a tubal pregnancy. The procedure for diagnosing an ectopic pregnancy has changed dramatically in the past few years. It is now possible to locate a tubal pregnancy in its early stages, which means that an ectopic pregnancy can often be found before it ruptures. A ruptured tube can cause excessive loss of blood and possible death; in addition, rupture of the tube may make surgical removal of the tube necessary.

If you have a positive pregnancy test but the doctor cannot detect anything in either fallopian tube or in your uterus, a quantitative HCG test may be ordered to measure the amount of pregnancy hormone in your body. The test will be repeated in forty-eight hours because in a normal pregnancy the amount of HCG present in your bloodstream will double every forty-eight-hour period. If the HCG has not doubled, you are having a very early miscarriage or an ectopic pregnancy. An ultrasound may be ordered. The doctor may then scrape some material out of your uterus. If there is no pregnancy tissue in your uterus, the pregnancy is present somewhere else and the most likely place is a fallopian tube (ectopic pregnancy). The doctor will then do one of the following procedures.

*Culdecentesis.* In the office, the physician can take a small needle and push it through the upper vagina up inside your body behind the uterus. If you have a tubal pregnancy and are bleeding inside, blood will collect in the space behind the uterus. The doctor can find blood there just by inserting the needle into that space. A local anesthetic will keep this from hurting too much. The presence of blood strongly suggests the presence of an ectopic pregnancy, and the doctor will proceed with an operation to remove the ectopic pregnancy tissue. Occasionally the presence of blood can be from a bleeding ovary; surgery would still be warranted in this situation.

*Laparoscopy.* By looking through a laparoscope at the inside of your abdomen, the doctor can see whether or not there is a tubal pregnancy. (See Q. 907.)

## 349 What will my doctor do if an ectopic pregnancy is found?

What is done depends on the doctor's training, at what point the ectopic pregnancy is discovered, and on its location.

**Early tubal ectopic pregnancy.** Ideally, you will have gone to your doctor early in your pregnancy, and your doctor will suspect right away that a tubal pregnancy exists. If from a laparoscopy he or she can determine that the tube has not ruptured, and may be able to use the laparoscope to make a small incision on one side of the tube, suck out the tissue, cauterize the edges of the incision, and thus avoid major surgery.

More commonly though, the doctor will have to open the abdomen to cut out the portion of the tube that contains the ectopic pregnancy tissue. Some physicians sew the tube back together; others leave the tube tied off, coming back later, if necessary, to repair the tube. Statistics are not yet conclusive as to which is the best method of treatment.

It is possible that the laparoscopy will reveal a ruptured tube and, if so, it will be necessary that the damaged portion of the tube be cut out. If the tube is badly distorted, the entire tube will probably need to be removed. Occasionally also the ovary will have to be removed.

If your doctor does not know how to do a laparoscopy, and does not have a consultant that can do one, you should allow him to operate through a regular incision if a tubal pregnancy is diagnosed.

**Late tubal ectopic pregnancy.** All tubal ectopic pregnancies are not detected early. Some patients will have mild early symptoms that they hardly notice, and doctors can easily miss the significance of the early signs and symptoms of ectopic pregnancy. When these early warnings are missed, the fetus and/or placental tissue will grow until finally the tube ruptures, pouring blood into the woman's abdomen and throwing her into shock.

The doctor will proceed immediately with a major incision in the woman's abdomen to remove the fetus and/or placental tissue as quickly as possible to save her life. He will not even wait to get blood ready for a transfusion. When a tube ruptures, it is usually ruined. Frequently the ovary and surrounding tissues become scarred together. Removal of both the tube and the ovary is occasionally necessary. When the portion of the tube affected is the part that goes through the wall of the uterus, a hole may have been blown out of the uterus at that site. This means a hysterectomy is necessary. This is, indeed, a life-or-death situation.

**Ovarian ectopic pregnancy.** Ovarian pregnancies do not occur very often, but when they do, they mimic a tubal pregnancy in almost every respect. The tube is not involved unless scarring and blood clots have affected it. The ovary will usually need to be removed entirely, but it is occasionally possible to save part of it.

**Abdominal ectopic pregnancy.** An abdominal pregnancy usually results when the tube ruptures and the placenta continues to grow from the tube to other organs. The baby, still enclosed in the sac, continues to grow. Finally, because the woman bleeds and experiences pain, surgery will be recommended and will reveal the ectopic pregnancy.

Normally the doctor will open the sac, remove the baby (which is rarely developed enough to live), and leave the placenta in place. Attempting to remove the placenta is extremely dangerous; bleeding will occur at every spot where the placenta is attached. The incision is closed. After a few days or weeks, the placenta will have separated and further surgery can remove it. This is safer than trying to remove the placenta at the time of the initial surgery. If infection occurs in the abdomen containing the placenta, surgery is necessary to remove the placenta and clear up the infection.

*Cervical ectopic pregnancy.* Cervical pregnancies are extremely rare. Because the placenta actually grows into the tissues of the cervix, it is almost impossible to remove the placenta without taking the cervix. The cervix, of course, is part of the uterus; removing the cervix, therefore, means removing the entire uterus: a hysterectomy.

## 350 What are the long-term effects of a tubal pregnancy?

The effects of a tubal pregnancy are both statistical and emotional.

There are some statistical effects on the woman's future ability to have a child. About 50 percent of women who have had an ectopic pregnancy later develop infertility problems. Then, even if a pregnancy does occur, the chance of carrying the baby to term is less than average.

There is also a 10-15 percent risk of having another ectopic pregnancy, probably because if one fallopian tube is so abnormal that it traps an egg, the other tube is probably also abnormal.

Deep emotional response to an ectopic pregnancy is not only reasonable but normal. First, for a pregnancy to end like this is, at the least, a disappointment. Second, you realize from the statistics that an ectopic pregnancy does affect your future chance of having a normal pregnancy. Finally, you must cope with the depressing effects of anesthetics and pain medications.

If you remain depressed and bothered following a tubal pregnancy, I strongly encourage you to get counsel. Certainly you, your husband, and your doctor need to talk about the way you feel. Don't let yourself go into a downward spiral emotionally. Help is available for you.

## General Medical Disorders During Pregnancy

## 351 Are there any specific medical and surgical problems related to being pregnant?

Yes. There are a few medical problems to which you may be more susceptible during pregnancy, such as infections in your urinary tract, but generally any medical or surgical problem that might affect you when you are not pregnant can also affect you while you are pregnant. Some of these problems can have a specific effect on your pregnancy and perhaps on your baby. Pregnancy may worsen some existing medical problems.

In this series of questions, we will be looking at two groups of problems: those conditions that pregnancy aggravates for the mother, and those problems of the mother that may affect the baby.

## 352 What is the most common medical problem during pregnancy?

Infections of the bladder and urinary-tract infections in general are probably the most common problems that you might encounter during pregnancy, other than the common cold.

Pregnancy causes the bladder to empty more slowly and drainage of urine from the kidneys is likely to be more lethargic, because of both hormonal changes and pressure of the pregnancy on the organs. Also, the urethra—the tube that empties your bladder—is short, so it is easy for germs to get from the vulva into your bladder and from there into your kidneys.

Because the urine is moving slowly, the germs have more time to start growing in the urine and to cause infection. As this is a common occurrence, most doctors routinely use a dipstick to check your urine on each visit to the office. This test also checks for diabetes and albumin.

When infection is found in the urinary tract, it is important that it be treated and then rechecked to be sure it has cleared up. Otherwise a kidney infection may result. A severe kidney infection can cause premature labor.

Your doctor should not treat you with tetracycline after the third month of pregnancy (it can stain the baby's teeth and bones). It is also important that you not use sulfa drugs during the last few weeks of pregnancy. If the baby is born while you are taking sulfa, any jaundice the baby might develop in its first few days of life can be more dangerous.

## 353 Is it safe to become pregnant after having had a kidney transplant?

I have taken care of two women who became pregnant after they had kidney transplants. Both did quite well during pregnancy, and most physicians report the same success in like situations.

The worry has been that the immunosuppression drugs taken by those who have had such transplants, which must be used even during pregnancy, could have some long-term effect on the baby. At this point, however, it seems that babies born to mothers who have had kidney transplants are usually normal.

## 354 What is anemia? Why is it so frequently a problem during pregnancy?

Anemia merely means that you have a low concentration of hemoglobin, the compound in your blood that carries oxygen. Normally hemoglobin should be 12 grams (or more) per 100 ml of blood. It is normal for

pregnant women to be a little bit anemic because the increased amount of fluid in the blood-vessel system dilutes the hemoglobin, making the actual count a little lower than twelve.

Almost all doctors recommend that their patients take iron during pregnancy. The baby absorbs iron from the mother's blood stream and it is a good idea for the mother to take supplemental iron to replace that loss.

If a mother is at all deficient in folic acid, she will not be able to make enough hemoglobin even if she has adequate iron in her system. For this reason, almost all prenatal vitamins contain some folic acid. If you develop a significant anemia in spite of taking adequate iron and folic acid, you need to see a hematologist, a specialist in problems of the blood.

## 355 What is sickle-cell anemia?

Anemia may be produced by abnormal hemoglobin, and the most common cause of this is sickle-cell disease. A pregnant woman with sickle-cell disease may have attacks of pain, greater anemia, more frequent and more serious infections in the body, and a greater chance of having miscarriages and premature babies.

It has been shown recently, however, that women with sickle-cell disease can tolerate pregnancies better and have healthier babies than was thought possible in the past. To accomplish this, expert medical care is necessary. The care includes careful treatment of infections and treatment of the anemia, perhaps even with transfusions throughout the pregnancy.

In the past this problem has been felt to be severe enough to warrant an abortion, but abortions are done less commonly now because of better care and better results.

## 356 Is it dangerous to become pregnant if I have heart disease?

The chance of a heart patient doing well during pregnancy depends on how serious the heart problem is and the quality of her medical care. Generally, if the heart disease is not severe, these patients need not worry when they become pregnant.

Heart disease is divided into four classifications:

*Class I:* patients with cardiac disease who have no limitation of physical activity

*Class II:* patients with cardiac disease who have slight limitation of physical activity

*Class III:* patients with cardiac disease who have marked limitation of physical activity

*Class IV:* patients with cardiac disease who are unable to perform any physical activity

Patients who have Class I and Class II cardiac disease can usually deliver normally. Ordinarily they will be admitted to the hospital a few days before their delivery date for stabilization of their heart condition.

Patients with Class III heart disease must be cared for very carefully. Abortion is usually considered, but if the woman wants to take the risks of pregnancy and delivery, and she has excellent medical care, it is probably safe to allow the pregnancy to continue. It is, of course, extremely important that she obey precisely her physician's instructions. She likely will need to spend many weeks in the hospital during the pregnancy.

Pregnancy for a woman with Class IV heart disease is extremely dangerous and has a high death rate for both mother and baby. In this situation a therapeutic abortion is indicated. Only if surgery can be done to decrease the severity of a woman's Class IV heart condition should pregnancy be considered. This is a complicated medical problem, and the solution comes only after consultation with specialists in the care of heart disease. Use of contraception is mandatory until such consultation and treatment has been completed.

## 357 What other common problems might be aggravated by pregnancy?

Respiratory problems and respiratory-tract infections are common in pregnancy. These range from the common cold to asthma and include allergies that involve the lungs, nose, and sinuses. A woman who suffers from any of these ailments may have more difficulty during pregnancy, mainly because the use of medication should be restricted. The general rule in pregnancy is to use as few medications as possible. With the common cold it is best to use no medication or, at most, drugs to decrease the amount of congestion.

Saline irrigation is one of the best things you can do for nasal congestion. Mix a teaspoon of salt with a cup of water. Use a baby's nasal syringe to irrigate the nose with this solution. Manufactured solutions, such as Salinex or Ocean Spray, may be used. Additionally, a WaterPik can be used to irrigate the nostrils most effectively; I recommend it.

## 358 What about using nose drops and nose sprays for nasal congestion?

These may be safely used. Afrin, for instance, is a drug that can be used because it is not absorbed into the body if used in proper amounts. It works locally, on the lining of the nose, and is safe during pregnancy. This, of course, is assuming that you are not using too much. If you use too much Afrin, it can be absorbed into your body and cause you to have a slow pulse and low blood pressure, causing dizziness and weakness.

Dependence on Afrin and similar drugs may develop. I suggest that you stop using nose sprays or drops after three days. If you continue using them, your nasal lining may become dependent on them and, from that point on, any time you stop using them you will become congested again, even though the infection is gone. I recommend using these nasal congestion sprays three days on, then three days off.

## 359 What drugs can I take orally to help with congestion during pregnancy?

There are several. Sudaphedrine is a good drug to use during pregnancy. For sneezing and runny nose, PBZ is an antihistamine that is useful and quite safe in pregnancy. Entex is a drug I prescribe a great deal, and it is one that my patients find quite effective.

Remember, though, it is probably best not to use any medication during the first three months of pregnancy because of the possible effects on the baby. After the first three months it is unlikely that these relatively safe drugs could cause a problem.

## 360 Is it advisable for me to take allergy shots during pregnancy?

If a woman who is already taking allergy shots when she becomes pregnant is not having fever, rash, or other problems when she takes her shots, it is fine for her to continue the shots if they are beneficial to her.

If you have not been taking allergy shots, you should not start taking them while you are pregnant. When these shots are given for the first time, a woman does not know whether or not she will have a bad reaction to them. A bad reaction carries a slight risk of causing a miscarriage.

## 361 How is asthma best treated during pregnancy?

Asthma should be treated in such a way that you are comfortable, can sleep well, and are not allowed to become too ill. This will prevent your baby from being affected by your asthma. Your obstetrician and your allergist will work together to insure that your treatment is safe and effective.

## 362 Does labor make asthma worse?

No. As a matter of fact, for some reason asthma during labor is unusual. If a pregnant woman in labor has had a recent asthma attack, though, drugs that she has been taking should be continued. In other words, if she has been using oral theophylline and inhaled cromolyn and dexamethasone, she should continue to do so while she is in labor. If a patient has been taking cortisone prior to labor, she should continue that drug during and after labor.

## 363 Is tuberculosis a problem during pregnancy?

Unless tuberculosis has already produced extensive damage to the body, or unless it is widely disseminated in the body, the pregnancy will usually progress well. As far as it is known, drugs used for tuberculosis can be given during pregnancy without hurting the baby. It is important that if there is any suspicion of active tuberculosis, it should be treated during the pregnancy.

## 364 I have problems with my adrenal glands. How will this affect my pregnancy?

If a woman has had her adrenal glands removed, or if she has disease of her adrenal glands, she needs to be observed carefully during pregnancy, labor and delivery, and after the delivery. If she does not have adequate production of hormones from her adrenal glands, these hormones will need to be supplemented while she is pregnant.

## 365 How does hepatitis affect pregnancy?

Hepatitis can be caused by more than twenty different viruses. The hepatitis that most people develop, however, is caused by either the hepatitis A virus or the hepatitis B virus. In the United States in 1981, hepatitis A occurred in 10 out of every 100,000 people, and hepatitis B occurred in 8 out of every 100,000 people. If a woman develops hepatitis during her pregnancy she will normally recover without any major problem. However, if she is malnourished or does not avail herself of good medical care, the hepatitis can damage her liver extensively and can even be fatal.

If you become sick, begin passing urine that is dark brown (Cola colored), pass stools that are very light gray in color, or if the whites of your eyes become yellow, you need to notify your doctor so that you can be tested for hepatitis and properly treated. Care consists primarily of bed rest and good diet.

If you will be traveling to a country where there is a great deal of hepatitis, you should receive a shot of gamma globulin to prevent being infected.

What we have said to this point applies to both hepatitis A and hepatitis B. If you have hepatitis A the baby is not affected and you will be allowed to breast feed.

If you have hepatitis B, your baby can become infected at the time of delivery. If your baby becomes infected, he or she has an 80–90-percent chance of becoming a carrier of hepatitis for the rest of his or her life. This would be a terrible burden for both you and your child to bear. Since someone can have hepatitis B without knowing it, it is best that all women be tested during pregnancy and before delivery, to see if they have this disease.

A woman who has hepatitis should be tested to see what type of hepatitis she has. If she has hepatitis B, it is important that the baby be given gamma globulin against hepatitis B within one hour of delivery and be started on immunization shots against hepatitis B soon after delivery. Such immunization is quite effective in keeping the baby from developing hepatitis B, and the importance of this treatment for the baby cannot be overemphasized.

A mother may nurse her baby even if she has hepatitis B.

## 366 What is jaundice of pregnancy?

Jaundice of pregnancy is a rare problem. A pregnant woman with this problem becomes jaundiced, but tests show that she does not have hepatitis. One of the primary complaints is itching. After delivery the itching and the jaundice disappear—until the next pregnancy. This problem is a result of the body's inability to handle properly the hormones of pregnancy.

## 367 What is the effect of pregnancy on ulcerative colitis?

Ulcerative colitis, or chronic inflammation of the colon, can be affected in two ways by pregnancy. As many as half of the women who are not having trouble with their ulcerative colitis develop difficulties during pregnancy. A smaller, but significant, number of women, however, have *less* trouble with their ulcerative colitis during pregnancy.

If a colectomy and ileostomy (removal of the colon, with the small intestine made to open to the outside through the abdominal wall) has been done in the past for the treatment of ulcerative colitis, it almost never interferes with pregnancy or delivery.

## 368 How should influenza be treated during pregnancy?

Pregnant women seem more susceptible to influenza, which is one of the reasons proper health care—good food, exercise, vitamins, and rest—should be stressed during pregnancy. The treatment of influenza in pregnancy is similar to that of the common cold. It is important that a woman who has a cold or the flu get adequate rest, plenty of fluids, and, if she develops a more severe cough or has signs of infection in her sinuses, that she begin taking antibiotics. If a woman is working (inside the home or out), it is important that she stop work and rest. A pregnant woman will tire more easily and be more susceptible to illness if she pushes herself too hard. Flu shots are recommended only for pregnant women who have some special medical problem, such as heart disease, lung disease, or some other chronic disease.

## Thrombophlebitis

## 369 Are blood clots in the veins a problem during pregnancy?

Blood clots in the veins occur five and a half times as often in a pregnant woman as in a woman who is not pregnant. This is called thrombophlebitis. These clots are three times as likely to occur during the month after delivery as they are before delivery.

Three things contribute to the development of blood clots in the veins.

*Slower blood flow*. In pregnancy, because of the pressure of the enlarged uterus on the veins, blood flows more slowly from the legs back to the upper body. During the last three months of pregnancy the blood flow in the veins of the legs is only half as fast as the flow in the veins of nonpregnant women.

*Damage to blood vessels by infection.* There is an increased chance of infection developing in the body during and after delivery. If such infection develops, there is an increased chance of blood clots developing in the pelvis. For example, infection can develop in the uterus, even after a normal delivery. A cesarean section can damage the uterine tissue and make it more likely for a woman to have infection in the uterus, ovaries, and tubes.

*Increased tendency to clotting.* In pregnancy the blood clots more easily because of hormonal changes. This is obviously a God-designed mechanism to protect the woman during this period. Immediately after delivery the clotting of the blood inside the uterus, and in any vaginal tears that might be present, keeps a woman from bleeding too much.

This increased tendency to clot can also cause blood to clot in the veins of the legs or of the pelvis.

## 370 What is the danger of blood-clot formation in the veins?

When blood clots form in the large veins of the legs and pelvis, they are very soft. Portions of the clots can break loose, pass through the heart into the lungs, and block blood flow to the lungs, thus causing serious medical problems or even death.

## 371 How often do blood clots break loose? Can this be treated?

One-fourth of the women who develop these blood clots in their veins have some of that clot break loose and go into the lungs if no treatment is given for the clots.

Even if blood clots in the veins are detected and treated, 5 percent of such patients will still have the blood clots break loose and go into the lungs; 1 percent will die of this problem.

It is crucial, obviously, that thrombophlebitis be found and treated. You should tell your doctor if you see any signs of this problem.

### 372  What are the signs and symptoms of thrombophlebitis?

There are several signs of blood clotting in the veins:

Pain and tenderness over the veins where the clot is located.

Swelling of the leg that is involved. That leg will often be more than an inch bigger around than the other leg.

Pain on raising the big toe of the leg that is involved.

### 373  Do these signs always mean that dangerous blood clots are present?

No. Half of the time there will be no blood clot present, even when the above-mentioned signs are present. The problem may be caused by several other factors.

On the other hand, people do occasionally die suddenly, having had no known problem with their veins. An autopsy reveals they have died from such blood clots. (This, of course, happens *rarely*.)

### 374  What tests are used to determine whether or not I have a blood clot in a swollen, tender leg?

There are several tests, two of which are:

*Venogram.* This test is done in an X-ray department. Dye is injected into a vein and an X-ray is taken to see if any part of the vein is blocked by a clot.

*Radioisotope tests.* Tests of this type are also done in an X-ray department. Drugs that will go into the blood clots are injected into the body. Attached to these drugs are radioactive particles. After these drugs have been given and allowed to disperse throughout the body a scan of the body is done. This scan will show where the radioactive material is concentrated, which shows where the blood clot is. Because the radioisotopes used for this technique would pass through the placenta into the baby, this procedure cannot be done during pregnancy. Since material also passes into the milk, the procedure cannot be done if a mother is breast-feeding.

### 375  How can I know if a blood clot has broken loose and gone into my lungs?

Fast breathing, shortness of breath, anxiety, pain in the chest on breathing, fast heart rate, and coughing blood are symptoms that accompany a pulmonary embolism (the passage of a blood clot through the veins into the lungs).

The problem with these symptoms, though, is that they can also occur in a person who does not have a pulmonary embolus. A woman who has had a cesarean section, for instance, will occasionally have a faster heart rate, shortness of breath, and pain in her chest during the normal recovery from that operation.

The important thing to remember in this matter, as in others during pregnancy and postdelivery, is to tell the nurse or the doctor if you notice unusual or disturbing symptoms of any kind. If a pulmonary embolism is suspected, the doctor will order tests to determine whether or not this is the case.

## 376 How are blood clots in my legs treated?

Bed rest and anticoagulation drugs are the primary techniques for treatment of thrombophlebitis.

*Bed rest.* You would be put to bed with your legs elevated so that the blood would drain from your veins, rapidly decreasing the chance of more clot formation. Elastic stockings would be recommended for the same reason. Application of heat to your legs and pain medication will be a part of your care and will make you feel better.

*Anticoagulation drugs.* The most important treatment is the use of heparin to stop blood coagulation. This drug prevents the clot from getting larger and allows the body to take care of the blood clot that is already formed. Although the body will often absorb the blood clot, sometimes the blood clot will be walled off, becoming scar tissue. This obstructs the vein, but blood returning from the leg will take an alternate route through other veins going in the same direction.

## 377 How is heparin given?

Initially the drug would be given intravenously (through your veins), but after the problem is under control you would need injections of heparin. You or someone else could administer these shots at home.

## 378 How long is heparin used?

The length of treatment has decreased over the years. In the past, heparin was admin-istered for three months. Now we know that the blood clot starts healing after two weeks, so heparin is often used for only three to four weeks. If there is a major complicating factor, though, you might be treated until the end of your pregnancy. If your problem develops after delivery and you are started on heparin then, you might be treated with it for as long as six months.

## 379 Why can't I take a pill to keep my blood from clotting, instead of having injections?

There are some situations in which you can use a pill, Coumadin. One time that it must not be used, though, is during pregnancy.

Coumadin used during pregnancy has been found to cause the baby to bleed while it is in the uterus. About 10–12 percent of pregnant mothers who use Coumadin will lose their babies either during the last three months of pregnancy or during labor and delivery.

Further, it has been found that Coumadin can cause abnormalities of the brain in the fetus, resulting in mental retardation, seizures, and a spastic body. If you are taking Coumadin while pregnant, the chance of these abnormalities developing in your baby is about 20 percent.

An additional problem with Coumadin is that if you were on Coumadin when you got pregnant, there is a great chance (about one in five) that you will miscarry. People who raise cattle know this. They do not let their bred cows into sweet clover, because they miscarry when they eat it. Coumadin comes from sweet clover.

It is best, obviously, to be anticoagulated with heparin during pregnancy. If the blood-clotting problem develops during the time following delivery, then, after heparin has been used for a while, you can be switched to Coumadin.

## Diabetes and Pregnancy

### 380 Is diabetes a special problem in pregnancy?

Yes. Every pregnant woman's body tends to handle sugar more like a diabetic's than a normal person's. When a diabetic has this added stress during pregnancy, it makes her diabetes even more of a problem.

### 381 Why does my pregnant body handle sugar like a diabetic's?

The hormonal changes in the body cause this. Some of the hormones that are produced during pregnancy are produced in astoundingly large amounts. For instance, one hormone, human placental lactogen, is produced by the placenta so that the baby can have good carbohydrate metabolism. This will provide it with the glucose that it needs to feed its high-energy needs for rapid growth. Without the human placental lactogen the baby's needs would not be met and its growth would be inadequate.

If the mother is a diabetic, the effect of her diabetes plus the diabeticlike effect in her body of the human placental lactogen can cause some real problems for the baby. It is up to the doctor and the mother to regulate the diabetes and yet allow the baby's metabolism to be adequate.

Other hormones that are produced in large quantities in the mother's body during pregnancy and which affect carbohydrate metabolism are progesterone, estriol (a form of estrogen), and free cortisole (a form of cortisone). All these hormones increase the diabeticlike metabolism of the normal (nondiabetic) woman.

### 382 Should I be tested for diabetes as a routine procedure if I am pregnant?

Doctors are coming to the conclusion that all pregnant women should be tested for diabetes. Studies have shown that half of the women who are pregnant diabetics are not detected during their pregnancy by the now routine practice of watching their urine for sugar. Because of this it is recommended that a blood-sugar test be done on every pregnant woman from the twenty-eighth to the thirty-second week of pregnancy. If your doctor has not started doing this, you must realize that it is a very new idea. You might diplomatically request that you have such a test, even if your routine urine tests for sugar are normal.

Some women are diabetic when they get pregnant. Other women are not diabetic when pregnancy begins, but they become diabetic during pregnancy. This is called gestational diabetes. Both groups of women are treated the same way during pregnancy. After pregnancy gestational diabetics will usually return to their nondiabetic state, although they often become true diabetics later in life.

Several factors would make it especially important for you to be tested for diabetes during pregnancy. If you have had a baby prior to this pregnancy that was very large (over nine pounds), you should be tested for diabetes. Other indications for careful testing would be if you have had diabetes in a previous pregnancy, if you have had an elevated blood-sugar level, or if you have had sugar in your urine with this pregnancy or in the past.

### 383 When should the test for diabetes be done? How is it performed?

You should be tested during the twenty-eighth to the thirty-second week of your pregnancy. This is the time when the production of hormones peaks; therefore the testing for diabetes is more reliable this late in pregnancy.

The test for diabetes involves a simple blood test done two hours after you have eaten a big meal, or after drinking a bottle of sugary substance called Glucola. If the blood test is questionable, the doctor will probably want to do a three- or four-hour glucose-tolerance test, which will allow him or her to see if your body is handling sugar as a diabetic or as a normal, nondiabetic person.

## 384   What blood-sugar level would indicate that I am a diabetic?

Any blood sugar test that is over 200 mg percent of sugar indicates that you are a diabetic. If you have been fasting (eating nothing since midnight the night before your blood test), and your blood-sugar test is above 140 mg, you are a diabetic.

If you have a three-hour glucose-tolerance test, your blood sugar level should be:

Fasting: 110 mg percent of sugar or below

One hour after meal: 200 or below

Two hours after meal: 150 or below

Three hours after meal: 130 or below

## 385   What will the doctor do if I am diabetic?

If you are a Class A diabetic, you will be handled differently than if you are a true overt diabetic. A Class A diabetic is one whose fasting blood sugar is under 110, but who shows two or three elevated levels on a glucose-tolerance test.

The risk of your baby dying before you deliver, which is the major potential risk of being a pregnant Class A diabetic, is no greater than if you did not have diabetes at all. The problem, however, is that you may

convert during pregnancy to a more severe form of diabetes.

Your doctor will probably want to see you more often than he would a nondiabetic pregnant woman, probably every week from the thirty-fourth week on. Your blood sugar will be tested frequently, and if your fasting blood-sugar level becomes greater than 110, you will be treated as a Class B diabetic. About 10 percent of women who have class A diabetes will become class B diabetics before the pregnancy is over.

The one exception to a Class A diabetic being treated differently from a true overt diabetic is if she has previously had a stillborn child. If she did, she will be treated as a Class B diabetic despite a normal fasting blood-sugar level.

If you are a Class B, C, D, or F diabetic, you are in greater danger of having problems with your baby during pregnancy since you have more severe diabetes. The more severe the diabetes, the more likely your baby is to have problems and the more necessary it is that your medical care be careful and precise. Even if the doctors do a good job and you follow their directions, a good outcome cannot be assured. The following questions will give you some idea of what to expect during pregnancy if you are diabetic.

## 386   How is my diet managed if I am a pregnant diabetic?

The ideal diet is a normal, healthy one. This includes doing without cakes, pies, and soft drinks. The purpose of excluding these sweets is not to limit calories, but to help your body handle sweets properly.

The goal is proper management of the sugar in the blood, not weight loss. As a matter of fact, doctors do not want pregnant diabetics to lose weight and generally ask diabetics to eat a diet that contains fifteen calories per pound of body weight per day. The diet suggested includes 50 percent complex carbohydrates (excluding concentrated sweets), 20 percent protein, and 30 percent fat.

## 387 As a diabetic, do I need a specialist other than my obstetrician to handle my pregnancy?

Ideally, the patient who is pregnant and has diabetes is cared for by both a specialist in internal medicine (an internist) and an obstetrician. The internist cares for the diabetes; the obstetrician does the obstetric management. This team approach results in good care and, most of the time, a good outcome for the pregnancy. Cooperation is necessary between the patient and her two doctors, but this is usually achieved quite well.

I feel that it is important to have an internist who is interested in diabetes, and particularly in diabetes and pregnancy. This specialist needs to understand how important it is that the diabetes be carefully controlled. He or she will probably instruct you in how to watch your blood-sugar levels at home, which will allow very careful control of those blood-sugar levels to the great benefit of your baby!

Your obstetrician must also be alert to the special needs of pregnancy in a diabetic mother. It is important that you have a physician you trust so that, because of that trust, you will follow all instructions.

Diabetics are often like people who are overweight; they try to act as though the problem does not exist. If you do this while you are pregnant, and let your blood sugar get out of control, you can seriously harm your baby. *A few days of undisciplined behavior can cause your child to die before birth or be abnormal for the rest of its life.* (See Q. 487.)

## 388 How is my baby cared for during pregnancy if I am a diabetic?

Special care is required for the unborn child of a diabetic mother. This care includes:

Early detection of intrauterine distress. Various tests will be done to evaluate the health of the baby during the last six weeks of pregnancy.

Prevention of prematurity by careful individual management. Prematurity cannot always be prevented because there are times when the baby of a diabetic mother must be delivered early.

Avoidance of birth injuries from difficult deliveries. Babies born to diabetic mothers are often more fragile, and early delivery is often necessary. Cesarean sections, therefore, are more frequently done on diabetic mothers.

Detecting fetal abnormalities. The number of babies born with major abnormalities is higher if the mother is diabetic during the pregnancy.

Between the thirty-second and the thirty-sixth weeks, your doctor will want to do certain tests. These may include the measurement of estriol, either in your blood or your urine, and may also include a nonstress test or a contraction-stress test. If estriol tests are going to be done during your pregnancy, they must be done almost every day because the estriols can change rapidly. Some doctors have found that it is more reasonable to do the nonstress tests as a proper evaluation of the baby of a diabetic pregnant woman.

These and other tests are further discussed in Q. 435–499.

## 389 What kinds of abnormalities most commonly occur in babies of diabetic mothers?

These abnormalities are primarily heart defects, the most common being a hole between the two major chambers of the heart (ventriculoseptal defect).

Another common defect is a neural-tube defect, an abnormality of the spinal cord, brain, or skull. An unusual defect that is seen almost exclusively in babies born to diabetics is the caudal regression syndrome, a condition in which the lower end of the spine does not develop normally.

Some studies have shown that these abnormalities develop because the baby is exposed to high levels of sugar during its early development. This would suggest that if you are a diabetic before pregnancy and want to increase your chance of having a normal baby, you should control your diabetes before becoming pregnant, as well as while you are pregnant, so that the baby is exposed as infrequently as possible to high levels of sugar from your blood.

## Thyroid Disease and Pregnancy

### 390 How often is thyroid disease a problem during pregnancy?

Thyroid disease is not a common problem in pregnancy. If it does occur, it can cause a mother to have preeclampsia (toxemia) and cause the baby to have low birth weight, or even to die.

Some studies have shown that if thyroid disease is not treated, as many as 45 percent of pregnancies will end as miscarriages, stillbirths, or deaths. It is important, if the expectant mother has abnormal thyroid function, that she be diagnosed and treated.

The diagnosis of hyperthyroidism in pregnancy is somewhat difficult because pregnancy itself produces signs that are typical of increased metabolism, such as excessive warmth, nervousness, and slight tremor. If a pregnant woman develops a fast heartbeat (especially while sleeping), if her eyes become a little protuberant, and if she is failing to gain weight normally, she should be tested for excessive thyroid function. If she is found to have increased thyroid function, this should be treated.

### 391 How is excessive thyroid function, or hyperthyroidism, treated during pregnancy?

A woman with this problem may be treated in one of the following ways: (1) Surgery to remove part of the thyroid after treatment with medicine to "quiet down" the thyroid; (2) Antithyroid medicine plus thyroid medication; or (3) Antithyroid medicine alone.

The treatment best for you depends on what your doctors think and on much more specific testing.

Although antithyroid medication does cross the placenta, the chance of this damaging the baby is small. This is fortunate, because it is necessary that a woman be treated if she has thyroid disease. (See Q. 486.) An obstetrician would normally refer such a patient to an internist for care of her thyroid problem.

## Arthritis and Pregnancy

### 392 What about rheumatoid arthritis? Does it get worse or better during pregnancy?

It gets better! Why this happens no one knows. It may be because of the increase of cortisone in the body during pregnancy, or due to a change in the immune system.

An interesting fact is that a physician at

Mayo Clinic discovered cortisone years ago because he noticed that patients with arthritis got better during pregnancy.

### 393 Are pregnancy and delivery affected by arthritis?

Unless the hip joints are severely affected, the pregnancy proceeds normally, and a woman may have a normal vaginal delivery. If the hip joints are severely affected and stiff, a woman may need a cesarean section for delivery because her legs cannot spread far enough for normal vaginal delivery.

### 394 How is arthritis treated during pregnancy?

Treatment is the same as when a woman is not pregnant, except that careful consideration must be given to any drugs involved. The treatment of arthritis involves a balance between rest and exercise, application of heat, and drugs. The use of aspirin is a mainstay in the treatment of arthritis in the nonpregnant patient, but the pregnant patient should not use aspirin during pregnancy. If a drug of this type is necessary and Tylenol helps, it should be used instead of aspirin.

### 395 Should aspirin be used during pregnancy?

The use of aspirin during pregnancy should be avoided. Aspirin can cause a pregnant mother to become anemic; it can increase her chance of bleeding, both before and after

delivery; and because it is an antiprostaglandin (prostaglandins are involved in the labor process), can stall the start of labor, and then cause it to be abnormally prolonged.

Aspirin does pass through the placenta to the baby, and many physicians think it can cause the baby's ductus arteriosus (located just outside the heart, it connects the aorta and the pulmonary artery) to close before delivery. The ductus arteriosus is an essential part of the baby's circulation prior to birth. It must not close until after the baby has been delivered or the baby will die in the uterus. Aspirin has also been associated with intrauterine growth retardation and a higher incidence of stillborn babies.

In addition, aspirin can keep the baby's blood from clotting properly. This is particularly significant in premature babies. Premature babies whose mothers use large amounts of aspirin during pregnancy have a greater chance of having bleeding into their brain after delivery. Full-term babies of mothers taking aspirin can bruise and bleed after delivery more easily than they would have otherwise.

It is obviously best that a mother not use aspirin during pregnancy. Every pregnant woman should read medication labels to make sure that no drug she takes contains salicylic acid. That is aspirin, and many drugs contain this without stating that they contain aspirin. (See Q. 481).

### 396 What about other drugs used for arthritis, such as chloroquin, gold, and cortisone?

There probably is no danger in using chloroquin during pregnancy. However, gold should be used with caution; it can pass through the placenta and *may* affect the baby. Studies are not conclusive.

As for cortisone, its use during pregnancy is discussed in Q. 399 and 400, in connection with lupus erythematosus. It is safe in pregnancy.

## Lupus Erythematosus and Pregnancy

### 397 What is lupus erythematosus? Does pregnancy make it worse?

Lupus erythematosus (lupus, or L.E.) is a rare disease of the connective tissue or collagen that causes a person to feel tired, to run a low-grade fever, and to have anemia and other symptoms. Many women have noticed that their lupus erythematosus began just after they delivered a baby, but why this happens has not been explained.

More than half of the patients with lupus will have some worsening of their symptoms during pregnancy. If the lupus gets frighteningly worse during the first three months of a pregnancy, an abortion will not alleviate the symptoms; they will intensify following the termination of the pregnancy. It seems wise, therefore, to let a patient continue her pregnancy, deliver the child, and then treat the symptoms after delivery. In this way, the woman can avoid the trauma of an abortion *and* the worsened lupus. The disease will remain either way.

The most common time for a pregnant woman with L.E. to have trouble is during the last three months of the pregnancy.

### 398 If lupus erythematosus develops during pregnancy, what will the symptoms be?

The symptoms of lupus may mimic those of preeclampsia. A woman suffering from high blood pressure and protein in the urine may be mistakenly diagnosed as having preeclampsia (toxemia of pregnancy).

It may not be possible for the doctor to know for sure that the problem actually is L.E. until after the pregnancy is over and a biopsy of the kidney proves that L.E. is present.

### 399 How is lupus erythematosus treated?

First, a new and exciting use of prednisone (cortisone) has been found. It has been shown that the use of cortisone during labor, and for four weeks after labor and delivery, prevents the worsening of L.E. that so often follows delivery. It seems to prevent skin, blood, or kidney changes from L.E. that can cause such sickness the month after delivery.

### 400 Does prednisone hurt the baby while I am pregnant?

No. Prednisone is an inactive form of cortisone. When you take it, your liver changes it to prednisolone, which is the active form of the drug. If you are pregnant, part of the prednisolone will circulate through the placenta into the baby, but the placenta changes the prednisolone back to the inactive form—prednisone.

If the baby has prednisone, an inactive drug, in its body, it will not be affected.

### 401 Does having lupus affect the course of a pregnancy?

Yes. Even before a woman finds out that she has lupus, she may have had several miscarriages.

Women who have lupus also have a greater chance of premature labor, of poor growth of the fetus during pregnancy, and of fetal death in the uterus during the last three months of pregnancy.

A recent discovery has given hope to lupus victims. An unusual antibody called circulating lupus anticoagulant has been identified as the substance responsible for such miscarriages. If a pregnant lupus victim takes an adequate amount of prednisone beginning early in pregnancy, a miscarriage may be prevented.

## 402 If the mother has lupus, will her baby get it from her?

No. The antibodies that cause lupus can pass into the baby through the placenta and cause a rash on the baby or some changes in the baby's blood count. This happens less than 5 percent of the time and is almost always of brief duration. It does not damage the baby at all, but the pediatrician should be made aware of the fact that you have lupus.

## Epilepsy and Pregnancy

## 403 How does pregnancy affect epilepsy?

Epilepsy is generally not affected by pregnancy. If an epileptic pregnant woman becomes so nauseated or sick from the pregnancy that she cannot take her medicine, she may have an increased chance of having a convulsion. Otherwise there is not an increased risk of a convulsion while she is pregnant.

An occasional mild convulsion in pregnancy will not hurt the baby. It would take a fairly prolonged seizure episode, or multiple

seizures, to damage the baby. A woman cannot breathe properly during convulsions and a diminished oxygen supply can adversely affect the baby.

The main problem with epilepsy during pregnancy is the effect of anticonvulsive medications on the baby. It is especially important, therefore, that if there is any question about the diagnosis of epilepsy that the diagnosis be confirmed before a woman stays on any drugs during pregnancy. The ideal situation would be that, if a woman expects that she is going to become pregnant, she consult with her neurologist. Together they can pick a drug that is safe in pregnancy and try it before the woman gets pregnant.

It is best, when possible, that an epileptic use only one drug during pregnancy. The drugs commonly used have a small risk to the baby, except for trimethadione and paramethadione. These drugs sometimes result in cleft lip and cleft palate, heart abnormalities, growth retardation, and mental deficiency. About 80 percent of babies born to mothers who take these drugs are affected to some extent. (See Q. 488.)

Dilantin (diphenylhydrantoin) carries about a 10-percent risk to the baby. The problems that can develop in babies born to mothers who are taking Dilantin are abnormal-looking face, cleft lip, heart abnormalities, or abnormal sex organs. It is obvious that if possible a woman should avoid taking Dilantin during her pregnancy.

## High Blood Pressure and Toxemia of Pregnancy

## 404 Why does my doctor check my blood pressure every time I go to the office?

The doctor is checking to see that your blood pressure is not too high. If your bloodpressure is elevated it can cause problems for you and your baby during the pregnancy.

An elevated blood pressure is usually associated with spasm of the blood vessels to the uterus and a corresponding decreased flow of blood through the baby's placenta. This limits the amount of nutrition and oxygen the baby can get from you and can affect the baby, even causing it to die before delivery. If your blood pressure gets high enough, it can cause a convulsion, which is obviously not good for you or the baby.

Your high blood pressure is treated during pregnancy to prevent your having convulsions, to enable you to deliver a healthy baby, to accomplish those goals with as little damage to either of you as possible, and to prevent your having high blood pressure later on. These four goals are clearly presented in the fifteenth edition of *Williams Obstetrics*, (New York: Appleton Century Crofts, 1976) written by Drs. Jack Pritchard and Paul MacDonald of the University of Texas Southwestern Medical School in Dallas.

---

## 405 What is toxemia of pregnancy?

Toxemia is an ill-defined metabolic disorder of pregnancy, characterized by hypertension (high blood pressure), edema (swelling), and albuminuria (protein in the urine). Toxemia is sometimes referred to as "poisoning" of pregnancy.

Toxemia is the general term for this disorder. Doctors, however, make two distinctions: (1) preeclampsia is toxemia without convulsions, and (2) eclampsia is toxemia with convulsions.

---

## 406 What causes toxemia of pregnancy to develop?

No one really knows what causes it, but there are some suggestions. One is that the trophoblast cells in the placenta seem capable of causing toxemia. For example, a woman who has a hydatidiform mole will sometimes develop toxemia. The presence of the placenta, rather than the presence of the baby, must be the cause of toxemia.

An additional interesting fact is that toxemia will develop if a hydatidiform mole develops in a woman's abdomen, outside her uterus. This is an important consideration, because some theories suggest that toxemia is due to stretching of the uterus in pregnancy. This cannot be true, since toxemia can develop in women whose pregnancy is not in the uterus.

One thing is definite: toxemia does not occur except when a woman is pregnant.

---

## 407 Do some women have a high-risk for developing toxemia of pregnancy?

Although any pregnant woman can have toxemia of pregnancy, there are individuals in whom this disorder is more likely to occur:

Women who have high blood pressure at the time they become pregnant

Teenagers or older women who become pregnant

Women who are having their first babies

Women who are carrying twins (or more)

Diabetics

Women who have hydatidiform molar pregnancy

Women whose family members (mother, sisters had toxemia of pregnancy

Women who have had toxemia with a previous pregnancy

## 408 How will my doctor check for toxemia of pregnancy?

There are three significant indicators.

*Hypertension.* A blood-pressure reading is written with one number over the other, such as 120/70. The upper number is the systolic pressure and the lower number is the diastolic. If the systolic pressure (the upper number) is 140 millimeters of mercury (mm Hg) or higher, or if, while you are pregnant it rises by 30 points, you have high blood pressure.

If the diastolic pressure (the lower number) is 90 or above, or if during pregnancy it increases by 15 points, you have high blood pressure.

A one-time reading of your blood pressure showing one of these abnormalities is not necessarily anything to worry about. Your doctor would want to check the pressure again, probably the next day, to see if it continues to be elevated.

*Protein in the urine.* During each office visit your urine will be tested for protein. A trace of protein can merely be the result of vaginal secretions or a temporary, normal spill of protein from the kidneys into your urine. If the urinalysis shows a 3 + or 4 + reaction on the dipstick, you have an abnormal amount of protein in your urine. This is probably due to toxemia.

If you have protein in your urine, but your blood pressure is normal, your doctor would probably suggest an evaluation by a kidney specialist to make sure that you do not have a kidney disease. If you have 3 + or 4 + protein in your urine and also have high blood pressure, you almost certainly have toxemia of pregnancy.

*Swelling.* Years ago doctors felt that any significant swelling was a sure sign of developing toxemia. There is now a much more relaxed attitude about edema. If a woman's blood pressure is normal and she does not have protein in her urine, we accept swelling as a normal part of pregnancy.

Diuretics are given only to women who have so much swelling of their feet that they actually hurt and who feel that they must have something to make the swelling less. Some doctors feel that it is unsafe to give diuretics even then. (See Q. 306–I.)

If there is elevated blood pressure plus significant swelling, then the presence of swelling is obviously more ominous, suggesting the presence of the toxemia process.

## 409 What if my blood pressure was high before I got pregnant? Will I develop toxemia?

If your blood pressure was high when you became pregnant, you will probably continue to have high blood pressure throughout your pregnancy. You will not necessarily develop toxemia.

The higher your blood pressure is—even if you are not toxemic—the greater chance there is that your pregnancy will be affected. It has been shown that if a woman's blood presure is 200/120 or greater when she becomes pregnant, she can expect to have her baby die (either before or directly after delivery) 50 percent of the time. Of those babies that don't die, many will be affected by poor growth during the pregnancy.

Most doctors feel that if the high blood pressure is below 150/100, no immediate medical treatment is required. They would want to watch the growth of the baby carefully if the blood pressure were mildly or markedly elevated during pregnancy. This is to be sure that the baby is growing adequately.

If you are taking medication for high blood pressure when you become pregnant, it is probably best that you stay on that medication throughout pregnancy. There are some blood pressure medications, however, that a woman should not take while she is pregnant; your doctor would want to evaluate the medicine to be sure it was proper for you to use it while you are pregnant.

If you are not on blood pressure medicine, and your blood pressure is not too high, it is probably best that you not take any medication unless your blood pressure starts rising.

### 410 What if I do develop toxemia with my chronic high blood pressure?

A pregnant woman who already has chronic high blood pressure, whose blood pressure goes up even higher, and who develops protein in the urine is developing toxemia. In this situation the woman would be treated for toxemia, but she would be watched especially closely because her toxemia and its effect on her baby might be worse than in a woman who does not have chronic high blood pressure.

### 411 How is toxemia treated?

If your toxemia does not seem to be severe (your blood pressure and the albumin level in your urine are not unduly elevated), the doctor will recommend rest. I normally have my patients go home and go to bed. They should stop caring for other children that they may have. I want them to stop cooking, going to the grocery store, and doing car pools. It is important that they actually go to bed and stay in bed except to get up to go to the bathroom, or perhaps to move to the couch to watch television.

If a woman will do this and keep her appointments with her doctor carefully, she may be able to avoid having to go to the hospital. In spite of good care at home, though, women will occasionally have worsening toxemia and need to be admitted to the hospital.

In addition to bed rest, it is important that a woman with toxemia limit her salt intake to only the salt that her food is cooked with.

She should eliminate pork from her diet because of its high salt content, and stop eating canned vegetables because of salt preservatives in them. Decreasing the salt helps decrease the amount of swelling and, therefore, helps control a woman's blood pressure.

If her toxemia worsens, or if initially her blood pressure is fairly high and she has a high concentration of albumin in her urine, she needs to be admitted to the hospital where she can be observed carefully. This insures that she will stay in bed, which is extremely difficult to do at home.

If the doctor is fearful that a woman is about to have a convulsion due to the toxemia, she may be injected with magnesium sulfate to prevent the convulsions, and possibly Apresoline to keep her blood pressure from getting too high. Doctors will be careful about giving too much medicine to lower the blood pressure, because if blood pressure gets too low, it can limit the amount of blood and, therefore, of oxygen, getting to the placenta and the baby.

### 412 Is there a cure for toxemia?

The cure for toxemia is delivery. When your baby is born, or your pregnancy is terminated, your toxemia will soon vanish.

If your toxemia is severe early in pregnancy, the doctor will insist that the baby be delivered so that you will not progress to convulsions. If you have already had convulsions, the baby must be delivered, regardless of the stage of the pregnancy. This must be done, because once severe toxemia develops, and once convulsions start, it does not stop until the baby is delivered. There are few situations in pregnancy in which the lives of both the baby and the mother are endangered, but this is one of them. Even if the baby must be delivered so early that its death is inevitable, this should be done. At least the life of the mother can be saved.

# Toxemia of Pregnancy

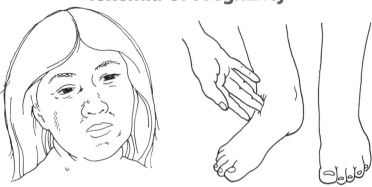

***Toxemia of pregnancy.*** Two signs of worsening toxemia are increasing weight gain and swelling especially of face and ankles.

Fortunately toxemia usually does not get severe until later in pregnancy. Delivery of a premature baby will often require cesarean section. You should certainly give your consent if your doctor recommends delivery of a premature baby by cesarean section. Most babies can be put into a good intensive-care nursery where they will be better off than in your uterus if you have toxemia.

Do not be surprised if the doctor wants to monitor your blood pressure, urine output, and urine albumin for the first few days after delivery. During this time there is a chance of your developing very high blood pressure and even of having a convulsion. In every patient toxemia does not immediately vanish after delivery.

---

**413** **What are specific symptoms of worsening toxemia?**

You definitely should notify your doctor if you notice any of the following signs:

*Severe, persistent headache.* This can be a sign of elevated blood pressure and should be reported to your doctor right away.

*Trouble with vision.* Your vision may be blurred or you may have trouble focusing.

*Pain in the upper abdomen.* If you start having really bothersome pain in the upper part of your abdomen, especially on the right

side, you should notify your doctor immediately. This can indicate swelling of the liver.

*Weight gain and swelling.* If you notice a significant weight gain, accompanied by swelling, you may have worsening toxemia.

*Convulsions.* If your toxemia is bad enough to cause a convulsion, you need to be treated immediately and expertly.

---

**414** **How is my unborn baby cared for if I am toxemic?**

If you have toxemia, your baby can be affected. The doctor's treatment will seem to be directed toward you rather than the baby. Actually the doctor is carefully considering the baby's health. As your toxemia is controlled, your baby will be less adversely affected.

Eclampsia is one of the most dangerous conditions you can have as a pregnant woman, not just for you but also for the baby you are carrying. The doctor's treatment of preeclampsia (toxemia without seizures) is to prevent its progression to true eclampsia (toxemia with seizures). In so doing, he or she will be protecting your baby.

Your doctor will be watching the baby's development as your toxemia is treated. He or she will be carefully measuring the baby to be sure that it is growing properly. Failure to grow adequately can indicate intrauterine growth retardation, which could result from inadequate oxygen and nutrients getting to the baby. This occurs because toxemia causes spasm of the uterine blood vessels.

The doctor may want you to have tests done to make sure the baby is developing properly. (See Q. 435–443.) If there are signs that the baby is not developing well, the doctor will want to consider delivering your baby, even if it requires a cesarean section.

## Diseases and Abnormalities of the Reproductive Organs

**415** **Are there diseases and abnormalities of the female organs that might cause problems or complications during pregnancy?**

Yes, there may be ovarian cysts, fibroid tumors, cervical irregularities, venereal warts, and herpes. These problems are discussed in the following questions. General discussion of these and other disorders will be found in chapters 10 and 13.

**416** **My doctor says that I have a cyst of the ovary. Does this endanger my pregnancy, and do I need surgery?**

The cyst your doctor found may be the corpus luteum cyst of pregnancy, a normal product of your pregnancy. When your ovary released the egg that was fertilized to become this pregnancy, it immediately formed a corpus luteum cyst. A corpus luteum cyst of pregnancy is responsible for producing progesterone, the hormone that maintains your pregnancy during the first few weeks.

Your doctor can occasionally feel this cyst during the pelvic exam early in pregnancy; if you have an ultrasound scan done early in pregnancy, the cyst will often be found.

Such cysts may become as large as two to two and a half inches in diameter and may persist for several months into the pregnancy. These cysts are usually normal and will gradually disappear during the pregnancy. In fact, pregnancy could not exist without them. A conservative approach to cyst surgery is warranted.

It is, of course, possible for you to have a growth on your ovary during pregnancy. If an enlargement of your ovary develops during your pregnancy, the doctor may feel that it should be removed. If possible, the doctor would perform the surgery during the middle three months of your pregnancy; this is the time least likely to cause premature labor.

Since a growth on the ovary has a 3 percent chance of being malignant, you and the doctor must make sure that you do not have such a malignancy present. Also, since ovarian growths can obstruct labor, a large one is best removed during the middle part of the pregnancy.

It is possible, although uncommon, for an ovary made heavier by an ovarian growth to twist around on itself and cut off its own blood supply. This will cause a great deal of pain and will necessitate immediate surgery, regardless of the stage of the pregnancy. About 12 percent of such ovarian growths will require surgery. During such surgery the doctor will occasionally find that the enlargement was not a growth but was merely a corpus luteum cyst on the ovary. If this could have been definitely determined beforehand, surgery would not have been necessary. However, whenever an ovarian enlargement continues to be present and seems suspicious to your doctor, there may be no choice but to have surgery. If you have any question about your doctor's recommendation, get a second opinion.

## 417 How will fibroid tumors in the uterus affect pregnancy?

Fibroid tumors usually do not cause pain or trouble in pregnancy. Occasionally, however, a fibroid will outgrow its blood supply. When this occurs it will begin degenerating and will then cause pain.

If you have a fibroid and are having pain in the area of the fibroid, you usually do not need surgery. The fibroid will probably cure itself, gradually scarring over. Sometimes a fibroid will be large enough to require a cesarean section because its size or location will interfere with normal labor. This is unusual.

It is, of course, possible for a woman to have fibroids that are inside the cavity of her uterus. If so, they can cause a miscarriage. In most cases, though, if a woman had fibroids growing in the cavity of her uterus, they would have caused bleeding or infertility and she would have had them taken care of before she became pregnant.

## 418 My doctor says that my uterus is retroverted. Is this a cause for alarm during pregnancy?

A retroverted uterus, one that is tipped or turned backward, is not abnormal; one-third of all women have a retroverted uterus. Rarely, however, a woman's uterus will stay in a retroverted position during pregnancy and not "lift up" out of the pelvis. The growth of the uterus can then force the cervix (the mouth of the uterus) up against the bladder, causing the woman to have trouble passing urine.

To correct this the doctor may need to push the uterus up and out of the pelvis. This usually produces immediate relief.

Sometimes a uterus can be so low in a woman's pelvis that the cervix will protrude from the vagina. This is not dangerous, but women who have this problem usually ex-perience a lot of vaginal and pelvic pressure in addition to the discomfort of feeling the cervical protrusion. Most women are not usually bothered much by this problem once the situation is explained, especially since, as pregnancy progresses, the enlarging uterus will usually draw the cervix back up into the vagina.

## 419 What are some abnormalities of the cervix that can cause problems with pregnancy or delivery?

There are four conditions of the cervix that can cause problems.

incompetent cervix

cervical stenosis

abnormal pap smear

cancer of the cervix

These conditions, as they relate to pregnancy, are discussed in the following questions.

## 420 What is an incompetent cervix?

An incompetent cervix is one that does not have the strength to hold the pregnancy. It relaxes and allows a woman to miscarry or to have a premature delivery. An incompetent cervix usually causes loss of the baby during the middle three months of pregnancy.

There is almost no way for the doctor to be absolutely certain that an incompetent cervix caused the pregnancy loss unless a woman had an earlier loss of pregnancy during the middle three months. Most doctors usually suspect an incompetent cervix if everything else is normal and a miscarriage has occurred in the middle three months. (See Q. 328.)

An incompetent cervical os may occasionally be caused by surgery on the cervix. Other causes may be previous abortions, D&Cs, or tears at earlier deliveries. Some women, however, have the condition without any previous history of cervical tearing or surgery. They were probably born with weak cervical tissue.

The woman who has had a previous loss of a pregnancy in the middle three months, and who does not have any other explanation, needs to be treated early in the subsequent pregnancy by having purse-string sutures put around her cervix to hold it closed. These sutures are put in through the vagina, and require that a woman have general anesthesia.

Doctors usually put in sutures that can be removed when labor starts. This is called a McDonald procedure. Occasionally, when cervical damage is extensive, a permanent strip of material is put around the cervix and left in place. Delivery is then by cesarean section. The surgery for strengthening the cervix with sutures or strips of material is called a cerclage procedure.

---

**421** What can be done if I have an abnormal Pap smear while I am pregnant?

Ideally you should have had Pap smears before you became pregnant so that you could avoid having to worry about abnormal cells in your cervix during pregnancy. If this was not done, however, and your doctor finds abnormal cells in your cervix during pregnancy, you will need to be evaluated.

Fortunately with the advent of colposcopy, an examination of the cervical lining by means of a magnifying instrument, it is easier to evaluate the cervix than it once was. The doctor will put acetic acid on your cervix. Acetic acid is in vinegar. It makes the areas of abnormality stand out more clearly. He or she will then look through your vagina at your cervix with a colposcope. Frequently

the doctor can tell whether or not the cells are anything to worry about just by looking. If there is any question, however, a very small biopsy (pinch of tissue) may be taken and sent to a pathologist for evaluation.

If you do not have invasive cancer on your cervix, the doctor will probably do a repeat colposcopy once or twice during the pregnancy just to make sure the growth on your cervix is not progressing, but he or she will not treat the area in any other way. You will usually be allowed to go through normal labor and delivery. You will probably need to return later for repeat colposcopy and treatment of the abnormal cells.

If your doctor, after finding abnormal cells in your Pap smear, recommends that surgery be done on your cervix without colposcopic diagnosis, you should ask to be referred to a doctor who does colposcopy. The only other way that a doctor can make an accurate diagnosis is to put you in the hospital, have you anesthetized, and do a conization of your cervix. This is a bloody operation that can cause you to miscarry or go into premature labor. And it is rarely necessary with the availability of colposcopy.

If, however, with colposcopy and biopsies, there is a suspicion that you might have invasive cancer of the cervix, then conization of the cervix would certainly be necessary.

---

**422** What if I am found to have cancer of the cervix while I am pregnant?

Fortunately cancer of the cervix in pregnancy is rare. If you are found to have truly invasive cancer early in your pregnancy, you should go ahead and have the cancer treated. This, of course, means termination of the pregnancy.

If you are far enough along in your pregnancy so that waiting another two to four weeks might give your baby a chance to live, it might be possible to wait that short time, have the baby delivered prematurely, and then have your cancer treated. Most doctors would want you to have a cesarean section for your delivery rather than deliver through a cancerous cervix. (See Q. 431.)

## Vulvar and Vaginal Problems

**423**  **What problems of the vulva or vagina might be present during pregnancy and cause problems?**

Two problems of the vulva and/or vagina that might cause trouble are venereal warts and herpes. These are discussed in the next two questions.

**424**  **What are venereal warts? What should be done if I have them?**

Venereal warts (condyloma acuminata) are warty growths that can exist in the vagina, on the cervix, on the external genitals, and on the anus. They are virus-caused and are not cancerous. (See Q. 1138–1144.)

It is a good idea to get rid of venereal warts before delivery, not only because they are irritating and bothersome, but because they can bleed and tear at delivery more easily than normal tissue. Also, pregnancy can cause them to grow extremely fast. As a result of this, a pregnant woman may have such massive venereal warts that a cesarean section is necessary.

Podophyllum, a solution that is often used on warts, can cause a pregnant woman to become sick and can cause the death of the baby. It should not be used in pregnancy. Four other methods of treatment are available. In my opinion, the best treatment is the laser which allows removal of the wart without damaging the tissue from which

the wart is growing; warts are less likely to grow back after laser treatment than they are with other methods. A second method of treatment is freezing. A third method is treatment with trichloroacetic acid. Finally, a different method of treatment (with local or general anesthesia) is for the doctor to cut the warts off and, at the same time, cauterize both the cuts and the smaller warts.

Doctors feel that it is possible for the venereal wart virus to be transmitted to babies and to produce small growths on their vocal cords called papillomas. If you have venereal warts at the time of your delivery, be sure your baby's pediatrician knows that fact.

**425**  **What if I have herpes and am pregnant?**

Herpes (an infection caused by herpes simplex virus) seems to strike more terror into the heart of a pregnant woman today than almost anything else that can happen to her. There has been so much bad publicity about herpes that many women are absolutely scared to death because of the problem.

Although there is reason to be concerned about herpes infections (see Q. 1148–1150 ), the danger to the child of a mother with herpes has been blown out of proportion. In Austin, Texas, a community of about 500,000 people, a local neonatalist recently said that he was aware of less than twenty cases suspected of being herpes infections of babies in the whole history of the city.

I am not saying that you and your doctor have no cause for concern or caution if you have herpes. I am merely saying that, even with the great amount of herpes that exists in a city such as Austin, herpes-affected babies are almost never seen.

If you have been diagnosed as having herpes, the pattern that you and your doctor will want to follow would probably be something like the following.

A cesarean section is necessary if there is

a herpes ulcer broken out anywhere on your vulva at the time of delivery.

If you have had a recent ulcer on your vulva from herpes, and if this was your first herpes sore, a cesarean section is necessary if the sore was present any time during the four weeks before delivery.

If a recent herpes ulcer was not your first, a cesarean section is not necessary unless the sore has broken out during the immediate two weeks before your delivery.

If you have an open herpes sore, or one that was recently open, and your bag of waters has ruptured more than four hours before delivery, there may be no need for a cesarean section. The herpes virus could have already infected your baby if it were going to do so.

If your baby does become infected by the herpes virus, there is a 70 percent chance of death or severe neurologic damage. As mentioned previously, though, the chance of the baby getting infected, even if you and your doctor ignore the above guidelines, is very small.

I suggest that if during pregnancy you have any kind of vulvar outbreak that might be herpes, have a culture for the virus done to find out for sure if you are carrying herpes.

## Surgery During Pregnancy

### 426 What problems might necessitate abdominal surgery while I am pregnant?

Problems that might require an abdominal incision other than C-section are the same as those that would necessitate surgery on a nonpregnant woman: an acute attack of gallbladder disease, appendicitis, intestinal obstruction, rupture of a blood vessel inside your abdomen, or other problems that cause what physicians sometimes term an acute abdomen.

Any of these problems that require surgery will give you definite signals that something is wrong. If you begin having unusual abdominal pain, don't delay calling your doctor.

If your abdomen is unusually tender when the doctor examines you, he or she may feel that immediate surgery is necessary.

It is sometimes difficult to diagnose an emergency surgery situation in a pregnant woman. Her symptoms may seem to be much less significant than identical symptoms in a nonpregnant woman. The obstetrician is the expert in knowing whether a problem in a pregnant woman is really severe enough to require surgery. Your doctor may need to call in a general surgeon for consultation if the area involved is not the female reproductive organs. This expertise, of course, is what will keep your condition from reaching the stage where you become seriously ill or lose your baby. If an obstetrician feels that a problem is severe enough to warrant surgery, have it done. To delay can be extremely dangerous.

### 427 Will surgery cause me to miscarry or deliver prematurely?

The surgery itself is not likely to cause you to miscarry or deliver early. The problem that is making the surgery necessary can cause your uterus to begin contracting and result in miscarriage or premature delivery.

There are drugs that can be given to relax the uterus to help prevent contractions. In spite of that, a woman will occasionally lose the pregnancy. Delaying the surgery, however, will not make you less likely to miscarry, since it is the problem that causes the miscarriage, not the surgery itself. The sooner you have the surgery, therefore, the less likely you are to miscarry or to deliver prematurely.

The overriding principle concerning surgery during pregnancy is that if surgery is necessary, have it done.

## 428 Will anesthetics during surgery hurt my baby?

Anesthetics that are given today apparently do not affect the baby at all. I have not been able to find any study or reference to show damage to a baby, miscarriage, or early labor because of anesthesia.

## Cancer and Pregnancy

## 429 Does cancer occur during pregnancy?

Cancer in a mother's body during pregnancy is rare, occurring in about one in a thousand pregnancies. The cancers that most often occur in pregnant women are, in order of frequency, breast cancer, cervical cancer, ovarian cancer, lymphomas, and colon and rectal cancer. Other cancers, of course, do occur during pregnancy, but much more rarely.

About 15 percent of the cases of breast cancer occur in women who are younger than forty-one years of age. Since more women are delaying childbirth until they are older, doctors are seeing breast cancer in about 3 percent of all pregnant patients.

It was felt in the past that breast cancer grew faster and was harder to cure in pregnant women. That may be true to a slight extent, but it has become clear that the major problem has been the tendency of both patients and doctors to ignore breast lumps during pregnancy because they assumed that the lumps were caused by hormones of pregnancy. This assumption, of course, delayed treatment, giving the cancer a greater chance to grow and spread.

If you have a mass in your breast that is new and different from anything you have felt before, whether or not you are pregnant, you must bring it to your doctor's attention, and he or she must pay attention to it! Further, you should get a second opinion if you continue to feel uncomfortable about the lump and your doctor does not seem to be paying close attention to it.

Your best chance of cure is to find a breast cancer when it is small, and to get it diagnosed and treated early. With prompt care you are as likely to have as good a prognosis from breast cancer as a woman who is not pregnant when her breast cancer is found. For further information on breast abnormalities, see Q. 851–883.

## 430 How is breast cancer treated during pregnancy?

Diagnosis and treatment of cancer during pregnancy are essentially the same as if you were not pregnant. There are a couple of differences, however.

First, there is a slight chance of miscarriage with any operation during pregnancy. The chance of miscarriage during a breast biopsy is extremely slight, and is still minimal even if a mastectomy is done. The chance of your baby being affected by diagnostic X-rays to the breast are also essentially zero.

Second, the other problem that might occur is if some of the cancer has already spread to the lymph nodes under the arm, or to other parts of the body. In this case you might need chemotherapeutic drugs, and chemotherapy can hurt the baby.

The complete situation must be carefully discussed with your doctors. If you are near

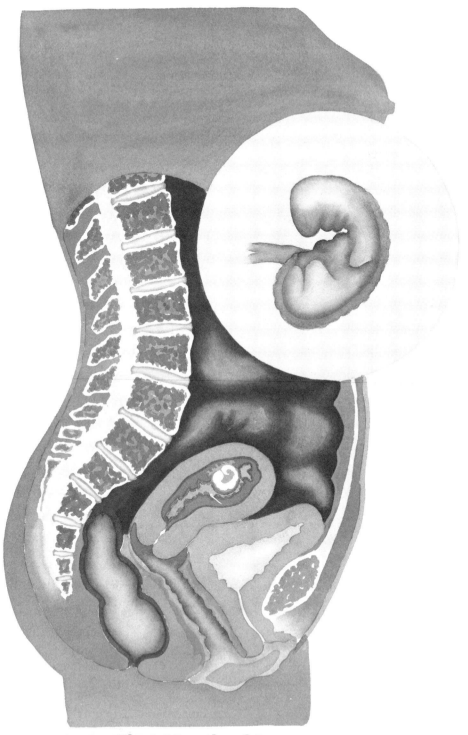

**First Month of Pregnancy**

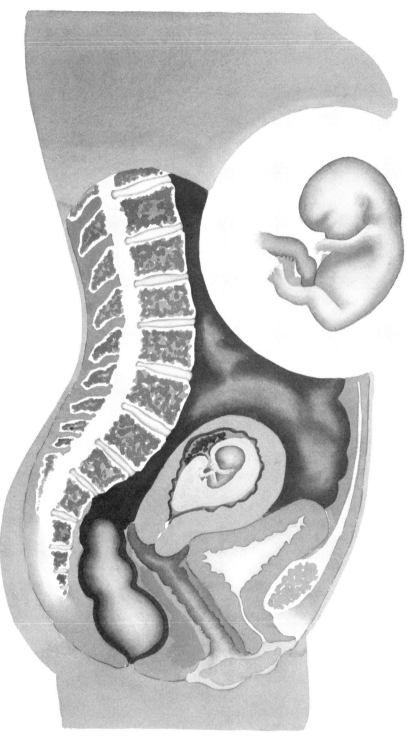

**Second Month of Pregnancy**

delivery, you might be able to delay the chemotherapy until your baby is mature enough for an early delivery. If your pregnancy has just begun, however, it might be too dangerous to delay taking the drugs.

You do not need to have an abortion done because you have been found to have breast cancer. Terminating the pregnancy will not give you a better chance of cure. The only reason for abortion would be if you were going to take chemotherapy, and it was felt, absolutely, that damage would be done to the baby. Even then, you are the one that makes the decision about an abortion.

One other concern is whether or not you should ever become pregnant again after having had breast cancer. Formerly, most doctors have advised patients not to get pregnant again because of the possibility of hormone stimulation to cancer cells, but statistics now seem to show that if you have gone five years without any recurrence of your breast cancer, it is "safe" to get pregnant again.

### 431 Can I develop cancer of the cervix while pregnant? How is it treated?

Cancer of the cervix can occur during pregnancy, as we discussed briefly in Q. 421 and 422. If abnormal cervical cells are discovered (from biopsy, colposcopy, or conization) but there are no cancer cells invading your tissues, you can have a normal vaginal delivery. This includes carcinoma *in situ*, a skin-cancer-type growth on your cervix often called CIN II.

If cervical cancer has already begun invading your tissues, and you are in the first two months of pregnancy, the cancer needs to be treated as though you were not pregnant. There are few medical conditions that a pregnant mother may have that make an abortion necessary, but this is one. If a cervical cancer is found when pregnancy has just begun, by the time delivery might occur

spontaneously, the cancer would probably have grown so much that it would no longer be curable. This type of cancer needs to be treated immediately, even if it means an abortion. A hysterectomy may be necessary (which, of course, would involve removal of the uterus with the baby in it) or your cervix may need radiation treatment.

Radiation will almost always produce a miscarriage. If it does not, your uterus must be opened by abdominal incision and emptied, because it is necessary for radium to be put up inside the cervix for proper treatment of the cervical cancer.

If you are in the last three months of pregnancy when the cancer is discovered, there is usually little risk in allowing your baby to grow to the point where it can be delivered early and yet be mature enough to live. The delivery must be by cesarean section, since delivery through a cervix with cancer might cause the cancer to spread. Pregnancy itself does not cause cancer of the cervix to grow any faster or to spread any more quickly than it would when one is not pregnant.

### 432 How are cancers other than of the breast and cervix treated during pregnancy?

Other cancers, as previously mentioned, occur less frequently in pregnancy. The general rule about treatment is that if the cancer is found in the later months of pregnancy, it is acceptable, and usually desirable, to avoid treatment until the baby is mature enough to survive premature delivery. If the pregnancy is not yet into the final trimester when the cancer is found, it is best to treat the cancer as though the pregnancy does not exist.

Since drugs and radiation can affect the baby, a decision about a therapeutic abortion must be reached by the patient and the doctors involved in treatment. This type of problem, of course, produces great emotional conflict. It is a time to have doctors who are very sensitive. It is also a time to have good counsel and comfort from friends, from professional counselors, and from pastor, priest, or rabbi. All these resources are available, and I strongly encourage patients to take advantage of them. This is not a time to try to go it alone.

## The Age Factor and Pregnancy

**433** **Does my being over thirty-five affect my chances for a normal pregnancy and delivery?**

Your age does affect your pregnancy. Your baby is more likely to have problems at birth if you are over thirty-five when you have your first child. You are more likely to have medical problems as a result of being pregnant at that age than if you were younger. The actual number of women who have medical problems or whose babies have problems at birth is fairly small. The major problem with delaying pregnancy until the latter part of the reproductive age (over thirty) is that fertility decreases. An excellent study done in France showed that up to the age of thirty, 74 percent of women were able to conceive. From age thirty-one to thirty-five, only 61 percent of women conceived. Over age thirty-five, only 53 percent of women conceived. The women in this study had artificial inseminations. The actual percentages are all too low but the trend the study shows is real.

A pregnant woman over age thirty-five may have the same problems that a younger woman may have but they occur more often. The death-rate from pregnancy doubles during every five-year increment from age twenty-five on. Because the actual death-rate from pregnancy is so low, this does not

involve many women, even those in their forties. The problems that cause death in older pregnant women are the same that affect younger women: infection, hemorrhage, and toxemia of pregnancy. The increased risk is apparently due to medical problems such as hypertension, liver malfunction, and diabetes of pregnancy which occur more often in older pregnant women.

Birth defects occur more often in infants born to older pregnant women. (See Q. 506.) Thirty-five seems to be the age at which the risk increases for delivering a baby that is sick or dies around the time of delivery. This may be caused by a placenta that does not carry oxygen and food to the baby as effectively as a placenta of a younger woman. Any woman over the age thirty-five who is pregnant for the first time must receive excellent medical care for herself. In addition, special attention must be paid to her developing baby's health.

For women over age thirty-five, there is a greater chance of having an irregular pattern of contractions and a longer labor than in women below that age. W. R. Cohen, M.D., L. Newman, M.D., and E. A. Friedman, M.D., of Harvard Medical School, reported this fact in a study published in 1980. They found that the patterns of irregularity were the same type of patterns that occurred in younger women; they just occurred more often in women over thirty-five. These doctors suggested that the irregular labors were somehow related to the muscle of the uterus being less efficient with increasing age.

Because of this change in labor patterns, there is a greater chance that an older mother will need a cesarean section for delivery. The obstetrician would not need to do a cesarean section just because of age; you should be followed along during your labor as would anyone else.

**434** **Are there any advantages to having children at an "older" age?**

Pregnancy among "older" women (over thirty-five) has greatly increased in popu-

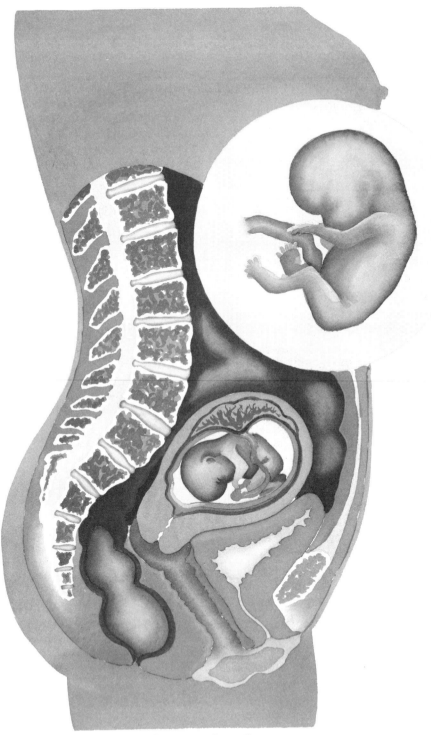

**Third Month of Pregnancy**

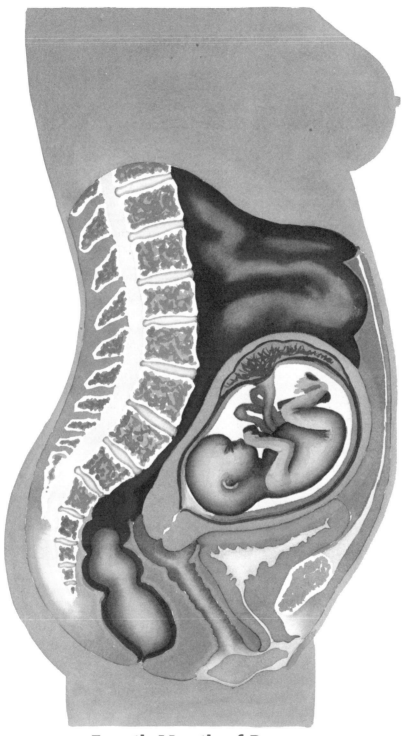

**Fourth Month of Pregnancy**

larity. The National Center for Health Statistics has reported that from 1975 to 1979 there was a 73 percent increase in first births to women in their thirties. Obviously some women feel there is an advantage to delaying pregnancy. These reasons usually include older ages at marriage, career desires, starting "second" families with another mate, economic considerations, and other factors related to modern society.

There also seem to be possible medical advantages to delaying pregnancy. Studies have shown that the children born to older mothers are less likely to die of sudden infant death syndrome (SIDS), and children of older mothers tend to develop better during the first few years of life.

## Monitoring the Fetus

### 435 What is the value of the techniques available to evaluate the condition of my unborn child?

Fetal testing has been mentioned in several places throughout this chapter. For example, pregnant diabetics must have their pregnancy monitored in many ways; toxemic and hypertensive mothers must also have their babies monitored; and if intrauterine growth retardation is suspected, fetal monitoring must be done. The techniques for monitoring are discussed in the following questions. The goal is to make sure that the baby is developing normally or, if it is not, to determine what needs to be done.

Every parent and every doctor wants to avoid the agony of delivering a stillborn or defective baby. Modern fetal monitoring makes it possible to avoid, alleviate, or at least anticipate problems.

If you or the baby has a problem that

might result in a stillbirth, the doctor would want to deliver the baby before the problem became dangerous. He or she would also want to avoid delivery of a baby so premature that it would have to be on a respirator for weeks or in intensive care for months. Fetal monitoring helps accomplish these goals.

Obviously parents and physicians are walking a tightrope when there is a problem that might affect the baby. During the past fifteen to twenty years there has been a major revolution in obstetric care that, in a sense, has provided a "long balancing stick" to help doctors and parents walk that tightrope between having a new baby that is sicker than it had to be (or one that is needlessly dead), and causing a baby to be born more prematurely than it had to be in an attempt to keep it from getting too sick inside the uterus.

The long stick that helps provide the balance and has produced this revolution is the testing of the baby that can be done even before it is born to determine its condition. This monitoring has saved many babies from death inside their mothers' unhealthy bodies; it has also allowed many a baby to remain in the uterus when other indications would suggest that the baby ought to be delivered early.

### 436 What tests can be done to determine whether or not the baby is developing normally?

Tests in this category are done to insure that the baby has proper growth inside the uterus, is not having trouble because the pregnancy has gone past the due date, or that the mother's diabetes, high blood pressure, or toxemia is not harming the baby. Tests done for these reasons include the following:

nonstress tests (NST)

stress tests (OCT—oxytocin challenge test)

estrogen tests

diagnostic ultrasonagraphy

---

### 437 What is a nonstress test?

A nonstress test (NST) is based on the heartbeat of a baby who is at least twenty-eight to thirty-four weeks along. When the baby moves, that movement should be followed by an increase in its heart rate. If the heart rate does not increase, the baby may not be healthy.

This is quite logical. When you exercise, you expect your heart rate to increase; if it does not, there is probably something wrong.

Studies have shown that as many as 40–50 percent of babies whose NSTs are not satisfactory will be sick when they are born; and about 3 percent of them will die either just before or just after delivery.

In addition to watching for an increased heartbeat after the baby moves, the NST checks the heart rate itself. The heart rate of a sick baby may also show other abnormalities. These are:

*A too-regular heart rate.* The heart rate should vary and not be absolutely the same minute by minute. When a baby's heartbeat is totally regular, it indicates a loss of the variations in the heart rate that are normal for any baby in the uterus (or for any normal person).

*Decrease in heart rate accompanying false labor pains.* It is normal for the heart rate to fluctuate, but if the baby's heartbeat drops and stays down for several seconds after the contraction, that baby is probably very sick.

*Occasional unexplained drop in the heart rate.* A baby whose heart rate occasionally drops significantly is a very sick baby, assuming the drop was not caused by a contraction.

*Absence or decrease in fetal movement.* Fetal movement, or lack of it, is hard for a mother to interpret, but if movement stops or decreases markedly and is accompanied by the loss of a variable heart rate and the presence of dipping heart rate, there may be a serious problem.

---

### 438 How is a nonstress test (NST) done?

The nonstress test is usually done in the labor and delivery department of the hospital. A nurse will place a fetal monitor on your abdomen to enable you to listen to and record your baby's heartbeat. She will then watch for the baby to move and will get a good recording of that heartbeat after the baby's movements. If the baby does not move, the nurse will try to wake up the baby by moving you around, by turning on a television or radio that might be in the room, or by giving you something with sugar in it. She will want to see at least two periods of increased heart rate of at least fifteen beats per minute, lasting for fifteen seconds.

If the baby does not have such accelerations of the heartbeat—or if there are any factors present that would indicate a sick baby (such as lack of variation in the regular heartbeat or the dip in the heart rate associated with contractions), the doctor would warn you that the baby is probably very sick and may suggest immediate delivery or an oxytocin challenge test (OCT).

---

### 439 What is an oxytocin challenge test?

The oxytocin challenge test (OCT) is also called a stress test. Since it is more accurate than the nonstress test, your doctor may occasionally feel that it would be wise to have an OCT to back up the nonstress test findings. If you are fairly close to your due date

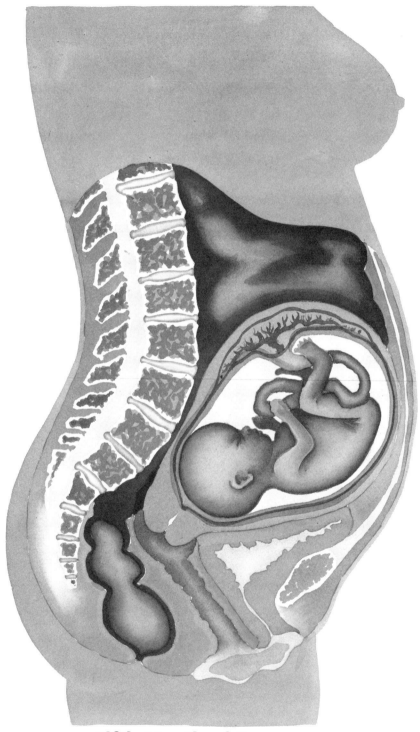

**Fifth Month of Pregnancy**

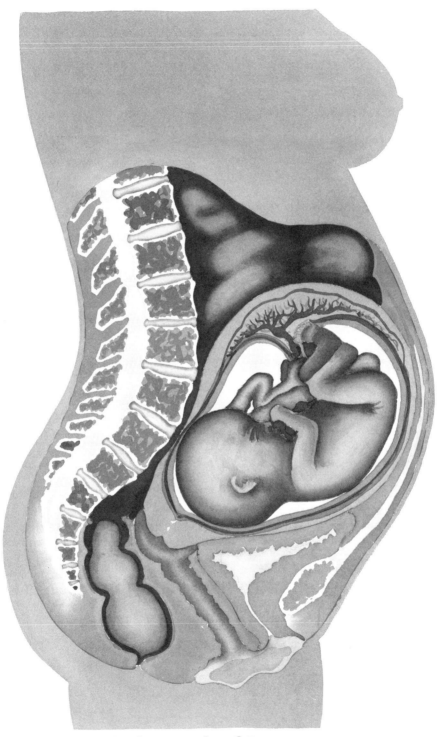

**Sixth Month of Pregnancy**

and your NST was abnormal, it would probably be easier for you to go ahead with delivery than to have the OCT done.

The oxytocin challenge test is merely a way of causing the uterus to have contractions to see if these contractions cause the baby's heartbeat to drop. During a contraction, blood flow through the placenta is decreased. This decreased blood flow through the placenta will allow less oxygen to get to the baby. This decrease in oxygen will cause an unhealthy baby's heartbeat to drop because of the stress.

## 440 How is an oxytocin challenge test done?

Like the NST, the oxytocin challenge test is done in the labor and delivery room of the hospital. After you are put to bed, a nurse will start an IV. Then she will put a heart rate monitor on your abdomen and record your baby's heartbeat for twenty minutes. After getting an initial heart tracing of the baby's beat, she will add Pitocin to the IV bottle and allow it to drip slowly into your vein. She will be trying to produce three contractions in a ten-minute period, with each contraction lasting forty to sixty seconds.

The baby's heart rate will be measured during those three contractions. If it does not drop during and right after the contractions, the baby is probably healthy. If, however, the baby's heartbeat drops after the contractions, and stays down for a few seconds, there is a fairly high chance that the baby is quite sick.

The problem with the OCT, though, is that at least 25 percent of babies who show a drop in the heartbeat after the contractions, if delivered, will be normal. The physician must evaluate the entire situation, taking into consideration both the NST and the OCT. After discussing the situation with you, a plan of action must be determined:

possibly immediate delivery, or maybe a repeat of the tests.

## 441 What is an estrogen (or estriol) test?

The amount of estrogen present in your blood and urine depends in part on the health of the baby that you are carrying. As amazing as this may seem, the baby is the source of most of the estrogen present in your body during pregnancy.

The baby's adrenal glands produce a hormone called DHEA sulfate (dehydroepiandrosterone sulfate). The placenta converts this DHEA sulfate to estrogen, which is passed into your blood stream and from there, into your urine. Doctors can test the amount of estrogen in your urine or in your blood and gain some idea of the health of the baby.

If the baby is getting sick, the adrenal glands will function poorly and will put out less estrogen. Also, if your baby's placenta is deteriorating, it will convert less of the DHEA to estrogen, decreasing the amount of estrogen getting into your blood stream.

When estrogen levels are being watched, it is most important not to depend on just one test as a sign that the baby is sick. Repeated measurements of the estrogen must be done.

An estrogen determination done on your blood is usually more reliable than one done on your urine, since the urine test can be thrown off by certain foods or drugs that you have taken, or by the fact that you did not collect all of your urine for the twenty-four-hour period being tested. The blood test is obviously also more convenient than the urine test.

## 442 Is the estrogen test reliable?

Because of the variation in the estrogen production in your body during pregnancy, the

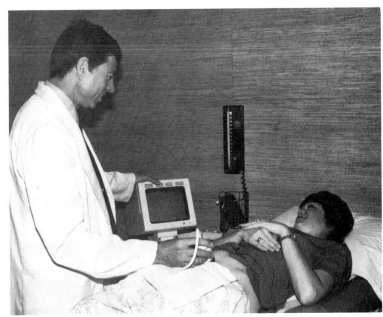

The use of the ultrasound scan has become a valuable tool in evaluation of pregnancy.

estrogen test is not a totally reliable one. It is helpful, however, in the following situations:

*Overly-long pregnancy.* In a pregnancy that continues past the estimated due date, if the estrogen level starts dropping the baby is probably getting into trouble and needs to be delivered.

*High blood pressure in pregnancy.* A low estrogen level may indicate that the baby faces some danger, indicating further need for evaluation, perhaps with the NST and OCT.

*Diabetes in pregnancy.* A stable, healthy level of estrogen may give you and your doctor some confidence that the baby is developing normally in spite of your diabetes. A low level can indicate trouble.

---

**443** **What is ultrasound and how is it used as a prenatal diagnostic tool?**

Diagnostic ultrasonography (ultrasound, scan, or sonogram) involves the use of high-frequency sound waves that are radiated into the uterus from a hand-held transmitter.

The sound waves bounce off the baby and the organs inside your body and back to the transmitting device. The echoes received are projected on a black-and-white television set for evaluation.

The use of the ultrasound scan has become a valuable tool in pregnancy evaluation. It is in no way related to X-ray, and in all the years of its use there has never been any report of damage to a baby from ultrasound.

Since ultrasound does not require the use of needles or other painful devices, it is a relatively comfortable procedure. The only discomfort is from the full bladder that is necessary for the test to be performed properly, and the only preparation for the test is drinking water so that your bladder will be full during the examination.

The usefulness of the ultrasound scan is in the following areas.

*Determination of length of pregnancy.* If an ultrasound scan is done about the twentieth to the twenty-fifth week, it can determine your due date accurately to within a week. This information can be helpful, especially in cases where a mother feels her pregnancy is further along than it really is,

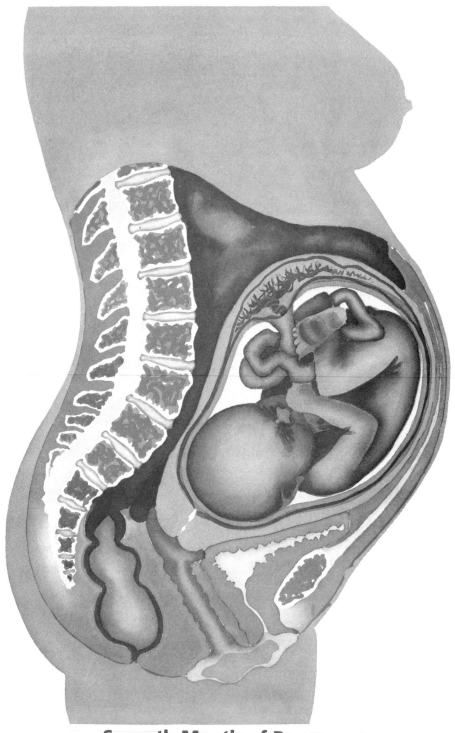

**Seventh Month of Pregnancy**

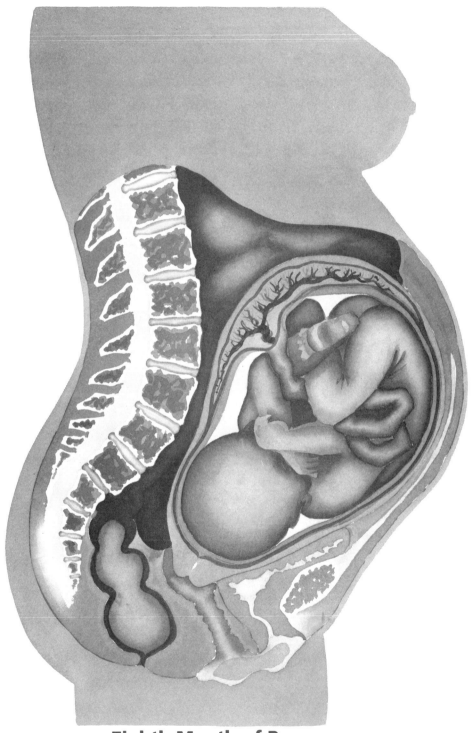

**Eighth Month of Pregnancy**

causing the obstetrician to think that the baby is not developing well because of its small size.

The scan can prove whether or not the baby is growing adequately by telling both you and your doctor your exact due date. By accurately determining your due date, ultrasound can help you both to know when it is safe for delivery of the baby.

I routinely have an ultrasound done on all my patients who have any question at all regarding the date of their last menstrual period. I also schedule an ultrasound scan between the twentieth and twenty-fifth week for all patients planning to deliver by C-section. Many doctors schedule their patients for elective cesarean section one week before their due date. The ultrasound scan helps pinpoint the exact due date so that the cesarean section is not performed prematurely and can be done before a woman goes into labor. A planned C-section has fewer risks than an emergency one.

*Evaluation of the baby's growth.* An ultrasound can show whether the baby's growth rate is slow or fast. This can be extremely helpful in knowing whether or not the baby needs to be assessed by a nonstress test or other techniques for fetal evaluation. Ultrasound would be used with a mother who has high blood pressure, diabetes, or other health problems.

*Number of babies in the uterus.* With ultrasound, the number of babies in your uterus can be determined by the time you are eight to ten weeks along in your pregnancy. This is helpful information, because if there is more than one baby, things can be done to help prevent premature delivery.

*Congenital abnormalities.* The ultrasound scan can detect certain abnormalities of the baby, such as those of the head, spinal cord, chest, or abdomen.

*Amount of fluid surrounding the baby.* The ultrasound can show how much fluid is present around the baby. This is important because it has been found that if the amount

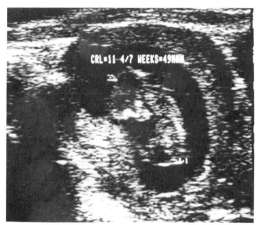

Ultrasound scan of a four- to seven-week fetus.

of fluid around the baby is small, there is a great chance that the baby is experiencing poor growth and needs to be further evaluated or perhaps delivered. Excess fluid is also a clue that something is wrong.

**444** **How is fetal movement used as a prenatal evaluation method?**

Checking fetal movement during the last three months of pregnancy is a technique that is not used much at present but may be used more frequently in the future. It involves the mother detecting and keeping a record of fetal movements on a daily basis. The most common technique recom-

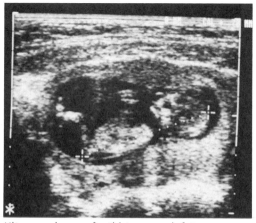

Ultrasound scan of a thirteen-week fetus.

mended is for the mother to record the fetal movements she feels during three separate hours each day: one hour in the morning, one hour at noon, and one hour in the evening. Most women who are carrying normal babies will feel more than three fetal movements in each one-hour period. If three or fewer fetal movements are felt in one of the hours of observation, the mother should observe fetal activity for from six to twelve hours a day until she and her doctor are assured that the baby is healthy, or until delivery. She should normally feel ten good movements in an eight-hour period if her baby is healthy.

An alternate technique is for a woman to start counting fetal movements at 9:00 A.M. The baby should move ten times by 6:00 P.M. If it doesn't, she should call her doctor.

It is interesting that most fetuses have a peak of activity between 9:00 P.M. and 1:00 A.M. (just what parents have always suspected). Most fetuses do show active periods alternating with quiet periods. If your baby is not too active in the morning, watch for activity late in the day.

It has also been found that a drop in the number of fetal movements over a three- or four-day period can indicate that the baby is getting into serious trouble. If this happens, the doctor would want to do further tests to check the baby.

### 445 Are there tests to determine the maturity of the fetus?

Yes. There are two ways to determine the baby's development: ultrasound and amniocentesis.

An ultrasound scan, done between the twentieth and twenty-fifth weeks of pregnancy, is the best way to determine whether or not your pregnancy is as far along as it is supposed to be. I have all my patients who have any question about their true due date have an ultrasound done. (See Q. 443.) Once

a pregnancy has gone into the last three months, the ultrasound scan is not as reliable in indicating when the baby is due.

If you were unable to get an ultrasound scan done earlier in your pregnancy, or if a problem makes it necessary to deliver the baby prematurely, an amniocentesis can be done. The fluid can be tested for certain chemicals that indicate whether or not the baby's lungs are mature enough for delivery. (See Q. 448.)

If the lungs are mature enough, even though the rest of the baby's organ systems may not be mature, it can live outside your body, breathing on its own and with less chance of medical problems than if it had to be put on a respirator. If the baby's lungs are still immature, then you and the doctor know that you will need to delay delivery until the lungs mature.

### 446 What testing can be done to determine genetic abnormalities?

Presently three different types of tests are done for such evaluation: ultrasound, amniocentesis, and AFP (alpha-fetoprotein) testing.

### 447 How is ultrasound used in genetic testing?

The use of ultrasound is technically the same in all situations. (See Q. 443.) It can be used for "seeing" certain abnormalities of the fetus that might be genetic in origin, such as anencephaly or meningomyelocele (abnormalities of the head or spinal cord) or abnormalities of the chest or abdomen.

### 448 What is amniocentesis, and how is it used in genetic testing?

Genetic amniocentesis is a test which is usually done when you are sixteen weeks along in pregnancy counted from the day you conceived. The doctor puts a local anesthetic in your skin and inserts a needle through the wall of the uterus into the sac that holds your baby. Some of the amniotic fluid is drawn off and sent to a laboratory, usually to have the cells cultured. Many different types of tests can be performed on that fluid in addition to those having to do with evaluating the baby's chromosomes for the purpose of genetic amniocentesis.

By looking at the baby's cultured cells under the microscope, the doctor can see if they show normal chromosomes. If normal chromosomes are present, the baby does not have Down's syndrome (mongolism). This possibility is the primary reason that this type of amniocentesis is done.

The use of ultrasound scan to insert the needle has decreased the chance that the needle will touch the baby. It also has decreased the chance of the needle going through the placenta and causing bleeding into the sac. One thing that continues to be a problem, however, is that as a result of amniocentesis about one in two hundred pregnancies will miscarry.

I know of an "older" couple who, despite an infertility problem, finally managed to achieve pregnancy. Without adequately considering the consequences, they had genetic amniocentesis performed. It resulted in the loss of a healthy boy and great heartbreak to these parents. My point is that the consequences of amniocentesis should be carefully considered, and it should not be done routinely or without good reason. For example, if you were to be fairly certain that if you were carrying a baby with a congenital abnormality you would not have an abortion done, then there is no reason to have the genetic amniocentesis in the first place, especially since it could cause you to lose a healthy child.

A woman does not have to have an amniocentesis done. And even if she has an amniocentesis done and learns that her baby

# Amniocentesis

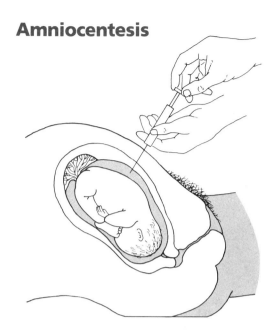

has an abnormality, she does not have to have an abortion. Unfortunately there are doctors who imply that a patient is legally required to have both an amniocentesis and an abortion if certain abnormalities are found. This is absolutely untrue! I have had patients who were told by a previous doctor that if they did not have an amniocentesis, they would have to find another doctor. Any patient who has a doctor who would say this, and who does not want an amniocentesis and/or abortion, should change doctors. (See Q. 495–516.)

---

### 449 What other tests can be done on the amniotic fluid?

In addition to doing chromosome studies on cells cultured from the amniotic fluid, other tests can also be done. The most common such test is having the amniotic fluid tested for alpha-fetoprotein (AFP). If the alpha-fetoprotein level in the amniotic fluid is elevated, the baby may have a neural tube defect such as anencephaly or spina bifida. Other congenital abnormalities, such as

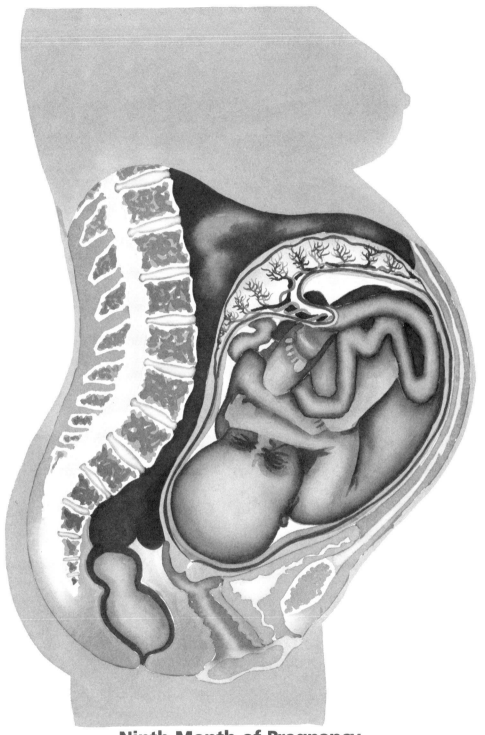

**Ninth Month of Pregnancy**

omphalocele, cystic hygroma, and congenital nephrosis, can also produce an elevated alpha-fetoprotein level.

Amniotic fluid can be tested for signs of genetic metabolic disease (See Q. 508 ).

## Intrauterine Growth Retardation

### 450 What is intrauterine growth retardation?

Intrauterine growth retardation (IUGR) is a term applied to babies who are born significantly underweight. Normally only their growth is retarded, not their brains.

Babies will usually have intrauterine growth retardation if they are within the smallest 10 percent by weight of all babies born at the same stage of pregnancy. If, for example, you delivered an eight-month baby that is very small, it would be considered to be intrauterine growth retarded if it is in the smallest 10 percent of babies born eight months along.

### 451 Doesn't this just mean my baby is premature?

No, since no matter at what stage your baby is born, if he or she is in the smallest 10 percent of all babies born at that stage, he or she would probably be intrauterine growth retarded. Many babies are born small; one-third of these small babies are growth retarded and two-thirds are small because they were born prematurely.

### 452 What is the concern about intrauterine growth retardation and its effect on babies?

IUGR babies have a stillbirth or immediately after delivery death rate that is eight times higher than normal. Their deaths frequently occur during labor, delivery, or during the first four weeks of life. They seem even more fragile as they get closer to term, unlike normal babies who become stronger, and they are more likely to die during the last month of pregnancy than they were earlier in pregnancy.

### 453 What causes intrauterine growth retardation?

To understand this problem it must first be stated that normally your body and your uterus provide a healthy environment for the growth of the baby during pregnancy. Because of this the overwhelming majority of babies are born healthy and normal, following healthy and normal pregnancies.

However, just as the environment in which you live can become unhealthy for you, so the baby's environment can become unhealthy. The effect of this bad environment on the baby is to limit its growth, occasionally making the baby so unhealthy that it dies before or soon after delivery.

Fortunately we have a greater understanding of these problems today and, with the testing that we discussed in the previous section, are better able to monitor the baby inside the uterus. When tests indicate that the baby is becoming unhealthy, it can be delivered before it is endangered by the bad environment inside the uterus.

Unfortunately, some of the things that cause the baby's environment to be "bad," and which have been present throughout the pregnancy, can cause the baby's body to be so affected that it is not normal or healthy. The best we can hope for in a pregnancy of this type is to get the baby delivered alive, so that it can grow to its greatest potential outside the uterus. Examples of things that can affect a baby in this way are alcohol, German measles, malnutrition, and cigarettes.

## 454 What things on the mother's part might cause IUGR?

Not only can you have problems that can cause your baby to be growth retarded, but you can also do things that can cause the baby to have poor growth.

*Hypertension and toxemia.* If you have chronic hypertension or prolonged toxemia, your chance of having a baby with IUGR is greatly increased.

*Chronic kidney disease.* This can affect the baby's growth.

*Sickle-cell anemia.* This, or other chronic anemia, causes the baby to be deprived of the normal amount of oxygen and can result in poor growth.

*Anorexia nervosa.* This problem, a personality disorder manifested by an aversion to food, results in a life-threatening weight loss for the mother and is disastrous for the baby.

*Medications.* Mothers who take Coumadin (a blood thinner that should not be used during pregnancy), Dilantin (a drug given for seizures that sometimes must be used in pregnancy), and certain other drugs, can have babies that are smaller than they otherwise would be.

*Smoking.* Women who smoke are not able to carry the normal amount of oxygen from their lungs to the baby. This causes the baby to be starved for oxygen and, therefore, not to develop adequately. This can be illustrated by holding your nose and covering your mouth with your hand so tightly that you can barely get enough oxygen to survive. This is a horrible thing to do to a baby. A mother who continues to smoke while pregnant is extremely selfish. If you are a smoker, I suggest that you go to any extent necessary to stop smoking. (See Q. 470–473.)

Studies have shown that if a mother stops smoking while she is pregnant, the baby will then start growing in a normal way, as though it is no longer being smothered.

*Drinking.* Alcohol consumption definitely affects a fetus. Babies of alcoholics are always affected to some extent. Although it is unlikely that a few sips of alcohol during pregnancy will hurt the baby, there is a proven relationship between the amount of alcohol taken in (as little as two drinks a week) and the health of the baby. My suggestion is to drink rarely, or not at all, during pregnancy and to avoid binge drinking completely. (See Q. 474, 475.)

## 455 What problems with the baby can cause IUGR?

Problems with the baby that can cause it to have IUGR include:

*Twin (or multiple) pregnancies.* The incidence of growth retardation in twins is about one in five.

*Abnormalities.* Often babies will have abnormalities, including chromosomal abnormalities, which will cause them to grow poorly.

*Placental abnormalities.* If a blood vessel from the baby to the placenta is missing, the baby can be receiving an inadequate blood supply. If a portion of the placenta pulls loose (and stays loose) it can limit the nutrition of the baby. If there is a large area of the placenta that has been "stopped up" (a large placental infarct), the placenta is less able to provide nutrition to the baby.

*Infections.* Certain infections, such as German measles, (see Q. 520–523) toxoplasmosis, (see Q. 517, 527–529) or cytomegaloviral (see Q. 517, 524) infections, will cause a baby to grow poorly. Fortunately these problems occur rarely.

*Prematurity.* A premature baby is sometimes poorly nourished. Prematurity and IUGR can coexist in a baby.

*Naturally small babies.* Some babies are small just because their mothers and fathers are small. Such babies must be watched just as carefully as babies that are small for other reasons.

If you have had a baby with IUGR in the past, you have a ten times greater chance of having another baby with this problem.

If you and your doctor watch for these indications (plus some of the things we have mentioned in previous questions), you have a good chance of anticipating a baby with IUGR. If you find that one of these situations exists, you can then watch your pregnancy more carefully than you otherwise might, to the great benefit of the child.

## 456   Does IUGR have different patterns in different babies?

Yes, some babies have what is called asymmetrical growth retardation. They have normally developed brains, but the rest of the body will grow more slowly and show signs of malnourishment. Fortunately the body selectively supplies adequate blood flow to the brain at the expense of other parts of the body. These babies will apparently develop normally later on.

On the other hand, babies with symmetrical growth retardation have growth retardation of both the body and the brain. These babies are more likely to have brain damage that could result in learning disabilities, seizures, or other problems. This type of growth retardation involves an overall decrease of the number of cells in the baby's body and usually begins early in pregnancy, whereas asymmetrical growth retardation rarely shows up before the seventh month of pregnancy. Symmetrical growth retardation, fortunately, involves only about 20 percent of the babies who have IUGR.

## 457   What will my doctor do if he or she suspects that I am carrying a baby with IUGR?

There are several different ways in which the doctor can evaluate the baby; some of them are not very reliable. The ones that are used most reliably are:

*Measuring the growth of the uterus.* Your doctor will measure your uterine growth each time you come in. The actual numbers don't matter; what is important is that there be continued growth. If growth seems to slow down or stop, the doctor will usually have an ultrasound scan done.

*Ultrasound.* The use of ultrasound has revolutionized the care of women who are suspected of having a baby with IUGR. Using the scan, a baby can usually be diagnosed as normal or as having retarded growth. These techniques involve measuring the baby's head or other body parts, as well as the amount of amniotic fluid around the baby, since the amount of fluid is usually less if the baby has growth retardation. The placenta will also usually be abnormal in pregnancies where the baby suffers from growth retardation.

## 458   If IUGR is diagnosed, what will the doctor do first?

After evaluation the doctor will want to treat you; the treatment will depend on what is causing the problem. For instance, if you smoke or drink, the doctor will encourage you to get help in stopping these habits. If you have high blood pressure, this will be treated.

There are some common-sense things that you will want to do to help improve your baby's growth. If you are a jogger, it would probably be best for you to walk instead. This would allow more blood to flow through your uterus and less to flow through your muscles. Resting an hour in the morning and an hour in the afternoon during the last half of pregnancy has been shown to result in a baby growing better. If your diet is poor it should be improved, perhaps with the help of a nutritionist.

You and your doctor must use ingenuity, common sense, and dedication to try to improve the baby's health. What you do does affect the growth of your baby.

---

**459** **What else will my doctor do if my baby has IUGR?**

Your doctor will try to establish a proper time for delivery. Using the techniques for evaluating the pregnancy that were mentioned in the previous section of this chapter, the doctor will monitor the baby. The goal is to allow the baby to stay in the uterus as long as it is a healthier environment than the intensive-care nursery would be.

Making that decision is difficult. You do not want to leave the baby in the uterus too long, nor do you want the baby delivered too prematurely. The nonstress test, stress test, estriols, and ultrasound are techniques that can be used to help watch the baby until it is getting into trouble, at which point delivery is necessary.

Unfortunately there are times when the baby will be so sick inside your uterus that it will have to be delivered too prematurely to live. Then, too, sometimes the baby will seem to be doing well and yet, when delivered, it will be too sick to live.

On the positive side, though, the techniques now available for evaluating babies before birth are much better than they were several years ago. Even if your baby does start developing IUGR, it has a much better chance of doing well than it would have had even a few years ago.

## Postmature Pregnancy

---

**460** **Is there a problem if my pregnancy goes longer than two weeks past my due date?**

A pregnancy that goes over forty-two weeks, or two weeks past the due date, must be watched carefully. This is calculated as forty-two weeks from the first day of the last menstrual period.

Only one-tenth of all pregnancies will persist more than two weeks after the expected date of delivery and one-third of those pregnancies will result in a baby who has postmaturity syndrome. (See the next question.) Of those babies with the postmature syndrome, 60 percent will have medical problems of some type.

The medical problems of postmature babies can be quite severe; 15 to 30 percent of these babies can die after delivery because of the effects of the prolonged pregnancy. In fact, the deaths of one half of all stillborn babies are due, at least in part, to postmaturity. This is almost as serious a problem for the baby as prematurity.

---

**461** **What symptoms might indicate postmature syndrome?**

The symptoms or effects of postmaturity are categorized by three stages.

*Stage 1.* In the first stage the baby's skin tends to be dry, cracked, and peeling. The baby looks malnourished—a little skinny, and without the fat, robust appearance of a normal newborn—but has an alert, open-eyed appearance.

*Stage 2.* In this stage the baby also looks malnourished and has an open-eyed look, but he or she is covered with a green film called meconium.

Meconium is bowel movement from the

baby, but since he or she has ingested no food, the material has no odor or germs. The baby sometimes passes this material from the colon when under stress. The meconium mixes with the amniotic fluid surrounding the baby and then coats its body.

Meconium staining is especially significant if the baby, the umbilical cord, and the placental lining are all green-stained. The coating itself does not hurt the baby, but a large amount of staining indicates that the baby was under a great deal of stress before birth. Frequently, however, normal babies will pass meconium into the amniotic fluid. When they do it is a normal, healthy event and is neither dangerous nor a sign of danger.

**Stage 3.** In Stage 3 (which includes all of the previously mentioned changes), the meconium is yellow, actually producing yellow staining of the baby's fingernails and toenails. This indicates that the stress was of long duration and the baby is sicker than a Stage 1 or Stage 2 baby.

---

**462** How does a prolonged pregnancy produce postmaturity syndrome?

The placenta can become too old and no longer able to support the baby. Just as your physical body has a life span of about eighty to ninety years, so the placenta seems to have a life span of about nine months or a little longer. When the placenta becomes too old, it seems to become less able to transfer nutrients and oxygen to the baby from the mother's body and to remove waste products from the baby. All of this can produce a sick baby.

---

**463** What causes a postmature baby to die before it is born (stillbirth) or to become very sick right after delivery?

There are several problems, but two specific ones are these:

*Inhaling the meconium-stained amniotic fluid.* As the postmature baby gets inadequate oxygen and food inside the mother's uterus, it becomes stressed. This stress is what causes the baby to have a bowel movement inside the uterus. The stress also can cause the baby to gasp and draw the meconium into its lungs. When the baby is born, its lungs cannot expand properly because of the plugs of meconium, causing severe health problems, and even death.

*Depletion of fetal sugar.* If the baby has not been getting adequate sugar through an "old" placenta, it cannot develop good sugar stores in its own body. Born without these stores of sugar, or glycogen, the baby becomes severely hypoglycemic, characterized by a severely low blood sugar level. This lack of glucose can cause seizures, brain damage, and death. Because glucose is the one and only fuel that the brain will operate on, the baby must have glucose to grow and function.

---

**464** If I go over two weeks past my due date, is it not possible that we have just miscalculated the time?

Yes, but that should not happen. The due date should have been definitely established early in the pregnancy. It is vital that a woman and her doctor determine the date she is actually due. If there is any question, an ultrasound scan should be done between the twentieth and twenty-fifth weeks of pregnancy. When done at this time in pregnancy, the ultrasound study can give a due date that is accurate within four or five days.

---

**465** Is it really that hard to tell when a pregnancy actually reaches term, even though the dates may be off and I have not had an ultrasound done?

Yes, sometimes it is quite difficult. I once had a physician's wife come to me as a patient when she was well into her pregnancy. Since her referring physician was a medical school professor, we all thought they had an accurate date for delivery of the baby.

We picked a day to do her repeat cesarean section, but when the baby was delivered its prematurity startled us. The baby was at least five weeks early.

This experience, which occurred several years before we had ultrasound for evaluating the actual stage of pregnancy, has made me extremely careful about due dates. When the patient is not absolutely sure of her last menstrual period, or when she has had irregular periods around the time that she got pregnant, or if she is going to have a cesarean section, I think a twenty- to twenty-five-week ultrasound study is imperative.

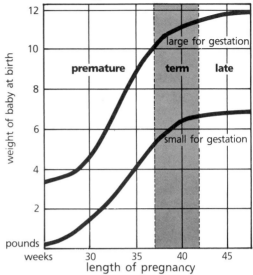

## Birth Weight and Length of Pregnancy

---

**466** **What should be done if my pregnancy is going past my expected date of delivery by more than two weeks?**

Most doctors feel that when a pregnancy has progressed two weeks past the due date, labor should be induced if the cervix has dilated and is soft, and if the baby is in good position. Normally a good obstetrician will be able to predict whether or not induction will work.

If your cervix does not seem to be "ripe," then it is probably best that you do not have induced labor. In this case tests should be done to be sure that the baby is staying healthy. These tests are the same ones discussed earlier in the previous section on "monitoring of the fetus." Regular testing should be done until your cervix is ready for induction or until there are signs that the baby is not doing well. When those signs develop, the baby should be delivered either by induction or by cesarean section.

Even if the baby appears healthy and your cervix is still not ripe, when you are starting the fourth week past due, most doctors feel that the baby should be delivered. Induction might work. If it is obvious that it will not or does not work, a cesarean section should be done.

Some postmature pregnancies might be avoided by instructing such women to stimulate their breasts. The technique is to gently rub the nipple with a finger for an hour at a time, three times daily, for three days. This exercise stimulates the release of enough natural oxytocin (from a pregnant woman's pituitary) for significant effacement and dilation of the cervix. Stimulation must be stopped when uterine contractions last one minute or longer. Do not try this technique without checking with your doctor to make sure such stimulation will not cause premature labor and delivery. If you have delivered a premature baby and you and your husband tend to use breast stimulation a great deal in sex play, it would be wise to discontinue use of that technique until your pregnancy is full term.

**467** Does anything need to be done for my baby immediately after birth if it has developed postmature problems?

Yes. If there are signs that the baby has inhaled the meconium from the amniotic fluid into its lungs, the doctor would use a laryngoscope (lighted viewing instrument) to look at the opening to the baby's trachea or main breathing tube. The doctor, while looking into the trachea, can use small suction instruments to remove the meconium. If this thick, jelly-like material is not extracted, it can clog the lungs and cause further trouble with the baby's breathing.

If the baby's sugar stores (glycogen) have been depleted because it was not getting enough sugar from its mother, the doctor will probably insert a small plastic tube into a blood vessel in the umbilical cord through which sugar water and drugs may be given, and to provide a way to do frequent testing on the baby to make sure that it is progressing well.

## Drugs, Smoking, and Alcohol During Pregnancy

**468** Why is there so much talk about the danger of taking drugs during pregnancy?

Prior to the discovery that thalidomide and DES (diethylstilbestrol) caused abnormalities in babies, there was little concern about the prenatal effects of drugs. That has now changed. Since the overwhelming majority of drugs that are now being used during pregnancy have not been thoroughly tested for their effects on babies, most obstetricians and many patients are concerned about the possible consequences of any drugs taken during pregnancy.

Most drugs that are given to you during pregnancy cross from your blood stream through the placenta into the baby's blood stream. In spite of this knowledge, drugs continue to be prescribed for the majority of pregnant patients at some time during their pregnancy. Some of the time this is necessary. Often it is not.

The National Collaborative Perinatal Project is a large study that was done with the cooperation of several hospitals and many physicians in this country. The project was set up to evaluate the pregnancies, deliveries, and subsequent development of children from 51,000 pregnancies. Much interesting and useful material has been discovered already from these records, and more is coming along as these children are now growing up. This study showed that more than 900 different drugs were taken by the 51,000 women during their pregnancies. The average patient took at least four drugs (not counting iron and vitamins). About 40 percent of the drugs were taken during the first three months of the pregnancies, which is, of course, the most sensitive time in the baby's development. A fair number of women took drugs before they even knew they were pregnant. It is obvious that the use of any drug by a woman of childbearing age who is not using contraception must be carefully considered, keeping in mind the possibility of pregnancy.

**469** What do you, as a physician, feel is the proper approach to drugs during pregnancy?

My routine advice to a patient is that it is preferable that she take no drugs except iron and vitamins, and then only the usual and accepted one or two prenatal vitamins a day. I always suggest that if they can possibly do so, women should get by with no drugs at all during pregnancy. A pregnant woman taking drugs that are medically necessary, should consult with her family practitioner or internist to determine that there are good reasons for continuing such drugs during pregnancy.

My concern is that, despite the warnings posed by thalidomide and DES, the use of drugs by pregnant women has not decreased. The problem is that it cannot be determined conclusively whether or not a drug hurts a baby until that drug has been used for a long time in many human pregnancies. Testing on animals does not help, and testing on human beings is not legal—nor is it a good idea!

Thalidomide is an example of the difficulty in knowing whether or not a drug taken during pregnancy affects the baby. No drug given in normal dosages has been proved to have as dramatic an effect on the fetuses as thalidomide, the drug that caused babies to be born with major problems, including no arms or legs. Yet this drug was sold for four years before its terrible consequences were confirmed!

In summary, my position is this: if drugs are necessary for the health of the mother, this is to the benefit of the baby and the mother should take such drugs. If the drug she is taking poses potential danger to the baby, perhaps another drug may be substituted.

If you want further information on specific drugs, there is an excellent book that has been published by Williams & Wilkins (Baltimore, 1983) *Drugs in Pregnancy and Lactation, A Reference of Fetal and Neonatal Risks*. The authors are Griggs, Bodendorfer, Freeman, and Yaffe. In addition to this book, *The Physician's Desk Reference* published by Medical Economics (Oradell, N.J.) annually, has information about drugs and their effect in pregnancy with occasional references to drugs during nursing. If you want more information about drugs, you might first try this book, since it is available in almost every physician's office and every library. (See also Q. 477–492.)

---

**470  Is smoking harmful during pregnancy?**

Yes. It has been proven that smoking during pregnancy is not only hazardous to the health of the unborn baby, it is also a factor affecting its condition during birth, immediately after birth, and also its future development. These problems include an increased chance of the baby being very sick or dying before it is born, during birth, or right after delivery. The chance of the baby dying around the time of delivery is increased to about 25–30 percent over normal. Because these babies are frail, they often do not tolerate labor as well as normal babies. Because the fetal monitor will show that they are in danger of dying before delivery, this necessitates getting these babies out by C-section more often than would otherwise be necessary.

In addition, a smoking mother is more likely to have a premature baby. Studies have shown a considerably higher rate of premature delivery for women who smoke during pregnancy. One report even states that up to 14 percent of all premature deliveries in the United States may be due to the mothers smoking while pregnant!

Studies have also shown that a child's physical growth and intelligence can be affected by the mothers' smoking during pregnancy. For instance, the attention span of such children has been found to be shorter, causing them to do more poorly in the early years in school, a bad way to start off such an important phase of life.

It appears quite obvious that children of smoking mothers may never "catch up" in certain phases of development with the children of nonsmokers. If you want your child to be the best he or she can be, you will not smoke while you are pregnant. Your smoking during pregnancy can affect your baby's future for the rest of his or her life.

### 471 How does my smoking affect the baby after birth?

In addition to the greater chance of death, there is also a greater chance of having a baby who develops sudden infant death syndrome (SIDS) if you smoked during pregnancy.

One study has shown an association between SIDS and smoking after delivery if a mother nurses her baby. If you smoke while nursing, your breast milk will contain nicotine. This may explain why smoking mothers who nurse are more likely to have a SIDS baby. Smoking has also been shown to interfere with the production of milk from the breasts, causing breast feeding to be less successful.

Smoking during pregnancy has also been found to be a cause of hyperactivity in children. In one study of twenty hyperactive children, sixteen had mothers who smoked. The nonsmoking mothers of the other four hyperactive children reported complicated deliveries.

Up until at least the age of five, the death rate of children is higher among those born to smokers than among the children born to nonsmokers.

### 472 Exactly how does smoking affect the baby?

When you smoke, your blood stream absorbs carbon monoxide from the smoke in your lungs. This carbon monoxide interferes with the ability of your blood to carry oxygen, and this lack of oxygen (anoxia) literally strangles your baby. This oxygen shortage for your child occurs during the most important time of growth in its entire lifetime, a time when the baby needs as much oxygen

as it can get to grow to its maximum, rather than just enough oxygen to "get by."

An additional mechanism limits the amount of oxygen that reaches the baby; the nicotine actually causes constriction of the blood vessels that normally carry large amounts of blood to the uterus during pregnancy.

The decreased oxygen supply to the babies of smoking mothers causes such babies, on the average, to weigh about one-half pound less than the babies of nonsmokers. Imagine someone squeezing your neck, limiting the amount of oxygen so much that you lost about one-tenth of your body weight! This is a strong illustration, but what a smoker does to her unborn child is a strong act of selfishness and irresponsibility. Just because you cannot see the baby while you are inflicting this damage to it does not relieve you of the responsibility for what you are doing to your child.

### 473 What can I do about my smoking? I want to quit, but it seems almost impossible.

First, of course, you must truly want to stop. The knowledge that you may be inflicting permanent, irrevocable damage on your helpless baby should give you the motivation you need to quit. I suggest that you do not try to do it on your own; get every available help that you can. (See Q. 1224.)

### 474 What about alcohol and pregnancy?

Simply stated, when you are drinking, your baby is drinking too. When the alcohol that you drink gets into your baby (and it always does), its body is affected as it develops. Problems produced in babies born to mothers who consume a lot of alcohol are so common that these problems are now called the fetal alcohol syndrome.

Fetal alcohol syndrome occurs, to some extent, in every baby born to an alcoholic mother. Following are some of the abnormalities associated with this syndrome.

*Mental retardation* About 44 percent of babies born to alcoholic mothers have IQs of less than eighty.

*Growth retardation*

*Facial appearance changes* Abnormal growth of the facial bones of babies born with this syndrome result in changes in facial appearance.

*Small head*

*Abnormalities in the growth of the arms, legs, and the joints of the arms and legs*

*Muscle abnormalities*

*Additional problems* Many of these babies show extreme nervousness and hyperactivity; many have poor attention spans that limit their ability to learn.

*Heart and blood-vessel abnormalities*

These abnormalities occur so regularly in children of alcoholics that it has even been suggested that alcoholic women who become pregnant should have abortions. My personal feeling is that "two wrongs don't make a right." Compounding an alcoholic's problems with the abortion of her baby does not help her. Rather, an alcoholic mother should use her pregnancy as a reason for doing everything in her power to stop her addiction. This would mean taking advantage of Alcoholics Anonymous, or any type of community help that is available in breaking the alcohol addiction.

## 475 I am a social, or occasional, drinker. Will this small amount of drinking affect my baby?

We still don't know the whole answer to that question, but recent studies suggest that babies of mothers who consume as few as two alcoholic drinks a week may experience neonatal withdrawal syndrome (tension, restlessness, stomach upset, inability to be comforted). Other studies have demonstrated that if a woman drinks two normal-sized drinks a day, her baby will weigh, on the average, six ounces less that the baby of a mother who drinks rarely or not at all. In light of these studies, I would strongly recommend that women abstain from drinking during pregnancy.

## 476 Does marijuana hurt the baby if used during pregnancy?

Some recent studies have indicated that using marijuana during pregnancy exposes the fetus to psychoactive chemicals that result in tremors, easy startling, and visual imperfections. It also seems to increase the chance of going into premature labor (which is always dangerous for the baby), and may produce growth retardation of the baby or certain congenital abnormalities. Marijuana is a much stronger drug than tobacco. This means that marijuana can produce its ill effects in the baby even though a woman thinks she is not smoking all that much. It seems quite clear that it is best to use absolutely no marijuana during pregnancy.

## Medications During Pregnancy

## 477 What about medications and pregnancy?

Almost every medication that humans have taken has been associated in some way with abnormalities in babies, including the time-honored intake of iron, the use of aspirin, sleeping pills, and antibiotics.

I personally do not feel that the studies implicating some of these drugs show strong enough evidence to make their moderate, occasional, and physician-prescribed use unwise. For instance, I still prescribe the usual prenatal vitamins and iron for my obstetric patients. The best approach, however, is to take as little medication during pregnancy as possible.

In the next series of questions, I will deal with fourteen classifications of drugs. These are:

sex hormones

nausea medications

pain pills

antibiotics

tranquilizers and antidepressants

cortisone

intestinal drugs

thyroid drugs

drugs for diabetes

drugs for epilepsy

blood-thinning drugs

diuretics

vitamins and iron

acne drugs

---

**478** **What affect might sex hormones taken during pregnancy have on the fetus?**

Sex hormones, which include Provera, birth-control pills, progesterone products, DES, androgens, and estrogen, have varying effects on the fetus.

*Provera, birth-control pills, and other progesterone products.* A few years ago an unusual congenital abnormality, referred to as VACTERL syndrome, was associated with the use of sex steroids during early pregnancy. The abnormalities included those of the vertebrae, anus, cardiovascular system, trachea, esophagus, renal systems, and limb buds. The association was weak, however, and most physicians feel that the chance of abnormalities in your baby from the use of these drugs is small.

The one exception would be the use of Provera. This could make a baby girl develop female organ changes such as a larger clitoris than normal or a vagina that does not quite open up.

In spite of the fact that there is only a weak correlation between taking sex hormones and congenital abnormalities, most doctors feel it is best not to use most of these drugs during pregnancy.

Pure progesterone suppositories, some progesterone rectal preparations, and some injectable progesterones are semisynthetic progesterone. Most doctors feel that a woman's body cannot tell the difference between semisynthetic and natural progesterone, and their use is not dangerous for the baby. The use of these preparations is sometimes necessary to avoid miscarriage.

*DES.* This hormone, although not used anymore during pregnancy, was used for many years to help prevent miscarriages. We know now that it did not prevent miscarriages, but that it did produce abnormalities of the female organs in some little girls. And some boys born to mothers who took DES also have abnormalities of their sex organs. (See Q. 208–218.)

*Male hormones (androgens).* Drugs such as testosterone and Danocrine can cause a female baby to be born with a larger-than-normal clitoris, or with the labia grown together (fused labia).

*Estrogen.* Even the female hormone estrogen, if given in large dosages during pregnancy, can cause some masculinization of the female fetus (a large clitoris and fused labia).

## 479 Is it safe to take the "morning-after" pill as a contraceptive?

No. The morning-after pill is not a reliable contraceptive. Therefore many of the women who use it will still become pregnant. Since morning-after pills consist of either DES or some type of estrogen, the problems discussed in the previous question could occur in the children of these pregnancies. These babies would have been exposed to large doses of hormones at the very earliest and most sensitive period of their existence.

## 480 Is it safe to take medication for nausea?

Bendectin, a drug that is now off the market, has been shown to be safe in pregnancy. Through the years, however, there has been an infrequent suggestion that this drug might be associated with an occasional abnormality. This has been so rare that it was probably only a coincidental finding.

If Bendectin can be implicated as "dangerous," then certainly any other drug given for nausea in pregnancy is probably more dangerous. Because of the problems with Bendectin, and because any drug for nausea will most often be given during the first three months, I am hesitant to prescribe any medication for morning sickness.

If, however, you are so nauseated that you are losing weight, and obviously not getting an adequate amount of nourishment for your baby, then I feel it is safer for your baby for you to use some nausea medications. Also, to my knowledge, no specific abnormality has been found with Combid, Phenergan, Tigan, or Emeticon. (See Q. 306-I.)

## 481 Can I take pain medication while pregnant?

The discussion of the safety of taking pain pills during pregnancy can be divided into four categories.

*Aspirin and Tylenol.* Excessive intake of aspirin has been associated with a baby being born with anemia and bleeding problems. Aspirin also appears sometimes to delay the onset of labor. Low birth weight congenital abnormalities of some babies have been attributed to excessive amounts of aspirin. There is some theoretical possibility of aspirin causing a change in the blood flow through some of the major blood vessels in the baby's body (premature closure of the *ductus arteriosus*) prior to delivery, resulting in a stillbirth. It is my opinion, therefore, that it is best not to take any aspirin during pregnancy. (See Q. 395.)

Tylenol, on the other hand, does not seem to produce any of these problems if taken for a short time in a normal dose. If Tylenol is taken in excessive amounts it can cause the mother to have severe anemia and the baby to have kidney damage, severe enough to cause death. The usual recommended dose seems permissible in pregnancy.

*Narcotics.* If taken shortly before delivery, narcotics can hinder a baby's ability to breathe. And if a mother is addicted to narcotics, her baby may be born with that same addiction. Narcotics are drugs such as Demerol, morphine, and "street drugs" such as heroin and cocaine. The baby's withdrawal from narcotics after birth can cause extreme illness and even death.

*Codeine.* I have been able to find only occasional mention of problems caused by taking codeine during pregnancy. Personally I feel fairly comfortable in giving moderate amounts of codeine to pregnant patients. I certainly would not prescribe to any patient enough of the drug to cause addiction. It is a narcotic but one with weak addictive powers.

*Nonsteroidal anti-inflammatory agents.* These drugs, such as Motrin, Nuprin, Advil, Anaprox, or Naprosin, have been used in the past for arthritis, but are now being given frequently for pain relief, especially for relief of menstrual cramps. Occasional one-time use of these drugs during pregnancy probably does no harm. Continued use, however, can theoretically produce some abnormalities of the circulation in the fetus (as with aspirin, premature closure of the *ductus arteriosus*). It seems wise that these drugs not be used often in pregnancy, if at all.

## 482 Is it permissible to take antibiotics while pregnant?

Obviously, antibiotics are needed at times during pregnancy; unfortunately, there are problems associated with most of them.

*Penicillin and cephalosporin-type drugs*. No problems during pregnancy have been associated with these drugs.

*Erythromycin*. Certain forms of this antibiotic have been shown to affect the liver in pregnant women, and they should not be used in pregnancy, specifically the estolate form of erythromycin.

*Tetracyclines*. These antibiotics can cause permanent staining of the baby's teeth and bones and should not be used after the third month of pregnancy.

*Sulfa*. Although sulfa itself does not cause any damage to the baby, if you go into labor immediately after taking a sulfa drug, a baby's jaundice may be complicated by any residual sulfa in its body. If you stop taking sulfa a day or two before delivery, the baby will be totally safe.

*Chloramycetin*. This drug is not used much anymore because of certain rare, but deadly, effects. It should not be used in pregnancy.

*Flagyl*. There may be a slightly increased rate of abnormalities in babies born to mothers who take Flagyl in the first three months of pregnancy. This would suggest that it is best not to take Flagyl during that part of pregnancy. Taking it during the last six months of pregnancy probably is not harmful.

*Streptomycin*. This drug can damage a baby's hearing and should be used in pregnancy only with careful dosage calculation. There are several other drugs in this category and the same precaution applies to them.

## 483 Are tranquilizers and antidepressants safe during pregnancy?

Valium, Librium, meprobamate, Thorazine, antidepressants, and barbiturates such as phenobarbital and pentothal have not conclusively been shown to have any bad effect on the baby. Babies born to mothers who have been taking these drugs regularly will sometimes show withdrawal symptoms, such as irritability. This suggests that there is a problem with the use of these drugs in pregnancy and that the best approach is not to use them unless it is absolutely necessary. I almost never give these drugs to a pregnant patient.

An additional consideration is that tranquilizers taken during pregnancy may result in an irritable, colicky baby. The frustration new mothers normally experience in dealing with these problems, combined with your own "anxious" nature, may lead to physical abuse of the child.

Lithium, however, is another story. About 15–20 percent of babies born to mothers who take lithium during pregnancy have abnormalities of their hearts. Therefore it is best, unless absolutely necessary, that lithium not be used during pregnancy.

## 484 Is cortisone safe during pregnancy?

Cortisone (and prednisone, and other drugs of this type) has been used without any sign of abnormalities in babies. This drug has been used in thousands of patients for many years, and most studies indicate that it is quite safe. Studies on rodents did show development of cleft palates, but the development of the palate in mice is different from its development in humans. There is no correlation between the two.

## 485 What about the use of drugs for intestinal problems during pregnancy?

Drugs for nausea were already discussed (see Q. 480). Other drugs used for intestinal disease are:

*Laxatives and antidiarrhea medications.* None of these have been shown to cause abnormalities in babies.

*Antacids.* One study, which included a number of different drugs of this type, showed an increase in the number of congenital abnormalities in the babies of mothers who had used these drugs excessively. Most physicians seem to feel that there is little chance of there being a problem with the moderate use of any antacid preparation, but perhaps cautious use is wise.

*Antispasmodics* (e.g., Librax, Donnatal). These drugs, given for the irritable bowel syndrome, have been only occasionally associated with a congenital abnormality. It seems that they are probably safe in pregnancy, but they should be used with respect.

## 486 Is the use of thyroid drugs dangerous during pregnancy?

Thyroid medication should be carefully prescribed during pregnancy. Some types should not be used at all.

*Propylthiouracil.* This drug of itself does not seem to affect the baby in pregnancy. If the proper dose is given to the mother, it is unlikely to hurt the baby in any way. An excessive dose can suppress the baby's own thyroid function and even produce cretinism.

*Tapazole (Methinazol).* Severe scalp deformities have been seen in babies born to mothers using this drug. It seems best not to use it unless absolutely necessary.

*Inorganic iodides.* These compounds can cause your baby to develop a goiter so large that it pushes the baby's head back, making a normal delivery difficult. Compounds of this type can also produce cretinism, a disorder of low thyroid function, and mental retardation in the baby.

*Radioactive iodine.* If given late in pregnancy this may cause fetal defects, including damage to the baby's thyroid gland. It should not be used in pregnancy unless absolutely necessary. (See Q. 390, 391.)

## 487 Can I continue to take my medication for diabetes?

Insulin, a naturally found hormone, is the only drug that should be used to regulate diabetes during pregnancy. The drugs that can be taken by mouth for diabetes control do not provide sufficient control in patients who are pregnant, although these drugs do not seem to cause any abnormalities in the baby. If insulin is not used and as a result diabetes control is poor, studies indicate that a mother is more likely to have an abnormal baby than if she had maintained good control of her diabetes. (See Q. 380–389.)

## 488 Are drugs for treating epilepsy safe to use during pregnancy?

Epileptics who are not taking drugs for their epilepsy have a slightly increased risk of having babies with abnormalities; epileptics who are on drugs for their epilepsy have a greater chance of having an abnormal baby. The question is, does the epilepsy cause the abnormalities or do the drugs? (See Q. 403.)

### 489 Are blood-thinning drugs safe to use during pregnancy?

Coumadin should not be used during pregnancy. It can cause mental retardation, brain abnormalities, deterioration of the eyes, and flattening of the nose (so much so that the baby cannot breathe through its nose after birth). This fact is important because newborn babies cannot breathe through their mouths and could suffocate if their noses are totally stopped up.

Heparin is such a large-molecule drug that it cannot pass through the placenta into the baby. Therefore, it has no effect on the baby and can be safely used in pregnancy. (See Q. 369–379.)

### 490 What about the use of diuretics during pregnancy?

Thiazide diuretics have been found to depress the formation of blood-clotting factors (platelets) in the fetus, causing hemorrhage when the baby is born. Use of these diuretics in the first three months of pregnancy seems to be associated with a slightly increased chance of congenital abnormalities in babies. Diuretics can decrease the blood volume of a pregnant mother enough to lower the flow of blood through the baby's placenta. This can be especially dangerous during the last three months of pregnancy. It seems best, therefore, to use diuretics as little as possible in pregnancy, and unless necessary, not at all in the first three months. (See Q. 306.)

### 491 Is it a good idea to take vitamins and iron?

Although one study has shown an increased number of congenital abnormalities in women receiving iron during the first fifty-six days of pregnancy, most studies have not

confirmed that. Not taking iron until after the fifty-sixth day would be an extreme precautionary measure, but probably not necessary.

It seems wise for women to take supplemental iron and vitamins during pregnancy because most women are somewhat deficient in folic acid and iron while pregnant. Without the supplement a mother may become anemic during pregnancy, causing problems that are much more dangerous to the baby than any risk that might be present from using iron and folic acid.

Almost all researchers feel that it is necessary for women to take 200 to 400 mg of folic acid a day, and most prenatal vitamins now include that. Excessive doses of vitamins A, D, and E should not be taken during pregnancy.

### 492 Can I safely use acne drugs?

A new drug, Acutane, is being used for severe acne; it should not be used during pregnancy. Studies have shown that it can produce abnormalities in animals. Because it is new and because of this suggestion from animal studies, it is best not to use it in pregnancy. Tetracycline should not be used during pregnancy either, but drugs applied to the surface of the skin of the face are absorbed in such small amounts that their use probably will not affect the fetus.

## Environmental Concerns During Pregnancy

### 493 Are X-rays harmful during pregnancy?

Diagnostic X-rays, such as X-rays of the chest, intestines, or the pelvic bones, do not produce nearly enough radiation to hurt your baby. Studies have shown that exposures of up to ten rads of X-ray is quite safe for a fetus. X-rays of the colon (barium enemas) or of the kidneys (IVP) produce only about one and a half rads; chest X-rays and pelvic X-rays produce even less than that.

Unfortunately, a number of unnecessary abortions have been done because of X-ray exposure. Naturally, if a pregnant woman had X-ray studies done before she knew she was pregnant, she would ask the radiologist or her doctor about the effect of the X-ray on the fetus when she learned she was pregnant. Knowing that there is a 3 percent chance of any baby being born with major abnormalities whether or not it was exposed to X-ray, and to protect his or her professional image, a doctor might suggest an abortion. The doctor might fear that if this particular mother happened to have a baby with an abnormality she would blame the X-rays, even though the X-rays had nothing to do with the baby's condition.

An abortion in such a situation might eliminate a potential problem for the doctor, but it would have been an unnecessary abortion for the woman and her baby. It is totally inappropriate to have an abortion done because the mother had been exposed to diagnostic X-rays.

**494** **Do environmental substances to which I am exposed affect my baby?**

This is one of the most common questions asked of obstetricians. Unfortunately, studies are not conclusive about the consequences of exposure to most environmental material. As in all matters related to the pregnant woman, being overly cautious is the safest measure.

*Household chemicals.* No studies have been done on these agents. No one really knows whether there is any effect on your baby of exposure to paints, lacquers, or cleaning compounds. A pregnant woman should have good ventilation, with open windows, whenever she is exposed to any of these chemicals.

*Chemicals at your place of work.* The same warning is in effect here. If you are constantly exposed to chemical fumes or agents at your place of employment, it would be best if you change jobs during the time of your pregnancy.

*Anesthetic gases.* Female anesthetists and anesthesiologists have been shown to have an increased incidence of miscarriage and of babies with congenital abnormalities. As operating rooms are now more conscientiously watched for gas leaks, I feel it is acceptable for pregnant doctors and nurses to continue working there. In spite of these precautions, time may show that there is still a risk to pregnant mothers who work in operating rooms day after day. This also applies to dental offices.

## Genetic Problems and Diseases

**495** **What about genetic problems?**

Read Q. 447–449 for a brief introduction to this subject.

The terms *genetic problem* or *genetic disease* are used in reference to certain diseases that are carried in the genes. This means that they are, in part, hereditary in nature. An example of a genetic disease is cystic fibrosis. The terms are also used in reference to the larger genetic unit called the chromosome. An example of chromosome abnormality is Down's syndrome, or mongolism.

As mentioned in chapter 6, each chromosome carries thousands of genes. Some chromosome disorders can be inherited; others can result from a single chromosomal accident in which too much or too little chromosomal material is present in a particular baby's cell make-up. (See Q. 499.)

**496** Can I know before I become pregnant whether I might produce a baby with a genetic problem? Can I know if the baby I am carrying has a genetic problem?

There are three main ways to determine the possibility of genetic problems.

*Genetic counseling.* Counseling is available to couples who suspect they might have a problem producing normal offspring. Genetic counseling is usually done when couples already have had a baby that is abnormal, but it is also frequently done when couples know that some family member has a hereditary disease.

*Tests before pregnancy.* If a couple suspects that they may be carriers of a genetic problem, such as Tay-Sachs disease (see Q. 509), or sickle-cell anemia, tests can be done to determine whether or not one or both of them is carrying such a congenital disease.

*Prenatal diagnosis.* Amniocentesis, as stated earlier in this chapter, is a prenatal test in which a needle is inserted through the abdominal wall into the fluid that surrounds your baby. This fluid is tested for chemicals, or some of the living cells which have sloughed off the baby can be evaluated.

Chorionic villi sampling is a new test that is only recently being done in the United States. It is not now widely available. The test involves inserting a tube into the uterus and withdrawing some of the placenta for testing. If the baby has a genetic problem, the tissue from the placenta will show the same abnormality. The problem with this test is that it can cause miscarriage of the pregnancy being tested.

**497** What does "prenatal diagnosis" mean, and why is it important?

The term diagnosis means "to find out what is wrong with," and prenatal diagnosis means "to find out what is wrong with a baby before it is born."

As 2–3 percent of babies that are born alive have some major abnormality, doctors and patients have become interested in trying to find out about the health of the baby before the baby is born. Congenital disease has become the major cause (25–35 percent) of infant mortality.

**498** Why would the doctor or the patient who is pregnant want to know if the baby has an abnormality?

They would want to know for three reasons: to make plans for the care of the baby when it is born; to be able to perform some type of medical care for the baby before birth; or to perform an abortion.

Modern medical technology has made many things possible. We can now find out a lot more about the baby before it is born than we could have in the past. We can now also do some types of treatment on the baby before birth. Although very new and still experimental, some prenatal surgery is being done for fetuses with certain specific congenital abnormalities. Certain technical developments have made it possible to do abortions at any stage of pregnancy, but there is always some risk. (See Q. 223–236.)

**499** Most newborn babies I've seen look normal. Are some of them really abnormal?

About 2–3 percent of newborns have an abnormality. Half of the major abnormalities a baby might have will show up at the time of birth; the rest do not show up until later in the child's life.

A child with a cleft lip or with an extra finger or toe will be identified immediately on delivery. Most of the diagnoses that are made before a baby is born are based on an evaluation of the baby's chromosomes. Many of these chromosomal abnormalities do not make the newborn look different, but they do show up during the baby's later development. Most of the abnormalities discovered during prenatal testing are traceable to the chromosomes.

## 500 Is amniocentesis dangerous to me?

The procedure does have some risks.

Risks for the mother from amniocentesis are extremely low. For instance, there has only been one maternal death from amniocentesis reported in European literature. I have never seen a mother have any complication from amniocentesis. Occasionally a mother will cramp or bleed after the procedure, but this usually stops after a few hours. The most likely thing that could occur would be mild infections where the needle is inserted through the abdominal wall, or in the fluid around the baby. An infection might require antibiotics for the mother.

## 501 Is amniocentesis dangerous to my baby?

Risks to the fetus are greater than the risks to the mother. There is about a 0.5 percent chance of miscarriage as a result of amniocentesis. This means that one out of every two hundred babies who undergo amniocentesis will be miscarried. These babies are usually normal and are lost as a result of the procedure.

During the procedure the needle can poke the baby but normally does not damage or hurt it. The baby will merely move to avoid the needle. Before the use of ultrasound during amniocentesis there was a greater possibility of damaging the baby's eyes, puncturing the umbilical cord and causing it to bleed, or perforating the baby's lungs. Such risks have been virtually eliminated today.

## 502 What abnormalities does amniocentesis not detect?

There are many abnormalities that amniocentesis cannot detect. Remember, about 3 percent of all pregnancies produce a baby with an abnormality. Some of the problems that amniocentesis would not detect are:

Isolated body defects not associated with genetic or chromosomal problems, such as absent or shortened fingers and toes, cleft lip, club foot, or absent or shortened arms and legs

An infant whose growth is affected by its mother's smoking or alcohol intake

Dwarfism

Siamese twins

Abnormalities produced by drugs the mother has taken

Heart defects

## 503 Is there a "balanced" approach to amniocentesis?

If you are one who would consider aborting your pregnancy if the baby were abnormal, be sure that the advantages of finding out if your baby is abnormal outweigh the risks to a normal baby that you might be carrying. The key factors to consider are these:

Do not have the test done if you would not have the pregnancy aborted in any event. If you are so worried about having an abnormal baby that you are having amniocentesis done just to find out if the baby is normal, and you know that you have little risk of having an abnormal child because your doctors tell you that you do not really need an amniocentesis, I suggest that you get some good counseling about handling your anxiety rather than endangering the probably normal baby inside you.

If you were to find out the baby is abnormal, be absolutely sure you would consider using that information in deciding to have the baby aborted. In other words, be realistic about how "abnormal" the baby would be, remembering that no one is perfect.

Remember that there are risks to a normal baby from amniocentesis and that the baby any woman is carrying is going to be normal most of the time.

## 504  What are the problems that justify amniocentesis and/or abortion (in the view of those who favor such abortion)?

There are four major categories to consider. They consist of situations where there is:

A previous child with chromosomal abnormality

A mother whose age is advanced

A mother or father whose chromosomes are abnormal

The possibility of a metabolic disorder, a neural-tube defect, or an X-linked disorder

## 505  If I have had a previous child with a chromosomal abnormality, what are the chances of this happening again?

In the past, a mother whose previous miscarriage or live baby showed abnormal chromosomes of Down's syndrome (mongolism

or trisomy) has been counseled that there is a 1–2 percent chance of having another baby with the same disorder. Newer studies reveal that if a woman is over twenty-four years of age she does not have a greater chance of having a baby with Down's syndrome than the woman who has not had a previous child with the abnormality. In the woman below the age of twenty-four, there is only a 0.7–1 percent increased chance of this happening a second time.

The facts from these studies mean that a woman who has had one baby with Down's syndrome does not need to have amniocentesis done to evaluate future pregnancies unless she is younger than twenty-four, and even then there is not as much chance of it happening a second time as had previously been thought. The exception to this is if the mother has had a baby with Down's syndrome caused by chromosomal translocation. There then is a greater chance of having another baby with Down's syndrome. If the translocation came from the father, there is a 5-percent chance of the couple having another baby with Down's syndrome. If the translocation came from the mother, there is a 15–20 percent chance of having a baby with Down's syndrome with a subsequent pregnancy. This means that if a person below the age of thirty has had a baby with chromosome abnormalities, both the mother and the father should have their chromosomes checked to see if they are carriers.

Other chromosomal abnormalities, such as Turner's syndrome (a baby girl born without ovaries because of having only one X chromosome), have no known risk for recurrence and are much less common than Down's. There is no reason for amniocentesis in future pregnancies even if this problem was present in a previous child.

## 506  At what age does a mother's chance of having a baby with Down's syndrome increase?

A mother who is over thirty-five will often be advised to have amniocentesis to test her baby for Down's syndrome. Many people have the mistaken idea that at age thirty-five suddenly there is higher risk of having a baby with abnormalities. This is not true. What the geneticists are saying is that thirty-five is the earliest age at which it is reasonable statistically to do chromosome testing with amniocentesis. Before the age of thirty-five such abnormalities do not occur often enough to warrant testing; the occurrence rates at age thirty-five barely make such testing reasonable (except possibly when an earlier baby had Down's).

Starting at about age thirty, there is a gradual increase in the chance of conceiving a baby with Down's syndrome. The risk figures I usually quote are:

Mother's age, thirty: 1-in-1,000 chance of a Down's baby

Mother's age, thirty-five: 1-in-400 chance

Mother's age, forty: 1-in-100 chance

A woman is twice as likely to give birth to a defective child at age forty than she was at age twenty-five; she is five times as likely to have an abnormal baby when she is forty-five than when she was twenty-five. Almost all of these age-related abnormal babies have Down's syndrome.

The father's age may have something to do with the baby's being born with Down's syndrome. It has been shown that approximately 30 percent of Down's syndrome births resulted from the father's sperm rather than the mother's egg. The statistical rate of risk with the father's age has not been determined as it has with the mother's age.

Most geneticists at this point do not consider the father's age that much of an issue. One significant point is that fathers should not blame the mother of a baby with Down's syndrome; the abnormality could have come from either parent.

## 507 How do we know if either my husband or I have abnormal genes and should undergo genetic testing?

A couple cannot really know that they carry and could pass on a genetic abnormality unless they have testing done. They would not ordinarily have such testing unless they have produced several miscarriages or have had a baby with some abnormality. It is usually during an evaluation of a couple who has a problem in producing a normal baby that a genetic abnormality is detected. When this type of abnormality is found, consultation with a geneticist is very helpful. A geneticist can give a couple some idea of their chance of producing a normal baby in the future.

When a parent has a genetic abnormality, the chance of producing an abnormal baby is theoretically high. In actual practice, however, far fewer abnormal babies are born to parents with genetic abnormalities than would be expected. When the father is the one with the abnormal genes, the risk of producing a baby with a genetic abnormality is far less than if the mother is the one who has a genetic abnormality.

## 508 What are metabolic diseases?

There is a large group of these genetic diseases; most are carried by recessive genes. For the baby to be affected both the mother and the father must carry the same abnormal gene.

Metabolic diseases are diverse and rare. The normal couple who has not had children and do not have a strong family history for one of these metabolic diseases would not have testing for any of these, with the exception of Tay-Sachs (see next question).

Very few laboratories are able to do the testing for more than one particular disease. Usually physicians in different locations become interested in specific metabolic diseases, setting up a laboratory for that particular disease. This means that a mother might have to travel a great distance to be tested for a particular problem that her baby might be carrying.

The tests are time-consuming, and testing for metabolic disorders must usually be started in the early months of pregnancy.

If there is a question about the possibility of there being a metabolic disorder in any child you bear, you should make plans before you get pregnant or at the beginning of your pregnancy, so you will know who will do your studies, where they will be done, and what the testing will require.

## 509    What is Tay-Sachs disease?

Tay-Sachs is a metabolic disease (a deficiency in the enzyme necessary to metabolize fatty substances for proper functioning of the nervous system) that occurs at a high frequency in one particular population group. Tay-Sachs is carried by one in thirty Ashkenazic Jews, the Jews of eastern Europe who are the ancestors of most of the Jewish population of the United States. If two Ashkenazic Jews marry and both carry the genes for Tay-Sachs disease, they have an extremely high chance of having a baby with that disease. Such babies seem to be normal at birth but soon show signs of slow development, paralysis, blindness, and other disorders of the nervous system. Tay-Sachs is usually fatal by age three or four.

Since the gene is also carried by both Sephardic Jews and by gentiles, or non-Jews at the rate of one in three hundred, it is possible for a baby to have the Tay-Sachs gene and have a gentile or Sephardic parent who is carrying the gene. This does not happen very often, but it is possible.

When only one partner is an Ashkenazic Jew, the chance of that couple producing a baby with Tay-Sachs is very small. Scientifically, it is probably unwise for them to

have amniocentesis and testing done, because there is a much greater chance of damaging a normal baby by amniocentesis than of identifying Tay-Sachs in their unborn baby.

The best approach to this problem is for any Jewish husband and/or wife to delay pregnancy until chromosome studies are conducted to see if either or both carry the gene for Tay-Sachs disease. The reason for this approach is that there is such a mixture of genes in the world's population that Jewish people cannot know for certain that they are not part Ashkenazic, and gentile people cannot know for sure that they are not part Jewish. When such a Jewish or Jewish/gentile couple later achieve pregnancy, they do not need to worry about their baby having Tay-Sachs disease unless both were found to be carriers of the disease.

## 510    What is a neural tube defect?

These defects are problems in which the baby can be born with most of its brain absent (anencephaly, which is incompatible with life) or with spina bifida, in which the spine has a defect that exposes the spinal nerves (these babies are often paralyzed from that part of the spine down).

One or two babies per thousand are born with such problems. If you have previously had a baby with anencephaly or spina bifida, your chance of a future baby having this same problem is about two per hundred. For some reason, if you have had the same abnormality and you live in England the chance of this happening to a future baby is about five per hundred.

If you would like to know more about spina bifida, contact:

Spina Bifida Association of America
Suite 317, 343 S. Dearborn St.
Chicago, Illinois 60604
800-621-3141

## 511  What causes a neural tube defect?

These problems can be caused by one of two things: the abnormal function of several genes working together or by the baby being born with a whole group of abnormalities, one of which happens to be spina bifida or anencephaly.

Although one of those two factors can cause neural tube defect, it is important to know for future reference which one caused the problem. If your previous baby had only spina bifida or only anencephaly, then the chance of recurrence is only 2 percent. If the baby had several different problems, and one of those happened to be spina bifida or anencephaly, then there is a 25 percent chance of another baby having a neural tube defect.

In calculating your chances for a normal birth the next time, it is important to make sure that your medical records are clear, and that you keep a set of them to show to any future doctor in order to intelligently discuss further pregnancies.

## 512  Which tests are available to determine whether or not my baby has a neural tube defect?

Two tests are available. The first is amniocentesis, to test for an increased amount of alpha-fetoprotein in the amniotic fluid; the second is ultrasound.

When amniocentesis is done to check for elevated alpha-fetoprotein levels in the amniotic fluid, almost 100 percent of the babies with anencephaly can be detected and 90 percent of babies with spina bifida can be detected.

A sonogram can detect almost all cases of anencephaly and most cases of spina bifida. The procedure is painless but not totally accurate. (See Q. 443.)

It is possible that neither the sonogram nor amniocentesis would show the baby as being abnormal when it does indeed have an abnormality. The sonogram does not relia-

bly indicate when the baby has spina bifida low in the spine near the tailbone; when the baby has that lesion and the skin is completely covering it, the alpha-fetoprotein level in the fluid might not be elevated.

## 513  Can the mother's blood be tested for an elevated alpha-fetoprotein (AFP) level instead of having amniocentesis done?

When the baby's alpha-fetoprotein level is elevated, enough of this material gets into the mother's blood for her alpha-fetoprotein level to be elevated too. Because of this many doctors are now screening all pregnant women to detect this elevation.

The sequence in the screening program is as follows:

Alpha-fetoprotein is produced in excess by a baby in a mother's uterus if the baby has a neural tube defect.

By the time the baby is fifteen to seventeen weeks along, the level of AFP in the mother's blood is high enough to be detected as abnormal.

All women would have their blood tested around the sixteenth week. The women who have a positive test would repeat the test. Only 4 percent of the women whose first test was abnormal will have a second abnormal test.

Sonograms would then be done on this 4 percent of these women who had a second abnormal AFP level. Half of this group would be shown to have another reason (other than neural tube defect) for having an elevated level, such as a dead fetus, twins, or inaccurate pregnancy dates. Any one of these things could explain an abnormal AFP level.

An amniocentesis would then be done on the 2 percent of women who did not have one of the above explanations for the abnormal alpha-fetoprotein.

One in ten of these women who have amniocentesis would have elevated AFP in the fluid surrounding the baby. *This means that 0.2 percent of the entire group that you started with would have an abnormality on the amniocentesis.*

Following the above sequence would allow the doctors to find 90 percent of the women who are carrying a baby with anencephaly and 80 percent of the women who are carrying a baby with spina bifida.

There are several problems with screening all pregnant women for AFP.

First, 4–7 percent of all pregnant women in the group being tested will be told that they have an abnormal level of AFP in their blood, yet only 0.2 percent of the entire group will actually have an abnormal baby. This results in scaring an extremely large number of pregnant women about a major complication their baby might have, when only a very few of those women will actually be carrying an abnormal baby.

In addition, this testing is demanding. It requires that physicians and laboratory personnel be well-trained and careful as they do these tests. Otherwise abnormalities would be missed, or women would be told they had babies with abnormalities when they did not.

Finally, the initial testing cannot be done until after the sixteenth week. By the time all the tests are performed, several weeks will have passed. An abortion—if that is the decision—this late in pregnancy carries increased levels of risk for the mother.

If you are sure that you would want to abort an abnormal baby or if you want to know if something might be wrong with your baby and your physician suggests that you have AFP screening done, I would encourage you to follow that advice. Be aware, though, of the problems associated with this type of screening.

## 514 What are the advantages of genetic testing for neural tube defects?

There are two major reasons for the testing. First, the testing will find babies who have an abnormality that is incompatible with life, so the mother may go ahead and have an abortion for that complication. A baby with anencephaly, for instance, is totally incapable of living. In my opinion it is better to have the baby aborted than for the mother to be pregnant nine months with a baby who cannot live.

Second, the testing can reveal abnormalities that need to be handled immediately after delivery. When spina bifida is found to be present in the fetus, the mother can be transferred to a hospital that will have a team of neurosurgeons standing by in the next room, ready to repair the baby's defect as soon as it is born. This will decrease the danger of infection and paralysis that could develop in the baby from this problem.

## 515 Where can I get more information about genetic abnormalities and testing?

This is a complex subject and one that is approached with a great deal of concern and emotion by both patients and doctors. The American College of Obstetricians and Gynecologists has an exellent booklet titled *Causes and Treatments for Genetic Disorders.* You can order it from:

The American College of Obstetricians and Gynecologists
Suite 2700, 1 East Wacker Drive
Chicago, Illinois 60601.

The United States Department of Health,

Education and Welfare also has an excellent book containing pictures of the amniocentesis technique and a short discussion about this subject. You can obtain this booklet by writing to:

Center for Disease Control
Attention: Chronic Disease Division
Bureau of Epidemiology
Atlanta, Georgia 30333.

---

**516** **All of this discussion on genetic problems is frightening and sad. Is there any other perspective one can take?**

None of us is totally normal, and I would hate to see the day when we judge everyone by some arbitrary degree of "normality." Just because children are born with limitations does not mean that they are "nonpersons" or worthless. These children do have limitations, but then so do you and I.

I have frequently referred my patients with babies who were not normal to the book, *Angel Unaware* by Dale Evans Rogers. Dale and Roy had a child with Down's syndrome and Dale wrote this book as a result of that experience. I believe her perspective is helpful.

No matter how much testing we do on pregnancies or how many abortions are done, we will never be totally able to prevent the birth of babies with some of these problems. I believe it is important to point out that with the development of infant-stimulation and early-intervention techniques, retarded babies are able to function more normally as they grow up than was previously thought possible.

In addition, these babies are greeted with more opportunity in our society than they have been in the past. They are no longer shut up in state schools where they cannot develop to their fullest potential, but are being treated as persons who do have worth.

Since Down's syndrome is the most common abnormality problem, there has been a great deal of interest in this subject. If you desire to learn more about Down's syndrome, you can write:

National Down's Syndrome Congress
1640 West Roosevelt Road
Chicago, Illinois 60608.

This group has a twenty-four-hour hotline for information, (312)-226-0416. They also publish a paper called *The Down's Syndrome News.*

It is important to note that Down's babies, although limited in their ability to function in various areas, are persons. It is important that we approach them—before birth and after—with the dignity, compassion, and thoughtfulness that we ourselves would want to be afforded. I realize that there are tremendous problems and expenses involved when you are faced with the care of one of these individuals, but I believe our entire society is elevated a notch when we care properly for individuals less fortunate than ourselves.

In thinking of this subject, my mind always turns to the autobiography of a Dutch woman named Corrie ten Boom. During World War II, this fifty-two-year-old watchmaker was arrested by the Nazis in Holland and held in the German concentration camp at Scheveningen. In *The Hiding Place* (Lincoln, VA: Chosen Books, 1971) written by John and Elizabeth Sherrill, Corrie gives an account of an interrogation by a German lieutenant:

"Your other activities, Miss ten Boom. What would you like to tell me about them?"

"Other activities? Oh, you mean—you want to know about my church for mentally retarded people?" And I plunged into an eager account of my efforts at preaching to the feeble-minded.

The lieutenant's eyebrows rose higher and higher. "What a waste of time and energy!" he exploded at last. "If you want converts, surely one normal person is worth all the half-wits in the world!"

I stared into the man's intelligent blue-gray eyes: true National-Socialist philosophy I thought, tulip bed or no. And then to my astonishment I heard my own voice saying boldly, "May I tell you the truth, Lieutenant Rahms?"

"This hearing, Miss ten Boom, is predicated on the assumption that you will do me that honor."

"The truth, Sir," I said, swallowing, "is that God's viewpoint is sometimes different from ours—so different that we could not even guess at it unless He had given us a Book which tells us such things."

I knew it was madness to talk this way to a Nazi officer. But he said nothing so I plunged ahead. "In the Bible I learn that God values us not for our strength or our brains but simply because He has made us. Who knows, in His eyes a half-wit may be worth more than a watchmaker. Or—a lieutenant."

Lieutenant Rahms stood up abruptly. "That will be all for today." He walked swiftly to the door. "Guard!"

I heard footsteps on the gravel path.

"The prisoner will return to her cell."

(p. 166)

## Infections During Pregnancy

### 517 What infections are common in pregnancy and how are they treated?

Infections in pregnancy may be divided into five groups:

viral
toxoplasmosis
malaria
venereal disease
Group B Streptococci infections

We will discuss the infections most common—or most asked about—during pregnancy, and also some of the least known. We will also discuss the treatment that is best for both mother and baby.

Before proceeding with the discussion, however, I must tell you that the information regarding three of the infections—toxoplasmosis, cytomegalovirus disease, and Group B Streptococci infections—will sound rather vague. This is because the knowledge we have concerning them, especially the latter two, is confusing. The symptoms are vague or nonexistent; the treatment is unclear; and opinion on diagnosis, prevention, and incidence is ambiguous.

Fortunately, the diseases are not common. I have never had a patient's baby affected by cytomegalovirus disease or with toxoplasmosis. I mention these diseases only because they do exist, and you may read about them in newspapers and magazines.

### 518 What problems do you include in the "viral infections" category?

Our discussion of viral infections will include the common cold and influenza, German measles, cytomegalovirus, mumps, and chicken pox. Herpes, a common and much-feared viral infection, was discussed in Q. 425.

### 519 Can my having a cold or the flu affect my baby?

There is no evidence that the common cold virus or an influenza virus can affect your baby. Pregnant women, however, seem to be a little more susceptible to developing pneumonia from a cold or from the flu. I tend to give antibiotics for a cold and/or flu more readily if a woman is pregnant than if she is not, because I often see women with those illnesses develop bronchitis or a long-lasting cough. I believe that these episodes are less severe and do not last as long if a woman takes antibiotics sooner than she might otherwise do to prevent secondary infections.

Since influenza does not affect the fetus, it seems sensible not to expose a pregnant woman to the risk of the influenza vaccine. Although studies have shown that the flu vaccine does not damage either the mother or the baby, any medication can have some side effects.

Most doctors feel that influenza vaccines in pregnancy are reasonable only for high-risk women, such as those who have heart disease, respiratory disease, asthma, or some other medical problem that would make flu dangerous.

## 520 What do I need to know about German measles?

The measles you need to be concerned about while pregnant is the German measles (rubella)—the three-day measles, a mild infection for the mother. Many people confuse rubella with rubeola, the seven-day or "red measles," which is not a problem for pregnancy but which can make the mother feel very sick.

Rubella is a mild, short-lived infection, and many women do not know whether or not they have ever had it. Women who get a mild rash and a little fever during pregnancy are often afraid that they have German measles but often they just have some other mild virus infection.

It is important to know if you contract German measles while you are pregnant. The best thing is to make sure that you do not get rubella while you are pregnant, by being vaccinated when you are not pregnant. It is important, if you do not know whether or not you have been vaccinated, that you have a test at the beginning of your pregnancy to see if you have protection against German measles. If you do then it is highly unlikely that you would develop German measles during your pregnancy.

Rubella vaccination has been available since 1969. Because of that most people were immune to German measles. Rubella epidemics became infrequent and a great deal of complacency has occurred. There are now many people who have not been vaccinated. They can, therefore, get the infection and give it to you.

If you are pregnant, and do not know whether or not you are immune, and you develop a fever, mild rash, enlarged and sensitive lymph nodes in your neck, and a little sore throat and cough, you should talk with your doctor. You may have German measles.

## 521 What happens if I get German measles while pregnant?

If you do get German measles while you are pregnant, there is at least a 50-percent chance of your baby having severe abnormalities. These abnormalities include cataracts, blood-vessel deformities, growth retardation, deafness, jaundice, and glaucoma. The abnormalities are more severe, and the chances greater for occurrence, if you have rubella during the first three months of your pregnancy.

Rubella infection of pregnancy can occur after the first three months, but the resulting abnormalities are much less likely to be severe problems for the baby. The baby is much less likely to have any problem, in fact.

**522** **Should I have an abortion if I contract German measles during the first three months of pregnancy?**

Because of the serious consequences stated above, many people feel that a woman should have an abortion if she has been infected during the first three months of pregnancy. The problem I have with that is this means that almost 50 percent of the babies aborted for that reason will have been normal babies, unaffected by the mother's German measles infection. Obviously, this is a very difficult problem, and I cannot tell you, or anyone, what to do if the situation occurs. I do believe that careful consideration should be given to the course of action that is taken.

**523** **What can I do to be sure I am in no danger from German measles?**

Prevent it. I suggest several courses of action:

Before you stop using birth-control methods, be sure that you are either immune or have had the shot for German measles.

If you are infertile and starting a fertility evaluation, be sure the doctor does a German measles test on you to see if you are immune.

If you become pregnant, insist that you have a German measles test at the start of your pregnancy so that if you do develop a rash later on, you can be sure that what you have contracted is just some other bothersome but unimportant virus.

If your children have not been vaccinated, have it done. You are more likely to pick up German measles from your unvaccinated children than from any other source. Even if you are pregnant, there is no danger to you from your child being vaccinated. Apparently the vaccine virus is not transferred from one person to another.

You should not be vaccinated while you are pregnant. However, if you do get vaccinated while unaware of your pregnancy, there is such a small chance of this hurting your baby that you should not consider abortion merely because of the vaccination.

**524** **What is cytomegalovirus disease?**

I have never had a patient who has had this type of infection, but it does occur. It has, in fact, been recently reported that as many as 30,000 babies are born each year in the United States with this problem. The virus can be passed from a mother to the baby during pregnancy, or it can be passed in breast milk to the baby while it nurses.

If a mother develops infection by cytomegalovirus, she would not know it. Most of the time there are no significant symptoms of such an infection.

There is no treatment for the mother or the baby, in spite of the fact that the effect on some babies is catastrophic: microcephaly (small skull), seizures, encephalitis, blindness, changes in the blood vessels, changes in the liver and spleen, and anemia.

**525** **What if I get mumps while pregnant?**

You can have mumps while you are pregnant. Some studies indicate that the mumps virus can cross the placenta and infect the baby, causing abortion or, if late in pregnancy, premature labor. Other reports seem to indicate that mumps does not increase the risk of these things occurring. Most physicians believe that a mother who develops mumps in pregnancy does not need to worry about such an infection.

## 526   What about chicken pox during pregnancy?

If a pregnant woman develops chicken pox (varicella), she may get a pneumonia from that virus that will be serious, and can even result in death. In addition, the chicken-pox virus can pass through the placenta into the baby, causing it to be born weakened and possibly to die after delivery. Apparently the chicken-pox virus will not cause congenital abnormalities in a baby whose mother has been infected.

I urge every mother to expose her little girls to chicken pox while they are young, so they will "get it over with" before they grow up and become pregnant.

## 527   What is toxoplasmosis?

Judging by the many questions I receive about toxoplasmosis in pregnancy, I would assume that every household in America has at least ten cats! This is one of the most common questions I get from my patients during pregnancy.

Toxoplasmosis is a disease caused by a protozoal organism called *Toxoplasma gondii*. This organism is present in raw or undercooked meat, and it can be present in the droppings of cats who are allowed outside where they can eat wild rodents or decaying meat.

A human can be infected by cat feces, not only by touching them but also by breathing the air that emanates from the feces that has the organism in it.

The *Toxoplasma gondii* organism is killed by dehydration, cooking, or freezing.

If you have had toxoplasmosis in the past, but do not have it now, your baby will not be harmed. If you get your first toxoplasmosis infection while you are pregnant, however, it might hurt your child, infecting the brain and the eyes. The baby born with toxoplasmosis can have hypotonia (weak mus-

cles), enlarged liver and spleen, small head (microcephaly), sleepiness, and inflammation of the retina and other parts of the eyes.

This type of infection is rarely severe when the baby is born, but it is important that a baby born with toxoplasmosis infection be treated as soon after birth as possible; the organisms continue to grow in the baby's brain and eyes after birth and can cause increasingly severe damage.

## 528   How is toxoplasmosis treated?

At the present time the treatment of toxoplasmosis has two directions. The first is the treatment of the baby born with the infection; the second is prevention.

There are tests for the infection. You can be tested at the start of your pregnancy to make sure you do not have toxoplasmosis antibodies. The problem here, though, is that symptoms of an infection by toxoplasmosis are so mild that every time you had a slightly stuffy nose or a low-grade fever, you would have to have a toxoplasmosis blood test to see if that little problem was a toxoplasmosis infection.

Because the methods of treatment of toxoplasmosis are untested and their effect on the pregnancy is unproven, some doctors believe that the only truly useful "treatment," if you get the infection while you are pregnant, would be to have an abortion. Since the infection in the baby at the time of birth is usually mild, it seems hardly worthwhile to have an abortion done for that reason. It seems wiser to treat the baby immediately after birth.

## 529   How can I prevent my being infected by toxoplasmosis?

The approach is fairly simple. First, pregnant women should not eat raw or undercooked meat. If you are at a restaurant and your meat seems to be poorly cooked, insist that it be taken back and cooked until it is well done.

Second, you should not handle cat droppings during your pregnancy. Let somebody else clean the litter box. In fact, I suggest to my patients that they not even handle the cat! It seems conceivable to me that some of the toxoplasmosis germs could be caught in the fur of the cat, and these could infect you. It seems best if you have an "outdoor cat," to have it stay outdoors during the time of your pregnancy. At the very least, don't handle an outdoor cat or its droppings.

A cat that is inside all the time and never gets out to eat, cannot cause you any trouble, provided it is not fed raw meat. More information on toxoplasmosis is contained in "Cat Owner's Guidelines," a brochure available from Toxoplasmosis/HL, NIAID Information Office, Building 31, Room 7a32, Bethesda, Maryland 20205, phone (301) 496-5717.

## 530 How does malaria affect pregnancy?

A discussion of malaria in this chapter may seem strange, as it is not a common disease in America. However, malaria is one of the most common diseases in the world. Because of widespread travel, especially to the Far East, some Americans do contract the disease.

Malaria organisms can pass into the placenta, but they rarely get into the baby. However, malaria can cause spontaneous abortion or premature labor.

There are two things that are important to know about malaria and pregnancy. First, malaria is more likely to occur during pregnancy or during the period after delivery than at other times in a woman's life. Second, it is not harmful for a pregnant woman to use most of the drugs that are given for malaria.

If you are going to be traveling to an area that has malaria, it is wise to take chloroquine to keep from contracting malaria while in that area of the world.

There seems to be no reason at all for an infected woman to consider abortion for malaria infection.

## 531 Will my having gonorrhea hurt my baby?

Gonorrhea does not affect the baby during pregnancy, but it can cause blindness in newborns if the baby is delivered through the vagina of a woman who has the gonorrhea germ. For this reason, most pediatricians use eyedrops (tetracycline, erythromycin, silver nitrate) to kill gonorrhea in the baby's eyes. There is a law that requires the use of some type of treatment of the newborn's eyes. The treatment does not have to be immediately after delivery. The mother may be allowed to spend some time with her baby, develop eye contact, and cuddle the newborn before the medication is used.

## 532 What problems does syphilis cause during pregnancy?

If you have syphilis and do not get it treated, the organism can infect the baby. About 30 percent of babies who are infected with syphilis will die before the mother goes into labor; 70 percent of the babies who are born alive will have some signs of infection by the syphilis germ.

Infection that the baby picked up before birth from its mother can result in its being anemic, restless, and feverish. The baby can also have a stuffy nose, skin eruptions, and moist sores around the mouth, the anus, and the genitals. The liver, spleen, brain, nerves, eyes, and teeth can all be affected quite severely. (See Q. 1177.)

## 533 What should I do if I think I might have syphilis?

If there is any possibility that you might have contracted syphilis during or shortly before your pregnancy, please tell your doctor. It takes about twelve weeks after being infected by syphilis for your blood to produce a positive syphilis test but it can be positive as early as four weeks. Your doctor will wait four weeks before having the test done, but may want to repeat it eight weeks later.

Do not expect the doctor to ask all through your pregnancy if you have had sex with someone who might have a venereal disease. Tell your doctor if you have such an encounter during your pregnancy.

If you suspect that your husband had intercourse with someone during your pregnancy who might have given him syphilis (which he, in turn, might pass on to you), tell your doctor so that a syphilis test can be ordered twelve weeks after your possible exposure to check your status.

## 534 How is syphilis treated during pregnancy?

Since syphilis has not become resistant to penicillin, this is the best treatment for it. If you are allergic to penicillin, there are a number of other antibiotics that will kill the germ.

Because syphilis can hurt the baby most states require a syphilis test early in pregnancy. In some states a syphilis test is also required in late pregnancy. Whether or not it is required, it is probably best that all pregnant women have a syphilis test done in both early and late pregnancy.

Syphilis occurrence has increased remarkably during the past few years. In spite of this I have had only a few patients in my practice who have had syphilis, and only one patient contracted syphilis during pregnancy.

## 535 What is a Group B Streptococci infection?

Intermittently during the past few years, there has been mention in newspapers and magazines of a bacterial infection in newborn babies by Group B Streptococcus.

As the incidence increases, many people ask why doctors do not routinely culture all pregnant women prior to delivery, and if the germ is present, treat it. There are several reasons why taking vaginal cultures on all pregnant women is not feasible. Even if a vaginal culture has shown this organism, and the patient is treated, she can get the germ again just before delivery and pass it to the baby. Also, vaginal cultures often will not show any Group B Streptococcus, and yet the baby will develop the infection. Although the mother may have the germ, the baby may be born without developing infection or not get the Group B Streptococcus infection until weeks after delivery.

No one knows where babies contract the germ. A baby may get it from its mother's vagina, but may also get it from personnel working in the hospital nursery. Because of this limited information, the procedure most obstetricians follow is to do cultures only on those pregnant women who have delivered a baby with this infection in the past. They do this culture when the mother starts labor or just before an induction or C-section. The culture information is sometimes useful to the pediatrician. Most obstetricians then go ahead and treat the mother with antibiotics while she is in labor or just before and during a C-section. The pediatrician will usually immediately treat such a newborn with antibiotics.

**536** **What is all the talk about "Rh negative" and "Rh positive" in pregnancy? How does it concern my baby and me?**

Before I tell you exactly what Rh factor is, let me explain some facts about it.

The term *Rh positive* means that a person's red blood cells have particles of a specific type of protein on their surface. About 85 percent of all people have that blood type. The people with Rh-negative blood do not have these particles of protein on the surface of the red blood cells and are therefore called Rh negative. They make up 15 percent of the general population.

If you are Rh positive (a blood test that is ordered at the beginning of pregnancy determines this), you do not need to worry at all about the Rh problem.

If you are Rh negative, your husband needs to be tested.

If both you and your husband are Rh negative, you do not need to worry about the Rh factor at all.

If, however, you are Rh negative and your husband is Rh positive, you could be carrying a baby that is Rh positive and this is the situation that can cause problems.

About 13 percent of the women with Rh-negative blood who are carrying an Rh-positive child will develop antibodies to Rh-positive blood; they will usually have a baby with some degree of jaundice from the Rh problem.

The process that occurs, if you are Rh negative, carry an Rh-positive baby, and are one of the 13 percent who develops Rh antibodies, is this:

During the later months of your pregnancy, or at the time of delivery, some of

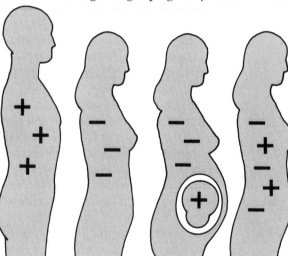
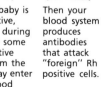
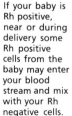
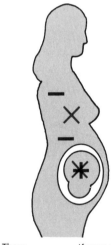

## The Rh Factor

Father, Rh positive

You, Rh negative

Your baby, Rh positive (possibly)

If your baby is Rh positive, near or during delivery some Rh positive cells from the baby may enter your blood stream and mix with your Rh negative cells.

Then your blood system produces antibodies that attack "foreign" Rh positive cells.

These antibodies become a permanent part of your blood stream and your next baby will receive them into its blood system.

If your next baby is Rh positive, these antibodies will fight to destroy the baby's Rh positive cells. Rh hemolytic disease results.

your baby's Rh-positive red blood cells leak from the placenta into your blood stream.

Your Rh-negative blood system reacts against these foreign Rh-positive blood cells by producing antibodies. Your body considers these cells as "foreign objects" that it must react against.

The antibodies that you form are then a permanent part of your blood system.

The next time you become pregnant with an Rh-positive baby, during the pregnancy your antibodies gradually pass through the placenta into the baby's bloodsystem, where they can destroy a number of the baby's red blood cells.

When a small number of the baby's red blood cells are destroyed, the baby may be born jaundiced, or develop jaundice after birth. When a large number of the baby's red blood cells are destroyed, the baby can die inside your uterus because of heart failure from severe anemia and an inadequate amount of blood in its blood stream.

If you are found to have reacted against Rh-positive blood in the past and you are pregnant again, your doctor will want to watch you carefully so that he or she will know if your baby is being affected. If the baby is affected, the doctor may need to give it a blood transfusion while still in the uterus or deliver it early so it will not be affected so severely. The shorter the time that the baby is exposed to your antibodies, the less severely affected the baby will be.

The scenario I just described happens rarely now. This is because we can now administer an immunization to prevent your body from reacting to Rh-positive red blood cells.

If you are Rh negative and your husband is Rh positive, you need to get a shot of Rh immune globulin (Rho-Gam) within seventy-two hours after delivery. You must do this whether you have an abortion, a miscar-riage, an ectopic pregnancy, or a normal delivery. If you have delivered a child, the baby's blood can be tested. If it is Rh negative, you do not need Rh immune globulin.

Even if you have a sterilization done after delivery, you should get your injection of the Rh immune globulin if your baby is Rh positive. A fairly large number of women return to their gynecologist to have their tubes repaired in later years in order to try to get pregnant again. You might do the same thing. Therefore you should go ahead and get the shot.

Additional protection for Rh-negative mothers with Rh-positive husbands is afforded if the pregnant mother gets an Rh immune globulin shot at twenty-eight weeks of pregnancy and also right after delivery. I feel that this is a wise procedure because 1–2 percent of women will become sensitized during the last months of pregnancy instead of after pregnancy. An Rh immune globulin shot at twenty-eight weeks prevents this.

The Rh immune globulin is a wonderful medical breakthrough! There is essentially no risk at all to receiving the Rh immune globulin and it almost totally prevents the possibility of the Rh problem affecting your future babies.

During my training program I did exchange transfusions on babies who had the Rh problem. We always worried that the babies would die during the transfusions. We also worried about the possibility of brain damage if the babies became too jaundiced, and about sticking the needles into their livers or other body parts if a transfusion was necessary before birth. These worries are almost a thing of the past, a miracle for which medical personnel, mothers, and fathers can be grateful.

## An Afterword

We have discussed a great number of things in this chapter, and many of them seem frightening. I think it is important at this point to come back to reality about pregnancy and newborns.

Most pregnancies and most babies are normal. If you walk by the nursery of a hospital you will see that almost all of the babies there are normal. In some fantastic way God has made us so that, in spite of the myriads of things that can go wrong, we and the babies we produce are usually normal.

We have discussed all the alarming things in this chapter primarily as a warning. Knowing these factors exist, and knowing what *can* go wrong, should help women be on the lookout for indications of a problem with their pregnancy or with their baby and help insure that they deliver a normal child.

If you suspect that any of the things that have been discussed in this chapter might apply to you, please tell your doctor. Today more and more mothers are able to participate in their medical care. Increased knowledge and better care can increase the probability that their babies will be healthy and normal.

I think it is important to mention that much of what we have discussed in this chapter could not have even been written twenty-five years ago. Many of these facts were not known. The techniques for following the baby in pregnancy were not available. Although knowing all these facts makes pregnancy seem a great deal more complicated, it certainly has added to a couple's ability to deliver a healthier baby.

It is my firm belief that God has given us the insight and the information that we now possess to help us in this whole process. He loves us more than we love ourselves and even more than we love our own children. He wants the best for us in everything.

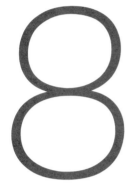

# Preparation for Childbirth

Prenatal training is widely accepted, readily available in most locales, and almost routine in America today. Although this training is one of the best things that has happened in obstetrics, it is a relatively new phenomenon.

When I began my practice in 1968, such things as childbirth classes, fathers in the delivery rooms, and deliveries without anesthesia were being done in only a few places. For instance, in Austin, Texas, in 1968, fathers were not allowed in any delivery room in the city, childbirth classes had been available for only two years, most women still wanted to be "put to sleep" or at least have a spinal for delivery, and doctors generally were not encouraging their patients to do differently.

When I suggested to my patients that they go to childbirth classes and plan to get by with as little anesthesia as possible, they would usually shake their heads in disbelief and say, "Put me to sleep! I don't want to know anything!"

Fortunately the attitudes of both patients and medical personnel have generally changed, and preparation for childbirth is now a widely accepted concept. I, and most other obstetricians, encourage all patients and their husbands to go to classes, whether or not they are interested in "natural childbirth."

Husbands who go to classes find to their surprise that they not only learn a lot but actually enjoy the learning. Such husbands are a

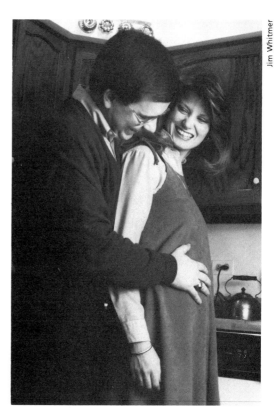

Producing a baby involves team effort—from conception to delivery.

great physical and emotional help to their wives during labor and delivery. With training mothers know more about the growth of the child in the uterus and are more aware of the danger signs that might indicate problems with their pregnancy. In addition, they are taught effective pain-control techniques that really do help during labor.

The team effort involved in producing a baby from conception to delivery helps a couple see the pleasure they can have in continuing as a team to rear the child they, and God, have produced.

I encourage patients who are going to have a C-section to go to cesarean section classes. By explaining to patients what takes place during a C-section, these classes help both a woman and her husband to relax during the last few weeks and days of pregnancy. Also, since it is impossible to predict what might happen in pregnancy, even though a cesarean is planned a woman may go into labor and deliver so quickly that there is no time for a cesarean. Classes will help a couple know what to do in that situation.

Many hospitals now offer more classes than patients can, or

will, attend. For instance, a recent circular from Austin's St. David's Community Hospital announced the following classes:

| | |
|---|---|
| Early Prenatal | Cesarean Birth |
| Lamaze | Breast Feeding |
| Lamaze Refresher | Child Care |
| Transition into Parenthood | Sibling Class |

I am delighted with the availability of these educational opportunities. I wish all patients had access to this training, since I believe that the better-informed patient is a better, healthier, happier patient, regardless of the medical situation.

## Training for Childbirth

### 537 How did the modern preparation-for-childbirth methods and training come about?

Three doctors were largely responsible for the popularity and acceptance of the preparation-for-childbirth techniques that are used today. In 1933 Dr. Grantly Dick-Read wrote his book, *Natural Childbirth* (New York: Harper and Row), followed in 1944 by his *Childbirth Without Fear*. His theory was that mothers who were educated about the labor-and-delivery process would not hurt from that process when they went through it. He also felt it was important that mothers not be left alone during labor.

In 1951 Dr. Fernand Lamaze brought his psychoprophylactic method to France. In 1958 his book, *Painless Childbirth* (Chicago: Contemporary Books, Inc.), was first introduced in English. Another book, *Thank You, Dr. Lamaze* by Marjorie Karmel (New York: Harper & Row, 1981), popularized Lamaze's approach. Lamaze's theory was based on his belief that a person can concentrate on only one thing at a time. If a woman concentrates her thoughts on something other than the pain of labor, the pain of labor will become peripheral in her mind and not be noticed. An example is the athlete who finishes a game with a broken bone, noticing the pain only after the game is over. Lamaze's approach also emphasized the importance of education beforehand and of the husband's involvement in the entire process.

Finally, Dr. Robert A. Bradley published *Husband-Coached Childbirth* (New York: Harper and Row) in 1965. His emphasis was on the presence and involvement of the husband during labor and delivery. Like Lamaze, he emphasized predelivery education.

Today few classes for expectant mothers teach a "pure" method. Most teachers draw from the many books that are available and in this way are able to tailor the material to a particular class or individual.

### 538 What information and training are given in childbirth classes?

Many books have been written about this subject, and it is beyond the scope of this one to include all that information. If you want further information on this subject, I suggest two things. First, enroll in childbirth classes. Some of the information about childbirth can be learned from books, but you will probably learn it more effectively in a series of classes. Second, read some of the books listed below. If you attend childbirth classes, you will probably be referred to other books by your instructor.

> *Six Practical Lessons For an Easier Childbirth* by Elizabeth Bing (Bantam, 1980)
>
> *Thank You, Dr. Lamaze* by Marjorie Karmel (Harper & Row, 1981)
>
> *A Lamaze Guide-Preparation for Childbirth* by Donna and Rodger Ewy (Formur, 1982)
>
> *Husband-Coached Childbirth* by Robert A. Bradley (Harper & Row, 1965)
>
> *Commonsense Childbirth* by Lester D. Hazell (Berkley, 1981)
>
> *Awake and Aware* by Irvin Chabon (Delacorte Press, 1969)
>
> *Moving Through Pregnancy* by Elizabeth Bing (Bobbs Merrill, 1975)
>
> *Childbirth Without Fear* by Grantly Dick-Read (Harper & Row, 1981)
>
> *Painless Childbirth* by Fernand Lamaze (Regnery, 1970)

Most of these books were written several years ago and represent the materials that popularized "natural childbirth" in the first place. I have omitted more recent books because most childbirth-preparation classes now have their own individual syllabuses. Many of them are excellent, and some of them are quite complete. The advantage of such individualized booklets is that they can be custom-fitted to the hospital where you deliver your baby.

---

**539** Aren't preparation-for-childbirth classes the same as "natural childbirth" classes?

To most people, the term *natural childbirth* implies the birth of a baby without any pain medication, or at most a local anesthetic for sewing up lacerations or for repairing a small episiotomy. But preparation-for-childbirth classes are not given to convince mothers that "natural childbirth" is the best way to have a baby.

Although there are some teachers who stress "natural childbirth," they do not necessarily represent the mainstream philosophy. If you are in a class in which the teacher seems to be trying to teach everyone in the class how to have a baby without pain medication, you probably are in the wrong class.

The goal of childbirth is to have a healthy baby, and the goal of childbirth classes is to produce an expectant mother/father team who can approach labor and delivery with the knowledge and attitude that they can handle whatever comes. The parents will have studied the anatomy and physiology of childbirth and learned techniques to cope with both the emotional and physical aspects of having a baby. The mother has learned that if she gets to the point where the pain is too uncomfortable, there are medications that can ease her discomfort without affecting her baby or interfering with a normal labor.

The mother and father also learn that if there is a medical problem, a cesarean section can be done. They know that if this occurs, it is not a "failed childbirth experience" but quite the opposite. It is a procedure which enables them to complete the childbirth process with the ultimate goal attained: the delivery of a healthy child.

---

**540** What are the advantages in going to preparation-for-childbirth classes?

There are many answers to this question, based on common sense and actual experience, but scientific studies have not proven any of them. The advantages that seem to be agreed on by physicians, nurses, and patients are the following.

*Reduction of anxiety for the father and mother.* Most women who have not experienced childbirth are at best uneasy about it, and at worst scared to death. Learning what will happen and how the process will affect them helps many women feel less anxiety as they anticipate labor. Many women find that knowing what is going on during the labor and delivery, and using learned techniques for dealing with pain, keeps them from being as anxious as they expected to be. The same is true for fathers: increased knowledge results in lessened anxiety.

*Parents have an active role.* With training the father can be involved in the process. Without training he is almost always just a bystander and observer. With training the mother and father can become a team during the childbirth process. Both actively participate in one of the most dramatic and exciting events of their lives: the birth of their baby.

*Expectant parents work better with the medical staff.* Prepared parents are better able to do the things suggested by the doctors and nurses that will help to ease distress. Most medical personnel enjoy working with patients who have some knowledge of what is going on and who want to be involved in the birth process.

*Prepared patients are ready for emergencies.* Simple things, such as knowing who to call if you start heavy bleeding, can save a baby's or mother's life. In the hospital, a patient's cooperation in the event of an emergency cesarean section can make delivery easier for the baby and thereby allow the birth of a healthier child.

*Prepared mothers utilize pain medications intelligently.* Although recent studies have shown that prepared mothers do not use less pain medication, I believe that prepared mothers are more knowledgeable in their requests for pain medication.

*Prepared parents are more alert at the time of delivery.* Patients who have not had any preparation for childbirth often seem to be so startled and even frightened during the entire birthing process that when delivery is accomplished, they are too agitated to appreciate the deliciousness of the moment of birth. Prepared mothers are often more alert and thus better able to enjoy the thrill of having given birth.

*Prepared mothers seem to have a better outcome.* This opinion is somewhat controversial, but some studies show that prepared mothers have fewer episiotomies, fewer cesarean sections, fewer episodes of fetal distress, fewer episodes of infection after delivery, and less toxemia. The reasons for this are neither proven nor clear. It may be that mothers who go to the trouble to take preparation-for-childbirth classes are also more likely to take good care of themselves and to choose doctors who are more sensitive, conservative, and careful.

---

**541** **What areas are covered in preparation-for-childbirth classes?**

All aspects of childbirth are covered in such classes.

*Educational.* You will study a woman's genital anatomy and the anatomy of pregnancy. You will also study the process of labor so that you will know what is happening as labor progresses. You will learn such things as how the cervix dilates and how the baby's head descends in the birth canal.

*Training.* You and your husband will practice breathing, positioning, and pushing techniques, and you will practice working together. He will learn how to time contractions and how to help you remember what to do during the different phases of your labor and delivery. This training reassures him that he has an important place during childbirth, you are reassured knowing he knows what to do, and you realize that there is more for you to do than lie passively and helplessly on your back during labor.

*Pain.* You will learn how breathing techniques can be used to help alleviate pain, and you will learn about drugs that can alleviate your pain without hurting your baby.

*Procedures.* You will be given information about entering and leaving the hospital. If your classes are affiliated with the hospital where you will deliver, you will probably tour the hospital, including the labor-and-delivery areas and the nursery.

*Practical suggestions.* You will be given many practical pointers through classroom teaching and discussion that will make labor and delivery easier and safer and will make the presence of a new baby in your home easier to cope with.

## 542 Are all preparation-for-childbirth classes equally good?

Of course not. Some classes are well planned, and some childbirth-class teachers are excellent. Others are not well planned and sensibly organized and are taught by less than successful teachers. Sometimes a teacher seems to suggest that you will be a failure if you do not make it through labor and delivery without any pain medication. This teacher has a warped view of the goals for preparation for childbirth. If what your teacher tells you does not seem to make common sense or if it seems to be unusually warped or biased, I would suggest that you find another class.

In an excellent article from *Clinical Obstetrics and Gynecology* (Vol. 24, No. 2, June, 1981), Drs. Arnolds, Anderson, and Sherline state:

The emphasis of prepared childbirth today has shifted since its conception. Whereas painlessness used to be the goal, psychological and emotional benefits are now stressed. Interpersonal relationships and the quality of the birth experience for each parturient are now more important than that the "prepared" mother understand that there are no absolute standards according to which she should judge her labor and delivery experience. If she requests pain medication, if an epidural anesthetic is given, if forceps are necessary, or if a cesarean section is required, the mother must not be made to feel as if she has failed. The only failure with regard to prepared childbirth occurs if members of the health care team have not made this option, in some form, available to all patients (pp. 575–585).

## 543 How can childbirth education help relieve pain?

Most women who have not experienced labor and delivery (and many who have) are afraid of the pain that labor will cause them. If this were not true, it is unlikely that Dr. Lamaze would have caused such a stir when he wrote *Painless Childbirth*. Without question, labor contractions are uncomfortable. It is also without question that pain can increase or decrease according to the way a woman perceives these contractions.

When a woman enters labor frightened, tense, and unaware of what is happening, she perceives her contractions as being much more painful than they really are. The beginning of a contraction signals to her that she should feel pain, even if the contraction itself is not very uncomfortable. Since she perceives contractions as very painful, as they become closer and stronger she envisions that they must hurt even more. She can become disoriented and exhausted as she perceives herself to be wracked with pain.

A woman in this condition is totally out of control and unable to cooperate as labor progresses. For her, the entire process of labor and delivery is such a wrenching experience that instead of enjoying the birth of the baby, all she can think of is getting relief from pain.

Although the situation just described is extreme, untrained women will generally experience similar problems with labor. We have all been conditioned to recognize pain as an indication that something is wrong. In labor, however, pain is a sign that things are right. Understanding that contraction pain is natural and good helps a woman relax and "go with the flow" of the contraction.

---

## 544 Will preparation-for-childbirth classes insure a pain-free delivery?

Not necessarily. Although many women who have their baby "naturally" receive no pain medication, experience very little pain during labor, and are up walking around the day of delivery, there are many who have a great deal of discomfort with their "natural childbirth." Even women who are well trained, unafraid, and enthusiastic about childbirth without medication can become so uncomfortable during labor that they require medication for pain relief and an epidural for the last part of labor and for delivery. Others enter labor without any preparation and progress through labor quietly and without any significant discomfort, delivering with only a local.

I think it is obvious that each of us is made with different thresholds of pain tolerance. No woman who has had a fairly painless "natural childbirth" should push this technique on another woman. The other woman may have nerves that are "hooked up" to be much more sensitive. She literally cannot tolerate labor pains, even

though she has the same resolve and education as the woman who had a good experience. Likewise, someone who has had a great deal of discomfort while trying to deliver without pain medication should not tell another woman how "terrible" it was. That other woman may have nerves connected in such a way that labor for her will not be so painful.

---

## 545 Do women who have had preparation-for-childbirth classes require less medication?

Several recent studies of medication and anesthesia given during labor have shown that medication rates have not been affected by childbirth preparation. This has surprised many of the strong advocates of such training, but I doubt that it was a surprise to most obstetricians.

My experience with women who have had childbirth classes is that most of the time they are able to go without Demerol through the early part of labor (from one or two centimeters on up to five centimeters of cervical dilation). At this point the contractions become stronger and more frequent. Those patients who are not able to tolerate labor comfortably will then request an epidural. (See next three questions.)

Whether or not less medication is used, however, childbirth classes make for an easier, healthier, and more enjoyable labor and delivery.

---

## Medication for Pain

---

## 546 Is it better not to use drugs during labor and delivery?

I believe that the less medication, the better—within reason. It is good if a woman can go through the early stages of labor without Demerol, but I do not see any medical reason why she should not have it if it helps her relax. Even if her relaxation is provided by Demerol, it is better for her to be relaxed than to be too tense. A woman would do well to attend childbirth classes and be as prepared as she can. Then, if she needs medication, she should go ahead and use it.

In my opinion there has been too much hysteria about drugs like Demerol and techniques like epidurals caused by well-meaning (but very biased) people who—without the support of medical research—make pregnant mothers feel they are damaging their babies by the use of these drugs and techniques. Since physicians stopped using large doses of Demerol (common prior to the mid-sixties), I have never seen a full-term baby affected in any significant way by Demerol, nor have I ever seen one affected in a negative way by an epidural.

## 547 What anesthesia options are available for labor and delivery?

There are eight anesthetics that we will discuss in the following questions:

| | |
|---|---|
| epidural | paracervical block |
| caudal anesthesia | pudendal block |
| spinal block | local anesthesia |
| general anesthesia | twilight sleep |

## 548 What is an epidural?

An epidural is an anesthetic given in the lower part of the back. It stops pain by numbing a woman from the waist down. The plastic catheter through which the drug is administered is left in place in the back for subsequent injections, and it does not interfere with a woman's movement.

An epidural seems to be ideal for a woman who decides during labor that she needs an anesthetic. It can be started when she is about five centimeters dilated, if the baby's head is far enough down in the birth canal.

In administering an epidural, a needle is inserted in the lower middle part of the back between the vertebrae. Since it does not penetrate the sac surrounding the nerves, the drug does not go into the spinal fluid. It is injected, rather, into the cavity between the bones and the sac that contains the nerves, anesthetizing the nerves as they come out of the sac from the spinal cord.

Because the nerves that control the muscles of the abdomen and legs are surrounded by a covering and are thus partially protected from the anesthetic agents, these muscles are not totally anesthetized. This allows some movement on the part of the woman. The nerves that carry the pain sensation, however, do not have a covering over them, and they are totally anesthetized.

A woman does not feel much pain when the epidural is working properly. Occasionally, however, accumulations of fat or connective tissue may result in uneven distribution of the anesthesia, or problems encountered in placing the tubes may prevent an epidural from working properly.

An epidural may be used for many hours, since the plastic tube is left in place in the back. The anesthesiologist will merely inject another dose of the anesthetic as the previous injection begins wearing off.

It is possible for labor to be slowed down by an epidural but, conversely, as some women relax with their epidural the cervix dilates faster and delivery is quicker than it might have been otherwise.

Even with an epidural in place, a woman can still push, although she does not feel the need for pushing. By following the techniques she learned in childbirth class and the instructions of the coach and the nurse who are helping her, she can be effective in pushing the baby down.

Forceps must be used more often with women who have epidurals than with those who do not. This, however, is not a bad thing, since forcep use in this situation is done when the baby's head is low in the birth canal and merely assists the baby's head out.

An epidural wears off within one to two hours after delivery, depending on the drug used.

One advantage of an epidural is that a woman who wants to undergo a sterilization procedure immediately after delivery can have it done with the epidural. Another advantage is that in the event of a sudden need for a cesarean section, it can be done with the epidural in place without any further anesthetic.

The epidural does not hurt the baby if the mother's blood pressure is not allowed to drop, a problem that is fairly easy to prevent. Complications for the mother from the use of the epidural are extremely rare and unusual.

Essentially, then, the epidural is a good anesthetic for labor and delivery; I encourage my patients to use it if they become so uncomfortable during labor that they feel that they need an anesthetic.

---

### 549  What is caudal anesthesia?

Caudal anesthesia is the same as an epidural, except that the catheter is threaded through a needle at the low end of the spinal column, right above the tailbone. All of the points stated about an epidural apply to the caudal. A caudal is a little less likely than an epidural to work properly, since it is given so low in the spinal canal where there are more variations in anatomy that can affect reliable placement of the caudal needle or tube. Because of this, caudals are rarely used today.

---

### 550  What is a "spinal?"

Spinal anesthesia is administered much like an epidural. Instead of stopping outside the sac containing the spinal nerves, however, the needle is pushed into that sac and the drug is injected into the spinal fluid in which the spinal nerves float. Because both the muscle and pain fibers are uncovered while inside this sac, both pain and movement are totally stopped by a spinal. A woman is numb from her waist down.

A spinal is not given until a woman is completely dilated, since it stops the contractions of the uterus. A baby must be far enough down in the birth canal so that, if the mother pushes, the baby will come out. Or it must be far enough down for the doctor to use forceps for delivery. A spinal is almost always given in the delivery room, unlike an epidural, which is usually given in the labor room. This is because the spinal stops labor and is not given until the doctor knows that delivery of the child can be completed.

A spinal is usually used these days only for special situations. For example, if a mother is completely dilated and her pushing is not effective, and a doctor believes he or she can deliver the baby with forceps if the mother's birth canal is totally relaxed, a spinal may be given to relax all the muscles in the pelvis. A spinal relaxes these muscles better than an epidural or general. Also, in certain situations, a spinal may be useful for a breech delivery.

Patients will often comment that since they are already ten centimeters dilated and the spinal is given when they are about to deliver anyway, why get a spinal? The truth is, even though a woman may be ten centimeters dilated, it frequently takes one or two uncomfortable hours of pushing to accomplish delivery. It is during this time that a spinal is often useful.

I have never seen a woman have any permanent paralysis from a spinal block. In the first half of this century, when less well-prepared anesthetics and larger needles were used, some nerve damage occasionally resulted from spinals, but this is not likely to occur with present-day medical techniques. Even the headaches that once accompanied spinals are much less likely to occur than they were when larger needles were used. Many anesthesiologists today do not even have patients remain flat on their backs for a long period of time after spinals as they once did.

If a woman does get a "spinal headache," several things may be done. She should take pain medication. These drugs will not harm a baby that is nursing and can give the mother a great deal of relief. She should stay in bed more and the amount of bed rest would be dictated by the severity of the headache. If the headache is fairly bad, the doctor may want the mother to drink a lot of fluids, and may even want to give her extra fluids in a vein to replace the spinal fluid that leaked out of the hole where the spinal was given, causing the headache.

If all these methods are not adequate, the doctor may want to do a "blood patch." This is a relatively simple procedure in which blood is drawn from the mother's arm and injected over the hole in the sac where the original spinal was given. The blood is injected through another spinal needle inserted in the same place as the original spinal needle, but not as deeply. The purpose of this is to "patch up" the hole and stop spinal-fluid leakage, thereby stopping the headache.

## 551　What is general anesthesia?

With general anesthesia a woman is normally first given pentothal in the veins to make her unconscious. Then a mask is put over her face or a tube is put in her trachea for administration of an anesthetic gas. With general anesthesia she is "put to sleep" completely.

Except for special situations, this type of anesthesia should not be used for a delivery. When a woman begins labor, her stomach stops working and any fluid or food in her stomach will still be there when she delivers the baby. If a woman vomits while under general anesthesia, the vomited material can get into her lungs and possibly cause death. An epidural anesthetic is much safer for a routine delivery.

A general anesthetic can be used with reasonable safety for a planned cesarean section. Ordinarily the anesthesiologist will put a tube into the woman's windpipe (trachea) and blow up a small balloon around that tube. With this in place, even if the woman vomits, that material cannot get into her lungs.

A baby can be delivered without any significant effect from the general anesthesia if it is given by an anesthesiologist who understands obstetric anesthesia and if the woman is being cared for by a competent obstetrician. The baby may be slightly sleepy, but it usually wakes within moments with a lusty cry.

## 552　What is a paracervical block?

This technique involves the injection of anesthetic drugs beside the cervix, at the top of the vagina. This deadens the nerves coming from the body into the uterus. It effectively stops the pain of contractions, but the drugs are injected near the blood vessels that flow into the uterus. The absorption of drugs into the baby's blood supply causes its heartbeat to slow and can, in rare cases, result in death. Because of this problem paracervicals are no longer used.

## 553　What is a pudendal block?

Pudendal blocks are used extensively for women who do not want or need epidural, caudal, or spinal anesthesia. The nerves to the lower vagina and the area around the opening of the vagina come up near the surface of the vagina, about halfway up the vagina. The pudendal is given by injecting an anesthetic agent first on one side and then on the other. A doctor competent in giving a pudendal can completely numb this area 75–80 percent of the time. When a pudendal is given, the doctor can use forceps, if necessary, with little discomfort for the mother, and the mother can have tears or an episiotomy sewn up without any discomfort. (See Q. 554.)

This type of anesthetic is given, of course, only after the cervix is completely dilated and when the baby's head is low enough in the birth canal that the mother's pushing will soon deliver it.

## 554 What is local anesthesia for delivery?

A local anesthetic is given in the tissues around the opening of the vagina. It can be given immediately before delivery, allowing an episiotomy to be cut, or it can be given after delivery so that tears can be repaired.

Because of the large number of blood vessels in the area around the opening of the vagina late in pregnancy, local anesthetic agents are often "carried away" quickly. Although a woman may be numb in that area when the doctor begins sewing, feeling may return before the stitching is completed. If this happens, the doctor will sometimes inject more local anesthetic agents. This in itself is so uncomfortable, however, that the doctor may just finish the repairs without it if there is not much sewing left to be done. The woman would probably be as uncomfortable from more injections of the drugs as she would be from completion of the sewing.

The only side effects from a local or a pudendal would be a mother's adverse reaction to the drug. It is possible for a woman to react to any medication, even the medication used for local and pudendal anesthesia.

When a patient tells me she wants to use a "local" for her delivery, I give either a local or a pudendal, depending on which seems best at the time of the delivery. The same amount of drug is injected, and the results are much the same.

## 555 What is twilight sleep?

Twilight sleep is rarely used anymore in this country. I mention it here merely as a matter of interest. First used in 1902, twilight sleep was a combination of morphine and scopolamine. Morphine was given for the same purpose that Demerol is now given, but it was used in much larger doses than we would give today, and scopolamine was given to make a woman forget that she had had labor at all!

The combination of these two drugs was quite effective in alleviating pain and taking away a woman's memory of her labor. It not only stopped her pain, however, but the large dosages of morphine made her baby very sleepy; in addition, she would not know that she had delivered a baby until hours later.

## Birthing Rooms

## 556 What is a birthing room? What is an LDR (labor, delivery, recovery room)?

*Birthing rooms*, also called alternative birthing centers, are now part of most modern obstetric units in the United States. They offer an alternative to the usual labor-and-delivery-room birth, providing a more casual, home-style setting.

There are both advantages and disadvantages to these centers. There are certain things that patients and their families may do in birthing centers that they cannot do in the regular labor-and-delivery unit. There are also certain things that patients may do in the regular labor-and-delivery unit that they may not do in the birthing room. We will discuss each situation separately.

*LDR rooms* are a new concept for obstetric care and are equipped so that all obstetric care can be given in one place. Women are allowed to labor, deliver, and recover in the same room without being moved. In contrast to birthing rooms, LDR rooms are set up for any obstetric care except for cesarean sections. Women who develop some problem in their pregnancy can be cared for, drugs or anesthesia may be given, and forceps delivery can be done. Also, a woman is normally allowed to have family or friends in for the delivery if she wants to.

*Things that may be done
in a birthing room*

More than just the father or a coach may be present during the labor and delivery. In most birthing rooms, family or friends may be present.

A woman may labor and deliver in the same bed. In the regular labor-and-delivery unit, labor takes place in the labor room and delivery in the delivery room.

Unless some complication develops, the mother and baby may go home as soon as the mother wants to. They can also go home as soon as she wants to from the regular labor-and-delivery unit, but for some reason patients often think they can "go home early" only from a birthing room.

*Things that may not be done
in a birthing room*

Some anesthetics cannot be administered. If a mother in labor needs more than local or pudendal anesthesia, she must be transferred to a regular labor room.

A woman may not labor with an established or an unexpected medical problem. If she has a medical problem or a high-risk pregnancy, labor must take place in the regular labor room. If she develops a problem during the labor, she must be transferred to a regular labor room.

Labor with a breech presentation is not allowed. If the baby is coming as a breech, the mother needs to be handled by the regular labor-and-delivery procedure.

Forceps may not be used. This might mean that if forceps are needed for completion of delivery, the mother must be transferred to the regular delivery room.

*Things that may be done
under regular labor-and-delivery care*

All anesthetics can be used.

High-risk pregnancies can be cared for. This includes problems with the mother and potential problems with the baby.

Some breech presentations can be allowed to labor.

A coach or father and some limited family can be present during the labor.

Forceps can be used for delivery if necessary.

*Things that may not be done
in the regular labor and delivery suite*

A woman may not labor and deliver in the same bed. She must be transferred from the labor room to the delivery room by stretcher.

She may not have more than one person with her for the delivery (other than authorized medical personnel).

My view concerning birthing centers and LDR rooms is that they have been developed by physicians and lay people who felt that labor and delivery in the United States had been "dehumanized." They believed that if there were a "special room," apart from the typical obstetric practice of a hospital, where the mother and father could be in a homelike, casual situation, they could have a more humanized hospital experience.

This type of pressure has caused most hospital labor-and-delivery units to respond to the expressed needs of mothers and fathers during labor and delivery. Although the improved sensitivity on the part of the regular childbirth units has not made birthing rooms extinct, it has made them less necessary.

When you look at the core of the situation, a woman may do everything she wants to in the regular labor-and-delivery area of the hospital—except have her family and friends with her for the delivery and deliver in the same bed she labors in.

---

**557** **Do you deliver your patients in a birthing center or a LDR room if they choose that route?**

I am happy to deliver those patients who desire it in a birthing center, except those who are having their first babies. With a first baby the mother is more likely to have large tears of the cervix or vagina, and she is also more likely to need forceps assistance for delivery. Because of that, I believe that first babies should be delivered in the regular de-

livery room. This gives the option of having a forceps delivery, if necessary, without a transfer from the birthing room to the delivery room. In addition, delivering on a regular delivery-room table makes it easier for the doctor to examine for and repair vaginal tears.

If a couple cannot accept the fact that regular labor-and-delivery care has become more sensitive and humane, and they are intent on "something different," I prefer to have them deliver in a birthing room and will attend them there rather than have them deliver at home. To me the major benefit of the birthing room is that it is often an acceptable option to those couples who would otherwise choose to deliver at home.

The sensitivity and humaneness of most doctors and nurses and many, if not most, labor-and-delivery units have changed dramatically in the past few years. A couple can expect to have the kind of experience they want for labor and delivery not only in a birthing room, but also in the regular labor-and-delivery rooms of a hospital.

The LDR room concept, while relatively new, is quite acceptable for the labor and delivery of any woman. These rooms are gradually becoming available throughout the country and perhaps in time they may replace the traditional labor room/delivery room set-up, or even the birthing room. Most physicians would readily accept such a change.

---

## The Leboyer Technique

---

**558** **What about using the Leboyer techniques for birth?**

In 1975 Dr. Frederick Leboyer wrote *Birth Without Violence* (New York: Knopf). In it he recommended delivering the baby in a warm, quiet, softly-lighted environment and, after the delivery, immersing the baby in a bath of warm water while allowing it to relax and become comfortable outside the uterus.

Dr. Leboyer's suggestions are good reminders to labor-and-delivery personnel, doctors and nurses included, to handle the delivery in a gentle way. His suggestion that babies are typically delivered in a rough fashion, however, is far from true.

A picture in Dr. Leboyer's book shows an angrily crying baby being held upside down by its feet, the implication being that this is a typical delivery. It is not! I have never held a baby upside down by its feet after delivery, nor have I ever seen an obstetrician who routinely spanks a newborn baby. Some stimulation of the baby may be necessary if the baby is "sleepy" when born, but certainly not to the extent that Leboyer suggests is routine.

Technically, it is interesting to note that studies have been done that show no difference between babies born with the rigid Leboyer technique and those born with conventional delivery handled in a gentle and appropriate fashion. The health and behavior of the two groups of babies were no different.

## Home Births

### 559  Is home birth a good alternative to a hospital delivery?

A doctor can hardly answer this question without being accused of bias. When I state that I feel home births are dangerous, I am not speaking for a nonexistent A.M.A. "fraternity," nor am I aligning myself *with* doctors and *against* patients. My only concern regarding this subject is the welfare of mothers and babies.

There have been incredible advances in labor-and-delivery care in the past fifteen years. Not only have the sensitivity and humaneness provided by health care professionals improved during these years, but the ability of doctors and nurses also has improved because of training and technical advances. If you choose to deliver outside the hospital, you cannot take advantage of these advances in the event that you or your baby have problems.

Normally a mother would not be hurt too badly in a home-birth situation. Although a mother could bleed to death before she could get to the hospital, it is more likely that a home-born baby might suffer. For example, something as simple as a plug of meconium getting sucked into the baby's lungs can damage the baby severely. In that event a suction machine with a laryngoscope, commonly available in delivery rooms, could remove the meconium in a matter of seconds, avoiding possible brain damage.

There are other and much more fearful problems that obstetricians often encounter that makes them realize how foolish home deliveries are. One in ten babies has some problem during the delivery process that requires expert medical attention. Midwives may say that you or the baby can be taken to the hospital by ambulance if an emergency does develop, but this reasoning ignores the fact that if a baby's brain is deprived of adequate oxygen for more than four minutes, it will be either severely brain damaged or dead. No emergency service in the United States could help your baby fast enough to make any difference in that case.

A recently released report of a seven-year study of pregnant women documents that mothers who do not receive obstetrical care have a much higher death rate and their babies are similarly affected. The study reported the death of twenty-one babies and six mothers in 344 deliveries. This was a much higher risk than for mothers in the same geographical district who received obstetrical care.

Certainly there is a statistical chance of getting by without having anything happen, but it is like playing Russian roulette. Once the unforeseen occurs, it is done. There is nothing you can do to change it or make up for it. If you make the choice to have a home birth, and your baby is brain damaged or dies because of that decision, you will regret your choice for the rest of your life. You can avoid the possibility of lifelong remorse and regret by going to the hospital for your care.

### 560 Would a home delivery be safe with a qualified nurse-midwife in attendance?

Certainly a home birth would be safer with a nurse-midwife than with a lay midwife or no midwife. Nurse-midwives generally have excellent training, whereas lay midwives generally have no medical background except for a couple of years of apprenticeship. Therefore, in my opinion there is no place in the care of a pregnant woman for lay midwives. Even a qualified and competent midwife, however, is not an obstetrician and cannot provide the expertise that an obstetrician can.

If you want to have a nurse-midwife care for your labor and delivery, and she can do that in a hospital where there is a doctor with whom she works to help if a problem develops, then I believe a nurse-midwife may safely be used. In the United States, however, there are few hospitals where nurse-midwives are allowed to so care for patients by themselves. The only place they can truly be "in charge" in the United States is in home deliveries.

Since they usually work in home situations, midwives will point out the "bright side" of delivering at home. They will assure you that it is uncommon for problems to develop with labor and will point out the pleasure of being in a home environment for delivery. They might also point out the economic advantage of delivering at home.

Nurse-midwives who deliver patients at home have a biased view of reality. This view is usually affected both by their egos, since it is a heady and exciting thing to participate in the delivery of a baby, and by the fact that they will be receiving the delivery fee.

As an obstetrician I too have my bias. I also find it heady and exciting to be present at a delivery and I receive a delivery fee. On my side, though, is the fact that I do my deliveries in well-equipped hospitals and with the training, knowledge, and experience in hospital techniques that help provide safe care.

The overriding principle of this entire discussion is that a woman who distrusts physicians and nurses, and who wants to have control of the entire birth experience, can let these emotions cause her to ignore the advantages that modern medicine has to offer. Following one's emotions instead of the mind can cause a situation that can damage her and her baby irreparably.

## Preparing for the Hospital's Routine

### 561 Aren't hospitals really just for sick people? Are they flexible enough to allow a program designed for healthy people, such as women in labor?

Just as it would be ridiculous to say that a doctor can take care of sick people, but cannot do routine annual physical examinations on healthy people, so it is absurd to say that a hospital can take care of sick people but cannot do anything properly for healthy people.

When you walk into the labor-and-delivery unit of a hospital or onto the floor where mothers stay after they have delivered, or when you peer into the nursery, you will sense a totally different atmosphere than exists anywhere else in the hospital. It is an upbeat spirit of pleasure, enjoyment, and contentment. These days there is also a sense of cooperation with patients, their husbands, and families.

There is a flexibility existing in most labor-and-delivery areas that is pleasant for both the patient and her family. When my patients ask about the possibility of doing things a little differently, I tell them that they can do anything they want to while they are in labor and delivery, unless a medical problem develops to prevent their carrying through with their plans, or unless there is something they want to do that would be medically unwise. This type of attitude prevails among most obstetricians today.

The nurses on most labor-and-delivery units are flexible enough not only to work with people who have had childbirth classes, but also with people who have had no preparation at all. I have seen nurses at our hospital care for many totally untrained patients in such a way that, by the time these people had finished their labor and delivery, they had had an amazingly complete course on how to breathe, how to relax, and how to push in order to have a baby with a minimum amount of analgesia or anesthesia.

Patients often ask if the hospital "requires" that they have an enema or some other medical treatment. It is important that patients realize that they receive no medication or treatment that has not been ordered by their physician. While hospitals have superbly trained staffs prepared to meet the needs of the patient, the attending physi-

cian is the one who orders the medication and treatments. The hospital does have certain regulations, but generally, the limitations on a patient and her treatment plan are set by the physician.

---

## 562 What should I take with me to the hospital?

It is a good idea to pack your suitcase for your hospital stay several weeks in advance of your due date. You might put these things in your bag:

For you in the hospital

2 or 3 nightgowns (front opening for nursing mothers)
robe
slippers
underwear
nursing bras (if you plan to nurse)
toothbrush
toothpaste
mouthwash
hair-care essentials
makeup
any special body-care items you use
reading material
thank-you notes
birth announcements
baby's book

For the baby going home

going-home outfit
disposable or cloth diapers
receiving blanket
heavy blanket, if necessary

For you going home

pants and top or dress
underwear
shoes and stockings
sweater or coat, if needed

Don't waste your time packing to go to the hospital if you suddenly begin bleeding heavily or develop some other medical emergency. There is nothing that you must have when you go to the hospital that it cannot provide. Once you get there and the emergency subsides, someone can bring the things you need.

## Do-It-Yourself Emergency Deliveries

### 563 What should I do if I start delivering on the way to the hospital?

This is, to say the least, a very exciting event. Most fathers have nightmares about such an occurrence, and few believe they could handle an emergency delivery. In such a situation they tend to step on the gas, a solution that not only fails to keep the baby from coming, but endangers the entire family!

It is wise to be aware that such an event can occur and be prepared for it. Prior knowledge in the "basics" of delivering a baby will be extremely helpful in an emergency birth. There are some clear "do's" and "don'ts" in this situation. For clarity of discussion, the husband will be addressed, but the advice is applicable, of course, to anyone who might need to help you deliver.

*Don't* panic. Even if you do absolutely nothing, your wife will almost certainly deliver with no problems. Deliveries have been taking place for thousands of years, and your wife's will occur whether or not you do anything.

*Don't* start driving faster. This merely endangers you, your wife, and your baby.

*Don't* stop the car and try to get the doc-tor on the phone. At this point there is nothing he or she can do.

*Do* listen to your wife. If she says the baby is coming NOW, it probably is. Stop the car in a safe place and help her!

*Do* help your wife remove her clothing from the waist down and assist her in lying back on the car seat.

*Do* tell your wife to push gently while you put your hand against the top of the baby's head. The head will look like a grapefruit pushing its way out of the vagina. The primary thing you can do at this time is to keep the baby's head from "popping" out of the birth canal. If it pops out without control, there is a possibility that some blood vessels inside the skull around the brain can tear, causing damage to the baby.

*Do* help ease the baby's head out. If your wife is pushing too hard, and you can see that it is likely that the baby's head will pop out, tell her to stop pushing. Keep gentle, but firm pressure against the top of the baby's head, letting it ease out over a few seconds' time.

*Do* "catch" the baby gently, then hold it face down to allow any mucus to drain from the mouth and nose. The baby will normally cough, gasp, and gag a little.

*Do* lay the baby on your wife's tummy, once it is breathing freely.

*Don't* take off your shoestring and tie the umbilical cord. Leave the cord alone and let the doctor or hospital personnel cut it later.

*Don't* worry about the placenta (afterbirth). It may deliver on its own while you are driving to the hospital or it may not. Either is fine.

*Do* wrap the baby gently in a blanket, or in anything you have handy, to keep it from being chilled.

*Do* assist your wife in lying back comfortably in the car. With the baby snuggled up on her abdomen, you can proceed to the hospital.

*Do* drive carefully to the hospital. After all the excitement, you will probably be a little "shook up." Go slowly so that you don't follow delivery with disaster!

*Do* congratulate yourself and enjoy the accolades of your friends! You are one of the select few husbands in the United States who has delivered his own child.

## An Afterword

While you are in the middle of the process, labor and delivery seem to be the focus of all of life. They are not. They are part of an event you will always remember, but they are still only one of many important events of a lifetime.

Those of us who observe pregnant women and their husbands are always saddened to see a couple focus so much on the birth experience that they almost ignore their baby. The whole process seems to have become a selfish program for them as parents.

I would urge you to keep the balance. Don't let your concept of the birth experience become a goal that you feel you must achieve. Many people seem to make completion of the birth process a frontier to be conquered, often to the detriment of their child. If they achieve that goal according to their preconceived plan, they are "successful." If they do not, they have "failed," even with a beautiful little baby resting in their arms!

Also sad, but probably of far greater consequence, is the couple who pour all of this effort into having the baby but fail to continue with the same zeal in providing for the child's future development. So often we see parents who form a great team in getting through childbirth, but who take the baby home to an environment of bickering, discontent, lack of moral direction, lack of discipline, and eventually divorce.

No matter how successful you are in the childbirth process, your baby will be a disadvantaged child if the environment in which you raise him or her is detrimental. I strongly encourage you not only to plan for the best delivery, but also to plan "the best" for the child's healthy future development. Both are absolutely vital to that child becoming a healthy, happy, complete adult.

# 9

# Labor and Delivery

When labor starts, the waiting is almost over. Soon that individual who has so completely filled your womb will fill your arms and your heart.

Your special baby really is a separate and unique individual, and a new baby shows that individuality from the start. Although we know approximately when the birth will take place, unless we do something artificial, the sex of the child and the exact time of its birth are beyond our control. It matters not that we want the baby to come on December thirty-first nor that we already have two boys and want a girl. The baby almost shouts aloud at birth, "See me! I am a separate creation of God. I came when God wanted me to. I am a boy or a girl as God wanted me to be. I am an individual before God, not an object to be manipulated."

So labor begins as the unborn baby issues the first of his or her thousands of untimely, unexpected, and usually selfish demands: "I want out!" Your bills may be piled up, your other children may have the chicken pox, your hair may be dirty, but the baby couldn't care less. Those first contractions herald the entrance of a brand-new person onto the stage of this world.

Ready or not, here the baby comes!

process is an extraordinary example of a functional design created by God.

## 564 What is labor? When does it start?

A basic definition of labor would be "contractions that produce progressive dilatation and effacement of the cervix." Incidentally, if the cervix does not dilate and thin out, the contractions are not true labor contractions. Labor, then, is the natural process which produces the birth of a baby.

No one knows why labor starts, even though extensive studies have been directed toward this question. In the practical sense, about all we can say is what was said of the virgin Mary in Luke 2:6 (NASV): "And it came about that while they were there, the days were completed for her to give birth." In other words, in normal circumstances when it is time for you to go into labor, you will go into labor.

## 565 How do uterine contractions—labor pains—bring about the birth of a baby?

Uterine contractions are unique. If the entire uterus were to contract in exactly the same way, producing exactly the same pressure in all parts of the uterus, nothing would happen except that the baby would be squeezed. This is not what happens, however.

The uterus basically has two segments—the upper and the lower. As the muscle of the upper segment contracts, it does not relax back to its original length, but gets thicker and thicker as labor progresses. The muscle of the lower part of the uterus thins out and is actually pulled into the upper segment and up around the baby's head. This explains why the cervix dilates. The whole

## 566 How frequent are labor contractions?

Labor contractions can occasionally be frequent even at the beginning of labor. I have had many patients whose contractions began three to four minutes apart. Generally, however, contractions will start ten to fifteen minutes apart, and gradually get closer and closer together.

During the active part of labor, contractions usually last about sixty seconds, with about one to three minutes between each contraction. After the cervix is completely dilated, contractions may last sixty seconds, with only sixty seconds between each contraction. At this point the body is really working to get the baby out.

## 567 Why are there periods of time between contractions?

Women in labor welcome the respite between labor contractions, but this "breathing space" is primarily for the baby's benefit, not theirs. During a contraction, there is almost no blood flow through the uterus. Periods of relaxation between contractions are essential for the baby's well-being, because the mother's blood can then flow into the uterus to provide the oxygen and nutrients necessary for keeping the baby healthy. This oxygen is transferred from the mother's blood, across the placental membrane, into the baby's blood. This allows the baby to tolerate the process of labor in a healthy way. Contractions coming too frequently could mean an inadequate oxygen supply for the baby and be one reason for immediate cesarean section.

## 568 When should I call the doctor if I think I might be in labor?

There are three primary indications of the onset of labor. You should call your physician if any of the following occur:

***Broken bag of waters.*** When your bag of waters ruptures, you may have a slow leak, a moderate flow, or an embarrassing gush of fluid from your vagina. When that happens, call your doctor immediately. After your membranes rupture, germs are likely to get up into the fluid around the baby and cause infection.

It is possible, however, that the fluid you are leaking is urine. The baby can "poke" your bladder, causing a squirt of urine which you may mistake for amniotic fluid. This happens fairly often.

It is important for you to understand that your bag of waters can break at any time during your pregnancy. When it occurs early in pregnancy (third or fourth month) the pregnancy ends as a late miscarriage.

If the bag of waters breaks after you are twenty-eight weeks along, your doctor will usually give you Pitocin to induce labor so that your baby can be delivered. If delivery is not achieved, your baby can get an infection from vaginal germs entering the uterus. Delivery this early results in a very premature baby. Therefore your doctor may want you to take your temperature to make sure you are not getting infected, stay in bed, and wait to see if you can keep the pregnancy a few more weeks before becoming infected or going into labor. The bag of waters almost never closes back up once it has ruptured.

***Contractions that are becoming hard and regular.*** I ask first-time mothers to call me when their contractions are about three to five minutes apart, unless they are more than an hour away from the hospital. Even if they wait until contractions are this close together, there are usually still several hours until delivery.

I ask patients who are having their second baby to call me when their contractions are eight or ten minutes apart, are coming regularly, and are getting harder.

Mothers with a third baby (or more) should call when they think they are in labor. By the third baby most women know what labor feels like. Also, labor can progress faster than with previous births. It is best, therefore, for a woman to call as soon as she thinks labor has begun, even if contractions are fairly far apart.

***Heavy bleeding.*** If you begin to bleed heavily at any time during pregnancy, you need to call your doctor. If you cannot reach your doctor, go straight to the hospital and leave someone at home to continue trying to notify the doctor that you are on your way to the hospital so that he or she can meet you there.

## 569 What if I have light bleeding or spotting?

One of the most likely causes of this type of bleeding during the last month of pregnancy is your doctor's pelvic examination. As the doctor examines your cervix, he or she will gently place a finger against the cervical opening to see how dilated it is. This can tear some of the delicate blood vessels of the cervix, causing light bleeding, which may be bright red and actually run out of your vagina. If it is not as heavy as a menstrual period, you do not need to worry about it and can go on about your business. Such bleeding may occur the night after an exam rather than immediately following it.

Bleeding not associated with this type of examination is called a "bloody show" and merely indicates that your cervix is beginning to dilate. The material that is passing is the mucus that has been plugging the cervix during pregnancy. In the later months of pregnancy the cervix will often stretch open a little, tearing small blood vessels and causing spotting, and passage of some of the cervical mucus. This can happen at least two or three weeks before you actually go into labor. You do not need to call your doctor because of this bloody show, unless you are also having contractions and think you may be in labor.

If you have a bloody show at any time other than the last month, though, you need to call your doctor immediately. It could be an indication of premature labor or a miscarriage.

## 570 What will the doctor do when I call?

If you have called because of the reasons discussed in the previous two questions, your doctor will probably do the following.

*If you are having contractions.* The doctor will examine you to see if you have dilated any since your last examination. If your cervix is thinning out (effacing) and opening (dilating), it means that you are in labor and should go to the hospital.

*If your water has broken.* If this has happened, the doctor will usually do a pelvic examination with a speculum. If you are definitely leaking fluid from the cervix, you will be sent to the hospital. If the doctor cannot tell if there is a definite leak of fluid, he or she will probably test some fluid from the opening of your cervix with pH paper. Since amniotic fluid is alkaline (the opposite of being acid) compared to vaginal secretions, pH paper will turn blue if there is a leakage of fluid through the cervix. If the pH paper indicates leaking amniotic fluid, the doctor will have you go to the hospital. Occasionally the doctor and you can tell without an exam that your bag of waters has broken because you are losing so much fluid.

The first sign of the onset of labor may be the breaking of the bag of waters, but the bag of waters can break without labor starting. If

this happens, your doctor may need to use Pitocin to start your labor.

Patients frequently ask me if their bag of waters will break with a second pregnancy if it broke with the first one. The answer is, "Not necessarily." One labor may be ushered in by breaking of the bag of waters and another with contractions.

*If you are bleeding heavily.* If this occurs the doctor will probably have you go immediately to the hospital. Once you have arrived at the labor-and-delivery unit, your doctor and the nurses will evaluate you to see if you can have a normal delivery or will need a cesarean section.

## 571 May I eat a last meal before going to the hospital?

If the doctor has asked you to go to the hospital, do not put anything into your mouth from that point until the time you are told specifically that you may have something to eat or drink. Any food or drink that you take in once labor has started will stay in your stomach for hours, because when the uterus starts working, the stomach seems to stop working. If you should suddenly need general anesthesia for a cesarean section, you could vomit while receiving your anesthesia, and such vomiting can cause aspiration of the food into your lungs, an extremely grave complication.

During labor your doctor may allow you to sip some water or eat some ice chips. If your labor is not progressing well, however, and a C-section may be necessary, he or she may require that you ingest absolutely nothing through your mouth.

Many obstetricians allow their patients to eat some hard candy and to use glycerin swabs, which are available in most labor-and-delivery departments, because these items do not add much to the contents of the stomach.

## 572 What is false labor?

Most women seem concerned about the "embarrassment" of being in false labor. You should not be embarrassed if you go to the doctor or to the hospital with some contractions and are told that they are not true labor contractions. Not even your doctor can tell whether or not you are in true labor without feeling your cervix. If the contractions you are having are not causing your cervix to thin out and to dilate, you are not in labor, no matter how strong they are. It is better to go to the doctor several times in false labor than it is to ignore significant contractions and risk having your baby at home because you thought you were in false labor.

We have all heard stories of women who were "in labor" for a week. These stories are almost never true. These women have usually had strong false labor contractions for the six days that preceded the onset of true labor on the seventh day!

A woman should not take any aspirin or prostaglandin inhibitors, such as Motrin, near the end of her pregnancy because they can interfere with labor.

## 573 Should labor be induced if false labor continues to occur?

After a patient has been examined several times and found to be in false labor, the question will arise as to why she cannot be "induced." Induction should usually not be done unless the cervix is adequately dilated (about two centimeters), soft, and the baby's head in good position. (See Q. 630.)

It is not safe to do an induction of labor, even if you are having numerous Braxton-Hicks contractions (false labor pains), if your body is not ready for induction.

## 574 What happens at the hospital if I am sent there in labor or with ruptured membranes?

Normal, routine procedures include:

*Admission to the hospital.* If you earlier completed procedures for preadmission to the hospital, you will merely pass through the admission office. They will lift the information from their computer or records and take you immediately by wheelchair to the labor-and-delivery section.

*Admission to labor and delivery.* Typically, the nurses who work in labor and delivery are pleasant and happy. They love helping women have babies! This attitude is contagious, and you will enjoy being in their competent hands while having your baby.

The nurses will make you comfortable in your labor room. Your history will be taken, including a record of past health problems, past pregnancies and labors, and of this particular pregnancy. Your blood pressure, pulse, and temperature will also be taken and recorded.

*Change of clothes.* You will be asked to undress completely and put on a hospital gown.

*Examination.* After you have changed clothes and gotten into bed, a labor-and-delivery nurse will examine you. Even if the doctor examined you in the office, the nurse may want to examine you too, to compare her findings with the earlier ones. Since labor can progress quickly it is important that the nurse know how fast you are progressing and how far along in labor you are when you are admitted to labor and delivery. The nurse will check your uterus for contractions and examine you to see if your bag of waters has broken.

A primary reason for this initial exam is to determine the position of the baby. If the baby is coming head first, then the nurse knows that it is safe for you to progress in labor. If she finds that the baby is not coming head first, she will call your obstetrician immediately.

*A call to your obstetrician.* After the nurse has completed the exam, she will call your obstetrician. If, as they discuss your situation, they feel that you are in labor, the doctor will ask the nurse to proceed with ordering your blood tests, the enema, the IV, and the application of the monitor, as described below.

If the nurse and the doctor are quite certain that you are not in labor, the doctor will ask the nurse to discharge you from labor and delivery. You will go home and probably go to the doctor's office the next day.

If it seems to them that you may be in false labor, but they are not sure, you may have to stay in the hospital for a couple of hours to be observed.

When a patient I have admitted to the hospital is in labor, I normally ask the nurses to call me when the patient has dilated to five centimeters. I then go to labor and delivery and stay in the hospital or in my nearby office until time for delivery. Prior to five centimeters of dilatation there may still be many hours of labor, and it is extremely rare for any unexpected problems to develop in that time. If, however, a patient has had a previous fast labor, or if she has already had several babies, I usually go to the hospital and then stay close by once I am certain she is in active labor.

*Blood and urine tests.* If you have had adequate prenatal care, you will need only to have a test for syphilis and a complete blood count drawn. If you have not had prenatal care, the doctors taking care of you will want to know if you are Rh negative or Rh positive. If it appears you might need a blood transfusion (some doctors like to have blood available if you are going to have a C-section), blood would be drawn in order to make arrangements to have the proper transfusion available. You will also be asked to collect a urine specimen to make sure

that you do not have a urinary-tract infection or other kidney abnormality.

*Enema and prep.* During the pushing phase of labor, anything loose in the lower part of your body is pushed out, including not only the baby, but also urine and stool. To avoid having both baby and stool passed at the same time, most patients and doctors prefer that an enema be given. I feel that having an enema is wise. In addition to preventing a messy birth, it also decreases contamination of vaginal tears and episiotomies and thus reduces the chance of infection. One additional advantage of an enema is that it can actually stimulate labor contractions to be more effective. Occasionally a patient will have her bag of waters rupture and yet have no contractions. Such a patient usually needs Pitocin to start her labor, but occasionally an enema will have that effect before the Pitocin is started.

Most doctors prefer some cleansing of the perineal area and having some of the vulvar hair shaved or clipped. Sometimes this is done soon after admittance to the hospital, and at other times it is done after you are moved to the delivery table. The purpose of shaving is to avoid any vulvar hair being caught in the sutures as the episiotomy or vaginal tears are sewn up. If that happens, the incision can become infected and break open.

*Intravenous fluid.* I like my patients to have an IV going. If sudden bleeding begins, or an unplanned C-section is necessary, the IV is immediately available for administration of medications or blood. A patient's sudden collapse into shock because of heavy uterine bleeding or a ruptured uterus or some other problem is dangerous enough by itself—but it could cause an even more serious problem if an IV were not already going, as it could be difficult to get one started under those conditions.

It is better to plan ahead, even though such complications do not occur very often. Your doctor wants both you and your baby to survive this whole process in a healthy fashion and thus may take certain precautions to insure that.

Some women worry about dislodging their intravenous needle. This fear is basically unwarranted because today most IVs are started with plastic needles that will not come out of the vein, even if the arm is moved around wildly.

*Fetal monitoring.* Modern fetal monitoring belts have become so comfortable that they do not seem to interfere with a patient's movement or freedom, and many obstetricians, myself included, now feel that continuous fetal monitoring is wise during every labor. It is the only way your baby can be adequately watched during the most dangerous passage it will have in its lifetime. If fetal monitoring is not done by a machine, the doctor or nurse who is taking care of you should be listening to your baby's heartbeat for a full minute every fifteen or twenty minutes. The difficulty with this is that if your baby develops a problem, it could cause the baby's death between the times the medical team listened for the heartbeat.

## The Stages of Labor

### 575 What are the stages of labor?

The stages of labor include Stage One, Stage Two, and Stage Three. These stages will be discussed in the following questions. (Childbirth classes label the stages differently. See Q. 579.)

### 576 What does the first stage of labor include?

This stage of labor includes the time from the start of true labor until the cervix is completely dilated. It is characterized by the following events:

*Gradually increasing strength and frequency of labor contractions.* Once the cervix is dilated five centimeters, the effectiveness of the contractions often increases. This is called the "phase of acceleration." Some women progress fairly rapidly from one or two centimeters up to five; others will take many hours to reach five centimeters of dilation.

Once the "phase of acceleration" is reached, the cervix often dilates much more quickly. Obstetricians expect the cervix to dilate at the rate of one centimeter an hour from five centimeters on; if progression is not that fast, the doctor will be watching carefully for a problem.

Most obstetricians rupture the bag of waters if the baby is coming down head first. This seems to make contractions more effective and, therefore, makes labor a little shorter.

*Descent of the baby's head in the birth canal.* During the first stage of labor, not only is the cervix dilating up to ten centimeters (complete dilation), but the baby's head is progressing down into the birth canal.

A woman's pelvic bones have some prominent projections called ischial spines, which are easily felt by the doctor on vaginal exam. When the top of the baby's head progresses down the birth canal to the level of the ischial spines, it means that the largest part of the baby's head has come through the ring of bone at the top of the birth canal and is probably going to deliver without a cesarean section, though many C-sections are still necessary even then. When the baby's head is at the ischial spines, the baby is said to be at "station zero." For each centimeter

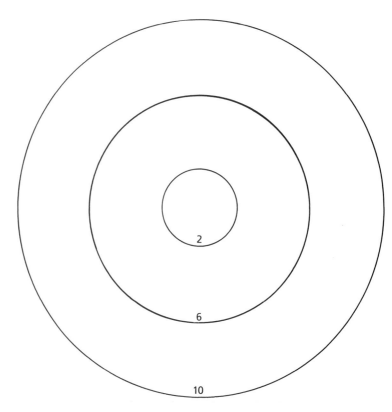

Cervical dilation in centimeters, shown actual size

10 cm = 3.9 inches

above the ischial spines that the top of the baby's head is, you are said to be at "minus one, minus two," and so on. For each centimeter that the top of the baby's head is past the ischial spines, you are said to be "plus one" or "plus two," as the case may be.

*Cervical dilatation.* The pregnant woman's cervix can be almost totally closed just before labor starts or it can be as much as three or four centimeters dilated before labor starts. The amount of dilatation of the cervix before labor starts does not cause the onset of labor. The changes in the woman's body that cause the start of labor are much more complicated than that. When labor starts, the cervix starts dilating (opening up). (See Q. 565.) The dilatation of the cervix enlarges the small round opening present at the start of labor to an opening big enough

for the baby to deliver through. For normal babies a dilatation of ten centimeters is required for delivery.

*Effacement.* Effacement of the cervix means the shortening of the cervix. The normal cervix is about one inch long, and during effacement the cervix gets shorter. This can happen during the last few weeks of pregnancy without any labor contractions occurring. A woman may go into labor with her cervix 100 percent effaced but dilated only a small amount. If the cervix is not totally effaced when a woman starts labor, the contractions of labor will result in the cervix being totally effaced by the time the cervix is completely dilated.

If a woman's cervix is about one inch long, it is not effaced (0 percent effacement) since the normal cervix is that long. If the

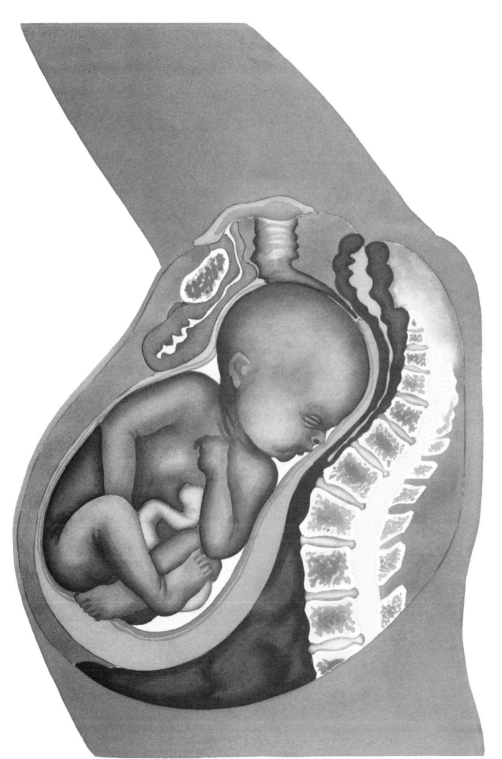

**First Stage of Delivery**

cervix is about one-half inch long, it is said to be 50 percent effaced. If the cervix is totally flattened out and amounts to no more than a circular opening with a paper-thin edge, it is said to be 100 percent effaced.

## 577 What does the second stage of labor include?

The second stage starts when the mother's cervix is completely dilated—ten centimeters—and ends with the delivery of the baby. This stage may be brief, because as soon as the mother reaches ten centimeters of cervical dilatation, the baby may progress immediately on out of the birth canal and be delivered.

During this stage of labor the lower part of the vagina is dilated and the perineum (the area between the lower vagina and the anus) is stretched out. An episiotomy may be done to keep the tissue of the perineum from tearing. Especially with the first baby the choice is almost always either tearing or episiotomy. After the first baby, episiotomies are sometimes necessary, sometimes not.

I am frequently asked by patients if I routinely do episiotomies. Few doctors "routinely" do episiotomies, but most agree that it is better for your tissues to have a clean straight cut as in an episiotomy, than ragged, bloody tears. Both of these, of course,

## Fetal Head Stations

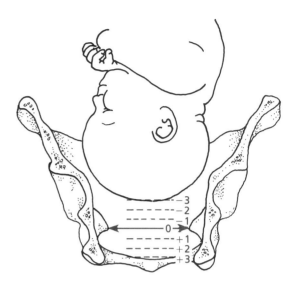

must be sewn up, but it seems that tissues heal more normally if they have been carefully cut than if they have torn (See Q. 590).

## 578 What does the third stage of labor include?

This stage begins with delivery of the baby and concludes with delivery of the placenta. As soon as the baby is born, the uterus continues to contract, eventually squeezing out the placenta. As the placenta is extruded

## Effacement

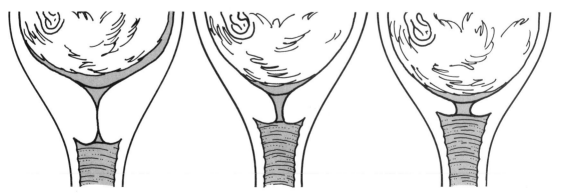

# Dilation

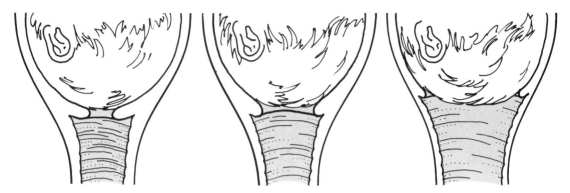

from the vagina, a gush of blood occurs. This happens because, as the placenta separates from the uterus, blood collects behind it, helping to make the separation complete. This loss of blood is not dangerous, and as the placenta leaves the uterine cavity, the uterus continues to "contract down," squeezing off its blood vessels so that little further bleeding occurs.

The placenta may be delivered quickly, spontaneously, or hours later if left alone. Usually if the placenta does not come out spontaneously, the doctor will put his or her hand up into the uterus, grasp the placenta, and pull it out.

Patients occasionally tell doctors that they want the placenta to deliver on its own. This is fine, except that it sometimes takes two or three hours and can heighten the chance of bleeding and infection. Most doctors believe that it is best to get the placenta delivered within ten or fifteen minutes after delivery of the baby.

Whether a placenta is removed by the

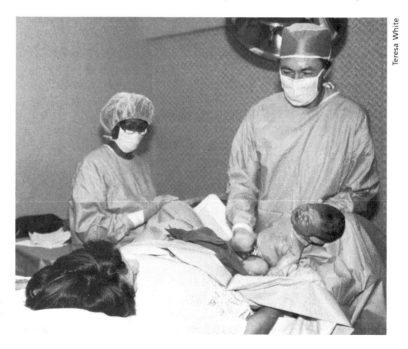

Teresa White

The second stage of labor ends with the delivery of the baby.

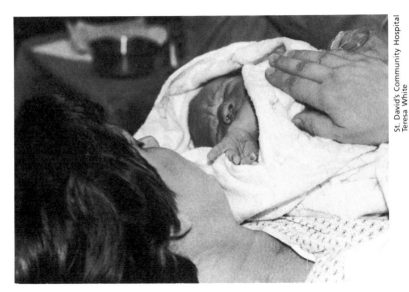

A separate creation of God
. . . a new individual . . . to
be loved and cherished.

doctor or is passed spontaneously, most doctors today carefully manually examine the inside of the uterus, making certain that all the membranes and placental tissue have been removed. In spite of this exam, however, it is fairly common for even large pieces of placental tissue to pass from the uterus a few hours or a few days later. The lining of the uterus and the placental tissue feel similar, and it is impossible to know for sure that all placental tissue is out.

Before the episiotomy or vulvar tears are sutured, most doctors will visually check the cervix and the vagina to make sure there are no tears of these tissues. If there are, these are repaired prior to the sewing of the episiotomy or the tears around the opening of the vagina.

first stage of labor (the time during which the cervix dilates from one or two centimeters up to ten centimeters) is made up of three different phases:

The first phase equals dilatation from zero to four centimeters; the second phase equals dilatation from four to eight centimeters (essentially the first part of the "phase of acceleration" that was discussed in Q. 576); the third phase transition equals dilatation from eight to ten centimeters (the last part of the phase of acceleration).

The reason the teachers of childbirth classes divide labor into these three phases is that progressively increasing amounts of effort and concentration are required. It is easier for the mother to anticipate what to expect if she considers labor divided into three segments.

**579** How does this account of the stages of labor correlate with the phases taught in childbirth classes?

Patients can be confused by the differing terminology used by their physicians and their childbirth class teachers. Obstetricians talk in terms of first stage, second stage, and third stage. Childbirth classes teach that the

## Practicalities in the Labor Room

**580** May I have visitors in the labor room with me?

Most labor-and-delivery units are now glad to have either the father or a friend or rela-

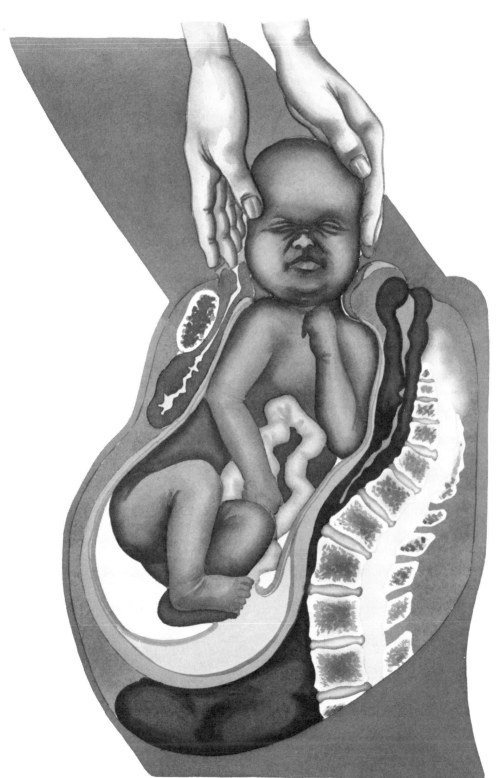

**Second Stage of Delivery**

tive in the labor room during the entire labor. I am in favor of this, since patients in labor are much more relaxed if they have a husband, friend, or relative present during labor. I encourage families, however, to send in only one member of the family at a time, in addition to the official "coach," while their relative is in labor. Too many people milling around in the labor room can be distracting to the mother.

### 581  How is monitoring done during labor? Why is it so important?

Monitoring of the fetus can be done with a fetoscope, a stethoscope designed specifically to hear the baby's heartbeat, or with an electronic monitor. The baby's heartbeat will normally be between 120 and 160 beats per minute, though it is normal for the rate to drop or to rise a little from those norms.

If the heartbeat develops an abnormal pattern of slow or fast rates, immediate delivery may be indicated, even if it involves a cesarean section. This is a situation in which the doctor's judgment is important. If you are in the second stage of labor, it may be possible for the baby to be delivered before it is damaged.

Monitoring of your contractions is also important. This may be done by the nurse's or the doctor's hand on your abdomen, or it may be done with an electronic monitor. Either way, both the intensity of the contractions and their frequency are evaluated. If the intensity suddenly becomes abnormally strong, or if the uterus is not relaxing between contractions, the baby might need to be delivered immediately, even if it required a cesarean section.

### 582  What examinations will take place during labor?

The nurse and doctor will be examining you throughout your labor. Only occasional examinations are necessary when you are less than five centimeters dilated, but more frequent exams are necessary when contractions increase in frequency and intensity.

These examinations are done for two reasons. First, they show the progress of dilation; second, they show the progression of the baby's head in the birth canal. If the baby's head is staying high, even with good contractions, you may have an obstructed labor and need a cesarean section.

The doctor will want your blood pressure, temperature, and pulse checked intermittently. Normally these are checked about every one to two hours.

The doctor and nurses will be watching your abdomen to make sure that your bladder is not too full. If your bladder is filling up, and you cannot urinate on your own, you will need to be catheterized. This involves the insertion of a hollow rubber tube through your urethra into your bladder for the drainage of urine.

### 583  How much will labor hurt?

The terms used to refer to the process of having a baby, *labor* and *pains,* should offer some clues to the woman who has never had a child as to how it feels.

The term *labor* indicates that the process is a lot of work. For this reason women should be in good physical condition as they approach the end of their pregnancy.

The term *pains* has been applied to the process of labor for thousands of years. Labor does hurt, but the amount of pain that women have with labor varies from individual to individual. A patient of mine described it as "like a gas pain that you cannot get rid of, which makes you feel like doubling over and bearing down." This is a good description of the pain of labor.

As labor starts, the pain is like a menstrual cramp. This cramping becomes increasingly more intense and more frequent, and about the time that a woman in labor is five centimeters dilated, the pain begins changing to a type of pain that she has never had before, similar to a severe gas pain that does not go away and that causes a great deal of discomfort.

Because each woman's nerves are "hooked up" differently, some women feel labor pains a great deal and others very little. I read a newspaper article several years ago about a pregnant woman who took a nap and awakened to find that she had delivered her baby! I suppose it would be wonderful if all women were like that, but few are.

One problem with "natural childbirth" classes is that to play down the pain aspect of labor, many teachers tend to imply that if a woman prepares herself adequately, she will not hurt during labor. This is untrue. Most women will have a great deal of discomfort during their labor, although usually this is a discomfort that they can tolerate. Women tend to "forget" about the severity of the pain. The fact that most women get pregnant again, shows that labor pains are not intolerably severe for most women.

## 584 What about pain relief during labor?

Many women in labor, whether or not they plan to have an epidural for delivery (see Q. 546–548), will want something in addition to their breathing techniques to help relieve pain. Most obstetricians (including me) normally give some type of narcotic in the vein through an IV tubing if the patient requests it.

The drugs usually given are 25 mg of Demerol with a mild tranquilizer. This is not enough to put a mother to sleep, nor can it hurt the baby. If the mother is still uncomfortable, that dosage can be repeated two or three times almost immediately without harming either mother or baby. The 25 mg

dose of Demerol can be repeated at intervals, and giving it every thirty to forty minutes is not excessive.

Some mothers feel that they "lose control" when they have been given Demerol. Those women should not receive a repeated dose of it. Many mothers, however, feel better with Demerol, and I strongly encourage its use.

## 585 Can regional anesthetics, such as spinal, epidural, caudal, be given during the first stage of labor?

In the first stage of labor, the only types of anesthesia that can be given are caudal or epidural. A spinal stops labor and therefore can be given only during the second stage of labor. An epidural is usually given when a woman having her first baby is dilated to five centimeters and the baby's head is at "plus one" (engaged). If the baby's head is higher than that, the doctor may not feel comfortable with the first-time mother's receiving an epidural even if she is six or seven centimeters dilated. (See Q. 576.)

If a woman has had a previous baby, she may be able to have an epidural when she is only three or four centimeters dilated. Most doctors feel that it is important, in an ordinary situation, that a good labor pattern be established before the epidural is given.

## 586 When and why is Pitocin given?

Pitocin (oxytocin) is normally given in the IV fluid when a woman is not having good contractions. The contractions in the first stage should gradually increase in intensity and frequency; if they are irregular and ineffective and the woman is dilating very slowly, it is probably best that she have Pitocin added slowly to the intravenous fluid. This is not given in an attempt to make contractions harder than normal con-

Third Stage of Delivery

tractions; it is given only to bring the quality of contractions and their frequency up to what is expected of normal labor.

The advantage of Pitocin is that it keeps a patient from staying in labor for a longer than normal time and prevents the woman and her uterus from getting weak, dehydrated, and tired. If a mother's contractions are monitored carefully by the medical attendants, there is almost no chance of any damage to her or her baby from Pitocin. (See Q. 643.)

Pitocin may also be given to cause labor to start. If a woman's bag of waters has broken, she needs to deliver the baby before germs from the vagina get into the uterus and infect the baby. Occasionally a woman and her doctor will want to induce labor because of convenience or because a pregnancy has gone more than two weeks past the due date. In these situations the doctor will usually break the bag of waters and start Pitocin.

## 587  What circumstances might indicate the need for a C-section?

During the first stage of labor, some problems may develop that make a cesarean section necessary.

*Placenta previa.* If the placenta is growing over the inside opening of the uterus, the baby cannot be delivered vaginally. You would probably know about this condition before you actually went into labor.

A woman with a placenta previa will normally have some bleeding from the vagina during the last few weeks of pregnancy. If she did not have bleeding before, she would probably start having heavy bleeding as labor started. If examination on admission to the hospital shows that the woman's placenta is covering her cervix, she would not be allowed to labor at all, but would be taken immediately to the operating room for a C-section.

*Abruptio placenta.* Occasionally, either before labor starts or during labor, a placenta will pull loose from the wall of the uterus. When this happens the uterus becomes tense and does not relax properly. Sometimes a pregnant woman in this situation will bleed from her vagina.

When abruptio placenta occurs, the whole placenta can pull loose and cause the baby to die immediately. More commonly the placenta pulls only partially loose, causing irritability of the uterus. When this happens an immediate cesarean section must be done. If only a very small part of the placenta has pulled loose, the uterus may not develop a great deal of irritability, and the baby's heartbeat may remain stable. Normally, however, a cesarean section is necessary if this problem develops.

*Fetal distress.* Fetal monitoring (observation of the baby's heartbeat) is done to detect any distress that the baby might experience. If your baby develops significant distress during the first stage of labor, you will probably need to have a cesarean section. Your doctor will usually be able to determine whether or not the fetal distress is a significant emergency or whether the baby can be watched further.

If the distress is seen on the monitor, and your bag of waters has broken and your cervix has dilated to at least three to four centimeters, the doctor can use a fetal scalp blood sampling technique in which the baby's scalp is pricked and blood is taken and examined. This examination can show whether or not the baby is getting adequate oxygen even though distress is indicated on the monitor. If the baby is getting adequate oxygen, then your labor will be allowed to continue. Repeat scalp blood sampling is usually done to make sure the baby's condition is not deteriorating. Because this test is not widely available, your hospital may not have such equipment.

*Obstruction to the progress of labor.* The term *cephalopelvic disproportion (CPD)* is normally used to describe this problem.

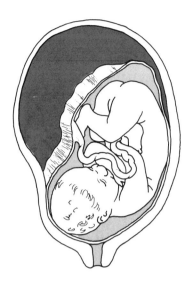

*Abruptio placenta*—internal bleeding

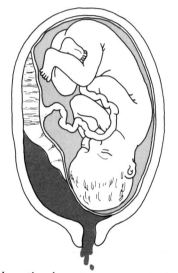

*Abruptio placenta*—external bleeding

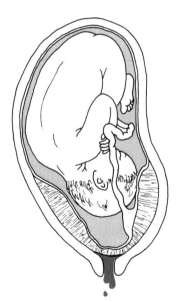

*Total placenta previa*

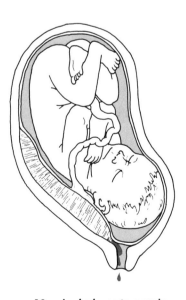

*Marginal placenta previa*

This basically means that there is disproportion between the size of the baby's head and the size of your pelvis.

If you have dilated to five centimeters and do not progress a centimeter an hour, your labor is going slowly. If your labor continues to be relatively slow but is progressing, the doctor will probably allow labor to continue to a vaginal delivery. If the labor is too slow, however, the doctor may feel that the baby's head is being compressed too hard by your contractions and that a cesarean section would be the wisest thing to avoid any damage to the baby. (See Q. 639–653.)

The decision in this situation is purely judgmental; there is no absolute criterion for the doctor to depend on. Fortunately, most of the time babies born by cesarean section because of obstructed labor are healthy and normal when the patient is being cared for by a competent, careful obstetrician.

## The Basics of Delivery

### 588 Does monitoring continue through delivery?

It is helpful if the baby can be monitored, either with the electric fetal monitor or with the fetoscope, all through the second stage of labor, which concludes with delivery. During this time the baby's head is being pressed by the birth canal. Contractions can become so forceful and prolonged that oxygen to the baby is compromised. If there is any indication that the baby is being affected, delivery can be quickly accomplished by the use of forceps. The problem is that at this stage of labor the mother is usually pushing hard with contractions, and the baby is so low in the uterus that its heartbeat can be hard to find. However, if monitoring can be done at least some of the time, it is reassuring.

### 589 When does it help for me to "push"?

Up to the point when you are completely dilated, you have probably been told that pushing would do no good. This is true. Finally, though, with your cervix completely dilated, pushing does help the progress of the baby through the birth canal. Many women find pushing to be a great relief; others find it uncomfortable and want to avoid pushing.

It is important, though, that you do push during this stage of labor. If you have an epidural, you will not feel the urge to push, but because of your childbirth-class training, your pushing will be effective in helping the baby come down.

The urge to push, when you do not have an epidural, feels like the need to have a bowel movement. This is because the baby's head is putting a great deal of pressure on the rectum.

Patients these days have learned to push so effectively that they put a great deal of pressure on the baby's head. I have seen babies born "depressed" (low Apgar score) after the mother had been allowed to push too long and too hard during this second stage. If you have been pushing for a length of time that the doctor feels is adequate, and the baby is still not ready to deliver, it would be safer to let your doctor go ahead with a forceps delivery than for you to continue pushing longer. Forceps almost never hurt a baby and their use can save many minutes of pushing. (See Q. 591, 592.)

### 590 What happens next if my delivery proceeds normally?

As you push and the contractions continue to be effective, the baby's head will cause your perineum and vulvar areas to bulge. The skin of this area will become tense, and a portion of the baby's scalp will show between your labia. If it is your first baby, you will almost certainly need an episiotomy at this point. If you do not have an episiotomy, the tissues all around the vaginal opening will usually tear in a jagged, irregular way. Some physicians feel that without an episiotomy, there is great stretching of the underlying ligaments of the vagina, making it more likely that you will need vaginal reparative surgery in the future.

If this is your second child, an episiotomy is less likely, and for each child thereafter there is a decreasing chance of your needing an episiotomy.

An episiotomy is a small incision cut from the back of the vagina toward the rectum (midline episiotomy) or cut to the right or the left from the lower vaginal (mediolateral episiotomy). It is not uncommon for an episiotomy to tear on into the muscular ring that is around your anus or even into the anus itself. This is not dangerous unless the physician doing the delivery is unaware that such a tear occurred. This type of tear must be sewn up so that you do not end up involuntarily leaking stool in the future.

As the baby's head progresses down through the birth canal, it will gradually bulge through the labia. At this point, progression is normally very rapid. The baby's head suddenly appears totally outside the vagina and the body quickly follows.

*It is important that the baby's head not "pop" out of the vagina.* While still in the vagina, there is pressure on the baby's head. The pressure decreases as the head emerges, and if this happens very rapidly, this decreased pressure and the expansion of the baby's skull bones can tear blood vessels inside the skull, causing the baby to have brain damage.

When the doctor tells you to stop pushing, it is important that you not push. If you are delivering the baby at home, in a car, or at someplace other than a hospital, the one helpful thing that a person can do is to hold the baby's head gently as it is coming out so that it does not pop out of your vagina.

---

## 591 How do you feel about the use of forceps?

Forceps have received an unwarranted bad reputation, one that resulted from the way they were previously used.

Forceps were invented in the early 1600s, making it possible for doctors to complete some difficult deliveries and save the mother's life. Until then the cesarean sections that were necessary for difficult births would almost always result in the mother's death. Prior to 1882 almost every woman who had a cesarean section died.

With the use of forceps, many babies were killed during difficult vaginal deliveries, or they were already dead at the time the forceps were used. Of the babies who survived, many were terribly brain-damaged because of either the long, difficult labor that had preceded the use of forceps or because of the forceps themselves. In these situations, however, without the use of forceps both mother and baby would have died.

The big difference now is that forceps are no longer used for difficult deliveries. Cesarean sections are done instead—safely. When forceps are used, it is merely to assist the baby's head in its completion of the passage through the birth canal.

Forceps tend to hold the walls of the vagina away from the baby's head, and they pull only on the strongest part of the baby's skull, the powerful facial bones of the baby that can almost not be damaged by the forcep's pressure. The forceps, therefore, actually protect the baby's brain to some degree from the pressure of the birth canal.

It is true that forceps can sometimes scrape or bruise the baby's skin, but any significant damage is unusual. For instance, in

# Episiotomy

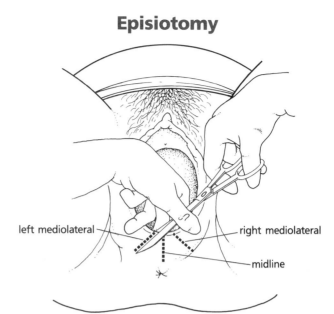

left mediolateral

right mediolateral

midline

# Cardinal Movements of Delivery

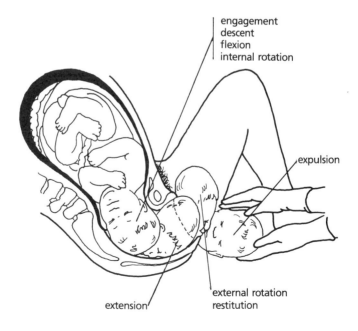

engagement
descent
flexion
internal rotation

expulsion

extension

external rotation
restitution

my years of practice I know of only one child in which my use of forceps produced a significant scraping of the facial skin, and this skin healed with very little scarring.

In my opinion, the use of forceps by a competent physician is extremely safe and almost never causes any problems. I encourage you to let your doctor use forceps if there is any indication that they would help your labor.

## 592 What might indicate the need for forceps?

As stated previously (Q. 587), contractions may become so forceful and prolonged that the baby's oxygen supply is threatened. In that situation a speedy delivery is important, and if you are ten centimeters dilated, forceps can help get the baby out quickly.

In addition, a baby delivers most easily face downward, looking toward your rectum. If the baby's head is in any other position, the doctor will probably want to rotate the baby. If this can be done with his or her hand, the doctor will do so; if not, forceps may be tried, because the head will sometimes fail to deliver unless it is turned. Normally the head is not stuck but has just been inadequately turned by your birth canal.

If the doctor cannot rotate the baby's head, it may be possible to deliver it with the baby facing up. If not, the only choice is to do a cesarean section.

## 593 Can the baby become stuck even after the head is delivered?

After delivery of the baby's head, the remainder of the body normally comes through easily. Occasionally, however, a shoulder will get stuck in the birth canal behind the mother's pubic bone.

There are various maneuvers that the doctor and the nurses can use to help, but it is a frightening situation and always leaves the doctors and nurses sweating when it is over.

If the doctor indicates to you that the head is out but the shoulders are stuck and then asks you to push, it is important that you push with all your might. The nurses will normally be pushing up above on your uterus, and the doctor will be doing his or her best to turn the shoulders into a position where they will deliver. If that is not working, the doctor may put a hand up into your uterus, grasping one of the baby's arms to pull it out of the birth canal. This allows the "stuck" shoulder to fall away from the pubic bone, allowing delivery of the baby.

Occasionally these maneuvers will result in some tearing of the nerves of one of the baby's arms, causing paralysis of that arm. Most of the time such paralysis is only temporary.

## 594 When is the umbilical cord clamped?

The cord is clamped after the baby is delivered, suctioned, and "plopped up" on the mother's abdomen. There have been long-standing arguments about the best time to clamp the cord. There are benefits to clamping it quickly, and there are benefits to delaying the clamping. Most doctors today feel that the time to clamp the cord is when they can get around to it, without adhering to a specific timetable.

Clamping the cord after some delay allows extra blood to get to the baby, but babies are almost always born with an excess of blood that must "break down." This breaking down of the excessive blood is what causes the mild degree of jaundice that almost all newborn babies have. Some doctors propose that if the cord is clamped immediately after delivery, there is a theoretical possibility that it might interfere, in some as yet undetermined way, with the baby's lung function and increase its chance of having respiratory distress. Currently this is only a theory.

## 595 Why does a newborn need to be "suctioned"?

As soon as the baby is delivered, whether by C-section or by vaginal delivery, a bulb syringe is used to suction the baby's throat and mouth and then its nose. This is important, not because the baby must breathe immediately, but because when the baby does take its first gasping breath, it could suck the material in its throat down into the lungs, causing breathing difficulties later.

## 596 What is done if the baby does not begin breathing immediately after birth?

Physicians and nurses are carefully trained in resuscitation of the baby, and this is done quickly and gently.

First, the baby will be suctioned again to make sure there is no material blocking its breathing tubes. If there is not, the baby will be stimulated by rubbing its back. These things often make the baby take a breath and become active.

If the baby is still not breathing after a few seconds of stimulation, the doctor or nurse will listen to its heartbeat. At this point the doctor may use the laryngoscope, a lighted instrument for looking at the baby's vocal cords. This allows direct suctioning of the area of the vocal cords and of the trachea for removal of meconium and mucus. It may be necessary to put a small tube into the trachea to give the baby oxygen directly. During this time the medical personnel would have already had pure oxygen flowing over the baby's mouth and nose.

The baby is in the delivery-room bassinet while these techniques are being performed. Most modern delivery rooms have an open bassinet, with an overhead heater that provides radiant heat to keep the baby warm. Being open, it allows medical personnel to work with the baby more easily.

With this care the baby usually begins breathing and crying spontaneously. If it does not, it would require continued close observation and care.

## 597 What is the Apgar score?

Up until several years ago, when the late Dr. Virginia Apgar, former professor of anesthesiology at Columbia College of Physicians and Surgeons, devised her scoring system, there was no standard way to determine the birth status of newborn babies. Dr. Apgar's special interest was the effect of anesthesia on labor. Using her system, based on five different signs, she began evaluating newborns, and the Apgar score soon came into routine use.

Most hospitals now give the baby an Apgar score when it is one minute old and another when it is five minutes old. Although the one-minute Apgar was the initial recommendation of Dr. Apgar, most physicians believe that the five-minute Apgar score tells more about the baby's condition.

The baby is given a number for each of the five signs; these numbers are totaled, and the baby has its Apgar score. It is uncommon, for a baby to have an Apgar of ten, because almost all normal babies have some blueness of their arms and legs or face. An Apgar score of eight or nine indicates a vigorous baby at birth, although any baby can have birth defects that do not cause a low Apgar score at birth.

## The Placenta and Other Considerations After Delivery

## 598 When is the placenta delivered?

Most doctors feel it is best to facilitate delivery of the placenta; this may be done by ap-

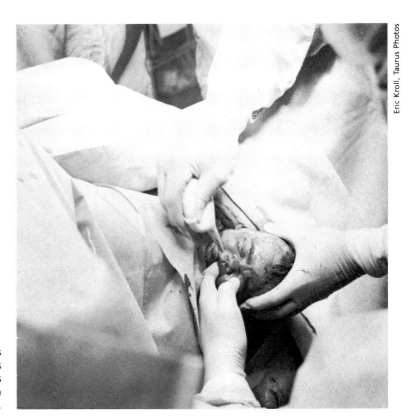

As soon as the baby is delivered, a bulb syringe is used to suction the baby's throat and mouth and then its nose.

plying moderate pressure on the uterus or by massaging the uterus while pulling on the umbilical cord. Normally, the doctor will ask the mother to bear down as when she was trying to push out the baby.

The placenta will come out fairly quickly about 75 percent of the time. In the 25 percent of situations where it does not, the doctor will ordinarily put a hand inside the uterus, grasp the placenta, and pull it out. The cord occasionally breaks off as the doctor is pulling on it, but that does not matter

## Apgar Scoring System

| Sign | Score of 0 | Score of 1 | Score of 2 |
|------|-----------|-----------|-----------|
| Heart rate | Absent | Slow (below 100) | Over 100 |
| Respiratory effort | Absent | Slow, irregular | Good, crying |
| Muscle tone | Flaccid | Some flexion (bending) of extremities | Active motion |
| Reflex irritability | No response | Grimace | Vigorous cry |
| Color | Blue & pale | Body, pink; extremities, blue | Completely pink |

since the placenta will come out easily without using the cord for a handle.

After the placenta and membranes have been removed, the doctor will often put a hand up in the uterus, feeling around to make sure that all the membranes of the placenta have been recovered. It is, however, very easy for a piece of placenta to be missed on that type of examination because the placenta can feel exactly like the wall of the uterus. It would not be good for the doctor to dig into the wall of the uterus to make sure that all of the placenta was out. The most that he or she should do is to feel for it, and if it is felt, take it out. (See Q. 578.)

---

**599** **After the placenta is delivered, what happens next?**

The doctor will probably ask the nurse to give you some Pitocin (oxytocin) and/or a shot of Methergine to make your uterus contract down. These drugs cause the uterus to contract better than it would on its own, and the contraction is more firm than without them. This decreases the amount of blood loss that you will have immediately after your delivery.

Nursing the baby immediately after birth also helps the uterus contract. This mechanism is real since the nursing causes the mother's pituitary gland to release the natural oxytocin which makes the uterus contract. Injection of the drugs works more quickly and effectively than nursing the baby, however, and does not in any way interfere with the natural contractions produced by nursing. The drugs just add to the effect of nursing.

---

**600** **Are there any problems that can develop soon after delivery of the placenta?**

Bleeding is a fairly common problem during the period immediately after delivery of a baby. This bleeding is usually caused by the uterus being so relaxed that the surface blood vessels remain open and continue bleeding. This is most likely to occur during the first hour or two after the placenta is delivered.

As mentioned in the previous question, Pitocin or Methergine is given to make the uterine muscle contract down and pinch off the blood vessels so they will stop bleeding. You should be carefully observed at this time and it is for this reason that you are usually brought to a recovery area instead of to your room. In past years patients occasionally died because they were sent to their rooms, not carefully watched, and bled heavily while no one was there.

If you have heavy bleeding, the doctor would give you more oxytocic drugs. If these drugs did not work, other techniques would be tried. These techniques might include packing the uterus, making an incision into the abdomen to tie off some of the arteries of the uterus, or even an abdominal hysterectomy.

This situation, of course, is frightening. The doctor never likes the thought of causing sterility in someone who might want to have more children. However, you would want to have a doctor whose primary concern is saving your life, one who would if necessary proceed expeditiously to a hysterectomy.

---

**601** **Can the uterus turn "inside out"?**

Yes, an inverted uterus can occur and always surprises the doctor and the nurses. The patient will often not even know what has happened.

It is important that the doctor push the uterus back into place before the mouth of the uterus can constrict down and keep the body of the uterus from going back up inside the abdomen. If the uterus will not go back into position, an abdominal incision may be necessary to pull the uterus back into proper position. An inverted uterus can cause hemorrhage and shock. It can require blood transfusions and aggressive resuscitation of the mother. Therefore, no matter what is required, the uterus must be put back quickly into its normal position.

## 602 What happens after delivery of the placenta and membranes?

There are several things that normally take place before you leave the delivery room.

***Removing placental membranes.*** As mentioned in Q. 598, the doctor will feel inside the uterus to make sure all the placenta and membranes have been removed. When the patient has had a local anesthetic for delivery, this may be such an uncomfortable procedure for her that the doctor will skip it if he or she thinks that all the membranes have been removed. This can be one of the disadvantages of having only a local for delivery.

Although a placenta can look intact, it is possible that a piece of the afterbirth is still inside the uterus and will cause bleeding later. (See Q. 578.) I do not believe that epidural anesthesia should be used merely to enable the doctor to feel the inside of the uterus, although I do often tell my patients that if they choose to have a local for delivery, they will have pain when the inside of the uterus is explored.

***Repairing cervical tears.*** The doctor will examine the cervix. If large tears are found, the doctor will use absorbable stitches to sew the cervix back together. It is hoped, of course, that this will allow the cervix to heal in such a way that it will be as strong as it was before delivery. In so doing, the doctor can prevent premature delivery of the next pregnancy due to a cervix so weak from a

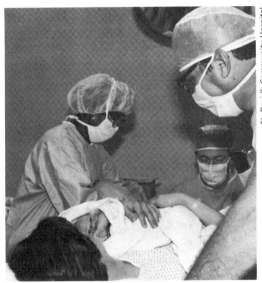

St. David's Community Hospital
Teresa White

While baby and parents become acquainted, the doctor delivers the placenta and membranes.

tear that it cannot hold the baby inside the uterus for the full term.

***Repairing vaginal tears.*** As the doctor explores the vagina, tears may also be found there. These too would be sewn with absorbable sutures to prevent bleeding and to prevent the vagina from being excessively scarred.

***Episiotomy repair.*** The doctor will explore the vaginal opening and will put sutures in any tears in the area that are at all deep. This suturing includes the episiotomy if one is done. Before sewing the episiotomy, though, the doctor will first see if there are any tears into the round muscle around the anus or into the anus or rectum, since episiotomies will occasionally tear all the way into the rectum.

Once the doctor makes sure of the extent of the episiotomy, it will be repaired properly so that you will be able to have normal bowel movements after proper healing. Occasionally episiotomy repairs will break open later. If this happens and it involves the rectal wall or the muscle ring around the anus, a future surgical procedure would be necessary to keep a woman from losing stool involuntarily.

## 603 When do the baby and I leave the labor-and-delivery section?

After the nurse "identifies" your baby (putting on its arm band, taking its footprints, and fingerprinting you), the newborn is given a royal ride to the nursery. After the doctor has sewn up your episiotomy, you will be taken to the recovery area, where you will be watched carefully until it is certain that you are not bleeding excessively and are having no problem from anesthesia. If your baby has not chilled too much and is healthy, it will usually be brought to you and your husband in the recovery room. Following this recovery period you will be taken to your room.

## Parent/Baby Bonding

## 604 What does the term *bonding* mean?

In this context, bonding usually refers to the attachment that develops between a mother and her baby, but it also occurs between the father and the newborn. Studies have shown that close contact between the new parents and the baby during the first few hours and days after delivery is very important. There seems to be a sensitive period during the first few hours after delivery when the bond between mother and father and their baby can be "cemented" if they can be together.

The best pattern seems to be for the mother, father, and healthy baby to be together for thirty to sixty minutes after delivery. Skin to skin contact between mother and baby seems to produce healthy emotional feelings in many mothers and may be important for the baby. Nursing the baby, of course, fits into this pattern, but nursing on

## Involution

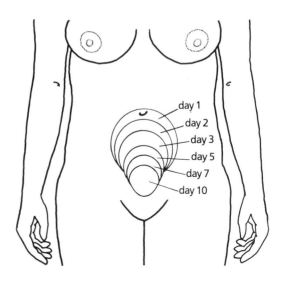

day 1
day 2
day 3
day 5
day 7
day 10

the delivery table immediately after delivery is usually a clumsy affair. It is probably best for this close contact between mother and baby to start in the recovery room.

## 605 Is "rooming in" a good idea?

There are indications that it is best for mother and baby to be together almost constantly during the first few days of life. This suggests that "rooming in"—having the baby stay in the mother's room rather than in the hospital nursery—is the best thing. With adequate help in the hospital, most new mothers can handle this. Being with the baby during her hospital stay can teach the new mother how to meet the needs of the baby.

Studies have indicated that spending this time together does appear to cement the bond between mother and baby. When mother and baby have spent time close together during the first hours and days of the baby's life, mothers will want to hold their babies more and will often kiss and look at them more than mothers who have not had a bonding time. These things indicate a good, healthy relationship and attachment between the mother and the baby. Babies who have had such close contact with the mother early in their lives seem to smile and laugh more, according to some studies.

## 606 Do most hospitals allow "bonding time" and "rooming in"?

Most hospitals are now aware of this need for parent-infant bonding and allow the baby to be brought to the mother in the recovery room. Incidentally, a brief time for the baby to go to the nursery to be weighed and cleaned up does not seem to affect this bonding process.

Additionally, most hospitals are now quite willing to provide "rooming in." More resistance to this arrangement comes from mothers themselves than from the hospital. Quite understandably, a mother may tend to see the two or three days in the hospital as a time of rest for her, not as a time for getting to know the new baby, especially if she has other children at home. Perhaps in the next few years we will see more education of mothers to the fact that the few days after delivery are not for rest, but for beginning the mothering process.

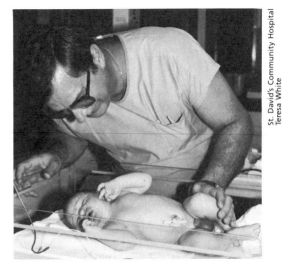

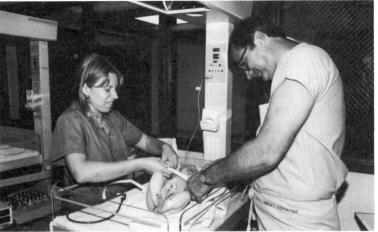

Today many hospitals allow the father to accompany the newborn to the nursery and to assist in giving the baby a bath and dressing it.

Up until the past few years, hospitals were so afraid of infection that they separated mothers and babies and visitors, particularly brothers, sisters, and fathers of the newborn. Fathers were kept out of delivery rooms and, until recently, mothers were often put completely to sleep for normal deliveries. Fortunately, up-to-date obstetric units in this country have realized the wisdom of having the father with the mother during labor and of allowing the mother, baby, and father to be together during the time immediately after delivery.

It is encouraging to note that intensive care nurseries are allowing even sick and premature babies to have their parents around them while they are in these units. Parents are being allowed to participate in the care of these babies. This, of course, probably helps the development of good emotional attachments between baby, mother, and father.

## Postdelivery Details in the Hospital

### 607 Are "the blues" normal after delivery?

Postpartum depression, or postpartum blues, has been reported in more than 80 percent of mothers. The problem, usually indicated by depression and crying during the hospital stay or soon after going home, is generally limited to a few days and goes away spontaneously. It has been suggested that this response may be partly produced by the habit many hospitals still have of separating the mother and the baby immediately after delivery, allowing them only short visits every four hours or so during the hospital time. However, I doubt that this is usually the cause today, since most hospitals no longer have those restrictions. Yet most mothers still experience some postpartum depression.

Most obstetricians feel that postpartum blues are caused by hormonal changes. Just before delivery there are amazingly high levels of estrogen, progesterone, and other hormones in the mother's body. Immediately after delivery these levels fall dramatically, and the mother's hormones do not return to normal for about two to three months. It seems reasonable to assume that these dramatic hormone changes contribute to a mother's feeling of depression.

In addition, the changes in a mother's life that the delivery represents must be considered. She may not be confident about her ability to care for the baby; financial concerns may be present; family problems may surface when a new family member arrives. All these things (and many more!) can certainly contribute to depression at a time when the mother is already "below par" from her delivery.

The depression usually clears up in just a few days. If it does not and you find yourself becoming more and more depressed, it is important to mention this to your physician. If it seems to be a bad-enough problem, your doctor will help you find a counselor to talk to so that this depression does not ruin this special time in your life.

### 608 Is infection of the uterus a common problem after delivery?

Uterine infections may occur after delivery. Most fevers that women develop after delivery are due to some degree of infection in the uterus.

Often this infection is due to the fact that a woman's waters ruptured several hours before delivery. The longer the bag of waters was ruptured prior to delivery, the greater the chance of uterine infection after delivery.

Also, the wall of the uterus is raw after delivery, and this entire surface is open to infection. The area of the uterine wall where the placenta was attached is especially raw, making this the area in which bacteria generally will grow after a delivery has occurred.

Infection in the uterus can become quite severe and can spread to the ovaries and tubes. It can extend into the large veins of the pelvis, and it can produce clots in those veins which can break loose and travel to the lungs. Infection of the female organs can also cause contamination of the abdominal tissues, or peritonitis.

Although infections of the uterus do not often develop after vaginal deliveries, even with the best of care they do occur. Such infections, especially the more severe forms, are much more common after C-sections.

---

## 609 Is circumcision advisable if my baby is a boy?

If you want to have your baby circumcised, have him circumcised. If you do not, don't have it done. There is no need to make a big deal of it, either in your own mind or because of what someone else says or thinks.

There are some advantages to having a baby circumcised. One study has shown that of males who were not circumcised as babies, 10 percent will need to be circumcised in later life for some medical problem. These include infections under the foreskin or a foreskin that is too tight to let the head of the penis out with an erection. Circumcision done when a man is older is not only painful but requires hospitalization, anesthesia, and significant expense.

Additionally, there is indication that men who have been circumcised as babies, are less likely to develop cancer or herpes of the penis and possibly less likely to get urinary tract infections.

If a baby has been circumcised, however, there is a slightly greater chance of a little infection at the opening of his penis. Though the penile opening may become a bit smaller following such an infection, it is easily opened. This problem does not happen very often and can also occur in babies who have not been circumcised.

There is some pain to the baby when the circumcision is done, but babies who are being circumcised cry as much from being restrained as they do from the actual operation itself. The pain produced causes no future psychological problems for the little boy.

Based on findings such as these, the American Academy of Pediatrics has stated that there are "no valid medical indications for circumcision in the newborn." Considering the things I have mentioned, I feel that this is too negative a statement toward circumcision. Many other pediatricians and obstetricians feel this way too.

Traditionally, the obstetrician rather than the pediatrician does the circumcision. However, some pediatricians do circumcisions. If you have a family practitioner or a general practitioner caring for both you and your baby, he or she would do the circumcision.

*Bris* or *brit* (the modern spelling) is a Jewish ceremonial circumcision usually performed by a *mohel*, a person who does such circumcisions as a profession but is not a physician. Conservative, Reform, and Reconstructionist Jews allow a Jewish doctor to perform the circumcision, provided a rabbi is in attendance. The ceremony is normally scheduled the eighth day after birth. The date may be changed if there are valid medical reasons. Usually held in the parents' home, the ceremony is a joyous occasion which includes the naming of the child.

---

## 610 What can I expect during my stay in the hospital?

If you have had a cesarean section, or if you have had an episiotomy, you will have some pain. You should take the pain medication that your doctor prescribes. Taking it will keep you from hurting, will allow you to sleep better at night, and will keep you from becoming tense. The less pain and discomfort you feel and the less tense you are now, the better you will feel later. If you are nursing, the pain medications you are given will not hurt your baby.

Some women will "break their tailbone" with delivery. If the tip of their spinal column (coccyx) curves forward toward the front of the body, as the baby's head delivers, the coccyx pops back (but does not break)

at one of the joints between the different segments of the coccyx. This can cause significant pain which continues to be moderately severe for many weeks. There is no treatment, except for pain medications and sitz baths; the condition usually clears spontaneously. If pain persists in the very end of the tailbone, check with your doctor.

Most hospitals these days have liberal visiting hours and will allow both your husband and your children to come frequently to visit. If your hospital does not allow this, I encourage you and others in your commu-

# Circumcision

Circumcision affects only the appearance of the penis, not its function.

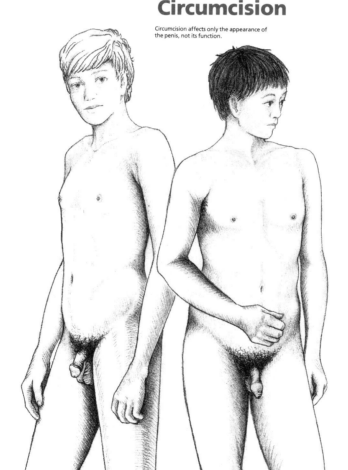

circumcised penis    uncircumcised penis

nity to talk to the hospital administration and show them statistics from hospitals that allow this type of visiting. Such statistics show no increased infection in the nursery because of family visitation, and the benefits from such visitation far outweigh any potential risks.

Most hospitals also allow "rooming in" and "feeding on demand." If at all possible you should go to a hospital that does allow these arrangements. If you have no choice of hospitals, go home as soon as you feel able to, even if it is the day after delivery. You cannot do this, of course, if you have had a cesarean section, but women now frequently go home only three or four days following a C-section. Then, later, you and others in your community should begin encouraging the hospital to update its attitudes about labor and delivery and to allow "rooming in" and "feeding on demand."

---

## Health Care Once You Are Home

---

**611** **What instructions do you give your patients when they go home from the hospital?**

My instructions are simple.

*Housework.* Have somebody else do the cooking, housekeeping, and other work around the house for two weeks. You can take care of the baby as long as you feel up to it, but if you get tired, let someone else do that too! I have found that my patients who follow this advice feel better a month or two later. Women who get too busy right after leaving the hospital, and who have a lot of responsibility and work to do, will often feel tired for several months after having a baby. The two weeks after delivery are a time when people want to take care of you. Let them!

*Constipation.* It is important that you not become constipated. I encourage my patients to use a tablespoon of Metamucil three times a day. Metamucil is basically fiber; it is not a laxative. When you are having bulky, soft stools, you can decrease the amount of Metamucil.

*Bleeding.* Bleeding can last as long as two months. It may come and go, and may be bright red or with clots, all of which is normal. You do not need to call your doctor unless the bleeding is heavier than a normal menstrual period and is causing you concern. You should not use tampons during the first three weeks following delivery, as their use could conceivably be uncomfortable or cause infection of the uterus.

*Intercourse.* Do not have intercourse for about three weeks. This allows any tears or the episiotomy to heal before you begin having sexual relations again. Do not douche during that three-week healing time.

*Exercise.* Women should not begin muscle-strengthening exercises until six weeks from the time of delivery because such exercise can cause muscle strain. The abdominal muscles have been stretched out of shape, but even without exercise they will shrink back to near-normal length. I feel it is best to let those muscles shrink on their own and then, six weeks after delivery, to begin exercising those now-shortened muscles. I certainly feel that it is normal and desirable for a new mother to go walking and climb stairs as soon as she gets home.

*Personal care.* It is fine to take a bath or shower and to wash your hair immediately. Being well-groomed and attractive is important at this time. The better you look, the better you will feel!

*Episiotomy care*. The episiotomy or tear repair requires no special care; normal cleansing and gentle towel-drying are all that is necessary. While heat lamps and spray medication are soothing to the area, neither speed healing. Care should be taken, however, in using heat lamps as leg burns result from careless use, considerably complicating your discomfort.

Occasionally the episiotomy will come open. This is not due to your doctor's negligence. In fact, it is amazing that this does not happen more often. When it does, the wound cannot be resewn. It will heal by itself. After healing, most women cannot tell it ever happened.

*Driving*. It is fine for you to ride in a car; in fact, getting out for a while will be good for you. I suggest that you refrain from driving, however, until you are confident that you can apply the brake quickly in an emergency situation.

*Iron and vitamins*. If you are nursing, continue taking your prenatal vitamins as long as you nurse. If you are not nursing, finish taking all your prenatal vitamins, then start taking an iron pill a day. Do this for six months. Most women need to make up for the iron they lost to the pregnancy. You do not need an expensive or prescription iron preparation. Ask your pharmacist for a reliable, cheap iron preparation that you can take once a day.

## 612 When will my doctor want to examine me again in the office?

I usually see my patients three weeks after delivery. If all is well at that time, I tell them that they can resume marital relations, and I discuss techniques for contraception, giving them whatever they need for that—information, a prescription for a diaphragm, a prescription for pills, or talk to them about an IUD. See Chapter 12 if you have questions on this subject.

When the baby is three months old, I see my patients again. At that time I do a Pap smear, a complete physical examination, and answer any further questions they have about contraception. After this three-month visit I have them come back to see me one year later, unless there is a special problem that needs to be rechecked sooner.

Other doctors may vary their schedules for seeing new mothers, but most of them have similar schedules.

## 613 When do menstrual periods begin again?

Women who are not breast-feeding will normally ovulate four weeks after they deliver a baby (or after a miscarriage or after stopping birth-control pills). A period will normally start two weeks after that. Most women, then, will have a period approximately six weeks after they deliver a baby. It is just as normal for a woman not to have an ovulation or a period for up to six months after delivery, although 90 percent of women will have started their periods within three months after delivery.

Many nursing mothers will not ovulate or have periods at all while they are nursing, but it is also quite normal to have menstrual periods while nursing, especially after beginning to supplement your baby's diet with other foods. Many women will have menstrual periods on a regular monthly basis even though they are having normal milk production (lactation).

It is important to understand that you can become pregnant even if you have not yet had a period. When ovulation occurs, which can happen even when you have not had a period, you can become pregnant. Therefore you cannot wait for a period to come and use that as a sign that you are fertile from that point on. You are fertile when you ovulate, whether or not you have had a period.

## 614 How long should I wait to become pregnant again?

I feel that a woman should wait at least three months after a delivery or a miscarriage (or after stopping birth-control pills) before she gets pregnant again. It takes about three months for most of the hormone effects from any of these events to be gone, and it is best to wait until that time before starting a new pregnancy. Of course, most women laugh when I tell them they can become pregnant three months after they have had a baby. For some reason, they are not yet quite ready to do it all over again.

A woman who becomes pregnant almost immediately after a previous baby needs to exercise more vigorously during that subsequent pregnancy to keep her body in good shape. Other than this, a pregnancy that closely follows a previous delivery can, in general, be considered and treated as a normal pregnancy.

## Breast-Feeding

## 615 Is breast-feeding my baby a good idea?

Yes! Without any question, breast-feeding is superior to bottle-feeding a newborn baby.

Studies show that babies who are breast-fed tend to be healthier, have a lower mortality rate, seem to develop better physically and mentally, and have fewer problems with allergies in later life. A recently conducted study indicated that mothers of infants born one to three months prematurely produce milk especially adapted to the needs of such preterm infants. Their milk is easily digested and contains a higher proportion of the nutrients that promote neurological maturation. I strongly encourage my patients to breast-feed their infants.

Millions of babies, however, have been bottle-fed, and if there is a difference in babies who are breast-fed and those who are not, it is not an enormous difference. A baby who is bottle-fed can be healthy and happy.

There are many things that can prevent a mother from breast-feeding, and no mother should feel guilty because she cannot breast-feed her baby. She may not be physically able, she may have to return to work, or she may become ill.

I believe that breast-feeding is the best of two choices, but that either choice is acceptable.

## 616 I have heard that breasts do not produce milk for several days after delivery. Is this true?

Yes. Breast milk does not "let down" for several days, but your breasts begin immediately to produce colostrum, a very important fluid for the baby. Some women produce colostrum even weeks before delivery. This is normal.

Because babies are born with excessive fluid in their bodies, just as your body had excessive fluid right up until the time that you delivered, they do not need fluid other than colostrum for the first two or three days. This thin, bluish fluid seems to have important antibodies and helps protect the baby from developing diarrhea and other intestinal illnesses. Although babies probably do not need anything but colostrum at first, most pediatricians will give babies water or formula by bottle until the mother's milk comes in.

**617** **My nipples are inverted—sunken back into the areola. Can I still nurse my baby?**

Yes. When a woman nurses, the nipple merely lies in the baby's mouth. The baby's lips and gums encircle the areola (the dark area that surrounds the nipple) and the sucking is concentrated on this area. It does not really matter, therefore, whether or not your nipple is inverted.

However, some women with inverted nipples or even with flat nipples have trouble nursing because of this. A simple remedy for this that almost always works is to use a breast cup. This is a dome-shaped plastic device with a hole in the middle. It is placed over the nipple, and the brassiere is put on over it. The pressure of the device around the nipple usually makes the nipple protrude. This protrusion makes it easier for the baby to nurse especially during the days soon after delivery when the breasts are engorged and firm. If your breast skin tends to get excessively moist and irritated with this device on, you can cut a hole in a nursing pad, put this around the nipple, and put the breast cup over this. One brand of this device available in our city is Nurse-N-Dri. Similar devices are made by other companies and marketed under other names.

**618** **My breasts are very small. Can I nurse my baby?**

Yes. The old wives' tale that suggests that small breasts cannot produce enough milk is unfounded and absolutely untrue. Women with such breasts have adequate enlarge-

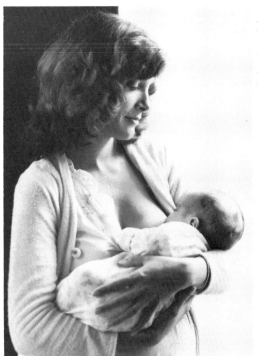

Breast-feeding is the best of two choices but either choice is acceptable.

ment of the gland tissue of their breasts after delivery and can usually provide an ample supply of milk for their babies.

**619** **Will I gain weight while nursing?**

I have found that most of my patients stay a few pounds overweight while they nurse. When they stop nursing, those pounds go away. I encourage my patients not to diet in an attempt to lose weight while nursing, though it is desirable for them to limit sugar, soft drinks, and desserts during and after nursing. A healthy, well-balanced diet is important during both pregnancy and nursing.

**620** **Do I need to eat differently while nursing?**

Certain foods that you eat may cause your baby to be irritable. Many women find that chocolate and some spicy foods will cause their baby to become a little cranky. This seems to be an individual factor. If you notice your baby is consistently irritable after you eat a certain food, common sense tells you to stop eating that food, not only for your baby's comfort but also for your own personal peace.

## 621 Is it normal to have cramping of the uterus during nursing?

Most women have some degree of cramping when they first begin to nurse, and some will continue to have cramping every time they nurse their baby. Most of the time, however, women do not feel cramping after the first few days.

It is normal to have severe cramps with nursing at first. One of the benefits of nursing is that it helps the uterus "contract down" and return to normal size. I encourage my patients who have this type of cramping to take a pain pill thirty minutes before they nurse. The small amount of narcotic that the mother would pass to her baby in her breast milk will not hurt the baby and will help relieve the uterine cramps caused by the nursing. Such cramps are usually worst in women with their second and third children.

## 622 May I take medications and smoke and drink while I am nursing?

Almost everything you eat, drink, or take by mouth or injection will be excreted into your milk to some extent. It makes sense, therefore, that a nursing mother exercise caution in this regard.

A modest amount of alcohol may not affect your baby adversely, other than perhaps to make it a little sleepy, but no one knows for sure. Consistent and more-than-modest alcohol intake is certainly not good for you or your baby.

Aside from the detrimental effects of smoking on you (see Q. 1222, 1223), cigarette smoking is dangerous for your baby and may increase the chance of the child getting cancer later. You might set your bedclothes on fire or ashes from your cigarette might burn your baby. Smoking may also decrease your milk production.

The same cautions about smoking and drinking pertain to drugs. It seems best for a nursing mother not to take any drugs unless necessary and suggested or prescribed by her doctor.

An excellent book on this subject that your doctor may have is *Drugs in Pregnancy and Lactation, A Reference Guide to Fetal and Neonatal Risk* by Griggs, Bodendorfer, Freeman, and Yaffe (Baltimore: Williams & Wilkins Publishing Company). It is the best book I have seen on this topic.

## 623 Should I take vitamins while nursing?

I have all my patients continue taking their prenatal vitamins during lactation. Many doctors feel that the folic acid is important during nursing. The iron in the prenatal vitamins can help the mother and the baby avoid anemia by replacing the iron lost from delivery bleeding, and it insures that the mother has enough iron to pass along to the baby.

## 624 What medical complications can occur during nursing?

In the first few weeks you may develop nipple soreness. This usually occurs because you let the baby use your nipples as a "pacifier" before your nipples become toughened to the infant's sucking.

A baby gets most of the milk from the

breast in four or five minutes. If the baby continues to nurse, that can cause your nipples to become sore. The key, then, is to let the baby nurse just long enough to get the milk, and then for you to use nipple cream (Masse or A&D ointment) to keep the nipples from becoming dry and cracked. Later you will be able to let the baby nurse as long as you want to.

Nursing mothers will sometimes have sore, red places develop on their breasts, and fever often accompanies these infections. The mother can usually continue to breast-feed, but she should call her doctor, who will ordinarily recommend antibiotics. In addition, warm, moist heat will help an area like this to clear up quickly.

The technique for providing heat treatment to infected breasts is to soak a small towel in warm water and place it on the reddened area of the breast. Put plastic wrap over the towel. On top of that place a heating pad or hot-water bottle. Keep this heat on the breast as much of the time as possible. It is common for nursing mothers to have several episodes of these infections during the time they nurse a baby.

## 625 If I nurse my baby, will my breasts become smaller, and will they sag more?

Most women will notice that their breasts are smaller and sag more if they have nursed a baby. This does not always occur, but you should be aware that it can happen and not be disappointed if you find a significant difference in your breasts after you nurse your first baby.

Breasts that have become smaller because of nursing can be augmented later with breast implants if the change is so significant that it becomes a real emotional problem for you. This breast implantation does not affect breast-feeding for a future child.

## 626 I have heard that nursing mothers cannot become pregnant. Is this true?

Absolutely not! It has been shown that it is the baby's hard sucking on the breasts that makes a woman less likely to ovulate and thus unlikely to become pregnant. After nursing for several weeks the baby and breasts usually form a pattern so that the baby does not need to suck as hard to get milk flow established each nursing. The less hard a baby sucks, the more likely you are to begin ovulation.

Since you will not know when ovulation has occurred, you can become pregnant if you have unprotected intercourse. This can happen even though you have not had any menstrual bleeding during the time you are nursing.

Do not use breast-feeding as a contraceptive! Use a barrier method, such as foam, rubbers, or a diaphragm, or have an IUD inserted. Most physicians feel that it is best that a nursing mother not use birth-control pills. No serious side effects have been found in babies whose mothers used birth-control pills while they nursed. Taking birth-control pills may cause a decline in milk production and nutritional value. There are no known side-effects from a progestin-only birth-control pill which can be used while a woman is nursing her baby. The possibility of pregnancy is higher than the rate for the usual birth-control pill.

## 627 After weaning a baby, is it common for the breasts to continue to secrete milk?

It is common for a mother to have milk coming from her nipples for many months (or even years) after she has weaned her baby. As long as the mother's menstrual periods are regular, this is not an indication of a medical problem.

If there continues to be fluid from the nipples after nursing has been stopped and the menstrual periods do not return to normal, a prolactin test (a simple blood test) should be performed. Fluid from the nipples with a failure to have periods may indicate a tumor in the pituitary. The prolactin test can show whether such a tumor is present.

**628** **I have many questions about nursing and my doctor doesn't seem to know the answers. What should I do?**

The LaLeche League has been of inestimable value to mothers who want to nurse; I encourage you to contact them for a copy of their excellent book, *The Womanly Art of Breast-feeding*, rev. ed. 1981 (LaLeche League, Intl., 9616 Minneapolis Ave., Franklin Park, Ill. 60131).

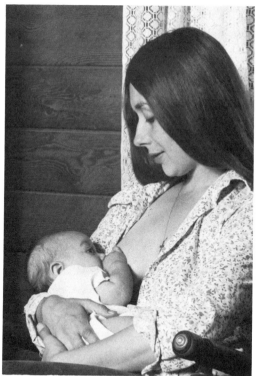

George Zucconi
Berg & Associates

After nursing for several weeks the baby and breasts usually form a pattern so that the baby does not need to suck as hard to get milk flow established each nursing.

## Special Labor-and-Delivery Situations

**629** **What are some of the special problems that need to be considered in relation to labor and delivery?**

Some special situations will be discussed in the next few questions.

Labor induction

Breech deliveries

Multiple-birth deliveries

Premature deliveries

Cesarean sections

*Labor Induction*

**630** **What is your opinion on inducing labor?**

I feel that the induction of labor in a woman who is certain of her due date and is "ripe" for labor is a safe process, and it is not likely to increase the necessity for cesarean section or to endanger the baby. It should not, however, be done flippantly.

Before an induction is done, certain elements must be considered.

*Due Date.* You must be absolutely certain of your due date. If a patient has any question about her due date, and I have not been able to determine a reliable date for her, I

374    Bearing a Child

will not induce her unless there is a medical reason for doing so. If a woman who is unsure of her due date sees her doctor by the twenty-fifth week of her pregnancy, the doctor can do ultrasound measurements of a baby's size and thus determine a reliable due date most of the time. If a woman does not see her doctor before the twenty-fifth week of her pregnancy, the doctor has no reliable way of establishing an accurate due date. For this and other important reasons, it is essential that a woman see a doctor early in her pregnancy.

*"Ripe" cervix.* Even if a woman is at term, she should not be induced unless the cervix is ripe. My own criteria are that a woman must be at least two centimeters dilated, with a cervix that has effaced (see Q. 576) at least 50 percent. The cervix must be soft and the baby's head down against it. The baby's head must be down because, if the doctor breaks the bag of waters and the head is not down against the cervix, the umbilical cord could be washed down through the cervical opening. This would precipitate the need for an immediate cesarean section.

*Medication risks.* The package information that comes with Pitocin, the drug used to induce labor, has a warning that it is not indicated for the induction of labor if there is no medical problem making the induction necessary. The warning states that the dangers of using Pitocin for inducing labor may outweigh the advantages of its use. This is because Pitocin, if improperly used, can cause the uterus to go into spasm. This can kill the baby and cause serious complications for the mother. However, obstetricians have been trained in the proper use of Pitocin and routinely use it for inductions.

To summarize my position, inducing labor should not be done as a matter of course or without due regard to all aspects. It should not be done unless there is a definite due date established, and the cervix should be "ripe" and the baby in proper position. If these criteria are followed, I feel that induction of labor is quite safe—even when there are no medical problems and it is done merely for convenience.

## 631 Is there anything I can do to start my own labor?

Not really. Unless it is time for labor to start anyway, physical activity such as washing walls or riding over railroad tracks, will not induce labor. Taking castor oil or an enema may produce contractions, but those contractions could be either intestinal or uterine. Hospitalization might be necessary to determine which type of contractions you are having.

Obviously, trying to stimulate labor is futile and possibly costly. Such endeavors result in frustration rather than delivery.

### Breech Deliveries

## 632 What about breech deliveries?

Breech babies (babies who come bottom first) occur in only 3–4 percent of all deliveries. Mothers always react with some degree of fear when I discover that their baby is "coming breech." This fear seems to be based on tales they have heard about the dangers and difficulties of breech labor and deliveries. I try to reassure them by telling them that I have never had a single dangerous complication or problem from a breech delivery. However, it is true that a woman who has a breech baby does have a greater chance of ending up with a C-section.

My advice is not to quibble with your doctor if he or she suggests that your breech baby be delivered by cesarean section. Let the C-section be done!

## 633 What is the problem in breech deliveries?

There are two. First, as the baby's bottom passes through the birth canal, the umbilical cord is dragged along behind and can then be pinched by the baby's head as it delivers. It is important, therefore, that once the baby's bottom has been delivered the remainder of its body be delivered quickly so that the umbilical cord is not compressed too long.

Second, the baby's head is larger in diameter than the rest of its body. This is especially true if the baby is premature. The birth canal may not be sufficiently dilated to allow passage of the baby's head without damage.

To avoid such damage, most doctors agree that it is "legitimate" (not mandatory) for a breech baby to be delivered by cesarean section if the following conditions exist (see also Q. 645):

It is a woman's first pregnancy

The baby is very large

The baby is premature

The mother's pelvic bones are small

The mother desires to have a sterilization procedure. Since she is going to have an incision in her abdomen anyway, this incision can be enlarged and accommodate both the delivery and the sterilization.

If your doctor is going to do a vaginal delivery of your breech baby, it is important that your pelvis be X-rayed to be sure that there are no deformities or constrictions of the bones that might cause problems.

## 634 Why not just do a cesarean section for all breeches?

A cesarean section should never be done unless there is a definite reason. There are risks involved in this major surgery. (See Q. 640.)

## 635 Can the baby be turned, either before or during labor, so that it will come head first?

This is an exciting technique because it can help women avoid cesarean sections. It can be tried and is a legitimate procedure. If you have a breech baby and are going to try this, you would be given medication intravenously to make your uterus relax (tocolytic agent). When your uterus is relaxed, the doctor would do an "external cephalic version." This means that with his or her hands on your abdomen, the doctor will try to push the baby around until the head rotates down into the pelvis. This procedure often works, and usually the baby stays down in the head-first position.

Many doctors will not do this procedure. In pushing the baby around, the placenta can come loose from the wall of the uterus—a dangerous thing for the baby. Even if this does not happen, manipulating the baby in this fashion can cause its heartbeat to drop, causing death, although this is extremely rare. These possible complications scare some doctors and some patients out of trying this useful procedure.

To avoid this happening, doctors who do this procedure carefully observe the baby with the ultrasound machine and fetal monitor as they rotate the baby. They do the manipulation very gently, with the woman's abdomen well-coated with oil.

Although your doctor may find your baby to be in the breech position before labor begins, and you are not going to have it rotated, the baby can still switch around on its own and be a head-first baby by the time you go to the hospital. Therefore, it is generally not advisable to have a cesarean section just because the baby is in breech position in your doctor's office. Wait until labor starts. If the baby is still in the breech position then, and the doctor believes that a C-section is the best thing for your baby, go ahead and get it done.

*Multiple-Birth Deliveries*

## 636 Are the deliveries of twins, triplets, and so on, managed in the same way as single babies?

No. Careful consideration must be given to the management of multiple-birth labor. For one thing, one of the two babies in a twin pregnancy will often come as a breech. Statistics show that the first baby is born head first 75 percent of the time, and the second baby is born head first 53 percent of the time.

Whether their delivery should be by normal vaginal delivery or by cesarean section depends on several factors. Since studies of twins born both ways do not show any significant difference in the health of the babies, you and your obstetrician must make the decision based on your individual situation.

Most obstetricians feel that it is usually fine for twin babies to be born vaginally unless they are premature. If your babies are more than four weeks early, it is probably best for them to be delivered by cesarean section. The reason for this is to avoid damaging the babies' heads or having to deliver the second baby by breech in case it got "stuck" in a difficult position after the first baby was born.

If you are in the last month of pregnancy, it is probably best to do the delivery vaginally unless some complication develops during the labor and delivery. It is sometimes necessary for the doctor to deliver one baby through the vagina and then, because of some problem, do a cesarean section for delivery of the second baby.

Some doctors would do cesarean sections on all triplets or more-than-triplet deliveries, and I believe that no obstetrician would argue with this approach. However, the one set of full-term triplets that I have delivered were delivered vaginally without any problem. Studies done of triplet deliveries show that with proper care, this is generally the case.

Mothers with triplets might like to contact Triplet Connection, Janet Bleye, 2618 Lucille Ave., Stockton, Calif. 95209 (209-474-3073). This organization publishes a newsletter and has triplet strollers.

*Premature Deliveries*

## 637 Are premature deliveries handled differently from normal deliveries?

Because a premature baby is more fragile than a full-term baby, it is normally delivered with great gentleness and extra care. Special consideration is given to such matters as making the episiotomy generously large in order to give the baby's head plenty of room, limiting the amount of pain medication the mother gets (to avoid depressing the baby), avoiding inductions unless necessary, and doing C-sections more freely (to provide a gentle delivery).

Although one would think that an episiotomy to deliver a premature baby would be unnecessary or quite small, most obstetricians do a liberal episiotomy so that as the baby comes through the birth canal it is not unduly pressed, or hurt, by the mother's pelvic muscles.

As for the pain medication for the mother during labor, the use of Demerol is extremely limited. I prefer not to use it at all during premature labor, as premature babies are more susceptible to the effects of drugs, which can cause the low Apgar score at birth. In the case of a premature delivery it is probably best that a mother use an epidural for her labor unless she has a medical problem that makes that unwise (for example, high blood pressure or uterine bleeding).

If there is a medical problem that has made it necessary for you to be delivered before full term, the doctor will most likely do a cesarean section rather than an induction before the cervix is ready, because an early induction can be dangerous for the baby. If you are not at the end of your full nine months, it is best that your baby be delivered by cesarean section.

A premature breech baby should be delivered by cesarean section because of its small body and proportionally large head, which can cause the head to become trapped after the delivery of the body.

---

**638** **How dangerous is it for a baby to be born prematurely?**

A baby born before the twenty-fifth week has only a slight chance of survival. From twenty-five to twenty-eight weeks there is an increasing chance of its living. Babies born at or after twenty-eight weeks of pregnancy will usually survive. However, they may have a difficult time for several weeks.

At least two things have improved the chances of healthy survival for a premature baby. The first is a revolution in intensive-care nurseries. In recent years technology in these nurseries has improved dramatically.

A second development has been the use of a cortisonelike drug given to the mother if she is expected to have a premature baby. If the mother is given a drug such as betamethazone before delivery, and delivery can be delayed for twenty-four hours, some premature baby's lungs will be more mature and better able to maintain life. Many obstetricians routinely use these drugs now if a mother is going to have a baby when she is less than thirty-four weeks along. Occasionally they are used when the mother is from thirty-four to thirty-six weeks along, but this may not be of any advantage for the baby. There is some evidence that these drugs are not helpful if a woman is carrying more than one baby.

If you have a "premie," these books may

help you: *Your Premature Baby—The Complete Guide to Premie Care During that First Crucial Year* by Henig and Fletcher (New York: Ballantine Books), 1983; *Premature Babies—A Handbook for Parents* by Nancy (New York: Berkley) 1982.

*Cesarean Sections*

---

**639** **Why are cesarean sections necessary?**

Cesarean sections can prevent some ghastly ordeals for the pregnant mother and her baby. They have become such a standard part of obstetric care that we tend to forget what labor and delivery were like when cesarean sections were not available. In those days, a mother having an obstructed labor, because the baby was too large to get out or the mother's bones were too small to deliver, could continue in labor for days. The baby would die because of the development of spastic uterine contractions and infection. Then the mother would die because of infection, a ruptured uterus, or blood loss.

When forceps came into use, they were used to deliver a baby that could not be born otherwise, but their use in that situation was a major undertaking and was delayed until the mother had been in labor for many, many hours. The forceps would often kill or maim the baby and could tear the mother's body, causing infection and bleeding.

A baby too weak to tolerate labor can be delivered safely by cesarean section. If the placenta comes loose, a baby can be delivered before it detaches completely, thus saving the baby. Likewise, if the placenta obstructs the uterine outlet, a C-section preserves the lives of both the mother and the child.

Cesarean sections are generally a very good thing, and both doctors and patients can be thankful that this operation is available. They have contributed more to health of babies and mothers than anything else in obstetrics. Because of this operation, we rarely find mother and baby in side-by-side graves in modern cemeteries, as we so commonly do in older cemeteries.

## 640 If cesarean sections are so beneficial, why are they not used routinely?

Although there is not a great deal of risk to cesarean sections, there is always some potential danger in any surgery. Various studies indicate that a mother's chance of dying is ten, twenty-five, or even a hundred times greater if she has a cesarean section rather than a vaginal delivery. Infections are also more likely with a cesarean section. These include infections of the wound in the uterus, the abdomen, or the urinary tract. The chance of such infections varies from as low as 12 percent to as high as 50 percent, the higher numbers usually occurring in indigent populations in large, public hospitals.

Because of these findings, it is important that neither the doctor nor the mother feel that a cesarean section is an option to be taken lightly. The doctor must not use it as an easy out from working with the patient in labor toward a vaginal delivery—and the patient must not feel that a cesarean section is a simple way to avoid painful labor or some other aspect of delivery she finds distasteful.

## 641 It seems to me that a great many cesarean sections are being done. Why is this?

It is true that some doctors are doing too many cesarean sections these days. The national average is about 18 percent of deliveries, but some physicians have cesarean rates as high as 50 percent.

It seems irrational that a God-designed mechanism for reproduction (pregnancy, labor, and delivery) should require cesarean sections half of the time. Indeed, most physicians who have studied this problem feel that a cesarean rate of more than 30 percent represents physician care that is not as good as it should be.

Most physicians do not know exactly what their cesarean section rate is, and many may not realize it is as high as it is. The one group of hospital personnel who does have an idea of which doctors do "too many" cesarean sections are the labor-and-delivery nurses. If your doctor's other patients seem frequently to end up having cesarean sections, perhaps you could phone the maternity department of your hospital, try to speak to one of the labor-and-delivery nurses, and ask if your doctor is one who does not do too many cesarean sections. I'm not sure you would get an answer to your question, but if you did it would be some guide to the reputation of your own personal physician.

I believe that some ingenuity in your selection and evaluation of a physician is a much wiser approach than to assume that all physicians are good or, conversely, that all are bad.

## 642 For what reasons are cesarean sections necessary?

There are many reasons, some of the most common ones will be discussed in the next few questions. These include:

failure to progress in labor

fetal distress

breech babies

prolapse of the umbilical cord

placental problems

problems of the mother

repeat cesareans

## 643 What causes labor to "fail to progress"?

There are two primary reasons for a failure to progress in labor, and they are the most common indications for a cesarean section to be done on a mother who has not had a previous C-section (primary cesarean section).

***Cephalopelvic disproportion (CPD).*** Some babies are too large to get through their mother's birth canal, and some women have pelvic bones too small to allow even a normal-sized baby through. Normally, if a woman has dilated to four centimeters in her labor and does not progress further (at the rate of about one centimeter of dilation per hour), she probably has cephalopelvic disproportion. If, after she is four centimeters dilated, she labors two hours and dilates only one more centimeter, she may have a problem of CPD. And if she dilates completely, spends from two to four hours pushing, and still the baby's head does not come down far enough for delivery, she may have CPD.

A woman who is completely dilated may get the baby's head down far enough for a forceps delivery. However, since "aggressive" forceps deliveries are not done anymore, if there is any question about the baby's inability to get through the birth canal, a cesarean section is preferable. (For an in-depth study on mid-forceps or low-forceps deliveries, see *Williams Obstetrics* by Pritchard and MacDonald, published by Appleton-Century-Crofts.)

Another cause of CPD can be the position of the baby's head. If the baby's head is coming into the birth canal "cockeyed," for instance, with the brow or chin coming first, a cesarean section may be necessary. This particular situation depends on which part of the baby's head is coming first.

***Ineffective contractions (uterine inertia).*** Although the uterus is a big muscle whose contractions push the baby out, there are times when it does not contract effectively. Some women begin labor with ineffective contractions (primary inertia); other women will begin labor with good contractions, only to have the uterus stop contracting effectively at a later point (secondary inertia). If the baby's position seems to be affecting the ability of the uterus to contract well, a cesarean section may be necessary. From 2–4 percent of mothers in labor will need a cesarean section for this reason. Normally, however, the baby's position is not a problem and a poorly contracting uterus can be stimulated to contract effectively by the use of Pitocin. Many C-sections have been prevented by the use of Pitocin for this purpose.

As a matter of fact, Pitocin is one of the most useful drugs a woman in labor has available. Pitocin is like the hormone produced by a woman's own body that makes the uterus contract. It is given through the veins in gradually increasing amounts, causing the uterus to contract longer and longer, and more and more often, until the contractions are occurring about every three minutes and lasting about sixty seconds, thus duplicating normal labor. When the uterus is made to contract effectively in this manner, labor will often progress as it is supposed to, concluding with a normal, healthy vaginal delivery. (See Q. 586.)

Note that doctors do not use Pitocin to cause stronger-than-normal contractions. When Pitocin is used, it is used to duplicate normal labor. Pitocin-stimulated contractions are no more painful than "normal" contractions.

Pitocin is a safe drug if it is used properly. If a woman's uterus contracts too hard, the IV (intravenous solution) that has the Pitocin in it can be stopped. The Pitocin in the blood stream is dissipated in just a few seconds and will not cause any more contractions. For labor and delivery Pitocin must always be given in an IV. After delivery a woman may be given it in the form of an injection.

**644** **When is a C-section necessary for fetal distress?**

Two important procedures help a doctor determine when a baby is in trouble during labor; monitoring the heartbeat and fetal scalp-blood-sampling. Both of these techniques help the doctor know when a C-section is called for.

A cesarean section because of fetal distress can help alleviate one of the most tragic problems that can face a mother and father: the death during labor of a baby that seemed to develop normally during pregnancy. (From 1.5 to 3 percent of mothers in labor will need cesarean sections for this indication.)

Continuous monitoring of the baby's heartbeat has increased the cesarean-section rate, but it has also decreased the number of babies that are born dead or terribly depressed (low Apgar score) because of some problem during labor.

Certain fetal heart-rate patterns indicate reliably that the baby is distressed and could die from continued labor. For these problems an emergency cesarean section is absolutely indicated. If you have a continuous fetal monitor during labor and your doctor and nurses see such a pattern developing, they would let you know right away.

One technique that is becoming more and more useful is fetal scalp blood sampling during labor. This is a technique in which the doctor pricks the baby's scalp with a small, sharp-pointed blade (just as your finger is pricked to check your blood count), collects a little bit of its blood from the scalp, and evaluates the pH of the baby's blood. If it is becoming too acid, it may indicate that the baby is in real danger and confirm the need for a C-section.

Your bag of waters must be broken and you must be adequately dilated before this procedure can be done. Also, the doctor must be able to see the baby's scalp with a speculum.

Fetal scalp testing will become especially useful when a technique is devised for continually watching the baby's blood pH instead of having to prick the baby's scalp every time a pH level is desired.

---

**645** **Why are cesarean sections needed for breech births?**

Studies of breech babies (or shoulder or other abnormal presentations) show that these babies have a greater chance of not delivering vaginally at all or of having more damage from delivery than babies born head first. Because of this, doctors are doing cesarean sections for many breech babies. Cesarean sections done for this problem involve from 1.5–3.5 percent of pregnant mothers. (See Q. 632–635.)

Many doctors feel it is best to deliver all women having their first babies as a breech by cesarean section, and most doctors also feel it is best to do a C-section if the baby's feet are coming first. This is in contrast to the baby's bottom settling down with the legs folded up against its chest. When a baby's bottom settles down into the birth canal, it keeps the umbilical cord from slithering down into the vagina when the bag of waters breaks; when the feet are coming first there is no "plug" to keep the umbilical cord from falling down into the vagina.

If labor has not started and the baby's shoulder is coming first, or there is some other unusual position of the baby, this may possibly be corrected by relaxing the mother's uterus with a uterine relaxative and then turning the baby. If, however, a woman goes into labor with the baby crossways in the uterus or the baby's arm comes through the cervical opening, an immediate cesarean section must be done. Labor with a baby in this position can cause twisting of the baby's body in such a way that the baby can soon die.

**646** **What causes prolapse of the umbilical cord? Why is a C-section necessary in this situation?**

If the baby's umbilical cord happens to slip by the baby's head (or its bottom, in the case of a breech position), an immediate cesarean section must be done. Labor in this situation is dangerous. It would push the baby's head or bottom against the umbilical cord, pinch off the flow of blood from the mother to the baby and kill the baby before delivery could be accomplished.

**647** **What problems of the placenta can necessitate a C-section?**

There are two.

*Abruptio placenta.* In this condition the placenta pulls loose, either partially or completely, from the wall of the uterus. If it pulls completely loose, the baby dies immediately. This can happen without any labor at all. In this situation a cesarean section to save the mother's life must be done immediately. A woman can lose a great deal of blood when the placenta pulls loose. Or a condition called DIC (disseminated intravascular coagulopathy) can develop. DIC has various causes (trauma, infection, serious medical problems), but the exact factor that triggers the condition has not been identified. When DIC occurs, the components that cause coagulation of the blood begin frenzied activity somewhat similar to spontaneous combustion. There is rapid clotting inside the blood vessels which continues until all the available blood-clotting components in the blood system are used. There are approximately 100,000 miles of blood vessels in the average adult human body so the blood clots that do form cause very little impact on that system. The problem that results from this clotting is that the blood loses all of its coagulation ability. A woman so affected becomes like a hemophiliac,

bleeding from every cut or raw surface on or in her body. This condition in its most severe form can be dangerous and even fatal.

If the placenta pulls only partially loose, an immediate C-section can be done and the baby can usually be saved.

An abruption is suspected when the uterus becomes irritable and begins frequent contractions, or when it becomes very hard and does not relax. This hardness is caused by a continuous tonic contraction with no relaxation of the uterus, a result of the irritating bleeding that is occurring between the uterus and the placenta.

*Placenta previa.* When a woman has this condition, it becomes evident that the placenta has been growing all through pregnancy in the wrong position: over the opening of the uterus through which the baby must be delivered. If the baby were delivered through the placenta, its source of oxygen supply from the mother is ruined, the torn placenta would gush blood and the baby would die during delivery.

When only a small portion of the placenta is low and the rest of it is higher up in the uterus, a vaginal delivery can occasionally be done. Usually with a definite placenta previa, a cesarean section must be done as soon as labor starts or whenever significant bleeding has occurred. (See Q. 587.)

**648** **What problems might the mother have that would make a cesarean section necessary?**

Problems the mother might have can be separated into three groups. Many conditions of this type were discussed in the chapter on pregnancy, and most of these problems are not commonly found to be causes of C-sections.

*Problems of the mother that could cause the baby to die before birth if delivery is not accomplished.* A good example of this is diabetes. Review the discussion of diabetes in

Q. 380–389. You will recall that when a mother is diabetic and pregnant, her baby can seem healthy one day and be dead inside her uterus the next. A well-timed C-section can usually prevent this. Another example of this type of situation is a pregnant woman who is in a coma from a stroke or accident.

*Problems of the mother that could cause her to die if the baby is not delivered.* One example of this would be an expectant mother who is critically ill with heart disease. Another would be a woman with cervical cancer that was found during the pregnancy.

*Problems of the mother that could cause the death of both mother and child.* Eclampsia is a classic example of this situation. Review the discussion of toxemia in the chapter on pregnancy, especially Q. 412–414.

**649** **If a woman has a C-section, do all future pregnancies have to be delivered this way?**

Many obstetricians feel that the standard dictum, "Once a cesarean section, always a cesarean section," still holds. More cesareans are done for that reason than for any other. This feeling is because, years ago, cesarean sections were done by making vertical incisions in the uterus, thereby cutting through the uterus in its thickest part. When healing occurred, it left a thin scar where there should have been strong, thick muscle tissue. When the patient became pregnant again and was allowed to labor, instead of the presence of strong muscle in the upper part of the uterus, there was strong muscle—but with a weak place in it. Occasionally this weak place ruptured. When that occurred, 50 percent of the babies and 5 percent of the mothers involved in this crisis situation died.

Most C-sections done in the past thirty years were done with a horizontal (trans-verse) incision low in the uterus. Recent studies have shown that there is very little chance of a uterus rupturing if a woman's previous cesarean was done this way. This portion of the uterus provides very little of its contracting power; it is a more passive area that thins out gradually during labor. Because of this passive nature it is much less likely to rupture during labor.

If a patient who has had a previous cesarean section does not go through labor, but simply has a repeat C-section, any risk of the uterus rupturing through the previous scar is eliminated. However, to avoid any possibility of uterine rupture, many doctors will still recommend a C-section for subsequent deliveries after an initial C-section.

**650** **I had a C-section for my last delivery. Is it risky for me to try to have a vaginal delivery with my next pregnancy?**

Recent studies have conclusively shown that it is safe for most women who have had a cesarean section (especially a low transverse C-section) to try to have their next child by going through labor and having a vaginal delivery. Not only is it safe to try this procedure, but from 50–80 percent of those women who try, are able to deliver vaginally. The National Institute of Child Health and Human Development Conference on Childbirth in *Cesarean Childbirth* (NIH publication #82–2067, 1981, U.S. Government Printing Office, Washington, D.C., pp. 351–374), reported on a 1980 study which indicated that having a vaginal delivery when a previous child had been delivered by cesarean section was a reasonable procedure for a woman to try.

In Western Europe women for years have been having vaginal deliveries after previously having a cesarean section. The safety of this procedure has, therefore, al-

# Cesarean Skin and Uterus Incisions

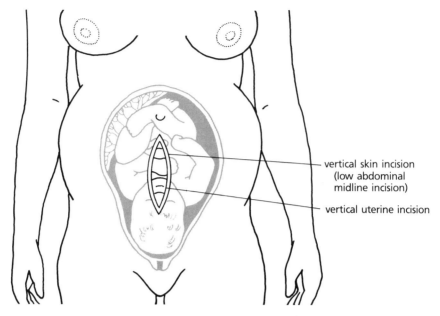

vertical skin incision (low abdominal midline incision)

vertical uterine incision

The skin incision does not have a bearing on whether or not a woman may labor with her next pregnancy; either uterine incision can be used, regardless which skin incision is used.

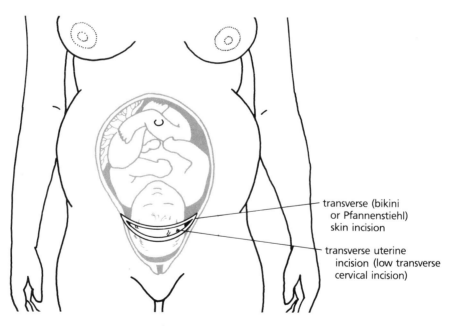

transverse (bikini or Pfannenstiehl) skin incision

transverse uterine incision (low transverse cervical incision)

If a woman has had this uterine incision she may be a candidate for labor with her next pregnancy.

ready been proven in these countries. It is not a new, untried procedure.

The advantages of having a vaginal delivery are numerous. There is no greater risk for the mother than having another cesarean section. There is no greater risk for the child who is delivered in this way instead of being delivered by cesarean section. Studies have conclusively proven the safety for both mother and child. It is possible for the mother's uterus to rupture when she is going through labor. Such a rupture can occur through the scar of the previous cesarean section. This is a rare event and is only minimally dangerous to either the mother or the child because of modern medical care.

Not all women should try to have a vaginal delivery after a previous cesarean section. Those who have had two or more cesarean sections should probably not try a vaginal delivery. Not enough women have done this to know whether or not it is safe. Women who have had a cesarean section and with the present pregnancy have a breech presentation should probably have another cesarean section. Not enough women have had vaginal deliveries of a breech after having previously had a cesarean section to know whether or not it is a safe procedure.

These guidelines were established in 1985 by the American College of Obstetricians and Gynecologists for attempting vaginal delivery after a previous cesarean section:

1. The woman and her physician should discuss fully, early in the prenatal course, the option of a trial of labor. This would allow for discussion throughout the pregnancy to make certain the patient is aware of the benefits and potential risks.

2. Absolute cephalopelvic disproportion *(a woman's pelvis being too small for the baby's head to come through)*, although rare, remains a contraindication to a trial of labor. However, studies show that subsequent trials of labor are successful in up to 70 percent of patients in whom the

indication for cesarean delivery was "failure to progress in labor."

3. A previous classical uterine incision remains a contraindication to labor. *A classical incision is a vertical incision in the uterus instead of across the uterus at its lower portion.*

4. There should be only one fetus and the estimated fetal weight should be less than 4000 g.: *8 pounds, 14 ounces.*

5. There should be continuous electronic fetal heart rate and uterine activity monitoring throughout labor, as well as staff and facilities required to respond to acute obstetric emergencies. (words in italics added by JSM)

Studies have shown that it is safe to use Pitocin carefully to stimulate labor if a woman is attempting to have a labor and delivery after a previous cesarean section.

Epidural anesthesia is safe for pain relief during such a labor. If a woman is in labor after having had a previous cesarean section, she should be in a hospital that has the capability of doing a cesarean section within thirty minutes from the time the decision is made to go ahead with the procedure. The physician should be one who is capable of evaluating her need for a cesarean section and for doing the surgery expeditiously when it is necessary.

No woman should be forced to go through labor and vaginal delivery after having had a previous cesarean section if she does not want to. I have found that many of my patients prefer having another cesarean section rather than trying to go through labor. I honor their requests and feel that it is a reasonable thing to do.

Avoiding the cesarean section will be successful for most women, will eliminate major surgery and post-op complications, and will shorten a hospital stay.

Subsequent vaginal delivery for previous C-section patients marks a major and dramatic change in the method of care for patients all over the United States. Many patients and doctors are still uncomfortable with the idea, but I feel that this procedure will become standard practice.

### 651 What does recovery from a cesarean section involve?

Recovery following a C-section takes about a week longer than it does after a vaginal birth. Patients are about a week slower in resuming normal activities at home and in "feeling good" again.

After a cesarean section is performed, the mother will go to the recovery room for a one- or two-hour stay. She is then taken to her room, where she is carefully watched. Fluids will probably be given intravenously for a day or two, and she will probably have a catheter in place for a day. A catheter is simply a hollow rubber tube that is usually inserted into the bladder just before a cesarean section is done. Urine drains through this catheter into a bag that is tied to the side of the bed. This is used for two reasons. First, with a C-section the obstetrician is cutting so near the bladder that it must be empty so the doctor can see where to cut and does not cut the bladder itself. Second, immediately after surgery a woman is often in too much discomfort to empty her bladder properly.

After a C-section the woman's diet will progress from a few sips of water to clear liquids, and then, by a gradually increasing schedule, to regular food over a period of about three days.

Most women can go home by the fourth or fifth day after the surgery.

A cesarean section does not interfere with nursing, but a woman will not want to be alone in the hospital room with her baby as long as she is taking strong pain medication. Pain medicine following a C-section is normally given by injection every three or four hours. I strongly encourage my patients to ask for pain medicine any time they hurt. As soon as a patient begins eagerly eating a liq-uid diet, she can usually start taking a pain pill. By this time a pain pill will usually be adequate to relieve pain.

When the patient goes home, I think it is best for her not to cook or keep house for two weeks, and I give the same recommendation to patients who have had normal vaginal deliveries. Though a woman may not feel quite as well as if she had delivered vaginally, at the end of three weeks from the day of surgery she will usually feel fairly normal and be ready to resume most normal activity.

Doctors generally allow patients to have intercourse about three weeks from the day of delivery, whether the baby was born vaginally or by cesarean section.

### 652 What if my C-section incision comes open?

Infections in the wound can occur, causing it to come open. Normally this opening is only in the skin itself. The strong sutures that hold the fascia (material surrounding your abdominal cavity that holds everything inside) are generally unaffected by such superficial openings in the wound. If the fascia does break loose, it must be sewn back together, requiring general anesthesia again.

Patients who have been in labor and had their bag of waters rupture always have some germs up inside the uterus. With a cesarean section, these germs can implant on the walls of the wound, start growing, and cause the wound to become infected and then to break open. If your wound comes apart superficially, it is inconvenient but not dangerous. It will, of course, leave your scar more irregular and "uglier" than if it had not come open. After about a year, healing is normally so good that there is not much difference in the scar's appearance.

### 653 Is a hysterectomy ever done following either a cesarean or vaginal delivery?

A hysterectomy may be necessary after delivery if a mother has bleeding that will not respond to any other procedure, such as receiving Pitocin through her veins or having her uterus packed with gauze.

Hysterectomy after delivery may also be necessary if there are tears in large blood vessels in the uterus, or if the placenta has so imbedded itself in the wall of the uterus that it cannot be removed.

Occasionally hysterectomies are done at the time of a cesarean section if the mother has developed precancerous cells on the cervix or wants to be sterilized and has something else wrong with her uterus.

Although the woman will be sterile after such surgery, the ovaries are normally left in so that she will not go through menopause nor have to take hormones.

A hysterectomy done immediately after delivery involves the loss of a moderately large amount of blood and will frequently require transfusions. Additional problems can occur if either the bladder or the ureters (the tubes that lead from the kidneys down to the bladder) are damaged at the time of a cesarean-hysterectomy, and such damage is much more likely to occur than after either a C-section or hysterectomy done separately.

Recovery after a hysterectomy done in this fashion is similar to the recovery after any hysterectomy or a normal cesarean section.

A cesarean-hysterectomy is major surgery and should not be undertaken lightly by a patient or her doctor.

## An Afterword

Having a baby is one of life's most interesting, exciting, and mysterious events. For nine months your body has been building toward the climactic event of delivering its precious burden. During all this time, changes have taken place in your body and in your baby's body, and while the most visible changes took place in your body before birth, your baby will steal the stage from now on with an amazing display of constant change and growth.

Your mind is now clear of some questions: Will the baby be all right? What will we name the baby? Should I have natural childbirth? Now it is cluttered with new ones: Cloth or disposable diapers? Breast or bottle? Why is the baby crying? Why am I sad? You long for form-fitting clothes. You can't wait to put on makeup and wash your hair. You wonder how soon you can play tennis!

Caring for your new child will be a series of constant contradictions—thrilling and trying, sweet and sad, fulfilling and empty-

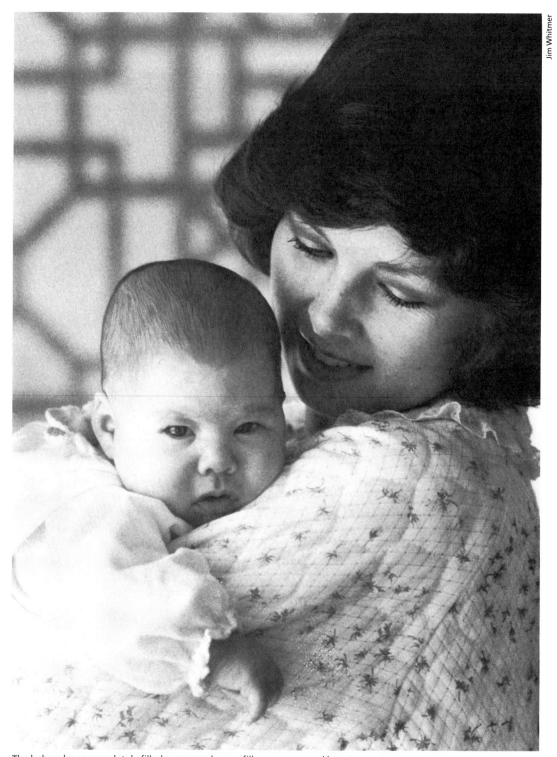

The baby who so completely filled your womb now fills your arms and heart.

Jim Whitmer

ing—yet you know that rearing this child from infancy to adulthood will be the most satisfying, rewarding, and challenging task of your life.

Pregnancy, labor, and delivery are in the past. The result is a truly miraculous "harvest."

Now the *real* labor begins!

# Part Three

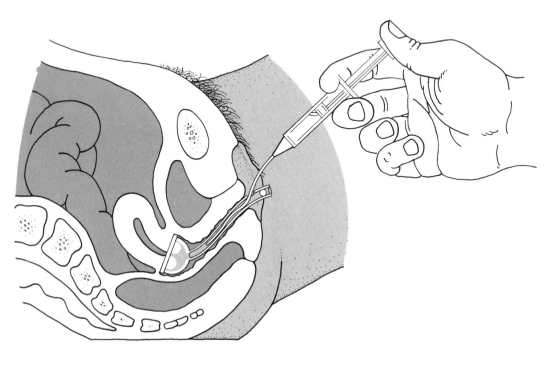

# Special Concerns

# 10

# Disorders of Sexual
# and Reproductive Organs

The female organs, like the women who have them, are a study in contrast. On the one hand these organs are intricate, sensitive, and delicate; on the other they are functional, sturdy, and hardworking. Remarkably, they are usually normal, performing efficiently and capably their extremely vital roles.

Sometimes things go wrong, resulting in a variety of problems for the female. Disorders of the female organs—vulva, vagina, cervix, uterus, fallopian tubes, ovaries, and breasts—are discussed in this chapter.

As background information, a review of chapter 1, "Basic Anatomical Facts," will be helpful. That chapter included a description of how the various female organs were formed during uterine life, the anatomy of these structures, and a broad overview of how they change from birth through the postmenopause period.

Chapters 2, 3, 4, and 5 continued a survey of the anatomical and functional changes of the female body, highlighting in turn four somewhat arbitrarily chosen age groups: childhood, adolescence, the reproductive years, and middle age and beyond. Although none of the health concerns discussed in those chapters can be isolated and specifically assigned to one particular age, many seemed to fall most easily into one chronological period.

In this chapter the emphasis will be on the disorders themselves as they relate to specific areas of the female body. Cross-referencing to other chapters should help you correlate the material to the developmental process; to pertinent segments in Part Two, which deal with conception, pregnancy, and delivery of a baby; and to the remaining chapters in Part Three which focus on infertility, birth control, sexually transmitted disease, and marital/sexual relationships. Consult the glossary and the index if you wish additional information and clarification.

## Problems of the Vulva

A woman's vulva—a term referring to the external part of the female genital organs—is an extremely important area of her body. It serves as guardian of the much more sensitive areas of her female organs, provides an outlet for the urine and stool, and is a source of a great deal of pleasure during sexual intercourse. In fact, the clitoris is the only organ of either male or female that is provided for no other purpose than sexual stimulation. Because of its location and functions, the vulva is subject to certain medical problems.

### 654 Does my vulva need any special daily care?

If you are having no problems with vulvar irritation or vaginal infection, you can continue the basic hygienic measures that you are now using. If you are not having any problems, you are probably employing a very good program of care. However, if you have episodes of vulvar irritation or infection, it will be helpful to consider the following recommendations:

*Bathe daily with a mild soap.* Some soaps marketed today are very strong and may contain perfumes and other chemicals that can cause irritation. Don't use these; choose a milder nondetergent, soap.

*Cleanse the vulva frequently if there is vaginal discharge.* At ovulation time and just before a period there may be increased vaginal secretions. During menstruation, blood that is not washed away may cause irritation. Merely cleansing the vulva with a moist washcloth as often as necessary during the day is usually adequate.

*Use tampons instead of pads.* Tampons absorb menstrual flow internally and do not hold moisture against the vulva as sanitary napkins do. If you do use pads, change as frequently as necessary to avoid the irrita-

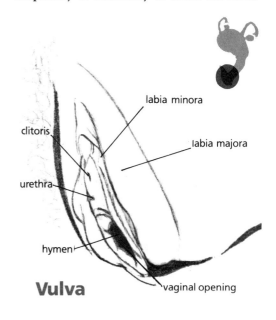

clitoris

urethra

hymen

labia minora

labia majora

vaginal opening

**Vulva**

tion a moist pad can cause. Absolutely do not use tampons or pads that have any deodorant or perfume, as these chemicals can be extremely irritating. (See Q. 118, 714, 717.)

*Wear cotton underpants.* If you do not have vulvar irritation, there is no need to change your clothing habits. If you do, however, cotton underpants are a big help. They absorb secretions and allow air flow, thus reducing moisture in the vulvar area.

*Don't wear panty hose or panty girdles.* Panty hose and panty girdles hold moisture against your vulva, greatly increasing the possibility of vulvar irritation, especially if you already have an infection. Panty hose with a cotton crotch are better, but these are not entirely satisfactory because they still inhibit good air circulation in the area. Women who feel that they cannot do without panty hose may have to pay the price by suffering the irritation that often accompanies the use of such clothing.

*Use no drugs, medications, or feminine-hygiene sprays on the vulva.* Unless your physician prescribes these things for a specific problem, do not use them. You can become sensitive to various drugs, chemicals, and medications; the best practice is not to use any of them except for a specific problem.

*Practice good toilet habits.* When you cleanse yourself after urinating or having a bowel movement, wipe from front to back. This avoids contamination of the vulvar area by urine or feces.

*Choose toilet tissue carefully.* Use tissue that does not contain deodorants or coloring. The chemicals in the dyes and deodorants can be quite irritating to your vulva.

*Wash your underwear with mild soap.* Avoid using detergents for your underwear. Detergents are likely to be more irritating than soap.

If you have an infection, these measures will not cure it but they will keep irritation

## Female External Genitalia

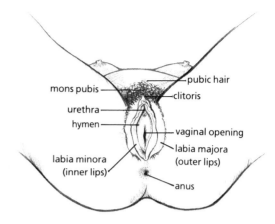

or infection from being quite so severe and will encourage faster healing when you do start specific treatment.

---

**655** **For what reasons should I see a doctor about a vulvar problem?**

I encourage you to have an annual physical examination or, at the least, an exam every eighteen months. In addition to a routine Pap smear, the doctor can also check your vulvar area for any growths or tumors that may have developed since your last visit. The doctor can record any changes and, by seeing you on a regular basis, he or she can more easily detect any change that might be important. Other than the routine physical, the following problems should prompt a visit to the doctor's office.

***Discharge.*** If you have secretions that cause you to wear a pad all the time, or if your secretions have an odor or cause itching, you should see your doctor. He or she can probably prescribe something that will clear up this problem. Some women, however, have enough normal discharge to require the constant use of small pads for protection. These women have no infection present, and there is no way and no reason to rid a woman of such discharge. Increased secretions at the time of ovulation, just before a period, and during pregnancy are normal. If you have discharge other than this, it may or may not be normal.

*Itching.* If you have vulvar itching, see your doctor so that he or she can determine the cause of the problem and treat you for it. If there is a spot on your vulva that itches "out of the ordinary," and there is no sign of infection, there may be a precancerous growth starting in that area. Such a precancerous growth can cause itching before it is visible. If you have itching that is persistent, continue to go back to your doctor until it is determined exactly why you have that uncomfortable spot of skin on your vulva. (See Q. 662.)

*Nodules or growths on your vulva.* Bumps in the tissues of the vulva are not usually malignant, but they can be. If you have a knot or a growth on your vulva, be sure to see your physician about it as soon as possible. (See Q. 669, 670.)

*Trauma.* See your physician if you have damaged your vulva in some way, unless you know for sure that it is no more than a mere bruise or slight tear.

*Other problems.* Other problems can develop in the vulvar area, such as pain, tightness or dryness with intercourse, and varicose veins. If you have any question about this area of your body, see your doctor. If the doctor is not sure what is going on or is not successful with his or her treatment, or if you have a spot that continues to itch, you may need to see a gynecologist for consultation. (See Q. 663, 664.)

---

**656** **Why does my doctor examine my *vagina* when I have a vulvar irritation?**

Infections of the vulva and vagina are so often connected that an infection of one usually indicates an infection of the other.

Most of the time, for instance, a vulvar irritation is caused by a vaginal infection. (See Q. 688–698.)

Vulvar problems caused by sexually transmitted diseases are discussed in chapter 13.

---

**657** **What might cause a lump or bump on my vulvar area?**

A lump or bump is the second most common vulvar problem that prompts women to see their doctor. The most common is irritation. A patient usually thinks of cancer when she discovers such a lump. Usually, however, the growth is not malignant. It can be one of a number of things, including epidermal inclusion cysts, venereal warts, or molluscum contagiosum. These and other vulvar growths are discussed in the next question.

---

**658** **What are epidermal inclusion cysts?**

These cysts prove to be the most common cause of a vulvar bump. They are rarely larger than a small pea and are located on the outer side of the labia majora.

The cause of epidermal inclusion cysts is undetermined, but it is most likely that some of the ducts in the skin become stopped up because of irritation or infection. When the duct is obstructed, a cheesy or gritty material builds up behind the blockage.

No treatment is necessary unless a patient wants it removed, it becomes infected, or it gets particularly big (three-fourths of an inch across). A doctor can use local anesthesia, slit the cyst open, and squeeze out the material.

## 659  What are venereal warts?

Venereal warts, or condyloma acuminata, can occur anywhere on the vulvar area, including the anus. These warts look like ordinary warts and can grow to a very large size. Some of my patients have had them as big as my fist.

Condyloma are generally a venereal disease caused by a virus passed by sexual intercourse. Occasionally however, they may not be passed this way, which is the reason they are mentioned here and not only in the chapter on sexually transmitted disease. A doctor can usually tell by looking that a condyloma is a condyloma. If there is any question, the doctor may want to biopsy the wart (take a small piece of it) and send it to a pathologist for confirmation. The doctor will probably put podophyllum on the wart. (See Q. 1142.) After a few applications, with a week between each treatment, these warts will usually go away.

Occasionally the warts will persist. The best treatment available for these persistent warts is the laser, which evaporates them. Repeat laser treatments may be necessary, but most of the time the warts can be cleared up much quicker this way than with anything else, even podophyllum. The disadvantage of laser treatment is that it is more expensive.

Venereal warts must not be treated with podophyllum during pregnancy, since the absorption of this drug during pregnancy has been associated with problems for the babies. (See Q. 1138–1145.)

## 660  What is molluscum contagiosum?

Molluscum contagiosum is an infection which causes dome-shaped bumps to grow on the inside of the thighs and on the vulva. These bumps are small, the largest ones are rarely more than an eighth of an inch across. They contain a pearly white core and do not hurt, although occasionally one of these bumps may become irritated and tender.

Molluscum contagiosum is caused by a virus that is spread primarily by sexual contact. Treatment is simple: scraping the core out of each bump stops its growth. If all are removed, these little growths normally do not come back. As this area is a little sensitive and difficult to reach, you will probably need to let your doctor scrape away the growths. This is not a dangerous problem and these growths do not become malignant or cause other problems.

## 661  Are there other nonmalignant growths and cysts of the vulva?

There are a large number of different types of growths and cysts of the vulva. It is important to realize that the doctor may not know and does not need to know exactly which one of these you have—he or she primarily wants to make sure you are comfortable and that you do not have cancer.

The usual medical approach is to inject a local anesthetic and cut out the growth or snip it off. The doctor will send the specimen to the lab so that a pathologist can check for cancer. If you have several of the same type of growths, the doctor may not feel it is necessary to take them all off if they are not bothering you too much. Some of these growths may be so large, so extensive, or so numerous, however, that your doctor may recommend hospitalization to have them removed, after a diagnosis has been made as to what they are.

Some of these growths may hang from your body on a thin, narrow stalk. Their removal is simple and can be done in the office. The doctor will merely inject some Xylocaine (a deadening agent) into the base of the growth, tie a suture around it, and cut it off.

A woman in her late teens came to see me once because of a five-inch long growth of tissue hanging from her vulva. At its tip, the growth was about three inches across. The woman had had to keep this tissue tucked into her panties all her life to keep it from hanging between her legs. Embarrassment and fear had kept her from seeing a doctor before. It took less than five minutes to remove the growth. When I saw her four weeks later, she was completely healed and totally free of what had been a bothersome and embarrassing problem for years.

## 662 What kind of growth can develop on my vulva and what will my doctor do if I have one?

If you have a growth on your vulva, your doctor will want to inject it with a local anesthetic and cut it off. If it is too large to take off in the office, he or she may still want to biopsy it in the office to make sure it is not malignant. Whether the entire growth is cut off or merely biopsied, your doctor will send the tissue to the pathologist for evaluation.

It really does not matter what kind of growth is present on the vulva, as long as it is not malignant. The pathologist may say it is any of the following type of growths if it is nonmalignant (benign). This following list is taken from an outstanding book, *Benign Diseases of the Vulva and Vagina,* by Drs. Herman L. Gardner and Raymond H. Kaufman, (Boston: G. K. Hall, 1981). If these growths are large, general anesthesia and a short hospital stay may be required to remove them.

acrochordion

seborrheic karatosis

nevus (mole)

hidradenoma

sebaceous adenoma

hemangioma

senile hemangioma

angiokeratoma

pyogenic granuloma

fibroma

lipoma

neurofibroma

leiomyoma

granular cell myoblastoma

pilonidal cysts

sebaceous cysts

syringoma

lymphangioma

## 663 I have a persistent itching of my vulva. What should I do?

As stated previously, if your vulva itches persistently and is not relieved by the usual treatment for vulvar infection, you must continue to see your doctor until the cause is discovered. This warning does not include women who have recurrent fungus infections which require intermittent treatment, nor women who have recurrent trichomonas infection, but rather those whose itching is unexplained and unrelieved.

If your doctor has not been able to give you a specific diagnosis and an organized approach for treatment, you probably need to see a gynecologist or seek another opinion if you have already seen a gynecologist.

There is a great deal of confusion, even in the minds of the best doctors, about the causes of this type of itching, and even the "best" treatment does not always give relief. Because of this I will merely give some general guidelines to help you understand what might be done if you have this problem.

## 664 What procedure will a doctor follow to find the cause of itching?

There are several basic steps that a doctor may take in an attempt to find the cause of persistent itching.

*History of the problem.* The doctor will want to know how long the problem has been present and whether or not you have been treated for infections of the vulvar area. He or she will also want to know if you have been using medications on the vulvar area and whether you have been using toilet tissue with perfumes or dyes in them or tampons or pads which contain chemicals.

*Treatment of infection.* The doctor will want to treat you for any infection found, to see if that will clear up the problem.

*Biopsy.* The doctor will look for any areas of abnormal tissue. In women under fifty there may be thickened vulvar tissue present, and in women over fifty there may be areas that have become thin and sensitive. The doctor will want to take several biopsies if there are areas that look the least bit abnormal. Occasionally a cancer of the vulva will first show up as itching.

*Further treatment.* If you do have pre-malignant or malignant tissue, the doctor will treat that. (See Q. 669–672.)

If you have any changes of the vulvar skin mentioned above, you need to continue seeing your doctor for regular checkups. He or she may want to do repeat biopsies of the tissues. If this is suggested, it means that your doctor is careful and conservative. Such conscientiousness may keep you from developing a malignancy.

---

**665** How will a doctor treat itching caused by thickened skin?

This is known as hyperplastic dystrophy. Cotton dressings soaked with cool Burrow's solution can be applied repeatedly to the areas of thickened skin. This helps clear up the irritation and oozing. In fact, Burrow's solution, a preparation available without prescription from a drugstore, is helpful for many skin problems. In addition, an antibiotic cream can be applied to the area if it seems infected at all, and cortisone-type ointments can be applied when the oozing and irritation have resolved. These cortisone preparations can be applied two or three times a day and may need to be continued intermittently for many years. Women tend to use it when they are itching and stop when the itching is better.

The thickened skin usually becomes much more normal-looking, but sometimes it does not. Occasionally the itching will not clear up either.

---

**666** My doctor did a biopsy of my vulva and said that I had LS and A. What is that? How is it treated?

LS and A (lichen sclerosus et atrophicus, now more commonly called lichen sclerosus) is a condition of the skin of the vulva of unknown cause. With this condition, part or all of the skin of the vulva gets thin, shrunken, white, and itchy. It is not an infection or a malignancy.

Your doctor will take a biopsy to confirm his or her impression of your problem and to make sure you do not have a malignancy. Once certain of your diagnosis, you can be given a prescription for medication. An application of 2 percent testosterone propionate in petrolatum, used two or three times a day for at least four weeks, has been found to be the best treatment. If the itching is intense, application of the testosterone ointment can be alternated with cortisone cream, or the two may be mixed together. It may be helpful to wrap a sanitary pad in plastic wrap and wear it to hold the ointment against the skin of the vulvar area more effectively.

After about a month most women will have much less itching and will be able to use the testosterone ointment less frequently. This less-frequent use is desirable because continued use of this male hormone can produce masculine changes in a woman such as increased hair growth, decreased breast size and increased sexual desire. But don't make a run on the pharmacy to get this drug just to increase your sexual interest! For most women, enough of this medication to increase libido would also be enough to give them a beard!

LS and A can cause shrinking of the vulvar tissues. Women who have shrinking of these tissues may find intercourse painful or impossible. In this situation, Premarin vaginal cream should be used in the vagina in addition to the testosterone on the vulva. One-half an applicator full of the Premarin cream in the vagina three times a week is the usual dose. If intercourse remains difficult, the doctor may be able to make a "relaxing incision" to open the vagina more widely. This would, of course, need to be done under anesthesia.

### 667 What if my vulvar itching does not respond to treatment?

If vulvar itching continues, injections of a cortisone-type drug (10 mg of triamcinalone diluted 2:1 with saline) directly into the itching skin may be given. If the cortisone injections do not work, an injection of an alcohol solution into the tissues to kill the nerves can be tried (under general anesthesia). This is effective only for itching. If there is burning in the vulva it will not help.

### 668 My doctor says I have leukoplakia on my vulva. What is this?

The term *leukoplakia* means "a white patch." Until recently, doctors were afraid that any time such a white patch was present it heralded the possible development of cancer. It has now been shown that this is not true and that leukoplakia is usually due only to thickening of the tissues.

If your doctor says that you have leukoplakia and suggests that a large part of your vulva be removed (a vulvectomy), you should generally refuse to have that done without expert consultation, unless you know that your doctor is a specialist in problems of this kind.

### 669 There is a growth on my vulva that itches. My doctor biopsied it and the report says it is premalignant. What does this mean and how should it be treated?

A premalignant growth contains cells whose chromosomes have changed in such a way that they no longer respond to normal growth controls. Somewhat like a skin cancer, the growth is not dangerous in its present form. However, if such a growth is neglected, it can become dangerous by growing down into the deeper tissues of the body. A premalignant growth, therefore, is at the stage doctors like to find a growth—before it is dangerous.

This type of premalignant growth of the vulva has been given many names in the past: Bowen's disease, erythroplasia of Queyrat, squamous cell carcinoma in situ, and Padget's disease. Presently specialists recognize only two different groups of this type of problem: squamous cell carcinoma in situ and Padget's disease. The symptoms and treatments for both are the same.

Once a biopsy has determined premalignancy, the doctor will suggest further treatment. It will be one of the following.

*Excision around the growth.* To insure getting all the growth, a doctor normally must cut wide of the outside edge of the growth by at least one-third inch. If the pathologist determines that the growth has actually extended to the edges of the tissue that the doctor has removed, the doctor will need to make a wider circle of incision around the area.

*Laser treatment.* The laser is now being used to vaporize these growths. Good treatment is afforded in this way, as the initial procedure is easier and there is less scarring. If the laser is used, it is easier to tell when a growth is coming back because there is less distortion of the vulva after healing.

*Chemotherapy treatment.* When 5 percent 5-fluorouracil cream (a chemotherapy drug) is applied to the surface of the vulva on a premalignant growth, it will frequently make the growth go away. The problem with this treatment is that it can cause a great deal of irritation to the tissues, and many women are unable to continue the use of this drug long enough for it to be effective. However, if a woman can tolerate it, it is often good therapy.

*DNCB treatment.* A new medication called DNCB (dinitrochlorobenzene) is being used for this type of growth. This cream, like 5-fluorouracil, can cause a great deal of irritation. With proper use, however, the irritation can frequently be avoided, and growths that cover even a large area of the vulva can be cleared up.

*Vulvectomy.* See the next question.

---

## 670 Is a vulvectomy ever necessary for premalignant growths?

Doctors in the past have felt that a woman with precancerous growths needed to have her vulva removed, a procedure involving the removal of both the labia majora and minora and often the clitoris and other skin. Very few doctors feel this is necessary today, unless the premalignant growths are extensive or severe, or unless these growths continue to recur.

A vulvectomy is not particularly dangerous, but it does occasionally require skin grafting to cover the raw areas. It changes the way a woman's vulva looks and also causes a problem with urination. Urine is normally guided by the libia into forming a stream; after a vulvectomy urine tends to splatter in a bothersome fashion.

Another problem with treating this type of growth with a vulvectomy is that the same type of growth for which the vulvectomy was done frequently regrows along the edges of the healed surgical incision. This requires further surgery.

---

## 671 What about cancer of the vulva?

Cancer of the vulva is usually squamous cell carcinoma of the labia majora. In other words, cancer of the skin of the labia majora is the most common cancer of the vulva, although vulvar cancer can originate in any of the other parts of the vulvar tissues: sweat glands, Bartholin's glands, clitoris, and urethra.

There has been a dramatic increase in the number of cases of both premalignant and malignant growths of the vulva in the past few years, many of these occurring in young, premenopausal women. Cancer of the vulva had always been considered to be a cancer of women of the postmenopausal age until this trend started a few years ago. During this same period of time, there has been a marked increase in the number of precancerous and cancerous growths on women's cervixes. Most researchers feel that both of these problems are related to infection by the same virus that causes venereal warts, or condyloma. (See Q. 1138–1145.) The increased presence of the venereal wart virus seems to be due to the increased number of sexual partners to whom so many young women are exposing themselves today.

It is important that both patients and doctors understand that if a growth is present on the vulva, or if there is an itching or uncomfortable area that persists, a biopsy should be done to make sure that no cancer is developing.

A cancer of the vulva is normally slow-growing, but after it has been present for a while, it will finally grow into the deeper tissues of the labial skin and from there spread inside the body to lymph nodes of the groin and the pelvis. Often, even then, this type of cancer will remain confined to these lymph nodes for a long time before it spreads on to other parts of the body.

## 672 How is vulvar cancer treated?

Treatment for this type of cancer is usually an operation which removes the labia, the mons pubis, and the lymph nodes of the groin and inner thigh. Skin grafting of the vulva, over the pubic bone, and of the groin is often necessary. This operation is called a radical vulvectomy.

If a pathologist studies all of the tissue removed at surgery and finds no lymph node involvement, which means that the cancer is growing only on the vulva, the patient has up to an 80-percent chance of being completely cured by the operation. If some of the lymph nodes are involved, however, the chance of complete cure drops to as low as 30 or 40 percent.

Because this type of cancer is occurring more often in younger women, and because the operation is so disfiguring to the external genital appearance, doctors are trying to determine ways to do a less radical operation. If you have a cancer of this type, be sure you are in the hands of doctors who are specialists in the care of female-organ cancer. In this way you will be able to get surgery and treatment that is custom-made to your particular needs, avoiding surgery that might be unnecessarily extensive.

If, after surgery for vulvar cancer, the cancer begins growing again, it is absolutely necessary that you be treated by a female-organ cancer specialist. There is still a chance for a cure, but only if it is handled with great expertise and care.

## 673 What does a biopsy of my vulva involve? How important is it for me to have such a biopsy?

Having read this chapter, you will have seen the common thread winding through all our discussions about vulvar lumps, bumps, growths, and irritations. That common thread is the vulvar biopsy—an absolutely mandatory part of the care of vulvar disease in women. A recent report on cancer of the vulva indicated that diagnosis of cancer of the vulva is delayed, on the average, by sixteen months. In other words, the patient went to the doctor with a complaint (usually itching), but the doctor did not make the diagnosis for another sixteen months! During that time the patient's cancer was enlarging and getting worse. All it takes to diagnose a cancer of the vulva is a simple biopsy.

If you have a small growth on your vulva, or an area that continues to itch and be uncomfortable, you should insist that your doctor do a careful examination of your vulva and consider doing a vulvar biopsy. I am talking about itching or pain that persists in a particular spot on the vulva, not the "all over" vulvar irritation of chronic vulvitis that so many women have.

The vulvar biopsy is not an extremely uncomfortable procedure for you. It is done in three simple steps:

The doctor injects anesthetic in the area to be biopsied.

The doctor twirls a small, round "punch" biopsy onto the numbed area of your vulva and snips away a small, round piece of tissue.

The doctor uses silver nitrate sticks to cauterize the bleeding from the walls of the small hole. This procedure eliminates the need for sutures.

The biopsied tissue is sent to a pathologist for diagnosis. If the report is "benign," the doctor can reassure you of that fact. If the report shows a malignancy, proper treatment can be started immediately.

## 674 What problems can affect the urethra?

A red, tumorlike growth can occur at the opening of the urethra, usually in women who have gone through the menopause. The problem is usually a caruncle, a condition in which the lining just inside the urethral opening protrudes from the urethra and is exposed to the irritation of underwear, intercourse, and other irritants. This delicate tissue, which is normally inside the urethra, cannot stand this type of trauma and becomes reddened and swollen.

Most of the time this problem, if not too bothersome, can be left alone. If the caruncle bleeds or is sensitive, an application of a vaginal estrogen cream or estrogen by mouth will normally clear it up. If it does not, the doctor may give a woman general anesthesia and cut out the irritated tissue. If a caruncle does not seem to be clearing up as quickly as it should, the doctor should certainly take a biopsy of it and send it to a pathologist. Carcinoma (cancer) of the urethra is possible.

Occasionally a reddish, bleeding urethra is caused by the inner lining of the urethra actually falling out. This problem, called urethral prolapse, can occur in young girls before they begin their menses and in women after the menopause. It rarely occurs in women of reproductive age. Urethral prolapse is not common. I have never had to treat a patient for this condition. Treatment for the problem is done with freezing (cryocautery), using the laser to evaporate the tissue, or with use of a catheter and sutures. In the latter method a catheter is put in the urethra and the suture tied down on the catheter, over the caruncle. After a few days the caruncle falls off.

## 675 What causes a cyst of the urethral opening?

There are glands at the entrance to the urethra (Skene's glands) that produce mucus that moistens the opening. When the outlet to these little glands gets blocked, they fill up with mucus and form small cysts. This may happen following an infection with gonorrhea, but it may also occur in women who have not had such an infection.

These urethral-opening cysts may cause discomfort during intercourse, or they may become infected and cause a great deal of pain. Occasionally they can block the opening of the urethra, making it difficult to empty the bladder.

When these glands are infected, they can be opened and drained. If these glands have become cystic and are being a problem, a urologist can cut them out in a simple but effective procedure.

## 676 My doctor said my Bartholin's glands are blocked. What does that mean?

Every woman has two Bartholin's glands, one on either side of the entrance to the lower vagina. These glands produce secretions that lubricate the vaginal entrance and are especially active during intercourse. They empty their secretions just inside the labia through two small tubes, or ducts.

If the ducts become obstructed, the gland, which continues to secrete mucus, will cause the duct to begin "ballooning up" from the pressure and presence of mucus.

The Bartholin's gland ducts may become blocked off for several reasons: infection from germs around the vaginal entrance (including venereal disease such as gonorrhea), underdeveloped ducts, and occasionally, stitches from episiotomies.

It is fairly easy for a doctor to tell if the swelling at the lower part of the vagina is a Bartholin's gland cyst or an infection. Once he or she has diagnosed the problem, treatment will be suggested.

## 677 How is a Bartholin's gland cyst treated?

If the cyst is not bothersome, it may be left alone. If it is bothersome, however, one of four treatments may be suggested. The doctor may want to open the cyst in an operating room and sew around the edges so that it stays open. This requires general anesthesia and is called marsupialization. A second alternative treatment suggested may be the use of the laser to make an opening in the cyst. Thirdly, the doctor may suggest the use of local anesthesia in the office so he or she can make a small nick into the cyst to insert a small rubber catheter called a Word catheter. The balloon on the tip of the catheter would then be inflated to keep it in place. Another alternative treatment is to cut out the entire Bartholin's gland.

When the Word catheter is removed after about four to six weeks, a sufficient opening is left to permit outflow of mucus allowing the duct to remain collapsed.

Intercourse may be difficult but is permitted with a Word catheter in place. The catheter hangs out of the Bartholin's gland about an inch.

I have been using the Word catheter for years and prefer it to sewing the gland open. The catheter can be inserted in the office, does not require general anesthesia, and patients tolerate it well. Patients are less likely to develop a subsequent Bartholin's gland cyst after use of a Word catheter than after marsupialization. Occasionally a woman finds the catheter too uncomfortable and must have it removed after only a few days, but this is uncommon. Using a laser to open a Bartholin's gland cyst is a new procedure. Time will tell if it is an effective method of treatment.

It is rarely necessary to cut out an entire Bartholin's-gland cyst. Cutting out the cyst leaves a big deformity of the lower vaginal opening, and it can be a bloody, messy operation. If, however, you have had a great deal of trouble with your Bartholin's gland and a competent doctor suggests that you have the gland removed, then it is probably best to follow that advice. By "a great deal of trouble," I mean many episodes of the recurrence of the cyst, with its presence causing persistent pain and problems. If a doctor suggests—on first seeing you for a cyst that has not been too troublesome—that you have the cyst cut out, it would be best to get another opinion before having this done.

### 678 How is a Bartholin's gland abscess, or infection, treated?

Occasionally a Bartholin's gland cyst will become infected. When this occurs, your lower vagina, either on the right side or on the left, will be inflamed and extremely tender. The doctor will usually cut open the abscess in the office under local anesthesia to allow drainage of the pus and relief of the painful pressure that has developed. Sometimes a Word catheter can be inserted at this time. I have been able to use the Word catheter with a number of patients at the time an abscess was opened. This saved their having to come back later to have a second procedure done. However, many times the infection will prevent anything more than just the opening of the abscess.

### 679 The blood vessels of my labia seem swollen and distended. What does this mean?

Swollen, distended blood vessels of the labia probably indicate varicose veins. Most women are surprised when this situation develops. Although varicose veins occur most often during pregnancy, they can occur any time. If the veins are not too bothersome, they can and should be left alone. If they do cause trouble, they may be treated.

If vulvar varicose veins develop during pregnancy, a woman may be able to make it through the pregnancy by lying down whenever the vulvar area becomes engorged and uncomfortable. A vulvar support (produced by Ortho-Vascular Products Company in Yonkers, New York) may help.

Vulvar varicose veins can bleed during pregnancy. If repeated bleeding occurs, surgery may be necessary. If it is necessary, it is probably best to have it done before the end of the seventh month of pregnancy.

If a person is not pregnant, the varicose veins can be ligated (tied off), just as they would be if they were present in a woman's legs.

### 680 How should injuries to the vulva be treated?

Most injuries to the vulva occur in children: falling on a bicycle seat, a fence, a toy, and so on. However, they do occur in adults too, usually as a result of water skiing, motorcycle or bicycle accidents, or because of some similar type trauma. (See Q. 59–61, 718.)

Injuries from intercourse also occur, but they are unusual except in rape cases. (See Q. 242–244.)

If an injury to the vulva produces a bruise, there is no need for treatment other than an ice pack during the first twenty-four hours, followed by sitting in a bathtub filled with warm water (sitz bath) several times a day until pain and swelling have subsided.

If the bruise includes a large accumulation of blood (hematoma), the area may need to be opened surgically. This is best done under general anesthesia in an operating room because, when the wound is opened, there may be bleeding from the raw area inside that requires suturing.

If there are tears of the vulva, these too will often require suturing. This, of course, would require anesthesia and treatment in an operating room. Tears of this type need to be washed thoroughly. Careful examination of the tissues is necessary to make sure that no foreign material is left embedded in the tissues.

If a vulvar injury happens to you or your daughter, it will not physically affect either of you sexually. If this area can tolerate delivery of a baby, which includes tears, bruising, and even hematomas, it can obviously tolerate other injuries. It was designed to heal well and to allow normal sexual function after trauma.

---

## Problems of the Vagina

The vagina is an important part of your body. Though you cannot see it, and you probably do not think of it often, the vagina performs several vitally important functions.

It serves as a passage for the menstrual flow.

It receives your husband's penis during sexual intercourse.

It serves as a receptacle for semen.

It serves as the walls of the birth canal for delivery of a baby.

It allows a doctor easy access to your cervix for Pap smears and permits easy examination of your uterus and other internal organs.

Most of the time a woman is as unaware of her vagina as she is of other internal body organs. Even when the vagina is diseased, she is primarily concerned with the blood or discharge or odor that comes from the vagina rather than with the vagina itself. These symptoms may indicate a vaginal problem:

abnormal discharge

abnormal bleeding

unusual odor

pain with intercourse

itching

tissue protruding from the vagina

In this section we will discuss ways to care for the vagina and problems of the vagina. Remember, however, that "our knowledge of the structure, function, physiology, and pathology of the vagina is still incomplete. The human vagina represents a complex eco system of epithelia, substrates, enzymes, secretions, and microflora."—*A Discussion of Vaginal Problems in Clinical Obstetrics and Gynecology* by Eduard G. Friedrich, Jr., M.D. (Philadelphia: Saunders) 1976. In other words, doctors do not know all there is to know about the vagina. It is a much more complicated organ than it appears to be. (See Q. 62–68.)

If it takes your doctor a while to help you get rid of a vaginal problem, be patient. The solution may not be simple! It may be reassuring to learn that the vagina rarely has a malignancy or a tumor or a problem that is dangerous to your health.

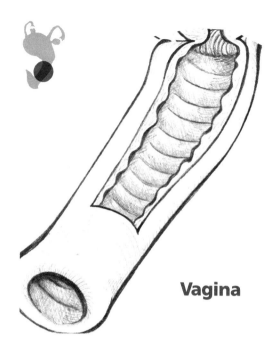

**Vagina**

### 681 Do I need to provide any special care for my vagina?

The best summary statement in answer to that question is: "If your vagina isn't bothering you, don't bother it!" If you are not having trouble with your vagina now, and have had no problems in the past, you are probably doing things right.

There are several topics I am frequently asked about by patients concerning the vagina and its care:

the use of tampons

lubrication with intercourse

avoiding sexually transmitted diseases

douching

intercourse after hysterectomy

first intercourse

### 682 Should I use tampons?

I recommend that women use tampons for absorption of menstrual flow. I also recommend that girls begin using tampons as soon as they begin having a menstrual flow. (See Q. 118.)

The advantage of internal protection is that it keeps the vulva drier, making it less likely to become irritated by moisture. However, although this is true for menstruation, using tampons throughout the month for vaginal discharge is not advisable because of the possibility of developing toxic shock.

An additional advantage is that if a young girl uses tampons, she becomes familiar with her hymen and with her vaginal structure. The tampons stretch the hymen a little, making her first pelvic exam and first intercourse easier. It is my impression that my young patients who use tampons are more relaxed about and comfortable with their bodies.

It is true that toxic shock syndrome has been associated with tampon use, but it has also been found in non-tampon users and even in men and small children. (See Q. 713–717.)

---

**683** **Should I use a lubricant during intercourse?**

I advise my patients to purchase a vaginal lubricant and keep it at their bedsides from the first night of marriage on. When women have times of poor sexual lubrication a little vaginal lubricant could help.

Vaginal dryness is not a sign of poor sexual response; it occurs under numerous circumstances in all women. For instance, lubricants are helpful for intercourse immediately after a menstrual period, or soon after a bath, or in cases of limited sexual excitement. Lubricants are especially important if you have gone through the menopause and find that you have less-than-satisfactory sexual lubrication. Because lubricants tend to kill sperm, you should not use one if you are trying to become pregnant.

There are several vaginal lubricants on the market, and they can be purchased without a prescription at a drug store. For example, the Ortho Company has one called Ortho Personal Lubricant; MaxiLube cream is pleasant to use because it is nongreasy and is quickly absorbed by bedsheets or by your skin. There are other good lubricants; any one should make you more comfortable.

---

**684** **How can I avoid sexually transmitted diseases?**

If only for the health of your vagina, it is best to have intercourse only with your husband. No matter what your personal moral stance, it is clear that you cannot contract a sexually transmitted disease if you have intercourse with only one person who has intercourse only with you. (See Q. 1145.)

Even if a man has not had intercourse with anyone else for two or three years (or who knows how long), he can still have sexually transmitted organisms from his last sexual contact that he can transmit to you during intercourse. The same applies to you in having intercourse with him.

For a more complete discussion of this see Q. 937, 946, 953, 962.

---

**685** **Should I douche?**

Douching is an artificial means of cleansing the vagina, a job the vagina is quite capable of doing on its own. Most gynecologists advise women not to douche unless specifically told to do so by a physician.

The vagina is "self-cleaning." If you could view the inside of your vagina immediately after a menstrual period, you would see that there is no blood left in it. The vagina rids itself of this material quickly, making douching after a menstrual period unnecessary.

The same is true following intercourse. Soon after intercourse, all the semen is absorbed or drains from the vagina.

Some women insist that they do not feel "clean" unless they douche. If you are one of those who insist on douching, I strongly encourage you to use a disposable douche nozzle and prepackaged douche solution. Re-using douche nozzles, or using one of the old-fashioned hanging bags for the douche solution, is not advisable because germs can grow in the bags. A douche nozzle cannot be completely sterilized without a sterilizer. Some fungus spores cannot even be boiled off a douche nozzle!

Douching can be useful for certain types of infection. If your doctor suggests that you douche with some medication, then you should do so. Douching can occasionally be useful for fertility problems, and your doctor might recommend that you douche with a sperm-nutrient solution. Other than for these two reasons, it is normally best for a woman not to douche.

### 686 Is my vagina open at the upper end after a hysterectomy?

No, there is no open upper end of the vagina after a hysterectomy has been performed. When the cervix is removed from the upper vagina, the front and back walls of the vagina are sewn together, closing it completely. When a doctor looks into your vagina after a hysterectomy, it looks the same as it did before, except that there is no cervix at the upper end.

A man cannot tell at intercourse whether or not a woman has had a hysterectomy. If anything, the woman's upper vagina is likely to be a little tighter, and perhaps a little more stimulating sexually because of that tightness.

### 687 Should I prepare my vagina in any way before I have intercourse for the first time?

The best preparation of the vagina for first intercourse is to have a doctor examine it. He or she can warn you of any existing problem, detect a hymen that is too tight and firm, and tell you if you have any kind of vaginal abnormality.

Even if you have been examined and found normal, you may still have some discomfort with your first intercourse. You are unlikely to have severe pain, but if you do, that pain is more likely a result of your tightening up your body out of fear of intercourse than it is of your hymen actually being resistant to intercourse.

If you have significant pain with your first intercourse, there are a couple of things you

might do to make it more comfortable the next time.

First, try to relax! If you are tensing up during entry of his penis, ask your husband to stop pushing in. Then consciously relax your vagina. You will be amazed at the amount of control you have over your vagina. As you tell your husband you are relaxed and that he can push in further, you can push down too, as though you are trying to have a bowel movement. This tends to open up your vagina a little, allowing further penetration. In addition, use a vaginal lubricant. If your pain persists, see your doctor.

It is normal to have soreness of the hymen after having intercourse the first time or two. If this occurs, refrain from intercourse for a few days to allow the irritation caused by the normal tears in your hymen to clear up.

It is also normal for you to have a little bleeding with the first intercourse, but it is just as normal not to, even if you are a virgin.

### 688 Is it normal to have some vaginal discharge?

It certainly is. As a matter of fact, it is remarkable that women do not have more discharge than they do. Secretions come from the sweat and oil glands of the vulva, and from the Bartholin's and Skene's glands; fluid oozes through the vaginal walls; cells slough off the vaginal walls continually; and the cervix, uterine lining, and fallopian tubes all contribute fluids to the vagina that are either absorbed by it or passed to the outside.

In spite of the secretion of all these fluids, most women do not require external protection for the vaginal secretions. Some women, however, have enough normal secretions to make them feel wet all the time, they will often be uncomfortable without some type of external protection.

Most women have increased secretions at

the time of ovulation (fourteen days before the next period is going to start) and just before a menstrual period begins. Some women may notice it only as a slight wetness at the opening of the vagina. Other women do not have any increased secretions at this time, also a totally normal situation.

Normal secretions produced by normal body function will usually be white or off-white in color. Their consistency will be "curdy." If vaginal secretions are milky or runny, they are usually not normal. The normal, curdy secretions cause some women to think they have a fungus infection even though they have no itching. If a woman has enough fungus infection to produce the typical "cottage cheese" discharge of such an infection, she will also have irritation.

If you are not sure that your secretions are normal, see your doctor who can check the acidity of your vaginal secretions. The acidity of normal secretions should be in the range of a pH of 3.8 to 4.2. If your secretions have this acidity, no odor, cause no itching, and have the normal off-white, curdy appearance, you have normal secretions.

---

## 689 What should I do if I have an abnormal vaginal discharge or odor or itch?

You need to see a physician for abnormal vaginal discharge, itch, odor, and so on. Your doctor will question you about your symptoms. Since problems of this sort almost always indicate a vaginal infection, he or she will ask you if the discharge causes itching or has a bad odor and will determine how heavy the discharge is and what color it is. Since the irritation might be caused by some medication or drug that comes in contact with your vulvar skin, you will be asked about materials or medications that have come in contact with that area. If you have had a vulvar irritation for a long time, for instance, you may have been using some

medication to which you have become sensitive. Your symptoms may now be due to the medication and not to the original irritant.

The doctor will examine you, checking the vulvar area to see if it is red, scratched, or has sores, and will look inside your vagina to see what the discharge looks like. Your physician will then take some of the secretions on a Q-tip, daub them onto a drop of saline (salt water) on a slide, and look at the suspension under a microscope.

On a wet mount of this type, a gardnerella (hemophilus) vaginal infection can be diagnosed. The gardnerella germs are small and stick to the normal vaginal cells seen under the microscope. A doctor can often identify gardnerella infection just by looking in the microscope for these normal cells with bacteria clinging to them ("clue" cells).

Trichomonas organisms can usually be seen quite easily in a saline preparation.

The doctor might do a KOH prep with your secretions: a drop of your secretions is placed on a slide and a drop of potassium hydroxide (KOH) placed on that. The potassium hydroxide will dissolve all the vaginal cells, leaving only fungus organisms, if there are any present.

The doctor may check the acidity of your vaginal secretions to help determine what type of infection you have. If the test shows a pH of 5.0 or higher, and you have an odorous discharge, you almost certainly have gardnerella vaginitis (formerly called hemophilus vaginitis); if you have an infection causing itching, and the pH of the secretions is 5.0 or above, you almost certainly have a trichomonas infection.

Since trichomonas and gardnerella are treated the same way—with Flagyl, a medication taken in pill form by mouth—the decision as to which drug you need could be made simply by testing the acidity of your vaginal secretions.

The doctor may feel it necessary, however, to take some of the secretions from your vagina for a culture. The culture can show whether or not you have fungus organisms in your vagina, even when you have such a minimal amount of infection that it cannot be directly seen on a microscope. Vaginal cultures can also identify infection by gonorrhea, chlamydia, or herpes.

Occasionally, poorly informed doctors will worry a patient about normal but unusual vaginal germs that they find on a vaginal culture. For example, it is normal to have an E. coli organism in the vagina, and it is normal to have a streptococcus organism in the vagina; if a doctor begins treatment for these organisms, he is treating you for a normal germ that cannot be the source of a vaginal infection. You should get further consultation if he insists on continuing treatment for such organisms. Of course, if infection is caused by gonorrhea, chlamydia, herpes, fungus, trichomonas, or gardnerella, treatment is usually necessary.

Treatment of gardnerella, trichomonas, or monilia infections is not necessary for purely health reasons because these infections will not damage a person's body. However, they will not usually go away on their own. These infections may stop bothering a woman temporarily only to start actively growing and causing discomfort later on.

---

## 690 What is *trichomonas* vaginitis? How is it treated?

This is an infection caused by a protozoan organism called trichomonas vaginalis and occurs only in the genital organs of men and women. Although it does not damage the people it infects, trichomonas can be extremely irritating, especially in women. If a woman is having a discharge that is irritating, she should be checked for "trich," as was described in the previous question.

Flagyl is effective in clearing up 99 percent of trichomonas infections. It is as effective for a person to take two grams of Flagyl all at one time as it is to take one-half gram twice a day for five days.

More important than which dosage schedule a woman follows is the fact that her sexual partner must also be treated. If a woman has trichomonas, her partner will also have it in his internal genital organs, even though he has no symptoms. If a woman is treated and her sexual partner is not, he will give the infection back to her as soon as they have intercourse again.

There is no doubt that this infection is transmitted sexually. As a matter of fact, if both partners are being treated, but infection recurs, it may be that one or the other of the two has an involvement with another sexual partner that is causing the reinfection. I would not want to cause unnecessary suspicion in a relationship between a couple, however. Even though trichomonas can be spread back and forth between two sexual partners, it does occur in people who have not had extramarital intercourse. Apparently the germ can be spread in other ways too. If you have developed a trichomonas infection, it does not necessarily mean that your husband has had sex with someone else. Also, 1 percent of trich patients do not respond to Flagyl because their infecting agent is a resistant organism.

If an infection seems to be resistant to Flagyl, both partners might try an increased dose of 500 mg of Flagyl taken four times a day for a week. Further treatment might consist of using Vagisect douches or Vagisect suppositories to try to clear up the local infection. Obviously, both partners will harbor the same resistant organism. To avoid such recurrent vaginal infections, your partner would have to wear a condom (rubber) with each intercourse to keep you from being infected. This is a frustrating problem, but fortunately it is uncommon for a person to have a trichomonas infection that does not respond to Flagyl.

---

## 691 What is *gardnerella* vaginitis? How is it treated?

Gardnerella (formerly called hemophilus) is the most commonly sexually transmitted vaginal infection. Though it is common and can cause an odorous discharge, the infection does no damage to the body of a woman. This type of infection has a discharge that is "fishy," foul-smelling, watery, and often heavy. It does not cause burning or itching. If itching is associated with the above symptoms, a mixed infection—gardnerella and fungus, or gardnerella and trichomonas—is probably present.

The doctor can make the diagnosis (as stated earlier in Q. 689), by putting a drop of the vaginal secretions in a drop of saline and looking at this under a microscope. The "clue" cells are the normal vaginal cells to which gardnerella germs have adhered.

The best treatment is with Flagyl, 500 mg taken twice a day for seven days. If you are also being treated for trichomonas, it might be wise to have the 500 mg–twice-a-day-for-seven-days regime instead of the one-time dose often given for trichomonas alone. This would insure that you will get rid of both gardnerella and trichomonas.

As with trichomonas, gardnerella is usually a sexually transmitted disease. For a woman to be free of it, her sexual partner must also be free of it. It is necessary, therefore, that both partners be treated. If the infection keeps recurring, it is possible that one of the couple has another sexual partner. But no treatment is perfect, and failure to eliminate gardnerella may not necessarily be due to outside exposure.

Also as with trichomonas, a man may not have any symptoms of the infection, but if a woman has it, her partner also does, and he must be treated too.

Gardnerella vaginitis can occur in women who have not (and whose husbands have not) had extramarital intercourse. If you have developed a gardnerella vaginitis infection, therefore, don't assume that your husband has been unfaithful.

## 692 What is *monilia* vaginitis? How is it treated?

Monilia vaginitis, also called fungus or yeast infection, is the most common vaginal infection. A woman who has a fungus infection will usually have itching, ranging from mild to severe. The vulvar area may be red and often thickened from the woman's scratching. Though this infection can be very irritating, it does no permanent damage to a woman's body.

Examination by the physician shows a cheesy, white discharge, which can be identified as fungus by putting a fleck of the white secretions in a drop of saline and looking at that under a microscope. What the doctor sees is an organism that looks like a tree branch with no leaves, and he or she may see small, round spores that look a little bit like holly berries stuck to the branches.

Occasionally a patient will have enough infection to cause her to have itching without the fungus showing up on a smear. In this case the doctor may want to do a culture to prove that monilia is the culprit. A culture is quite reliable for detecting the presence of the fungus organism.

Treatment for fungus infection is with a drug such as Monistat or Gyne-Lotrimin. Normally a seven-day course of nightly vaginal applications takes care of the infection. Patients can also apply some of this medicine over their vulva. This not only soothes the area but helps kill any infection that might be developing on the vulvar skin.

Some women have doggedly persistent fungus infections. Occasionally these recur because a woman is predisposed to the development of fungus infections. For example, pregnancy is a situation in which infections will often return soon after treatment has been completed. Diabetics and patients who have poor immunity because of being on immunosuppressive agents (such as a kidney recipient) or who have some other condition that affects their immunity will have problems getting rid of a fungus infection. Markedly debilitated patients, weakened because of cancer or old age, will also have trouble getting rid of fungus infections.

For many years physicians thought that women on oral contraceptives were more likely to develop vaginal fungus infections. Recent studies have shown that this is probably not true. In spite of those studies, if I have a patient who takes oral contraceptives and cannot get rid of her vaginal monilia, I suggest that she try stopping her oral contraceptives for a few months to see if she gets better; occasionally this seems to help.

Some women will continue having fungus infection, even though they have none of the above problems. Apparently the bodies of some women just grow fungus easier than the bodies of other women. A chronic fungus infection can be one of the most frustrating problems a woman can have. Some suggestions in the next answer may help if you have this problem.

Although a man may occasionally have penile or skin irritation (a form of "jock itch") from fungus infection, he does not develop it inside his body. If he has such an irritation, he can use some of his wife's medication on himself once or twice a day.

Monilia vaginitis is not a classic sexually transmitted disease, but a person with a severe monila infection can infect his or her sexual partner.

---

**693** **What is the treatment for persistent fungus infection?**

If a fungus infection does not clear up with regular treatment (see previous question), the following treatment techniques may be helpful.

Monistat or Gyne-Lotrimin can be used every day for four to six weeks, followed by the use of one of these drugs for two or three days at the beginning of the menstrual period for six months, or even indefinitely.

In addition, medication should be used for an entire week whenever there is any discomfort or itching.

If the irritation continues to be a problem in spite of the above-mentioned treatment, the woman can usually keep it under control by inserting fungus medication into the vagina every two or three days indefinitely.

If the woman is having external irritation, the medicine should be put not only in the vagina, but also on the vulvar tissues. The fungus medicine that the woman uses should be applied to the man's penis once a day. He needs to get it under the foreskin if he is not circumcised. One good technique is to have intercourse within a few hours of a vaginal application of fungus medication.

Any time antibiotics are taken, the same vaginal-fungus medication should be used during the entire time the antibiotics are taken. As far as is known, these medications are safe for indefinite use, even during pregnancy.

Additionally, there is a fungus vaccine available. The effectiveness of this treatment has not been confirmed by clinical studies, but the impression of those of us whose patients have used this type of vaccination is that it does help prevent fungus infections. I feel it is a good thing to try if the fungus is not responding to anything else.

Finally, since it is felt that fungus organisms are harbored in the rectums of some people, drugs should be taken by mouth to clear up such organisms. There are two medications for this: Mycostatin and Nizoral. Your doctor would need to give you a prescription for one of these if this seems to be a factor.

---

**694** **How is vaginitis treated if it is caused by a sexually transmitted disease such as gonorrhea, herpes, or chlamydia?**

The most important thing concerning such infections is that you tell the doctor if you think there is any possibility that you have picked up one of these diseases. You could have contracted it from intercourse with someone with such an infection, including your husband. If you think there is a possibility that your husband may have had intercourse with someone else, be sure to tell your doctor so that you can be checked for infection. Don't let embarrassment keep you from good medical care; such delay can cause your body damage.

Your doctor knows that neither you nor your husband is perfect and that occasionally you might do things which you regret. The majority of doctors wants to know if a patient has had an extramarital affair to make sure a sexually transmitted germ is not present. Most doctors will not be judgmental and will treat their patients compassionately. Their desire is for the patient's best interest: good medical care and treatment. If your doctor is not understanding, change doctors.

I often have patients who say that it is impossible that they could have a sexually transmitted disease because their sexual partner has not had intercourse with anybody for the past two or three months. Such a statement indicates ignorance of sexually transmitted disease. If you have intercourse with anyone who has had relations with anyone else, even several years ago, he can still give you the germs that can cause you to contract a sexually transmitted disease. If you have questions about this, read chapter 13.

## 695 My doctor says that my IUD is causing my discharge. Is this possible?

Yes, an IUD (intrauterine contraceptive device) can cause vaginal discharge. Some women can use an IUD for several years without any problems and then suddenly begin having a discharge. In this case it is best to remove the IUD. In some women, IUDs can set up an irritation of the lining of the uterus that causes discharge. This may actually be a low-grade infection.

If you develop this type of discharge and do not want your IUD removed, you may want to try taking a penicillin-type antibiotic or some Flagyl. Ask your doctor. If this does not stop the discharge, it may be best for you to have your IUD removed to stop the discharge. If such a discharge is caused by infection, then getting rid of the IUD would be the best thing, since it would allow the uterus to clear itself of such infection.

## 696 Is there anything other than infection or disease that might cause an abnormal vaginal discharge?

There are two other causes of vaginal discharge that should be mentioned, although both are relatively rare in the United States. These are discharges caused by a hole from the vagina into the rectum (rectovaginal fistula) or by a hole from the vagina into the bladder (vesicovaginal fistula). The discharge associated with these fistulas is irritating, bothersome, and offensive because of the continual drainage of urine or feces into the vagina.

## 697 What are the causes of vesicovaginal fistula? How is this treated?

In the United States a vesicovaginal fistula (hole from the vagina into the bladder) is usually a result of a hysterectomy or of surgery to repair a loose, relaxed vaginal wall. In undeveloped countries the most common cause is erosion of the wall between the vagina and the bladder from a baby's head in extremely prolonged labor.

If your gynecologist suspects a vesicovaginal fistula, he or she might suggest that you see a urologist. This specialist would look into your bladder to detect a hole and would order X-rays for the same reason. In addition, your doctor might have you wear a tampon, put colored water into your bladder, and check the tampon to see if the color comes through a hole into your vagina.

The treatment for a vesicovaginal fistula is surgery. It is important that the doctor who does this performs it carefully and with great expertise. Since this problem occurs rarely in this country, few doctors have extensive experience in repairing such fistulas. Good doctors can do a competent job, however, if they will study the available literature to determine the best approach to your particular problem.

### 698 What causes a rectovaginal fistula? How is this treated?

The most common cause of rectovaginal fistula (hole from the vagina into the rectum) is an episiotomy. No matter how well an obstetrician sews up an episiotomy, occasionally it will break open, either partially or completely. The opening can be through a part of the episiotomy, or the entire episiotomy can tear open into your rectum so that you have no control of your stool.

Other causes of rectovaginal fistulas can be from treatment with radiation for cancer of the cervix (this can occur up to ten years after the radiation treatment has been used) and from a diverticulum (an outpouching of the colon) eroding into the vagina.

If there is any suspicion of a stool leak into the vagina, your gynecologist will probably consult with a proctologist, a specialist in colon and rectal disease. This specialist will look up into your rectum to see if an opening can be seen, and X-rays will also be ordered in an effort to detect a hole. The gynecologist, of course, would have already looked into your vagina to check for a hole but sometimes an opening is so small that it cannot be seen.

The treatment for rectovaginal fistula is the same as for vesicovaginal fistula: surgery. It is important that careful, competent technique be used for repair of a rectovaginal fistula. The best chance of cure is for the surgical operation to be done correctly the first time. In spite of great care and skill, however, a fistula can break down after an operation and would then require further surgery.

### 699 Can my vagina be "too loose"? What causes this?

Yes, a woman can have vaginal looseness. It is almost always due to the stretching of the vaginal tissues from childbirth. There are several symptoms of this problem (See Q. 700). If you are not bothered by looseness of your vagina, however, it is not too loose or relaxed. Physicians will often recommend a hysterectomy with vaginal repairs, merely because the patient's uterus is positioned lower than usual in the vagina and her vagina looks loose at office examination. Surgery for looseness that is not bothering you is absolutely unnecessary. It does not matter how many children you have had nor how relaxed your vagina may appear to a physician nor that your uterus has fallen—you do not need surgery to repair it unless it bothers you!

Occasionally the uterus may lose its support and fall down far enough in the vagina so that the cervix will actually protrude. In some situations the entire uterus will come down and hang out of the vagina. At times the vaginal walls will bulge out of the vagina, causing a woman to actually sit on her prolapsed vaginal tissues when she sits down. When problems of this sort develop, it is best to have surgery. Women with this condition are almost always uncomfortable enough to ask for surgery.

**700** **What problems might result from vaginal looseness?**

There are several symptoms or problems with vaginal looseness.

*Looseness with intercourse.* This may result in too little friction for good sexual response. Such looseness often causes air to gush in and out of the vagina during intercourse (embarrasing but not dangerous). This looseness can also prevent adequate friction for your husband to have satisfactory sexual feeling or stimulation with intercourse.

*Pelvic pressure.* If you have a "falling out" feeling of the tissues of your vagina when you have been on your feet for several hours, you probably have vaginal relaxation.

*Loss of urine with cough, sneeze, or laugh.* It is normal for a woman to "wet her pants" occasionally with a strong, hard laugh or sneeze, but if this problem necessitates wearing a pad, if it makes her fearful to be around people, or if it keeps her from exercising because she might be embarrassed by urine on her clothes, there is too much vaginal looseness.

*Inability to have a bowel movement without finger pressure.* If a woman is "constipated" unless she inserts her finger into her vagina and pushes back on her rectum to help during a bowel movement (called rectal splinting), she needs a repair of the vaginal tissues.

*Pain with intercourse.* When the vaginal walls are very relaxed and the uterus has lost its support, it can tend to fall down or even "fall out" of the vagina. When the uterus is this low in the vagina, there may be discomfort with intercourse when the penis pushes against the uterus.

**701** **What is the treatment for vaginal looseness?**

If a woman is bothered by any of the problems mentioned above and she has had all the children she wants to have, the treatment is a vaginal hysterectomy with repairs of the front and back walls of the vagina. In some cases there might be no vaginal repairs or only one repair. Remember, though, the key words are *bothered by*. Any woman who has vaginal looseness and is not bothered by or concerned about it should not have surgery.

If a woman chooses to have corrective surgery for vaginal looseness, she should have it done by a physician who will do it carefully and properly. Some doctors are so proud of their ability to do surgery quickly that they do not take the time to carefully sew the bladder and urethra back in place or to meticulously rebuild the back wall of the vagina in such a way that the vagina has appropriate size for intercourse. If the surgery is not done properly, the tissues can quickly lose their support again and all the symptoms a woman had previously will recur.

If your tissues are healthy and you have a surgeon who knows what he or she is doing, you can expect excellent results from this type of operation. Although there is some discomfort for a few days after surgery, most patients do not find it a terribly uncomfortable procedure.

The surgical technique and recovery from this problem is described in Q. 171–173.

**702** **Why can't I have vaginal repair done without a hysterectomy?**

It is not ordinarily effective to have vaginal repair work done without a hysterectomy because repair of the bladder cannot be handled as well if the uterus is in the way during the operation. The bladder is attached to the uterus and this is what causes the problem. In addition to this practicality, if you became pregnant later and had a vaginal delivery, it would tear down the repair. A "re-repair" of the vagina is difficult and is more likely to be unsuccessful. If, however, you have enough problems with your vaginal looseness to warrant surgery, but you may still want children later, you could have a repair done and have a cesarean section for a later delivery.

### 703 I have heard of Kegel's exercises for vaginal looseness. What are they?

If a woman has symptoms of vaginal relaxation but does not want surgery, she can do Kegel's (pronounced Kay'-gulls) exercises. The late Arnold Kegel, M.D., clinical professor of gynecology at the University of Southern California School of Medicine, developed strengthening exercises for the pubococcygeus muscles. These muscles are shaped like a sling that goes from the front to the back of the pelvis and holds the abdominal and pelvic contents up in place. The urethra, vagina, and rectum are like tubes poking down through this sling of muscle to get to the outside. When these muscles become weak, the vagina, rectum, and urethra lose their support. Strengthening these muscles can give better support to those tissues.

The exercise consists of doing the same tightening movement (and hold it for a second or two) that you would make if you would purposely stop your urine flow. One does not need to be urinating to tighten these muscles, but to learn which muscles need to be contracted for Kegel's exercise it is helpful for a woman to begin urinating and then shut off the flow by tightening her muscles. Once she has discovered which muscles are tightened to stop urine flow, she has discovered how to do a Kegel's exercise! I encourage a patient to think in terms of tightening the muscles all the way around to her anus so that, in essence, she is tightening her whole "bottom" when she does the exercise.

Also, a device which gives battery-powered, electronic stimulation to the mus-

cles of the pelvis is available for use in strengthening these muscles. It is called Vagitone and is available through the manufacturer (Gyn-O-Tek, Inc., P.O. Box 29017, Portland, Oregon 97229-0017).

This stimulus to the pelvic muscles is not shocking or painful, nor is it administered with needles. The device consists of a tampon-shaped tube that can be inserted in a woman's vagina, stimulating her pelvic muscles to contract. The degree of involuntary muscle contractions can be increased or decreased with a dial. I have had only a few patients use this device, but it does seem to strengthen pelvic muscles effectively.

### 704 Are Kegel's exercises effective?

If a woman will do these exercises for twelve weeks, she will often gain the vaginal tightness she wants and will not have to do the exercises thereafter. It takes real commitment, however, to do the exercises effectively and consistently.

A woman needs to do three hundred contractions a day. I suggest to my patients that they do them in six groups of fifty each. These exercises can be done while riding in a car, watching TV, or even while having intercourse. Such contractions can be quite stimulating to a man but can be a distraction for the woman.

In all honesty, I find that most women will not do these exercises adequately and that many who claim they have done them do not get much improvement in pubococcygeal muscle strength. There are others, however, who find them a great deal of help, and I continue to recommend these exercises to patients.

Women who do Kegel's exercises often have an unexpected pleasure in store: better sexual responsiveness. Dr. Kegel became interested in this aspect of his exercises when some patients returned to him to say that although they had never had an orgasm before, after doing his exercises they became orgasmic. Therefore, books dealing with sexual problems will often be found to suggest Kegel's exercises as a partial solution to failure to achieve orgasm.

## 705 What types of growths can occur in the vagina?

There are a number of different types of growths which can occur on the vaginal walls. Premalignant and malignant growths can develop (see Q. 709–712) as can nonmalignant growths and cysts. None of these occur often, however. When they do, they are usually easily diagnosed and treated. The most common growths that occur in the vagina are: cysts and polyps, endometriosis, adenosis, and condyloma.

Any growth that is uncomfortable, protrudes from the vagina, or causes any problems can be surgically removed. Such surgery usually requires general anesthesia. After surgery the patient ordinarily has no discomfort and no problem with recovery. For further information on the above growths and treatment, see Q. 706–712.

## 706 What is a Gartner's duct cyst?

Of the cysts and polyps that can occur in the vagina (fibro-epithelial polyp, leiomyoma, dermoid cysts, and Gartner's duct cysts) the most common is the Gartner's duct cyst.

A Gartner's duct cyst seems to arise from tissue "left over" from fetal life that would have been part of the sperm-carrying tubes if the fetus had developed into a male. It has recently been found that many of these cysts come from remnants of female-type fetal tissue that lines the vagina rather than male-type tissue. These tissues generally lie dormant as mere fragments of tissue resting in the vaginal walls. Occasionally, though, enough of this tissue may be present to col-

lect fluid and form a cyst. This type of cyst is known as a Gartner's duct cyst.

Gartner's duct cysts are not painful, but they can be quite large and there can be more than one of them. They do not become malignant, and if they do not bother the woman, surgery is not indicated.

Your doctor can tell the difference between a polyp and a cyst by looking. If you are told that you have a polyp or growth in your vagina, you should have it removed even if you cannot feel it. However, if the doctor tells you that you have a "cyst" that needs to be removed, and it is not causing you any pain or discomfort, you should ask if it is a Gartner's duct cyst. If it is, you can feel quite confident in telling your doctor that you do not want it removed. If he or she insists, it would probably be best to get a second opinion.

## 707 What is endometriosis of the vagina?

The most common cause of this condition is endometriosis up inside the pelvic structures that has grown through the wall behind the uterus into the vagina. Such endometriosis can cause pain with intercourse, and a woman with this type of endometriosis will often have bleeding from this tissue. She would ordinarily not know this, however, because she would usually bleed only during her period, at which time she could not differentiate between endometriosis bleeding and the menstrual blood from her cervix. A woman with vaginal endometriosis may have more symptoms, such as pain with intercourse or pain with menstrual periods, than a woman whose endometriosis is contained inside her pelvic structures.

Occasionally a woman may have vaginal endometriosis because the endometrial tissue which comes out with her menstrual flow can "seed" an irritated area of the vagina, such as broken-down episiotomy or a tear in the vaginal wall, and start growing there. Such endometriosis would most easily be treated by the laser, a freezing instrument, or excision with scissors or knife.

If the endometriosis is perforating through the upper vagina from inside the pelvis, treatment is much different. The doctor may prescribe Danocrine, a hormone which will usually cause the endometriosis to stop growing. Or, if a woman is having a great deal of trouble with endometriosis and does not want any more children, hysterectomy, with removal of tubes and ovaries, is probably the best treatment. For further information about endometriosis, see Q. 174–179, 953–960.

If treatment with Danocrine is not successful and a hysterectomy is not desired, it is possible to have surgery to cut out the endometriosis and leave the uterus, tubes, and ovaries. But this is difficult for the surgeon to do, and such surgery does not always get rid of all the endometriosis.

---

## 708   What is adenosis?

Adenosis is a situation in which small areas of the normal vaginal lining are replaced by a lining that is like the lining of the inside of the cervical canal. Most of the time adenosis occurs in women who were exposed to DES in their mother's womb, but occasionally women who have not had such exposure can have small patches of adenosis in their upper vaginas. (See Q. 212.)

Most women who have adenosis are not even aware of its presence. The first indication they have of the problem is usually during a checkup when a doctor discovers it.

Most good physicians feel that no treatment is necessary for these small areas of adenosis. However, just as a doctor watches

your cervix for the development of cancer, so will he or she watch these small areas. You do not have your cervix removed just because there is a possibility of developing cancer of the cervix. Likewise you do not need to have adenosis taken out just because it is structurally similar to the lining of the cervical canal and thus capable of cancer.

Occasionally, however, adenosis can cause a discharge just as the cervix can develop profuse mucus discharge. If this does not bother a woman, she can leave it alone. If it does become a problem to her, she can get it treated. Treatment is most easily done with the laser. The laser can be used to "wipe away" this adenosis much like a pencil eraser can remove markings on a piece of paper. If your doctor does not have access to a laser, he or she can cut out the area or use a freezing machine to get rid of it.

If you are treated with a laser or a freezing machine, the doctor can do these procedures in the office. I prefer use of the laser for this type of abnormality. Since not all physicians have a laser instrument in their office, probably you would go to a hospital for such treatment. If the abnormality is at the top of the vagina, treatment does not usually cause enough pain to require any anesthetic. If it is in the lower part of the vagina, it would usually require a local anesthetic. Your doctor might suggest that you have a general anesthetic for the procedure. The laser is a machine which emits an extremely hot ray which vaporizes away the abnormal tissue and yet leaves the tissue that is immediately under that abnormal tissue undisturbed and undamaged. Healing is faster after laser treatment than after either freezing or surgical excision. Surgical excision definitely requires general anesthesia.

My principal warning concerning adenosis is that if you have it and are having no trouble with it, you can afford to be a little skeptical about any suggestion to have it removed. If a doctor insists on its removal, it would probably be wise to get a second opinion.

## 709 Are precancerous or cancerous growths in the vagina common?

Both precancerous and cancerous growths can occur in the vagina, but they do so rarely. Their frequency has increased during the past thirty years, however, just as the frequency of cancers of the vulva and cervix has increased, apparently due to the rising incidence of condyloma infections.

Precancerous changes of the lining of the vagina are called vaginal intraepithelial neoplasia (VAIN). Most often this precancerous type of growth is present in association with a woman's cancer of the cervix or the vulva. All these abnormalities are more likely to occur after menopause.

## 710 How is a precancerous or cancerous growth of the vagina discovered?

Precancerous (see Q. 669) or cancerous growths of the vagina might show up as abnormal vaginal bleeding—such as bleeding after intercourse, between periods, or after menopause—or as red or brown vaginal discharge. Most of the time, however, precancerous growths are found on routine Pap smears, with no symptoms at all having occurred.

If a woman has an abnormal Pap smear, the physician will do a colposcopy (see Q. 751) to magnify the cervix. As the cervix is viewed, the doctor will usually look carefully at the vagina with the colposcope and can then biopsy any abnormal area of the vagina, just as would be done with abnormalities of the cervix. Because the area is magnified, only a very small piece of tissue is necessary for an adequate biopsy; therefore such a biopsy is not very painful.

## 711 How is a precancerous vaginal growth treated?

If the doctor finds a precancerous growth of the vagina, treatment is necessary. The treatment that seems best at this time is laser therapy (see Q. 708), which can be used to wipe away this type of growth on the vaginal wall without penetrating the important underlying structures of the body. Other treatments are available. If the area is small, the doctor might want to use general anesthesia and cut it out. Or a doctor might suggest the use of a cream containing an agent (5-fluorouracil) that will kill cells. This cream can be quite irritating. If you use it you should also use a lot of Vaseline on the vulva to avoid irritation.

## 712 How are cancerous growths of the vagina treated?

If cancer is present, you should consult with a specialist in gynecologic cancer (gynecologic oncologist). If your doctor is not an expert in the treatment of vaginal cancer, he or she should refer you to an experienced physician in that field.

The main reason for great care in this treatment is that radiation is usually used, and if it is not given properly, it can cause holes between the vagina and the bladder or between the vagina and the rectum. (See Q. 696–698.) Also, surgery is occasionally indicated for this type of cancer. As it is major surgery and the decision as to whether or not to do surgery or use radiation is a critical one, it should be made by doctors who have a great deal of experience in this type of treatment.

Vaginal cancer has been found in women who were exposed to DES in their mother's uterus. Because DES affects several parts of the female organs, it is discussed in Q. 208–218.

Most vaginal tumors occur in women

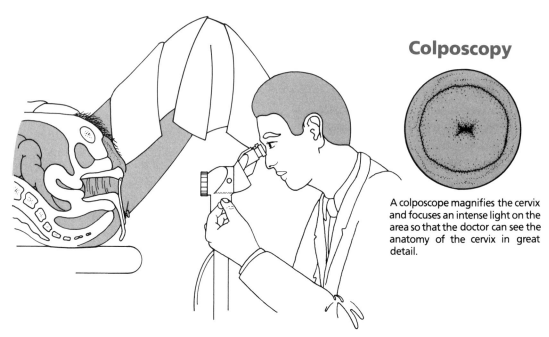

## Colposcopy

A colposcope magnifies the cervix and focuses an intense light on the area so that the doctor can see the anatomy of the cervix in great detail.

who have (or had) precancerous or cancerous cells on the cervix or vulva. It is important, therefore, that careful vaginal examination be done during each annual checkup, especially if a woman has previously had cancer of the cervix or vulva.

Also, if a woman has had a hysterectomy for precancerous cells (an abnormal Pap smear)—but her doctor did not do a colposcopy before surgery to find out exactly where the abnormal cells were on the cervix—she should be even more meticulous about having follow-up Pap smears. If the doctor did not look to see exactly where the precancerous cells were before the surgery, some precancerous cells could have already spread out onto the vaginal lining and have been left behind to continue growing even though a hysterectomy was done.

### 713    What is toxic shock?

Toxic shock is a condition caused by a bacterium called staphylococcus aureus. The most commonly held theory concerning toxic shock is that when this germ grows in the body of a person, either male or female,

who does not have natural immunity (antibodies) against the germ, it produces a chemical called a toxin which spreads through the body and causes severe illness.

Although 5 percent of reproductive-age women have staphylococcus aureus germs in their vaginas, the large majority of such women are immune to the toxin that these staphylococci can produce.

It is important to understand that the staphylococcus aureus germs occur in both men and women, and that their growth and release of toxin can affect them both. Toxic shock syndrome has been reported in both men and nonmenstruating women. Toxic shock has been identified in patients who have staph infections in burns and abrasions, lacerations, abscesses, insect bites, surgical wounds, vaginal deliveries, and abortions.

### 714    How are tampons related to toxic shock?

In 1983 the Texas Department of Health reported that tampon-related cases of toxic shock accounted for 89 percent of all such cases reported in the state.

*Rely* tampons were the most popular high-absorbency tampon when the toxic shock syndrome became most evident, as they had about 50 percent of the high-absorbency tampon market at that time. *Rely* tampons were removed from the market and no tampon with its fiber content is now available. But all types of tampons have been associated to some extent with the development of toxic shock syndrome. (See Q. 717.)

Since foreign objects such as vaginal sponge, diaphragm, and tampon are associated with toxic shock, it seems best that those objects not be left in the vagina any longer than necessary. One recommendation is that tampons be changed at least every six to eight hours.

In 1985 researchers identified two fibers, polyester foam and polyacrylate rayon, found in some super-absorbent tampons, as possible contributing factors to toxic shock syndrome. These fibers have amazing ability to absorb magnesium from the menstrual flow. When the magnesium level in the flow is low, staphylococci organisms (which cause toxic shock syndrome) grow abundantly. Presently this is only theory and must be confirmed by further investigation.

## 715   What symptoms might indicate toxic shock syndrome?

There are a number of toxic shock symptoms that a woman might have. She may

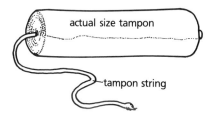

actual size tampon

tampon string

have all or only a few of them, and they may be severe or mild. The symptoms that a woman may watch for, especially during a menstrual period, are these:

| | |
|---|---|
| fever | fainting |
| chills | shockiness |
| vomiting | sore throat |
| diarrhea | sunburnlike rash |
| dizziness | |

In addition, a woman may have a rash on the palms of her hands and the soles of her feet. After a few days she will notice that her palms and soles are scaling (desquamating).

If a woman develops these symptoms, and if they go away and recur when she has another menstrual period, she should see her doctor and suggest that she might have toxic shock syndrome. About 3 percent of toxic shock cases reported have resulted in death. This figure should not alarm you unduly, however, because many of the milder cases are not even reported to doctors, and even when they are, the doctor often does not report them to the local health department.

## 716   What will the doctor do if I have symptoms of toxic shock?

If you report toxic shock symptoms to your doctor, he or she will want to take a culture from your vagina to see if the germ is present. Even if the doctor cannot culture out the organism, treatment with appropriate antibiotics may be prescribed. It may also be suggested—if the infection is not related to a sore in some other part of the body—that you stop using tampons. If women are treated with appropriate antibiotics and stop using tampons, toxic shock recurs only about 18 percent of the time. If the use of tampons continues, even when antibiotics have been given, there will be a recurrence 72 percent of the time.

If you are fainting, have a high fever, and are quite sick, the doctor will admit you to a hospital because it is possible that you will become severely ill or die from this infection. In the hospital, cultures will be taken of your vagina and other body parts. You will receive antibiotics in large doses through your veins and also fluids in your veins to help with any shock that you might be developing.

**717** **In view of the toxic shock syndrome, should I use tampons?**

Most physicians, including myself, do not advise patients to stop using tampons. (See Q. 682.) Though the toxic shock syndrome can occur, it certainly does not occur very often. The chance of a reproductive-age woman developing toxic shock syndrome is about 10 out of 10,000 per year. I have been practicing for almost twenty years and have had only one patient in whom I absolutely confirmed the presence of toxic shock.

My advice is that women continue to use tampons, but not high-absorbency tampons. Studies have shown that women who use the less-absorbent tampons definitely have a smaller risk of developing toxic shock syndrome.

I recommend that those women who worry about toxic shock, and who cannot get it out of their minds, either stop using tampons completely or alternate a tampon with a pad during menstruation, or perhaps use tampons during the day and pads at night.

**718** **Are vaginal injuries common? What things might injure my vagina?**

Although they can happen, vaginal injuries are relatively uncommon. They can occur in the following situations.

*Tampons.* Some women develop ulcers in their upper vaginas from the use of tampons. Usually they are not aware of such ulcers and learn of them only at the time of their routine exams. Occasionally a patient will have a little bleeding from such an ulcer and the ulcer will be found when she sees her doctor for the bleeding. Such ulcers do not seem to be dangerous and clear up when a woman stops using tampons. Once the ulcer is gone, a woman may resume use of tampons if she desires, but she needs to change the direction and depth of insertion. She should see her gynecologist after a couple of months to be sure she is not producing another ulcer.

*Intercourse.* On rare occasions a vagina can be torn during normal intercourse. Symptoms of such a tear are pain with intercourse followed by bleeding from the vagina. A doctor may or may not need to stitch the torn area.

*Rape.* Injuries of the vagina can occur with rape, but this is normally a problem only in young girls who have not yet begun their menses.

*Sharp objects.* Falling on a sharp object can cause vaginal lacerations. If this occurs, a woman would see her doctor for evaluation. He or she would suture any torn area, if necessary. Normally such suturing requires general anesthesia.

*Tears.* Tears of the vagina occur most commonly during delivery. This type of injury was discussed in Q. 602. A competent obstetrician will be able to repair any vaginal tear to insure good healing and minimal loss of blood.

If you (or your daughter) have a vaginal injury, it is important that you seek medical help and that the physician do a very gentle and complete examination. Such an exam, especially of a child, will often require general anesthetic. (See Q. 59–61, 680.)

Occasionally an injury to the vaginal area will result only in a large bruise, called a hematoma. It does not normally need to be drained since such blood will usually be absorbed. If the hematoma is too large, however, the doctor will need to open it and let it drain. General anesthesia may be required.

---

## 719 Is it normal to have pain during intercourse? Should I tell my doctor about it?

If you are having pain with intercourse (dyspareunia), it is important that you tell your doctor. This type of pain is probably not an indication of a serious problem, but it should be dealt with. Pain with intercourse can almost always be relieved.

Occasional pain with intercourse is normal. When your husband pushes into the upper part of your vagina with his penis, it may sometimes catch your uterus, your ovary, or your colon in just the right way to cause pain. This type of pain may be a sharp stabbing sensation, sudden severe cramping, or just a pain deep in your pelvis. The pain may persist for a while (a few minutes or a few hours), but usually goes away fairly quickly.

Often, all a man or woman needs to do to stop this type of pain is to shift position a little bit during intercourse. If the pain is more intense, more constant, and more bothersome than the above so-called normal pain, a woman should certainly have the problem checked.

A recent study showed that the most common age for women to have painful intercourse is from thirty to fifty-five years. The conclusion from this study was that as women fall into an intercourse routine through the years, they become less stimulated, have inadequate lubrication, and begin having dryness and superficial discomfort with intercourse. Women in this age group are often embarrassed by the fact that they are experiencing pain with intercourse, since they have been having intercourse for years and feel they should be able to have it

without pain. They should, however, tell their doctor of such pain. Intercourse should be a gratifying and pleasant experience; if you are having pain it cannot be all it should be. More importantly, if you are having pain with intercourse you will subconsciously avoid it. Such a problem can trigger conflict between you and your husband because he will feel that you are rejecting him, even though you explain the problem.

If you are having discomfort with intercourse, it is important that you discuss it with both your husband and your doctor.

---

## 720 What things can cause painful intercourse, and what can be done to solve these problems?

The problems that can cause pain with intercourse and the cures for those problems are discussed in the next nine questions. They are:

fear of intercourse

vaginal dryness

vaginal infections

physical problems

childbirth-related problems

pelvic abnormalities

pelvic congestion

intrauterine device (IUD)

The size of a man's penis does not cause continued painful intercourse. The vagina can stretch to accommodate whatever size penis a woman's husband has. This is illustrated by the distensibility of the vagina, allowing the passage of a baby's head in delivery.

Some women also believe, because they have been told so, that painful intercourse is caused by a tipped or retroverted uterus. One-third of all women have a tipped uterus. It is a perfectly "normal" position for the uterus and is almost never the cause of painful intercourse.

### 721 Can fear, or aversion, actually cause intercourse to be painful?

Yes. Some women have not dealt well with their sexuality and enter marriage with a distorted view of their bodies, sex, or men. There are many reasons why a woman might enter marriage unprepared for the cooperation with a man that is necessary for comfortable, happy sexual activity. The independence and self-assertiveness that is so valued by our society can be a factor in this. Distorting, and failing to understand, the healthy biblical view of sex can color a woman's attitude toward sex. Finally, a lack of adequate sex education can inhibit a healthy sex life. Doctors are finding more and more that women who have aversion to intercourse, with related problems, often have that aversion because of previous rape or sexual molestation.

Many experts who write about sexual problems often attribute such difficulties to a woman being "overly religious" and inhibited. Actually, it has recently been shown that the healthier a woman's relationship with God is, the happier will be her sex life. (See chapter 14.)

### 722 What can be done to help overcome fear of, or an aversion to, intercourse?

It is important that every couple planning marriage have premarital counseling and that every woman have a pelvic examination before marriage. Such counseling and exams can eliminate most of the concern about intercourse that couples have on entering marriage.

After marriage, if there is pain with each act of intercourse, even after several weeks,

you need some help. If you do not get help, you can end up with a serious marital problem. First, you should see your doctor and have another examination to be sure that you have no abnormalities in your pelvic structures. He or she may be able to suggest some logical approaches to the problem. One of these suggestions may include having your husband come to the doctor's office with you, so that the doctor can show him how to gently dilate your vagina with progressively larger vaginal dilators. As soon as you are able to tolerate the largest dilator, you may be able to resume intercourse comfortably.

If the doctor is not successful in helping you, or doesn't know how to help, you should be referred to a good sexual counselor. (See Q. 1199, 1210.)

### 723 If vaginal dryness is causing painful intercourse, how should this be treated?

Vaginal dryness can result from decreased lubrication. It is normal for a woman to have less lubrication immediately after a period, after menopause, and if she is not very sexually excited. If discomfort during intercourse is only a result of poor lubrication at those special times, you can assume that you are normal. Merely use a lubricant (Maxilube, or Ortho's Personal Lubricant) when you need it and don't worry about anything being wrong.

If such lubricants are not adequate for a postmenopausal woman, she may need to use some estrogen cream in her vagina. This is available as Premarin vaginal cream and requires a prescription.

### 724 When vaginal infection causes pain with intercourse, what should be done?

The vaginal infection that usually causes pain with intercourse is monilia vaginitis.

(See Q. 692.) Trichomonal vaginitis, which can cause itching in the vagina and vulva, can also cause pain with intercourse. In addition, venereal warts (condyloma) located at the entrance to the vagina can cause painful intercourse.

A vaginal infection should be treated by a doctor. When the infection is cleared, the pain normally stops.

## 725 What other physical problems might cause painful intercourse?

With first intercourse, the hymen separates into small projections of tissue that are left just inside the entrance to the vagina. These segments of hymenal tissue occasionally become irritated or tender.

A Bartholin's gland infection can also cause painful intercourse. (See Q. 676–678.)

Abnormalities of the hymen and vagina can cause pain, especially with first intercourse. It is problems of this type that a doctor can find at the premarital examination.

The treatment of a physical problem causing painful intercourse is, of course, based on the nature of the problem. The important thing is to see your doctor for a pelvic examination. If the doctor cannot see an abnormality and cannot tell exactly where you are hurting, you should feel around in your vagina until you find the spot that is uncomfortable and identify it for the doctor.

## 726 What problems associated with pregnancy and childbirth can cause painful intercourse?

Many women find intercourse during the last two or three months of pregnancy uncomfortable and at times even painful, but it is not dangerous. This is due to the swelling of the vaginal and vulvar tissues and the fullness of the pelvic structures because of the presence of the baby and the enlarged uterus.

Episiotomies or tears of the vagina heal with some scarring and this can cause pain with intercourse, usually worse if a woman is nursing. If such pain persists for more than a year or two, it might be necessary for the doctor to cut out an area of scar and try to sew it up in such a way that there will be less scar remaining in the area. This is unusual, however, and I have done it on only one or two patients in my entire time of practice.

One of the most common causes of painful intercourse related to childbirth is that which occurs when a woman is nursing. During lactation, the pituitary gland suppresses the production of estrogen from the ovaries and stimulates the production of milk from the breasts. This inadequate estrogen causes the vagina to become dry and sensitive. In fact, this happens so often that I warn every nursing mother that she will probably have painful intercourse and should use a vaginal lubricant.

## 727 How is painful intercourse related to pelvic abnormalities?

It is relatively common for a sudden onset of severe pain during intercourse to be the first major sign of an ectopic (tubal) pregnancy. Occasionally patients who have painful intercourse are found to have a growth on an ovary or in their uterus. There are three other pelvic problems that can cause painful intercourse.

*Loss of uterine support.* If the uterus has lost its support and is dropping down in the vagina, intercourse can be painful because the man's penis pushes directly on a uterus that is too low in the vagina.

*Congested uterus.* If the uterus becomes congested, swollen, or has adenomyosis, it can be tender during intercourse.

*Damaged uterine ligaments.* The ligaments that support the uterus can be damaged at childbirth. Subsequently those damaged tissues can cause intercourse to be painful. Such a situation is often called the "pelvic congestion syndrome." (See next question.)

The treatment for any pelvic problem causing painful intercourse is determined by the nature of the problem. Growths of the ovaries or uterus that are causing pain normally need to be removed; infections of the tubes can be treated with antibiotics; and an ectopic pregnancy must be surgically removed.

If painful intercourse is related to prolapse of the uterus, or to tears in, or varicose veins of, the supporting ligaments of the uterus, hysterectomy may be necessary. Such a hysterectomy is done only for comfort and only when the patient asks for it. A patient certainly should not have a hysterectomy for this reason alone until she has had all the children she wants. If a woman does not want more children, a hysterectomy is the best treatment for most of these problems, assuming the pain is severe enough to warrant it.

If a patient wants more children and does not want a hysterectomy, the doctor may be able to provide some less effective treatment that can at least be a stopgap measure. A fallen uterus, for instance, can be suspended; tears in the supporting structures of the uterus can be sewn up with surgery through an abdominal incision; and endometriosis can normally be removed, leaving the uterus and at least part of an ovary and tube intact. If the pain is only intermittent and does not come too often, pain pills can be useful and may be all that is necessary.

---

## 728 What is pelvic congestion? How does it cause painful intercourse?

Pelvic congestion usually occurs in women who have had several children. The supporting structures of the uterus, tubes, and ovaries have become weakened and have allowed the veins around the uterus to be-come swollen and distended. These varicose-type veins cause swelling and sensitivity of the tissues supporting the uterus. The treatment for this problem is normally hysterectomy. Most women are able to tolerate the problem of pelvic pressure and of painful intercourse one way or another until their families are complete. Then, if the problem is bad enough and they desire it, they can have surgery.

Another theory for the cause of pelvic congestion, and one often discussed by authorities on sexual problems, is a woman's failure to have orgasm with intercourse. The theory is that a woman's continued failure to have orgasm with intercourse causes congestion in the pelvic structures. The suggestion is that a woman should learn to have an orgasm. Supposedly, the contractions of the female organs during orgasm squeeze the swelling out of the tissues and allow them to return to their uncongested state. This may or may not be true, but the suggested treatment is beneficial for a husband/wife relationship anyway.

If a woman is having intercourse and not having orgasm, she is not experiencing the pleasure and joy of intercourse as fully as she could. For this reason, if for no other, she should consult her physician or sexual counselor to learn techniques for intercourse that will allow her fuller enjoyment of the pleasure that intercourse has to offer. See chapter 14 for some suggestions about this.

---

## 729 Can IUDs, or intrauterine contraceptive devices, cause painful intercourse?

Women who have IUDs will occasionally have pain with intercourse. Apparently, the IUD can make the uterus more irritable, and intercourse with an IUD present can cause the uterus to contract very strongly. These contractions are felt by a woman as pain.

If a woman knows that the IUD is the

cause of the pain and she can tolerate it, it is fine for her to keep it in. If the pain is bothersome enough to make her dread having intercourse, she should get the IUD removed and use some other method of contraception. Of course, if painful intercourse or low abdominal pain from her IUD is accompanied by fever, the IUD must be removed and antibiotics taken to prevent what is obviously a uterine infection from getting out of control.

## Problems of the Cervix

The cervix is the mouth—lower part, entrance—of the uterus. It is not just a "mouth," however. In newborn babies the cervix makes up five-sixths of the entire uterus! During adolescence, because of hormone stimulation, the upper part of the uterus (called the fundus) grows proportionately more than the cervix. By the time a girl starts her first period, the fundus is approximately equal in size to the cervix. When a woman reaches adulthood, and before menopause, her cervix represents the lower one-third of her uterus.

The cervix is not as passive a part of the body as it might seem. When the cervix allows the flow of menstrual fluid from the uterus it is being passive, but its production of cervical mucus is an active process. Cervical mucus is the fluid through which the sperm swim up into the uterus to allow fertilization to occur. Through a wonderfully selective process, sperm are allowed passage through the cervix while germs are not. Once the sperm are in the uterus, the cervical mucus becomes thick and sticky, sealing off the outside world so that, if a pregnancy occurs, it is safe from outside interference. (See Q. 91–95, 291, 292.)

When pregnancy does occur, the cervix is

# Cervix

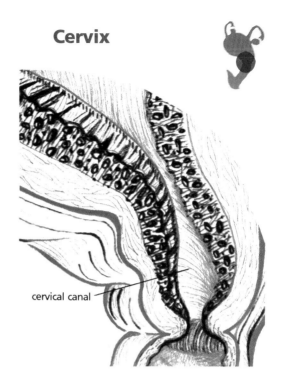

cervical canal

able to stay closed until labor causes it to dilate. Before dilation, the cervix is so small that nothing larger than a small straw can go through its opening. It is so elastic, though, that labor can stretch it enough to allow the passage of a full-term baby.

The elasticity of the cervix allows it to close back up after delivery so that within just a few days, nothing—not a tampon, a penis, or anything larger than one-eighth of an inch in diameter—can normally get into the uterus through the cervix!

Both before and after one's reproductive age, the cervix is relatively inactive; it does little more than protect the inside of the uterus by the small amount of mucus it produces. For more information on the cervix see Q. 19.

## 730 Do I need to do anything in particular to keep my cervix healthy?

There are three things you can do to help insure that your cervix stays healthy and normal.

Have a pelvic exam and Pap smear done on a yearly basis. The Pap smear is a screening procedure that can help prevent your developing cancer of the cervix, and the examination can make sure that you do not have polyps or growths on the cervix. (See Q. 741–752.)

Have intercourse with your husband only. Since precancerous and cancerous cells of the cervix, herpes, gonorrhea, and many other infections are sexually transmitted, you will probably not contract these if you or your husband have intercourse only with each other. (See Q. 747.)

Have your doctor leave your cervix alone if it doesn't need treatment! If treatment is necessary, make sure as little as possible is done to your cervix. See the next question.

### 731 What conditions of the cervix might better be left alone?

Three fairly common conditions that are better left alone are: cervical erosion (ectropion), leukoplakia, and Nabothian cysts. These three problems are discussed in the following three questions.

### 732 What is cervical erosion?

The technical terms are *ectropion* and *eversion*. When a doctor looks at your cervix, he or she will often see a reddish discoloration immediately around the opening of the cervix. This is most commonly called an erosion and is a normal finding, it is the lining from the inside of the cervix spreading out from the cervical opening onto the external surface of the cervix. The color of this epithelial lining from the inside of the cervix (columnar epithelium) is more red than the lining of the rest of the external cervix (stratified squamous epithelium) because it is more delicate and its small blood vessels are closer to the surface. The juncture of these

two linings (squamocolumnar junction) is usually a distinct and abrupt line that makes a circle around the opening, or just inside the opening, of the cervix. It is the red color of the columnar epithelium that led to this finding being erroneously named *erosion*. It is more properly an *ectropion* or, if a woman has had a baby in the past and the cervix tends to gape open, an *eversion*. However, erosion is in such common usage, even by physicians, that I am sure it will continue to be used.

Let me repeat, though, that this finding is normal and does not need any treatment so long as the Pap smear is normal and there is no cervical infection producing excessive, bothersome amounts of mucus.

It has been shown that if women have this area frozen or cauterized, there is a slightly lower chance of their developing cancer of the cervix, but such treatment can itself cause problems. At any rate, a woman still needs to have a Pap smear done every year, a procedure that would catch a precancerous condition if one should develop, whether or not she has had freezing or cautery of the cervix.

Routine treatment of a normal ectropion, therefore, accomplishes little, and most physicians who have studied this situation feel that routine freezing or cautery of a cervix that is otherwise normal is a waste of a patient's money and is not the best practice.

### 733 What is leukoplakia of the cervix?

Leukoplakia means "white patch." Occasionally a woman will have an area of the cervix that looks as though someone has painted it white. When this occurs, the same approach should be taken as is recommended for cervical erosion—nothing.

In years past, leukoplakia was thought to be premalignant, but we now know that it is not. A Pap smear will ordinarily be able to scrape off enough cells to assure you and your doctor that the white patches are normal. The doctor may want to use the colposcope (see p. 420) to look at the area, and may even want to biopsy it. This is good practice. Your doctor does not need to do a conization (excising a wedge of tissue) or hysterectomy because of these white patches. As a matter of fact, he or she does not need to do anything to get rid of leukoplakia permanently. At most, the patches just need to be evaluated each year.

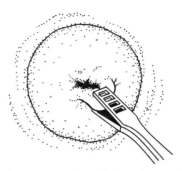

If the colposcope reveals an obvious abnormality of the cervix, small pieces of it may be removed for microscopic examination (biopsied).

### 734 What is a cervical Nabothian cyst?

It is fairly common for a woman to find a small hard nodule on her cervix. It may be discovered in feeling around in the vagina for a "lost" tampon, in checking for an IUD string, or in making sure a diaphragm is in the right position. If you feel a nodule, you can be fairly sure that it is a Nabothian cyst. I have never found a nodule discovered by a patient to be anything else except, rarely, a wart of the cervix.

Nabothian cysts on the cervix are extremely common. They are like acne of the face in that they are glands, in this case mucus glands, with their openings stopped up, trapping the mucus and forming small, round nodules. Since these are not precancerous, dangerous, nor painful, they do not need to be treated. They may vary in size from pea-sized to a half inch in diameter.

Cervical cancers, by the way, are usually soft growths that bleed easily. It is unlikely that a woman would be able to feel a cervical cancer until it had gotten extremely large, perhaps as much as half the size of a hen's egg. By this time she would have had abnormal vaginal bleeding for weeks.

### 735 Can my cervix become infected? What should be done if it does?

Yes, the cervix can become infected. Such an infection is called cervicitis. A persistent discharge of mucus (similar to what you might have from your nose with infected sinuses) might indicate a cervical infection. This type of discharge does not ordinarily cause itching.

The only way that you can know for sure whether or not you have a cervical infection is to see your doctor. When you are examined, it may be found that your cervix is slightly swollen, red, and producing infected mucus. Often when the doctor touches the infected cervix, it will bleed easily. In fact, you may have had bleeding after intercourse as a result of this infection.

The doctor will usually want to do both a Pap smear and a cervical biopsy. A biopsy is necessary because cervical cancer can look exactly like, and produce the same type secretions as, cervicitis. A Pap smear is occasionally not reliable when taken from a cervical cancer that is far enough along to be producing infected-looking discharge because the Pap smear will occasionally pick up only the mucus and no cancer cells.

After the examination, the Pap smear, and possibly biopsies, the doctor will probably treat your infection with a vaginal cream containing an antibiotic. If the infection persists, he or she may need to treat your cervix with an instrument that kills the infection by freezing the area (a cryocone). The doctor may prefer using the laser on your cervicitis, especially if you have not had all the children you want. This is because the laser leaves less scar on the cervix as it heals. Occasionally doctors will use cautery on the cervix. This is acceptable but slightly outdated treatment. (See Q. 740.)

If your cervix is markedly infected, the doctor would always treat you with medication first. To use the cryo, laser, or cautery on an inflamed cervix could cause it to flare up, producing a dangerous uterine infection.

It is possible for a woman to have a sudden onset of cervical infection. This situation would ordinarily be caused by a sexually transmitted disease such as gonorrhea or herpes. In this situation there would be a sudden onset of vaginal discharge, and there would be pelvic pressure or heaviness, perhaps with the feeling of needing to urinate more frequently. If you develop these symptoms, you should go to the doctor and have cultures done at the time the examination is performed. You will be treated according to the findings. See chapter 13, Sexually Transmitted Disease.

---

## 736 What types of benign (nonmalignant) polyps and growths can be present on the cervix?

There are four: cervical polyps, endometriosis, fibroid tumors, and venereal warts.

These conditions are discussed in the following four questions.

---

## 737 What is a cervical polyp? How is it treated?

The most frequent type of benign abnormality that occurs on the cervix is a cervical polyp. These polyps are usually small (up to one-fourth inch in diameter); they are red and usually bleed easily when touched; and they are not dangerous. Most of the time women do not even know that they are present, and the doctor may discover them protruding from the cervical opening at the time of an annual exam. Occasionally a woman will experience bleeding with intercourse as the first indication of a cervical polyp.

Premenopausal women seldom have cervical polyps that are malignant, although they can occur. A cervical polyp that is found in a postmenopausal woman is more likely to be a malignant growth because cancer of the inside of the uterus is more likely to occur in postmenopausal women and to show up as a polyp at the cervical opening.

Benign polyps of this type are normally a result of infection in the glands of the cervical canal. This type of infection does not need to be treated and is merely producing an irritation of the glands in that area of the cervix.

To treat a polyp, all a doctor needs to do is to grasp the growth with an instrument and twist it off. There is almost no bleeding with this procedure. Such polyps may or may not grow back. If they do recur, it is not a bad sign.

---

## 738 What is cervical endometriosis? How is it treated?

Endometriosis is uterine-lining-type tissue that is growing in the wrong place. Since that type of tissue responds to hormones, it builds up during the month. Then at menstrual time, as the hormone levels are lowered in the body, it bleeds. Endometriosis on the cervix will do the same thing. These growths are usually small—no more than one-eighth to one-fourth inch across—and usually look like "blood blisters."

Women normally do not know they have endometriosis of the cervix unless told so by their physicians.

Treatment consists of a biopsy, to be sure it actually is endometriosis. Such a biopsy usually removes the entire growth; occasionally a biopsy must be followed by use of the freezing machine, cautery, or laser to destroy all the abnormal tissue.

This condition rarely occurs and is usually not a problem, though extensive cervical endometriosis can be a factor in a woman's infertility.

## 739 What are cervical fibroid tumors? How are they treated?

If a woman has fibroid tumors growing inside her uterine cavity, the uterus will try to "deliver" that fibroid by contracting and working it down and out of the uterus, resulting in abnormal vaginal bleeding. The fibroid may even finally protrude from the cervical opening. When this happens, its blood supply may be partly pinched off, causing the fibroid to swell.

This type of problem frequently requires a hysterectomy. The fibroid may be attached so high in the uterus that it is impossible to take it out without doing a hysterectomy. Occasionally, however, a fibroid will be so small that the doctor may be able to put a wire loop around it, run the loop up to the base of the fibroid inside the uterus, and pinch the base off. This must be done under general anesthesia in the operating room. Bleeding can be so heavy from an attempted vaginal removal of such a fibroid that a hysterectomy is still necessary.

If your doctor suggests a hysterectomy for this problem and you have all the children you want, it is probably best to have it done to get rid of the fibroid without attempting partial removal. If you definitely want to remain fertile, the doctor can make an incision in your abdomen, split your uterus open, and usually safely cut the fibroid off at its base. (See Q. 770–777.)

## 740 What are cervical venereal warts?

Venereal warts (condyloma) can grow on the vulva, vagina, or cervix. Most of the time condyloma are a sexually transmitted disease, but sometimes a patient will have condyloma that are not transmitted by sexual intercourse. (See Q. 1138–1144.)

Treatment of condyloma of the cervix is the same as that of the vagina or the vulva except that podophyllum must be used with care on the vagina or cervix. Podophyllum can be put on a patient's cervical warts if the warts are small and do not require too much podophyllum. Too much podophyllum in a patient's vagina can be toxic to her. Of course, podophyllum cannot be used if a woman is pregnant. (See Q. 424.) The freezing machine can be used on cervical warts. If a woman is pregnant, the laser is the best treatment technique. Not only does it get rid of the condyloma, it also seals the blood vessels to prevent bleeding as the condyloma are eradicated. The cervix of a pregnant woman is quite vascular and bleeds easily, making it difficult to use any other method of treatment. The freezing machine (cryosurgery) can also be used to treat these warts, and it can be used during pregnancy. This technique involves the use of an instrument that many gynecologists have in their offices. The device has a probe which will freeze tissue. Although injection of a local anesthetic is necessary for treating vulvar warts by either freezing or laser, it is not usually necessary for warts of the vagina or cervix. If the freezing technique is used during pregnancy, it must be done carefully so as not to damage too much tissue and cause excessive bleeding.

## 741 What is a Pap smear?

A Pap smear is a scraping of a woman's cervix or vagina transferred to a glass slide. The scrapings are taken by the doctor with a blunt wooden or plastic stick after visualizing the cervix and vagina with a vaginal speculum. A chemical solution (fixative) is put on the smear before it dries and this preparation is sent to a pathologist.

There are cells from a woman's cervix or vagina in the material that was scraped off, preserved, and sent to the laboratory. If the surface from which the scraping was taken was normal, the cells will look normal to the pathologist. If the cells have been affected by infection such as trichomonas or fungus, or are inflamed by some other infection, the pathologist can usually tell that. If there is a premalignant (see Q. 669) or malignant growth, the pathologist can usually recognize this type of cell.

The Pap smear is named after the late Dr. G. N. Papanicolaou who found, in 1943, that cancerous and precancerous cells could be discovered with a screening test of this kind. The annual Pap smear became a reality for most women during the 1950s, and it has served to prevent a devastating cancer in many, many women since that time.

The surface cells of the body are continually sloughing off as new cells from underneath are growing. The cells that are sloughing off are the ones that are picked up by a Pap smear. If there is a precancerous or cancerous growth present, this area sloughs off cells at a much higher rate, perhaps ten or fifteen times as many cells as the normal tissue around it. This explains why even a small precancerous or cancerous growth on the cervix or vagina can be picked up by a Pap smear.

### 742 Will a vaginal or cervical Pap smear show if I have cancer in any other part of my body?

No. A vaginal or cervical Pap smear is useful only for identifying cancer of the cervix or vagina. Abnormal cells of the cervix almost always start at the squamocolumnar junc-

tion, where the lining of the vagina meets the cells that line the inside of the cervix. This small area, representing a ring of no more than one-half inch, is the origin of almost all the precancerous and cancerous cervical growths that women develop.

To understand the tremendous amount of cellular growth and activity going on there, compare the fact that this area (about the size of one of your fingernails) is responsible for cancer in 2 percent of the female population, while the breasts, which are many hundreds of times larger by comparison, are responsible for cancer in 7 percent of the female population.

### 743 Does a Pap smear hurt?

A Pap smear for many patients is painless. For some women a Pap smear will be painless one year and uncomfortable another year. For others, it will always be uncomfortable. Whether or not it is painful has more to do with the degree of sensitivity of a particular woman's cervix than it does with the technique that a doctor uses in obtaining the Pap smear.

It is important to point out, however, that a Pap smear is taken from both the outer part of the cervix and from the cervical canal that is the opening into the uterus. If the doctor does not scrape both places, he or she is likely to miss a precancerous growth. It is the scraping from the canal that is most likely to be uncomfortable, but it is a vital part of a good Pap smear. I might mention that an excellent newer technique for evaluating the cervical canal involves aspiration of the cervical mucus and smearing that out on a slide.

### 744 How often should a Pap smear be done?

A Pap smear should be done annually. If you have had a hysterectomy, however, a Pap smear every three years is adequate, because a hysterectomy removes the cervix, the most likely source of cancer detectable with a Pap smear.

If you had an abnormal Pap smear for which you were treated, your doctor may suggest that you have Pap smears more frequently for a while. For instance, if I have treated a patient for a precancerous Pap smear, I will have her get a Pap smear every three months until she has had three normal Pap smears. Then I will do one six months later and, if that one is normal, I will have the woman come back every year for a routine Pap smear. If I have a patient who had a precancerous growth on her cervix resulting in a hysterectomy, the same pattern will be followed. Instead of a Pap smear at every third annual exam, I do a Pap smear at every annual exam indefinitely.

If a woman has had a hysterectomy a Pap smear at least every third year is a good idea because it can detect vaginal cancer. If a patient has had a hysterectomy the doctor would scrape the upper vagina, an area much less likely to develop cancer than the cervix. In spite of a Pap smear being necessary only every three years after a hysterectomy, it is still important that you have a routine exam annually to help you know that you do not have breast or ovarian cancer, hypertension, and so on.

In 1980 the American Cancer Society recommended that Pap smears be done only every three years instead of yearly as they had always recommended before. They estimated that this would save patients a total of one billion dollars in the United States each year. While the Society stated that there would be some women who would develop invasive cancer in that three-year period, it felt that since this would not happen often the financial savings was worthwhile. This suggestion were not accepted by gynecologists or medical associations, and few authorities now suggest a Pap smear only every

three years. There are several reasons for this.

A Pap smear can be wrong! If you are getting one only every three years, that means a possibility of a six-year interval with an inaccurate Pap finding.

Having annual Pap smears is wise because the number of women developing abnormal Pap smears is increasing markedly, especially among younger women. This is directly related to the sexual mores of the country. (See Q. 747, 1145.)

About 5 percent of precancerous growths on the cervix will be aggressive, fast-growing tumors. This 5-percent group will be so aggressive that within a year or two these growths can progress from the very earliest precancerous stage to invasive cancer. In 1980 it was not appreciated that such a large percentage of patients could have such fast-growing tumors.

American Cancer Society doctors who recommend the Pap every three years seem to ignore the fact that many other things are accomplished at the annual exam. Most patients have a question about something—a pelvic pain, sexual relationships, contraception, or another aspect of their health care—when they see their doctor annually. In addition, doctors check their blood count and urine and encourage them to do breast self-examination, to exercise, and to eat properly. By seeing patients only every three years, these things could not be accomplished.

---

**745** **My doctor recommends a Pap smear every six months. Is that necessary?**

As mentioned in the previous question, even the fast-growing tumors take a year to two years to develop. An annual Pap smear, therefore, would pick up almost all the precancerous growths of the cervix before they become dangerous, even if they were the fast-growing kind. It is only remotely possible that there might be an occasional cancer that would grow so fast that it would not be found with an annual Pap smear.

Many doctors recommend an exam every six months after a woman has gone through the menopause. However, the chance of developing cancer of the cervix after menopause, if a woman has always had normal Pap smears, is much less than the chance of cervical cancer earlier in her life. There seems to be no reason for a woman to start having exams every six months after the menopause unless she has had abnormal Paps in the past or has some other problem with her cervix or other organs. It is true that as a woman gets older and passes through the menopause, her chance of getting breast cancer increases, but the protection against breast cancer getting out of hand is the breast self-examination and annual mammograms, not more frequent visits to the doctor.

## 746 Can a Pap smear be done while I am having my period or bleeding from the uterus?

Most of the time Pap smears are quite reliable if taken while a woman is bleeding. The fixative that is put on the smear breaks down the red blood cells so that they do not interfere with the pathologist's study of the slides. Because of this, if a patient is having her period when her appointment for a Pap smear rolls around, she can keep her appointment. Many women are a little embarrassed to see their gynecologist while they are having their period, but your doctor sees much more vaginal bleeding when a woman is having a miscarriage or having a baby than you have with your menstrual period. If you can tolerate an exam during your period, it surely will not bother your doctor.

## 747 Is cervical cancer related to sexual intercourse?

Yes, it is! Precancerous or cancerous changes of the cervix are usually a result of sexually transmitted disease. Most gynecologists now feel that the disease that is transmitted is the venereal wart virus (condyloma virus). Researchers are able to grow this type of virus out of many women's cervical cancers. There are many other facts that indicate that precancerous and cancerous growths of the cervix are due to this virus.

Once a woman has condyloma of her cervix, she has up to twelve hundred times greater risk of developing precancerous or cancerous cells in her cervix than a normal person! This is one of the highest risk factors ever described for any precancerous or cancerous growth of the body. It is probably best that if a woman has venereal warts (condyloma) of her cervix it be treated as though it were a precancerous growth.

The human papillomavirus (HPV) infection may be caused by one of several strains of this particular virus. No matter which strain it is, it is almost always passed by sexual intercourse. This explains what doctors have known for years about the character of cervical cancer: it is more likely to occur in women who started having intercourse early and who have had many sexual partners. Prostitutes, for example, have an 8-percent chance of developing cancer of the cervix as opposed to 2 percent for most women.

It has now been shown that the risk for a woman's developing cervical precancerous or cancerous change is directly related to the number of sexual partners that she has had. If she has had two sexual partners, she has doubled her chance of having this type of change of her cervix. If she has three sexual partners during her lifetime, she has three times the normal risk. This pattern continues up to as many sexual partners a woman might have, increasing the chance of having abnormal cells of the cervix by the number of sexual partners a woman has had.

Doctors are fairly sure, therefore, that if a woman never had intercourse, she would almost never develop an abnormal Pap smear due to precancerous or cancerous cells of the cervix. In addition, if neither a woman nor her husband ever had intercourse with anyone else, the woman would probably never develop an abnormal Pap smear due to such cells. If husband or wife had intercourse with someone else, however, he or she may have picked up the virus. Even if the exposure took place years ago, the virus may still be present in his or her body. From the man's body it can pass to his wife, causing precancerous or cancerous growths of the cervix; in the woman it can work in her body to produce that problem many years after exposure. (See Q. 1141, 1145.)

## 748 If I have not had intercourse, do I need to have a Pap smear done?

Virginal patients can develop a cervical cancer called adenocarcinoma occasionally. Therefore most doctors advise all women to begin having Pap smears at the age of twenty. If a woman becomes sexually active only with her husband, and he has never had intercourse with anyone else, she still does not need to worry much about developing precancerous or cancerous changes on her cervix.

I recommend a yearly pelvic exam and Pap smear for virginal women from age twenty on. We do not know all there is to know about this subject yet and there are always factors to consider, such as whether or not a partner is unfaithful or untruthful. In addition, the yearly Pap smear is a good reason to see your doctor on a regular basis. It is just one part of the complete physical examination that is recommended for maintaining good health.

All this information makes the biblical approach to human sexuality seem so logical! God says, on the one hand, that we are not to commit adultery (Exod. 20:14, Matt. 19:18). And yet, on the other hand, we are urged to thoroughly enjoy our marriage partner sexually with the bodies God gave us, with that purpose obviously in mind.

## 749 What can make a Pap smear "abnormal" other than precancerous or cancerous changes of the cervix?

It is true that a pathologist may report your Pap smear as "mildly abnormal" when there is no precancerous change on the cervix. Inflammation can cause your cervical cells to look somewhat abnormal. Trichomonas infection, for instance, can do this. If your cervix has had some inflammation present and a healing process is going on, the healing cells that are produced are growing quite rapidly and can appear to the pathologist to be somewhat abnormal.

The bothersome thing about this is that these slightly abnormal cells can persist. Most gynecologists feel that if such Pap smears persist, a patient should have her cervix evaluated by colposcopy.

## 750 Should I worry if I am told I have an abnormal Pap smear?

First, it is important to realize that an abnormal Pap smear does not mean cancer. The situation is totally different from breast cancer, where doctors are trying to get patients to find an actual cancer early so that it can be treated before it invades the body. With the cervix, we find the cells before they become cancer at all. The stage at which doctors can, and like to, pick up abnormal cells is during the precancerous stage. Obviously, however, malignant cells also can be found with a Pap smear.

Precancerous cells are called cervical intraepithelial neoplasia (CIN) and are graded as to the stage of the abnormality:

CIN I: mild abnormality

CIN II: moderate abnormality

CIN III: severe abnormality

CIN III is the classification that precedes the tissue turning into truly invasive cancer.

Most people are more familiar with another type of Pap-smear classification: Pap I through Pap V. Using that classification scale, Pap I is considered normal and Pap V refers to either dangerous precancerous cells or cells that have already turned into invasive cancer.

It is important to realize that if you have been having Pap smears yearly, an abnormal current Pap smear usually does not mean that you have invasive cancer. Whatever type of cells are on your cervix will probably be treatable, since cervical cancer usually takes several years to develop after the first abnormal cells show up on a Pap smear. Even though this is true, it is important that your doctor make sure that your first abnormal Pap smear be carefully evaluated and your condition be treated if necessary. This is to make sure it is not cancer and to keep it from becoming cancer.

If you have not been having annual Pap smears, an even mildly abnormal one could possibly indicate invasive cancer. A Pap smear taken from an invasive cancer can sometimes be masked by the mucus and infectious debris that often covers it. I say this to encourage you to get an annual Pap smear and also to have your doctor do a thorough evaluation and investigation of any abnormal Pap smear if you have not been having regular Pap smears. Your doctor should assume that even a mildly abnormal Pap smear can be "hiding" cancerous tissue. I have a patient who had a truly aggressive and invasive cancer whose Pap smear was only "mildly abnormal."

## 751 What should be done if I have an abnormal Pap smear?

Fortunately, today the investigation of an abnormal Pap smear is much simpler and involves surgery much less often than in the past. For an abnormal Pap smear, the following plan for diagnosis will be followed by most gynecologists and is the plan that I feel is best.

*Colposcopy.* (See p. 420) The doctor will insert a vaginal speculum and will swab your cervix with vinegar or acetic acid. The acetic acid will cause the abnormal areas of the cervix or vagina to become whiter than the surrounding tissue and make them easier to see. The doctor will then be able to find the area of your vagina or cervix that is producing the abnormal cells.

When this area is identified, the doctor will use biopsy instruments to take a small piece of the worst part of the abnormality and will also scrape the lining of your cervical canal (an endocervical curettage). This procedure checks for abnormal cells in the cervical canal, an area that cannot be seen with the colposcope.

There is usually some mild bleeding. The doctor will put a swab against your cervix to compress the area and slow the bleeding.

Colposcopy is not a very painful procedure for most women. Since the cervix is magnified so greatly, it is necessary to take only minute pinches (biopsies) of tissues. The endocervical scraping hurts a little, but it takes such a short time to do that most women can stand the brief discomfort.

*Conization.* Most of the time a colposcopy is all that is needed. There are several situations, however, in which a conization might be necessary:

If the doctor cannot see all areas of your

cervix adequately or has some question about what is actually seen.

If the squamocolumnar junction (where the linings of the vagina and cervix meet cannot be seen).

If there is any question on the pathologist's report following a colposcopy.

If the scraping from inside the cervical canal shows precancerous cells.

If there is any suspicion that invasive cancer is present.

All these things would make a colposcopy unreliable and make a conization necessary. (See Q. 754.)

---

**752** **If I continue to have abnormal Pap smears but the colposcopy and biopsy findings are normal, what should be done?**

Often when a woman's Pap smear is only slightly abnormal, the colposcopy will not show any abnormality and biopsies that are taken are normal too. In this case the problem is just inflammation. I often suggest to a patient that she let me freeze or laser her cervix to get rid of the inflammation. When this is done, and the Pap smear reverts to normal, she does not have to worry about the Pap smear coming back mildly abnormal year after year.

---

**753** **If my colposcopy is considered reliable and shows that I have a precancerous condition of my cervix, what should be done?**

In this case, the cervix can be treated with several techniques.

*Cryoconization.* This procedure is called a *"cryocone"* because the area killed with the freezing probe is similar to that which would be excised by knife with a conization,

as described in the next question. Cryoconization involves freezing the cervix for about seven minutes. This is done in the doctor's office without anesthetic and is a painless process for most women. After the cervix is frozen, there is a fairly heavy, messy discharge for about a month. I usually have patients refrain from intercourse for three weeks after cryoconization.

Occasionally, as a cervix heals from cryoconization, the cervical opening gets very small (stenotic). This tight cervical opening can make it difficult for a repeat colposcopy to be done in case abnormal Pap smears develop again. This can make it necessary for a surgical conization to be done if such abnormal smears develop in the future.

*Laser therapy.* This is called a "vaporization conization" because a cone-shaped area of tissue is removed from the cervix by vaporization with the laser, just as a cone-shaped piece of tissue is removed from the cervix with a knife with surgical conization. The laser seems to be the best method of treatment for the cervix. It leaves less scar and less chance of cervical stenosis. The disadvantage of the use of the laser is that laser therapy is more expensive and is not yet universally available in the United States.

I suggest that my patients who have precancerous cervical cells let me use the laser on them (if they have not had children or have not completed their families), whenever they have a CIN III, (severe dysplasia or carcinoma in situ: equivalent to a Pap III, IV, or V) or if they have a less severe precancerous growth which covers a large area of the cervix.

Vaporization conization (laser treatment) heals quickly. Normally there is very little discharge and a patient can usually begin having intercourse after two weeks.

I recommend that the husband use condoms during intercourse for the first two weeks after laser treatment of his wife. It seems reasonable that if some factor related to intercourse causes CIN, the cervix should not be exposed to a man's penis during the healing stage, perhaps decreasing the chance of any recurrence of such a growth.

### 754 If my colposcopy was unreliable, what should be done?

If the cells that were scraped out of your cervical canal at colposcopy were shown to be abnormal, or if there is any question about whether or not there is actually an invasive cancer, or if there exist any of the other problems mentioned in Q. 751, a conization should be done. This conization can be both diagnostic and therapeutic (can tell whether or not invasive cancer is present and, by excising the abnormal issue, can cure the problem).

A conization is done under general anesthesia, but it can be done on an outpatient basis, in which case you do not have to spend the night in the hospital after the procedure.

Conization (see illustration) is actually a simple procedure in which the doctor removes a cone-shaped wedge from around the opening of the cervix, including the cervical canal from the outer half to two-thirds of the cervix, and then sutures the cervix to stop the bleeding. To allow proper healing, it will probably be suggested that you not have intercourse for about a month following the procedure. Some doctors use the laser as a knife to cut out the cone. This requires fewer sutures.

The cone of tissue is sent to the laboratory for diagnosis. Ordinarily a doctor will do a D&C with a conization to make sure there is no cancer inside the uterus; that tissue is also sent to the pathologist.

About 10 percent of women who have a conization done will have some fairly heavy bleeding about two to three weeks after the cone is removed. Occasionally this bleeding will be heavy enough to require a transfusion and admission to the hospital for re-suturing of the area. Do not think your

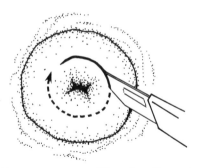

A conization removes a core of tissue from the cervix for microscopic examination. The core is taken from the area around the opening of the cervical canal.

doctor has done anything wrong if this happens. No matter how the procedure is done, nor who does it, a conization will occasionally result in postoperative bleeding. It is not dangerous and all you need do is let your doctor know if you start having heavier-than-normal bleeding any time after a conization. If you have bleeding heavier than the bleeding of a normal period, or if you have bleeding like a normal period that lasts longer than a normal period, consider your bleeding to be abnormal and call your doctor.

A conization can result in such tight scarring (stenosis) of the canal of the cervix that problems can develop. Occasionally this can even interfere with fertility, although this problem is rare. Such tight scarring can cause a slight problem with dilation of the cervix when a woman is in labor. Again, this is unusual and can normally be taken care of by the doctor stretching the cervix with his or her fingers during labor. Tightness of the cervix can also make it difficult to evaluate the cervix later if another abnormal Pap smear develops. In that case, a second conization may be necessary for a recurrent abnormal Pap smear.

After a conization is done, it is important that your doctor probe your cervix the next few times you are in the office to make sure it is staying open. There have been patients whose cervix scarred totally shut so that menstrual flow could not get through.

## 755 What if my doctor suggests a completely different approach to an abnormal Pap smear than what you have outlined?

Treatment by your doctor should be compatible with the methods of treatment listed in the previous question. If it is not, you probably should get a second opinion.

Cervical cancer is serious enough to warrant taking the necessary precautions to avoid it or to have it treated correctly. On the other hand, the cervix is an important part of your body, and it is best to have as little done to it as possible. You should not let a doctor do conizations or other treatments to your cervix unless they are done only after thorough diagnostic techniques (colposcopy) have been performed and a straightforward plan of treatment is outlined.

A study done in 1982 of women who had conization showed that one-fifth of them required suturing of the cervix to help retain subsequent pregnancies or needed a cesarean section at delivery because of severe cervical scarring. In addition, the chance of spontaneous abortion after the eighth week was seven times higher in women who had had a conization than in women who had not.

It remains to be proven whether or not this report is absolutely accurate for all groups of women who have had conizations. But it does serve to warn us that conization should not be done unless absolutely necessary.

## 756 What are some common errors that doctors make in relation to the cervix?

Because of their lack of understanding or because they let patients push them into doing things they do not want to do, doctors often make errors in their treatment of the cervix. Some of the most common of these are:

*Overtreatment of cervical erosion, ectropion, or "red spots."* Most of the time these areas are normal and need no treatment at all. Any doctor who has questions about them, should do a colposcopy to view the cervix, biopsying if necessary. Only if true abnormalities are found is treatment necessary.

*Allowing a Pap to stay abnormal.* Many doctors do nothing about a mildly abnormal Pap smear. Cervical cancer, however, can be present when an only mildly abnormal Pap smear is found because of the debris and mucus that often overlie it. If you have even a mildly abnormal Pap smear, you should have it evaluated and treated until it becomes normal.

*Treating for an abnormal Pap smear without prior colposcopy.* Without colposcopy, a doctor cannot know where or how bad are the cells that have produced an abnormal Pap smear. It is most important that you not allow a doctor to freeze, cauterize, or laser your cervix because of an abnormal Pap smear without having first obtained a reliable colposcopy and biopsies of tissue from your cervix to be sure that you do not have invasive cancer. If you do have an invasive cancer and have it frozen, cauterized, or treated in some way other than a conization, that can allow the cancer to spread farther in your body than it would if proper treatment is started without delay.

*Overtreatment of "severe dysplasia" or "carcinoma in situ."* In years past, any time a patient was found to have severe dysplasia or carcinoma in situ (CIN III), her doctor felt that she needed a hysterectomy. At that time colposcopies were not done, and conization was the standard diagnostic procedure for abnormal Pap smears. After a "cone," a patient would usually not have abnormal cells on her Pap smears anymore. It was believed that a hysterectomy was necessary because the cells had been on the verge of invasive cancer.

We know now that a woman is no worse off having so-called severe dysplasia or carcinoma in situ (CIN III) than she is having mild dysplasia (CIN I). Both need treatment and both can develop into true invasive cancer if not treated. But if either condition is adequately treated, there is no greater chance of recurrence on a woman's cervix than for the mildest precancerous condition (CIN I). A woman does not need to have a hysterectomy or a conization for the more severe forms of cervical intraepithelial neoplasia (CIN III).

*Hysterectomy for cervical intraepithelial neoplasia (dysplasia).* Hysterectomy is useful for a woman who has an abnormal Pap smear that has been reliably evaluated by colposcopy and biopsies, but only if she wants no more children and wants to have the hysterectomy. Such a woman can certainly request, and legitimately have, a hysterectomy. In any case, colposcopy should be done to make sure that she does not have invasive cancer and that her abnormal cervical cells have not spread off her cervix onto her vaginal walls. If she has invasive cancer, a simple hysterectomy is not adequate treatment. Even though it is not invasive cancer, if the precancerous cells have spread to the vaginal walls and a simple hysterectomy is done, the incision might cut across the area where the abnormal cells are, leaving some of them on the vaginal walls. With colposcopy the doctor knows exactly where the abnormal cells are growing and can either remove the lining of the upper part of the vagina at the same time he or she does the hysterectomy or use some other combined approach, perhaps the laser and hysterectomy.

## 757 What are the stages of invasive cervical cancer?

Once cervical cancer has become invasive, it is no longer a "skin cancer" of the cervix but has started growing down into the substance of the cervix. When this occurs your doctor will want to determine exactly how extensive this cancer has become in your body. There are four stages of cervical cancer.

Stage I. The cancer is confined to the cervix.

Stage II. The cancer has grown from the cervix into the surrounding tissues but has not yet extended out to the pelvic bones or into the lower third of the vagina or into the bladder or rectum.

Stage III. The cancer has grown to the pelvic bones or to the lower third of the vagina or into the bladder or rectum.

Stage IV. The cancer has grown outside of the areas involved in Stage III to involve other parts of the body, such as the intestines in the pelvic area or other distant parts of the body.

## 758 How is invasive cervical cancer treated?

The treatment of cervical cancer depends on which stage the cancer is in when it is discovered.

Most of the time the treatment for cervical cancer consists of radiation therapy. This is usually "combined therapy," which involves the use of radium in the cervix and uterus and then, either before or after that, external treatment with cobalt therapy or some similar source of external radiation given over a period of several weeks.

Radiation therapy of this type should be administered by someone well trained in its use. Even in the best of hands it can produce some annoying complications, such as a chronic irritation of the bladder due to the effect of radiation on the bladder wall. Irritation of the rectal wall can also occur. Even when competently used radiation therapy can produce some serious complications, such as holes between the vagina and either the rectum or bladder. The chance of this happening is much greater if you are not being treated by an expert in radiation therapy.

## 759 Is surgery ever used to treat invasive cervical cancer?

Surgery for cancer of the cervix is occasionally used, but only patients with Stage I or Stage II cervical cancer are so treated. The choice as to whether to use radiation treatment or surgery is made by a woman and her physicians. Normally the doctors will use radiation therapy, but they may have some good reasons for using surgery. The issues involved are so individualized and so numerous that it is impossible to discuss them fully here. Suffice it to say that it is vitally important that any woman with cervical cancer be in capable hands.

## 760 Is it possible to cure invasive cervical cancer?

Yes. A woman can be cured, meaning she is totally free of any cancer after treatment. Overall cure rates with radiation therapy vary from 55 to 60 percent. Stage I cancer has an 80-percent chance of cure; Stage II, 60-percent chance of cure. For Stages III and IV there is much less chance of cure.

In spite of the availability of Pap smears, colposcopies, biopsies, and all the early-detection procedures that we have talked about, cancer of the cervix is still the fifth-leading cause of death from malignant disease among American women. Approximately ten thousand women in the United States died in the year 1970 from this disease.

One of the saddest things about this statistic is that it could be much less if women were to be involved sexually only in mar-

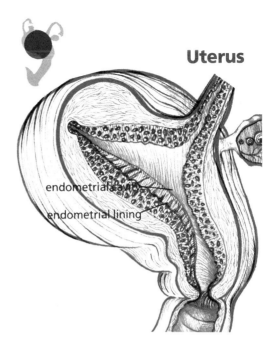

**Uterus**

endometrial cavity
endometrial lining

riages in which both they and their husbands were faithful—and if they would have annual Pap smears and appropriate treatment of any abnormalities found.

## Problems of the Uterus

The clearest way to think of your uterus is to imagine that it is a large paper sack whose sole purpose is to hold a baby while it develops! Thinking of the uterus in this way cuts through all the mystique about the uterus (womb) and its role in a woman's life.

The uterus performs its one job, childbearing, well. We can rightly be amazed at God's creative genius in producing a body part that functions so perfectly in the performance of its task. The lining of the uterus (the endometrium), for instance, must develop daily in a precise way during a woman's menstrual cycle in order to receive and nurture a fertilized egg. It must allow the fertilized egg to implant itself, and this must occur without excessive bleeding since too much bleeding could interfere with implantation. In addition, the uterus must be elastic enough to allow the growth of the baby and strong enough to perform the labor that will result in delivery of the infant. Further, the contractions that cause delivery must not start too early or too late, and after delivery the lining of the uterus must heal quickly, so that the whole cycle can begin again.

The uterus is a receiver of hormones. These hormones, produced by the ovaries, enter the body's general circulation and are brought back to the uterus after being pumped through the heart and blood vessels.

The uterus itself produces only two hormones: prostaglandins and prolactin. Prostaglandins produce many of the symptoms that women feel with their menstrual periods: uterine cramping, bloating, and irritability. God did not create hormones that are merely troublesome and unnecessary, however. Prostaglandins also produce the uterine muscle contractions that help control the amount of menstrual blood flow during a period and are also involved in the contractions of labor.

Prolactin, which is secreted by the lining of the uterus, is produced in significant amounts only during pregnancy. The function of uterine prolactin seems to be confined to the uterus for local action. No one knows exactly what it does, but it may be responsible for allowing implantation of the fertilized egg on the wall of the uterus. Since the body's usual source of prolactin is the pituitary, a blood test done for prolactin checks the amount of prolactin from your pituitary gland (located at the base of your brain), not the amount produced by your uterus.

As the uterus is involved in such varied activity, it stands to reason that it is subject to medical problems. We will discuss these problems in this chapter. (See also Q. 159–173. Because hysterectomies often involve operations on organs other than just the uterus, a discussion of that surgery best fits into chapter 4.)

---

## 761 Do I need to give my uterus any special care?

The uterus requires no special care. It is self-cleaning, self-regulating, self-programmed. If you are maintaining sound whole body health care and hygiene (including monogamous sex), if your menstrual periods are in the normal range (see Q. 763–767), and if you are conscientious about seeing your doctor for problems and annual checkups, you are doing all you need to do to keep your uterus in good working order.

---

## 762 Is there anything I should do for a tilted uterus?

There is only one thing to do about a tilted uterus—do not worry about it! One-third of all women have a uterus that is tilted back toward their backbone (retroverted); the other two-thirds have a uterus tilted forward. A retroverted uterus is no more different from a uterus that is tilted forward than a long nose is from a short nose; both are normal variations in the way a body can develop.

I frequently see new patients who are worried about a tilted uterus, usually because a previous physician told them their uterus was abnormal. I reassure them that this is neither an abnormality nor a medical problem.

You should not let a doctor operate on you simply because your uterus is tilted back. If you are having painful intercourse or pelvic congestion and have been told it is due to a tilted uterus, be skeptical about such a simple answer. These things occur whether or not a woman's uterus is tilted backward.

Pelvic discomfort can be due to a problem with the uterus, however, and you may need surgery. If this is the case, it is probably best for you to have a hysterectomy because the problem is almost certainly caused by something other than the position of the uterus. If you want more children and your pain is severe, you can let a doctor try a uterine suspension operation. But do not be surprised if it does not work.

Infertility is almost never caused by a retroverted uterus. Although during the years I have practiced I have operated on two infertile patients who had a retroverted uterus (to suspend the uterus), I did so after years of otherwise unexplained infertility. I made sure the patient understood that it was unlikely that the infertility was caused by the retroverted uterus but that I had no other reason to explain the infertility. One of these patients did become pregnant after such a procedure.

I believe the retroverted (tilted) uterus acquired a bad name in years past because some doctors used it as a catchall diagnosis for numerous unexplained problems. Women are occasionally infertile and do sometimes have pelvic pain and painful intercourse. Before the 1960s these things were difficult to diagnose, and doctors found it convenient to blame otherwise unexplained problems on a retroverted uterus. Physicians always like to come up with a reason for problems! None of us likes to admit our ignorance. Of course, patients want to be given a specific reason for a problem, too. As time went by, newer techniques for diagnosing pelvic problems were developed and a retroverted uterus does not have to be used as a scapegoat.

If you have a pelvic problem you can be 99 percent sure that it is not due to a retroverted or tilted-back uterus, even if yours is in that position.

## 763 Should I worry about irregular periods?

Do not worry about menstrual irregularities if they are within the "normal" limits described in the next three questions. If your bleeding pattern seems to be more abnormal than these guidelines suggest, see a physician.

Frequently patients ask if a cortisone shot will cause irregular periods. Several of my patients receive cortisone shots occasionally because of severe allergies; some of them will have irregular periods for several months as a side effect of that shot. Neither the woman nor her doctor should ignore this type of bleeding. If it persists beyond three or four months, the woman should notify her doctor and check if further investigation is warranted. Bleeding might be caused by a growth in the uterus.

## 764 How much blood loss is normal?

If the pattern of blood loss with your periods is consistent each month and you are not becoming anemic, you almost certainly do not have abnormally heavy bleeding.

The average woman loses from two to eight tablespoons of blood (30 cc to 120 cc) with each menstrual period, although it always seems more than this.

Some women must change sanitary pads every hour for two or three days and will even bleed through onto their clothes and bedsheets occasionally. If they do not become anemic, this is a normal menstrual pattern for these women.

Some patients who have always had very heavy periods, and do not want any more children, get tired of such heavy bleeding and want a hysterectomy. This is a legitimate request and I will comply with their request if I feel it is not frivolous. Most women do not need or want a hysterectomy for this situation but can use birth-control pills to make their periods lighter—up to the age of about forty when all women need to stop taking oral contraceptives.

If a woman has to use two large pads every hour, and if that protection is not enough to prevent staining of clothes or bed, she is having abnormal bleeding and needs to see a doctor. Also, if a woman with normally heavy periods becomes anemic, she should talk to a gynecologist about controlling her menstrual flow. Birth-control pills and hysterectomies are the only cure for such bleeding.

Some women have a light flow. Most gynecologists feel that if a woman has some spotting and bleeding for even one day she is having a normal period. This type of flow is often present if a woman is on birth-control pills. Women who have light periods should not worry or try to do anything to make them heavier. They should just enjoy having such little inconvenience with their menstrual bleeding.

---

## 765 How long is a normal period?

Menstrual flow can last from one to ten days and still be in a normal range. If a woman's menstrual pattern has become established and occurs every month, it is usually normal, no matter what length it is. However, if the pattern changes suddenly—a "three-day" woman has a period that lasts ten or twelve days, for instance—she should see a physician.

It is also normal for a woman to have spotting for two or three days before her period and/or spotting for two or three days after. Spotting that comes just before and just after a period is a part of menstruation and is not a sign of disease of the uterus.

---

## 766 What does the blood of a normal period look like?

Color or texture of menstrual blood do not indicate abnormalities. The color and consistency can vary from bright red blood to a muddy, brownish-black material. It is also normal for the blood to be in liquid form or in clots. Neither does a woman need to worry if her flow changes from one form to another.

## Positions of the Uterus

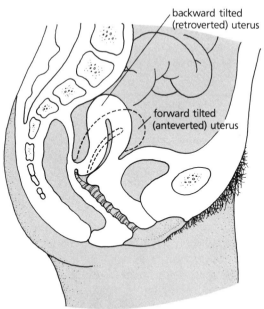

Positions of the uterus. About one-third of all women have a uterus tilted toward their backbone (retroverted). The remaining women have a forward tilted (anteverted) uterus. Both positions are normal.

The appearance of the blood does not indicate malignancy or abnormality in the uterus.

---

## 767 What should I do if my periods are infrequent?

It is normal for a woman's cycle, the days from the start of one period to the start of the next, to vary from twenty to thirty-five days. However, if a woman's cycle has become regular outside these guidelines, that too may be normal. For instance, I have some patients who have had menstrual periods every eighteen or twenty days on a regular basis for a long time. They have no sign of any medical problem and are obviously normal.

If a woman has menstrual periods further apart than thirty-five days, they are usually also irregular. They may be thirty-five days apart one time and fifty-five days apart the next time. If your cycles are of this type and you occasionally go for two to three months without a period, you should talk to your doctor. Everything may be normal but it is best to be checked out.

When a woman has a pattern of infrequent periods, farther apart than thirty-five days, that goes on for many years, she has a higher than average chance of developing cancer of the uterus later on in life. Because of this most gynecologists feel that such a woman should take progesterone (Provera) every other month if a period has not begun. This increased risk applies to women who skip periods repeatedly, not those who have this happen occasionally or who temporarily, even for a year or two, have such patterns. Provera must not be taken during pregnancy, as it might cause abnormalities in the baby.

When a woman in her forties starts having less-frequent periods, she may be entering premenopause. See Q. 258–264.

In summary, if your menstrual periods fall into a normal pattern, there is nothing you need to do unless some change occurs. If this happens you should talk to a physician to see if he or she feels that diagnostic tests need to be done. After this decision you and your doctor can decide whether or not to regulate your periods. Regulation can best be done with birth-control pills, but you should not use these if you are over thirty-five and a smoker, or if you are over forty.

See Q. 792–796 for a discussion of the problem of increased or excessive bleeding of the uterus.

---

## 768 Why do so many women have cramps with their menstrual periods?

Most of the time menstrual cramping, or dysmenorrhea, is a result of the normal function of the woman's body. It is occasion-ally true that women will have secondary dysmenorrhea—cramping caused by physical abnormalities, such as a cervical opening that is too small to let menstrual blood out, or because of some other abnormality of the uterus, or because of endometriosis. Most menstrual cramping, however, is primary dysmenorrhea—cramps that are present because of the normal function of the female body.

Prostaglandins are hormones normally produced by the inside lining of the uterus (the endometrium) as a result of the stimulation of that lining by progesterone. Secretion of progesterone from the ovary starts as soon as ovulation occurs and continues until the menstrual period begins. When the ovarian progesterone production stops the breakdown of the endometrium starts, prostaglandin production increases, and the prostaglandins are released into the blood stream of the woman's body. Prostaglandins cause menstrual cramps. Research physicians who injected pure prostaglandins into women found that all the symptoms of menstrual cramps resulted: uterine cramping, diarrhea, vomiting, headache, irritability, difficulty with concentration, and dizziness.

The prostaglandins produce uterine pain by causing the uterus to contract just as it does when a woman is in labor. Such contractions come and go. During a contraction blood is prevented from circulating through the uterus. This lack of circulation deprives the uterine muscle of oxygen, causing it to hurt. The woman senses this pain as cramping.

As mentioned, prostaglandins can affect various other body organs. For instance, they can affect the colon and cause diarrhea, or they can affect the brain and decrease the ability to concentrate. If a young woman has these symptoms and they are severe, she should see a doctor to be sure that no abnormality of her female organs is producing secondary dysmenorrhea. If she is normal on exam, she can be quite sure that her bad cramps are a result of the normal functioning of her body.

## 769 What can be done about dysmenorrhea?

There are several methods of treatment available. When I advise a woman about treatment for her cramps, I tell her that my goal for her is to be able to continue normal activities in comfort throughout her menstrual period.

*Exercise.* A woman who is in good physical condition and gets enough sensible exercise will occasionally have less cramps than if her body is in poor condition. If you have cramps, try to improve your physical condition to see if you feel better. Try to stay in shape, both for your general health and to decrease menstrual cramping.

*Pain medication.* Tylenol, aspirin, Midol, codeine, and other such medications can relieve cramps. Except for codeine, these can be obtained without a prescription and can provide sufficient relief from cramps in most women. They can be taken just when the cramps are painful, are not expensive, and are almost totally free of bad side effects.

*Prostaglandin inhibitors.* These medications were first used for people with arthritis. Later it was found that they relieved dysmenorrhea symptoms. There are several different forms of these medications. One of these is available (in a very weak strength) over the counter as Advil and Nuprin.

Theoretically one would think that these drugs would relieve all menstrual cramps, but that is not so. About half of my patients respond favorably to these drugs. The other half receive little or no relief. If your doctor gives you a prescription for one of these drugs and it does not work after one or two months, ask if you can have a prescription for a different form of this type of medication.

If you are one of the fortunate ones on whom these drugs work, you will probably have almost total relief of your discomfort, no matter how bad it is. It can be almost like magic. If the drug works, be certain to use it correctly: as soon as you feel any cramping with your periods, start taking the drug. Once you begin taking it, do not use it as you would aspirin, one here and one there. Take it regularly, just as the doctor has prescribed. These pills do not work the way you are accustomed to having pain pills work. Therefore, taking more than is prescribed will not help and could make you sick, although overall, these drugs are safe. If you have cramps that bother you, you should try this medication.

*Birth-control pills.* If other methods do not help, birth-control pills can be tried and will usually work. When a woman is taking birth-control pills, the lining of her uterus stays thinner than when she experiences her own normal hormone cycle. When she has a period, she will usually have lighter bleeding because there is less lining to shed. Since there is less lining, there is less prostaglandin production and less cramping.

See the discussion of birth-control pills in Q. 1007–1020. By reading that material you will see that birth-control pills are safe for most women, even teenagers. If you have dysmenorrhea, I encourage you to ask your doctor if you may try them.

*Heating pads or warm baths.* Many find that heat relieves cramps. No one knows why. It may be that heat to the pelvis improves the blood flow through the uterus during periods of cramping and in that way decreases uterine pain. The disadvantage of this treatment is that you cannot continue normal activities while using it.

*Fluid pills (diuretics).* Most women will not be relieved of their cramps by using diuretics, but they will be less bloated when using these medications. If you feel bloated with your periods, cut down on your salt intake, and drink more water. If this does not stop the problem, ask your doctor to prescribe diuretics for the time just before and during your period. They might make you feel better and just might help your cramps.

## 770 I have been told that I have fibroid tumors of my uterus. What are these?

Fibroid tumors, or leiomyoma, are not cancer, but growths made up of muscle tissue. No one knows what makes uterine muscle grow so abnormally. The most common current theory of the source of fibroids is that they grow from the small muscle cells in the walls of blood vessels in the uterus. Fibroids apparently grow in response to stimulation by estrogen from a woman's ovaries because they never appear in females before the onset of menstrual periods. After menopause, any fibroids that are present usually get smaller.

Fibroid tumors occur in from 5 to 10 percent of all women. Black women are seven or eight times more likely to have uterine fibroid tumors than white women. As a woman grows older, her uterus is more likely to have fibroids. As previously mentioned, uterine fibroids almost never occur in children, but they are present in 40 percent of women who are over fifty years old.

Fibroids can occur anywhere in the uterus. They can be present in the wall, they can protrude from the wall on a stalk, or they can grow into the interior cavity of the uterus and cause bleeding. Fibroids can even hang on a stalk out of the cervical opening and can grow from the cervix itself.

Since fibroids probably start from a single cell, they can be as small as only a few cells, much too small for a physician to detect on a pelvic examination. They can also get very large, filling the abdomen as much as a pregnant uterus.

## 771 What are the symptoms of a fibroid?

A woman is not usually aware of small fibroids. If and when they grow, however, they can cause several symptoms. If the fibroid is growing under the inside lining of the uterus (the endometrium), it can cause heavy periods or bleeding between periods; it can become so large that it puts pressure on the bladder and the rectum, causing a woman to feel the continual need to urinate or making her feel constipated. Large fibroids, by exerting pressure on the veins that come back into the body from the legs, can produce leg swelling.

A fibroid will occasionally outgrow its blood supply and start degenerating, causing a woman's uterus to become tender. This does not necessarily require surgery, but if the tenderness is too marked she may need to have surgery to make sure that it is a fibroid and not some other, more dangerous, problem.

If a fibroid is growing inside the cavity of the uterus, the uterus will try to expel it by contracting, working the fibroid down into the lower part of the uterus and "delivering" it through the cervix. When a doctor looks into the vagina of a woman with such a fibroid, he or she will see a reddish-purple, swollen mass protruding through the cervix. (See Q. 639.)

## 772 How is a fibroid diagnosed?

A doctor's pelvic examination is the most useful technique for diagnosing a fibroid. The doctor can tell if the uterus feels enlarged and irregular and if it can be moved around. In addition, a fibroid will not usually be tender on the pelvic exam. If a cancer is present, the uterus will usually be stuck to some inside organ and will not be movable.

An X-ray of the pelvis will sometimes be helpful in determining whether or not a growth is present in the pelvis but an X-ray cannot determine whether or not a growth is a fibroid. Although an ultrasound study is often wrong about the presence of a pelvic growth, once a doctor has found a pelvic growth, an ultrasound may help determine whether or not it is a fibroid. Since a uterus with fibroids can be enlarged because of pregnancy, it is important that you and your doctor consider the possibility that you may be pregnant. An ultrasound can be especially helpful for this. (See Q. 792.)

One technique that a doctor might use is to pass a probe up through your cervix into your uterus. If you have a large fibroid present, it often distorts the inner cavity of your uterus. A probe can tell that the cavity is enlarged and distorted, proving that there is a fibroid present. Such probing, called "sounding" of the uterus, must not be done if you are pregnant.

An X-ray of the uterine cavity (a hysterosalpingogram) can show the presence of fibroids if they are growing to the inside of the uterus. (See Q. 905.)

## 773 How are fibroids treated?

If you have small fibroids and have not yet had all the children that you want, you must make sure that your doctor examines your fibroids on a regular six-month basis. If your fibroids are large or are growing, you should have them removed. Such an operation is called a myomectomy. There is usually no real urgency, but if you let your uterus get as large as a three-month pregnancy before you have the fibroids removed, your chance of subsequently conceiving and carrying a normal pregnancy is greatly diminished. If you have the fibroids removed when your uterus is smaller (the size of a two-month pregnancy or less), your chances of becoming pregnant and carrying a healthy pregnancy are much greater. I took twenty-six fibroids out of a woman's uterus, following which she had two uncomplicated pregnancies.

If your fibroids are not growing very fast, are not as large as a three-month pregnancy, and you are not worried about pregnancy, you do not need surgery. You can have a pelvic examination done every six to twelve months to make sure that the fibroids are not growing too fast. Many women have fibroids for years and years with no problem; after menopause fibroids will usually shrink and become almost nonexistent.

If you are having heavy bleeding because of fibroids, you may need a D&C to be sure there are no premalignant or malignant cells in the uterus, especially if you are forty years old or more. If the D&C is normal but the bleeding persists, you need to have either a myomectomy or a hysterectomy. If your uterus has gotten to the size of a three-month pregnancy, it may be best that you go ahead with a hysterectomy, since the pregnancy rate is so low after a myomectomy done on a uterus that has gotten that large. Although I would advise a hysterectomy in this situation, and your own doctor probably would too, remember that you do not have to have one if that is not your choice. If you want to preserve the possibility of a pregnancy in the future, even though the chance may be small, don't consent to a hysterectomy: find a doctor who will do a myomectomy.

Having a hysterectomy for fibroids is not done because of the possibility of developing cancer, but because it becomes increasingly difficult to remove the enlarging uterus. Common sense would say that if you are going to need surgery, you may as well have it done at a time when it is easiest for the doctor to do. This can decrease the chances of complications from the surgery, although most competent gynecologists rarely have a problem doing a hysterectomy for fibroids.

## 774 What if a doctor cannot determine whether or not I have a fibroid?

Occasionally, in spite of your having symptoms of a fibroid tumor (see Q. 771), a doctor may not be able to tell for sure whether or not you have a fibroid. If the fibroid is growing out from the side of the uterus or in the supporting structures of the uterus, the doctor often cannot tell whether there is a fibroid growing or whether there is a growth on your ovary.

It is vital to make the differentiation between the two, because an ovarian growth can be malignant and a fibroid almost never is.

If this situation exists, a laparoscopy—viewing the internal organs through a small abdominal incision—is usually necessary. This procedure can be done in twenty or thirty minutes on an outpatient basis. At laparoscopy a doctor can look directly at the internal organs, will be able to see where a growth is coming from, and can usually tell what it is. (See Q. 907–909.)

## 775  What kind of surgery is done for fibroids?

The incision made for fibroid surgery is the same whether it is a hysterectomy or a myomectomy, which involves removal of the fibroids, leaving the uterus in place. That incision can be either bikini-type or up-and-down from the umbilicus to the pubic bone. Hysterectomy is discussed in Q. 159–173. Since the incisions are the same, it is necessary for you to be hospitalized for the same length of time either way.

If you are having a myomectomy, the doctor will make an abdominal incision and then cut across the surface of the uterus over the fibroids so they can be removed. He or she shells the fibroids out of the uterus, just as hardboiled eggs can be shelled. Sutures are used to close the holes and to stop the bleeding. This procedure is repeated over and over until all the fibroids are out. The doctor will close the incision in your uterus with small, delicate sutures to try to prevent

any adhesions, which could interfere with your future fertility.

If there are many fibroids, there may be fairly active bleeding from the uterus as the doctor is removing the fibroids. Transfusion may be needed to keep you from becoming too anemic after surgery. This does not mean that the operation is an unusually dangerous procedure.

A doctor cannot guarantee that all the fibroids have been removed, because there can be fibroids that are only a few cells in size. These cannot be found by a doctor who is feeling the uterus. As a matter of fact, the chance of developing fibroid tumors again is probably about 10 percent. Most women, however, are able to have all the children they want after a myomectomy, even if they eventually grow a few small fibroids again.

## 776  Will a cesarean section be necessary for delivery after fibroids have been removed?

If the doctor had to cut into the interior (endometrial) cavity of the uterus to get the fibroids out, a cesarean section would be necessary later. As this is not usually the case, most women who have had fibroids removed from the uterus do not need a cesarean section and can go through normal labor.

## 777  What are endometrial polyps?

A polyp is a piece of tissue that hangs from a stem. An endometrial polyp is an overgrowth of an area of the lining of the uterus that projects from the wall of the uterus. Such polyps do not occur too often. Fibroid tumors are by far the most predominant growth in the uterus.

Endometrial polyps may vary in size. They have been measured from less than one-eighth of an inch to more than three inches across.

## 778 What are the symptoms of an endometrial polyp?

Bleeding or spotting from the uterus between periods is the most common sign that a polyp is present, and bleeding after menopause can also indicate the presence of a polyp. Polyps are occasionally found when a hysterosalpingogram (see Q. 905.) is done, and polyps are sometimes found by the pathologist who examines the uterus after a hysterectomy. Obviously, polyps can be present without causing any problems at all.

## 779 How are polyps diagnosed?

If you have persistent abnormal bleeding, your doctor will probably do a D&C. The scraping of the uterus will frequently remove any polyps that are present. Occasionally, though, the instrument that is used in the uterus will merely push the polyp to the side and scrape the wall of the uterus without sensing the presence of the polyp. If a woman continues to bleed, the doctor may suggest that she have another D&C, or a hysterectomy if she does not want any more children.

If the woman does not want a hysterectomy, the doctor may suggest a hysterosalpingogram. Such an X-ray can show the presence of a polyp.

A newer technique—done with a small telescope inserted through the vagina, through the cervix, and into the uterus —is called a hysteroscopy. This procedure is quite useful in continued uterine bleeding situations. Hysteroscopy lets the doctor see inside the uterus so that he or she can identify not only polyps of the uterine cavity but also other uterine abnormalities that might be present. While doing the hysteroscopy,

the doctor can sometimes snip away polyps, avoiding more major surgery. The procedure may be done in a doctor's office by using a paracervical block or in a hospital under paracervical or general anesthesia (see Q. 919).

## 780 How are endometrial polyps treated?

A D&C will often get rid of any endometrial polyps that are large enough to cause bleeding. If not, hysteroscopy with excision of the polyps can often solve the problem. Although polyps usually do not recur once they have been removed, a hysterectomy is a good method of treatment for this problem when polyps become persistent and bothersome and the woman has had all the children she wants.

Endometrial polyps are not in themselves premalignant growths. However, just as premalignant or malignant cells can occur anywhere on the lining of the uterus, so they can occur on the surface of these polyps. Also, since cancer of the uterus can grow in such a way that it produces polyps, a polyp can be a sign of malignancy in the uterus. It is important, therefore, that a polyp growing inside the uterus be removed, the wall of the uterus be scraped, and all the tissue sent to a pathologist to make sure that none of it is malignant.

## 781 I have pressure and discomfort in my lower abdomen, and my doctor says my uterus is sensitive and a little enlarged. What can cause this, and what can be done for it?

There are three problems that can produce this kind of discomfort. The first two conditions, adenomyosis and pelvic congestion, have no danger potential at all and should be treated only if they are bothering a woman enough to be treated. The third problem, endolymphatic stromal myosis, an extremely rare condition, will cause uterine bleeding that is abnormal enough to require a D&C. Since the D&C will definitely confirm the presence of this problem, there is no danger of confusing endolymphatic stromal myosis with adenomyosis or pelvic congestion.

The ultimate treatment for all three problems is a hysterectomy. But, while a hysterectomy is absolutely necessary if endolymphatic stromal myosis is present, it is never necessary for adenomyosis or pelvic congestion unless the discomfort is bad enough to make a woman want the hysterectomy. (See Q. 180–189.)

## 782 What is adenomyosis?

Adenomyosis is endometriosis of the muscular wall of the uterus. (See Q. 174–179, 953–960.) I picture adenomyosis as a condition in which roots of the endometrium (lining of the interior of the uterus) grow down into the muscle of the uterus. Although these projections have been cut off from the cavity of the uterus, this tissue still builds up each month. Since this tissue is the same as that which lines the uterus, it bleeds at the time of the menstrual period. Adenomyosis, however, bleeds into the muscle of the uterus instead of out the vagina. This bleeding into the uterine muscle causes the uterus to be sensitive, especially at the time of a period. It can cause the uterus to be enlarged, although adenomyosis can be present when a uterus is totally normal in size.

The symptoms of adenomyosis are severe cramps, excessive uterine bleeding with periods, and spotting before or after the periods. Pain with intercourse can be present, and there may be an infertility problem associated with the adenomyosis.

Adenomyosis occurs in as many as 20 percent of women in the reproductive age. As

with endometriosis, it is active in women during childbearing years and becomes inactive as menopause occurs, subsequently causing no further discomfort.

## 783 How is adenomyosis treated?

Hysterectomy is the treatment that is best for this problem, but this is necessary only as a matter of comfort. If a doctor feels that adenomyosis is contributing to a woman's infertility, he or she may suggest a hormone called Danocrine. This hormone will suppress both endometriosis and adenomyosis and increase the woman's chance of becoming pregnant if these problems are causing infertility.

The doctor can never know for sure that adenomyosis is present until the uterus is removed and the pathologist has examined it. This can be frustrating for an infertility patient, but if adenomyosis is suspected the doctor will probably suggest taking Danocrine "just in case."

For patients who are having significant pelvic pain or bleeding problems, and who have all the children they plan to bear, it really does not matter whether or not the doctor can tell her for sure that she has adenomyosis. If she is having enough discomfort to need a hysterectomy, surgery is done because of the discomfort, not because of the possible presence of adenomyosis.

## 784 What is pelvic congestion syndrome?

Pelvic congestion syndrome is a condition in which the pelvic tissues are swollen, boggy, and congested with fluid. I describe this problem to my patients as a situation in which the veins in the supporting structures of the uterus become like varicose veins. These swollen veins ooze fluid into the tissues and cause tenderness. Dr. Masters of the Masters and Johnson team has described breaks in the tissues supporting the uterus. These have come to be known as "Masters windows." He feels that these breaks in the supporting structures allow the tissues to swell and are partly responsible for the pain of pelvic congestion.

A patient with pelvic congestion syndrome has discomfort low in the pelvis before and during menstrual periods and occasionally at ovulation. This may consist of pain or a feeling of pelvic pressure. The discomfort may be worse with intercourse. The patient may even have low backache associated with pelvic congestion.

### 785 How is pelvic congestion syndrome treated?

Treatment for this condition is normally hysterectomy. If a woman has not had all the children she wants, she may find that birth-control pills can help her symptoms.

Some doctors feel that a retroverted uterus is associated with pelvic congestion syndrome. In that case, a device called a pessary can be inserted into the vagina to hold the uterus out of the retroverted position. This is not often done these days because the device can be bothersome and often does not help. If a woman is having a great deal of trouble and wants no more children, she is better off with a hysterectomy. If she has not completed her family, a pessary might be worth a try. (See Q. 787.)

Some sex therapists feel that pelvic congestion is caused by repeated episodes of sexual arousal without orgasm. They feel that lack of orgasm allows the pelvic structure to become congested, and they encourage patients with the problem to see a sexual counselor and learn techniques for developing orgasmic intercourse.

### 786 What is endolymphatic stromal myosis?

This uterine growth is extremely rare; I have never had a patient with the condition. It is apparently an overgrowth of the connective tissue of the uterus. It produces heavy periods, bleeding between periods, and even bleeding after menopause. It can also produce discomfort in the low pelvis and cause the uterus to enlarge.

If a patient has these symptoms, she would almost always have a D&C done because of the bleeding. After studying the tissue scraped from the uterus, the pathologist would make the diagnosis.

The only treatment for endolymphatic stromal myosis is surgery. A woman must have her uterus, tubes, and ovaries removed. Although endolymphatic stromal myosis is not considered a true malignancy, the growths can spread to other parts of the body, and 10–15 percent of the women who have this problem die as a result. Therefore, after a hysterectomy for this condition, a woman should have continued medical observation and care. If there are further signs of the problem, specialized consultation will be necessary.

### 787 Can the uterus "fall down"?

The condition in which the uterus is "falling" is usually referred to by doctors as uterine prolapse or uterine decensus. This is a situation in which the ligaments that hold the uterus in place are no longer strong enough to hold the uterus up where it belongs. This is usually a result of stretching and tearing these ligaments during childbirth, but the ligaments can be abnormally weak in women who have never been pregnant, apparently an inherited weakness.

Often a doctor will tell a patient that her uterus has fallen when she has not been aware of it. In this situation, the patient does not need to do anything about it and can usually ignore any suggestions a doctor might have about surgery.

Occasionally a uterine prolapse will cause a patient to have low abdominal and low back pain. If a patient begins having trouble with uterine prolapse and has had all the children that she wants, she should consider a vaginal hysterectomy. Uterine prolapse is often associated with a prolapse (relaxation) of the vaginal walls known as cystocele and/or rectocele. If the vaginal walls are becoming weakened and these problems are bothering her and she has decided to have a hysterectomy, she should also have vaginal repairs. (See Q. 159–173, 699–702.)

If a patient wants more children or does not want to have surgery, she can either ignore the problem or have her uterus pushed back up the vaginal canal with a pessary. A pessary is a plastic or rubber device that is inserted into the vagina for the purpose of holding up the uterus on a temporary basis. With some pessaries a patient can have intercourse; with others intercourse is impossible.

If a woman has prolapse of the uterus, has not completed her family, and cannot wear a pessary, she needs to have an abdominal operation in which the doctor would make an incision, grasp the ligaments of the uterus and shorten and tighten them to hold her uterus higher up in the vagina.

Some doctors will fit a woman with a pessary when they feel that she is too old or too ill to have surgery. I have never seen a woman alert enough to be bothered by vaginal relaxation who was not also healthy enough to have vaginal surgery. Most women can have vaginal surgery because it does not stress a woman's body very much and can be done relatively quickly. Often older women who try to avoid surgery by using a pessary, get tired of it after a few months and go ahead with surgery.

## Prolapsed Uterus

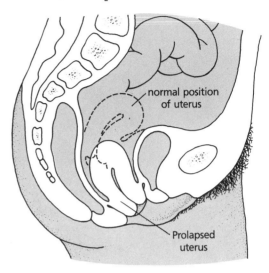

normal position of uterus

Prolapsed uterus

---

## 788   What is a D&C?

D&C stands for "dilatation and curettage." This means that the cervix is dilated, or stretched open, in order to introduce an instrument into the uterus to scrape out, or curette, the soft-surface portion of the lining of the uterus. A forceps is usually introduced into the uterus to explore the inner cavity of the uterus for polyps. If a D&C is being done with a suction instrument, this instrument will often suck a small polyp into the opening of the instrument and pull it out.

All removed tissue is sent to the pathologist to be examined for malignancy.

For this procedure a patient is admitted to an outpatient surgical facility or to a regular hospital and given general anesthesia. An alternative method is the office curettage discussed in Q. 789. There is only mild low-abdominal discomfort after a D&C, caused by the uterine cramping that often follows the procedure. The recovery time is related primarily to the anesthesia. Women are often tired and a little groggy for a few days after this has been done but they usually feel completely well again within a week.

After a D&C, if a woman develops fever,

## Dilatation

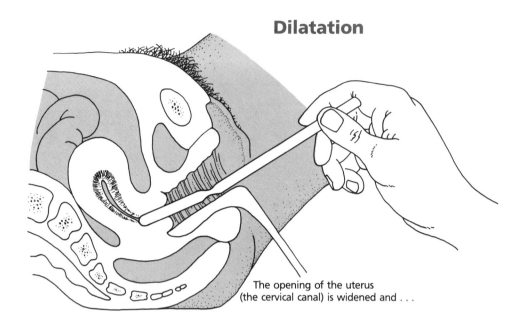

The opening of the uterus
(the cervical canal) is widened and . . .

increasing pain in the deep pelvis, or bleeding that is heavier than a menstrual period, she needs to call her doctor immediately.

This usually indicates an infection in the uterus from the D&C.

It is normal to have some bleeding or

## Curettage

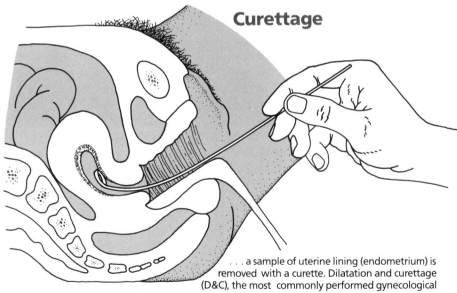

. . . a sample of uterine lining (endometrium) is removed with a curette. Dilatation and curettage (D&C), the most commonly performed gynecological procedure in America is used primarily to diagnose the cause of uterine bleeding or to empty the uterus after a miscarriage.

spotting for a week or ten days after a D&C. I recommend that my patients not have intercourse, douche, or use tampons for one week after a D&C. Exercise or regular activity, however, is fine if you have recovered from the anesthetic enough to do such things.

A D&C is a simple procedure that does not require any cutting of the woman's tissues, even though it does require a general anesthetic. (See Q. 789.)

---

## 789   Are there alternatives to a D&C?

Yes. These are:

*Endometrial biopsy.* If a woman is having bleeding that needs evaluation but the doctor does not suspect cancer, he or she will often suggest an endometrial biopsy. This technique, which can be done in the office, is not truly a D&C but is merely a sampling of the tissue that lines the uterus. From the tissue taken the pathologist can tell if infection, hormone imbalance, or some other problem is causing the bleeding. This technique is often used to see if a hormone imbalance is causing infertility.

A small round tube with an open end is inserted into the uterus, scraped around three or four times, and pulled out. The open end of the tube usually has a sharp lip that will scrape away tissue from the wall of the uterus. While scraping the doctor usually applies a little suction with a syringe to pull the tissue that is scraped off into the tube. This material is squirted into a preservative and sent to the pathologist for evaluation.

An endometrial biopsy is normally done without any pain medication. While it is a painful procedure, it takes only a brief time, less than one minute. Patients do not like this procedure and usually remember it for a long, long time.

*Office curettage.* A startling new technique, curettage in the doctor's office, is now being done by many gynecologists as a substitute for the traditional D&C. Along with many other gynecologists, I have always considered a D&C as a cornerstone of the practice of gynecology. Now I believe this new technique will eventually almost totally replace the traditional D&C for most patients.

For this procedure, an injection of local anesthetic (a paracervical) is given on both sides of a woman's cervix. This injection, which is only mildly uncomfortable, numbs the cervix and the uterus. After waiting thirty minutes for the paracervical to become effective, the doctor introduces a small plastic tube into the uterus. This tube has an opening in the tip, with a lip on it that will scrape the uterine wall as the device is moved back and forth. Powerful suction is applied with a large syringe or some other device as the doctor scrapes the uterus. The scraping is done much like it would be done if the patient were asleep in an operating room.

Studies have shown that the accuracy of this type of curettage is even greater than that of the traditional D&C. In addition, it eliminates the necessity for general anesthesia and the cost of the operating room, and of the anesthesiologist. The charge for this procedure would be less than the charge for a hospital D&C because it is a more efficient use of a doctor's time!

A further advantage of the office curettage is that a woman can return to work after leaving the office, and she can even resume marital relations the same day if she wants to. There is generally less cramping with this procedure than following the traditional D&C.

Finally, for the patient who has heart disease or some other reason for avoiding more major surgery or anesthesia, this procedure can be done with essentially no risk at all.

---

## 790   Why can't a Pap smear be done instead of a D&C if a doctor suspects cancer?

The Pap smear and the D&C are looking for two completely different disease processes in the body. The Pap smear detects precancerous or cancerous cells of the cervix, the mouth of the uterus. The D&C is looking for precancerous or cancerous cells or other abnormalities of the endometrium, high up inside the uterus. The D&C tells almost nothing about the cervix, and the Pap smear tells almost nothing about the part of the uterus above the cervix.

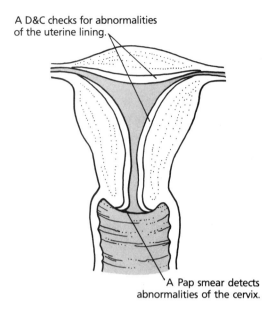

A D&C checks for abnormalities of the uterine lining.

A Pap smear detects abnormalities of the cervix.

### 791 What is meant by temporary irregularity of the menstrual cycle, and what causes it?

One of the most common reasons for women to see their gynecologists is because of temporary irregularity of their menstrual pattern. These women usually come in worried, complaining that they have never had an abnormal period before but that during the last month they have had irregular bleeding. Such irregularity may include any of the following:

Bleeding again only a few days after a normal period ends, with the "extra" bleeding being heavier and lasting longer than a normal period would.

Five or six weeks with no period, than a heavy and abnormal period (reported by a woman who knows that she cannot be pregnant).

A "normal" period that never stopped and is still going on at the time of the office visit.

These situations are almost always a result of failure of ovulation, and they can occur when a woman is in her teens or forties or in between. Almost every woman will have an episode of this type during the reproductive years of her life. If this occurs it is nothing to worry about. After about three months a woman's body will almost always stop this abnormal-type bleeding as normal ovulation

once again occurs. By the third month the woman will begin having regular, normal cycles again. In other words, a woman's body has done its own D&C.

Unless the bleeding persists for more than three months, or is so bothersome that a woman wants it treated, she needs no therapy. There is certainly nothing wrong with taking birth-control pills for two or three months to stop this bleeding and to regulate it—assuming that the woman is under forty years of age—but it is not necessary.

### 792 What should I do if I have truly abnormal uterine bleeding: much more in amount and/or lasting much longer than that mentioned in Q. 791?

If you truly have abnormal bleeding, outside the limits previously discussed, you need to see a doctor who will find out from you what the pattern of your bleeding is. He or she will then do a pelvic examination to check for abnormalities of your vagina, cervix, uterus, tubes, or ovaries.

In addition, since pregnancy is the most common cause for uterine bleeding in women in the reproductive age, the doctor will want to determine if you are pregnant.

These diagnostic tests will often follow.

*Pregnancy tests.* If there is any possibility of pregnancy, the doctor will want to do a pregnancy test to see if you are pregnant and whether or not your bleeding is a complication of that pregnancy.

*Sonogram of the pelvis.* A sonogram helps detect whether or not there is a tubal pregnancy, a growth on your ovary, or a growth in your uterus. Although a sonogram may help determine if there is a pregnancy in the uterus itself, a sonogram alone generally cannot diagnose a tubal pregnancy. (See Q. 195–201.)

A strong warning regarding sonograms is in order, however: they can present misleading information. They can look totally normal even though a woman has a large growth present in her pelvis or may even indicate that a growth is present when there is none. A sonogram is a lab test, and it is often inaccurate when relied on to find growths in the female organs. Don't let a doctor scare you or operate on you on the basis of a sonogram alone. The doctor's pelvic exam is more reliable in determining whether or not you have a growth in your pelvis. When the doctor has found a growth, the sonogram can be useful in helping decide what kind it is.

*D&C.* A D&C is done much like an endometrial biopsy but is more thoroughly and vigorously performed. It is done to evaluate the lining of the uterus not only for cancer but also for other problems that might cause bleeding. (See Q. 788, 789.)

*Other tests.* Various diseases and disorders of the body can cause uterine bleeding. For example, a woman who has a blood clotting deficiency can have abnormal and heavy bleeding; stress can cause a woman's periods to become temporarily irregular; and hepatitis can produce irregularity of the menstrual pattern. Other tests, therefore, would be directed toward any suspected disease process that might be going on.

---

**793** **How is abnormal bleeding treated? Should I be concerned about bleeding less often than every month?**

Once the uterus has been found free of precancerous or cancerous cells, and if no other body disease is found, the cause is almost always hormone irregularity produced by or producing irregular ovulation. Once this is known, treatment can be started. If a growth or other problem of the uterus is found, it would be treated as necessary. Check the index for the various uterine problems and their treatment. Remember, though, that treatment of irregular menses is necessary only if the irregularity has been going on for many months or if it is bothering a woman enough for her to desire such treatment.

Having a period as infrequently as every other month is not a cause for concern but if a woman has periods that are three months or farther apart for many years, she has an increased chance of developing cancer of the uterus sometime in the future. This is because the estrogen from the ovaries is produced on a daily basis, whether or not a woman has a period, and this continued stimulation of the uterus by estrogen from the ovaries without the balance of hormones provided by regular periods increases the chance of uterine cancer.

The most effective treatment for abnormal bleeding due to hormone irregularity is the use of birth-control pills, but if you are over thirty-five and a smoker or over forty you should not take them. (See Q. 1007–1021.)

An alternate approach to treatment may be recommended by a woman's doctor and is necessary for women who cannot take oral contraceptives. This treatment is the use of a progesterone pill ( usually Provera) to take the place of the progesterone that a woman's body should be producing each month starting with ovulation. If a woman with this problem will take 10 mg of Provera for ten days every other month, it will usually bring on her period. Provera, by producing regular bleeding in this fashion, reduces a woman's chance of developing cancer of the uterus in later years. A period every other month is often enough for this purpose.

## 794 Will a D&C stop my abnormal bleeding?

A D&C rarely stops abnormal bleeding, even though in years past it was used for that purpose. Prior to the development of the birth-control-type hormones that are now used to stop abnormal uterine bleeding, there was absolutely nothing to stop spotting and irregularity between periods, nor anything to stop heavy menstrual periods. Women who did not want a hysterectomy or could not have one for health reasons would often have multiple D&Cs. Doctors had nothing else to offer the patient, and occasionally a patient's bleeding would seem to be better after a D&C.

These days D&Cs are done for diagnosis: to find out if there is cancer or precancer present in the uterus or if there are other uterine abnormalities. If a patient has bothersome abnormal bleeding doctors handle that with hormones. When a D&C reveals no abnormalities, a hysteroscopy (See Q. 779.) can often spot a problem and thus save a woman from a hysterectomy.

The most efficient hormones for this purpose are birth-control pills. If these are not effective or if a woman cannot use them, Provera given ten days each month can sometimes regulate a woman's cycle. If these measures do not work and a woman is continuing to bleed heavily, hysterectomy is usually indicated.

## 795 What type of bleeding might signal cancer of the uterus and indicate the need for a diagnostic D&C?

Most women who have bleeding at the wrong time of the month worry about the cause being cancer, especially if it occurs when they are forty or over. It is important that a woman realize that the cause of such bleeding is not usually cancer. Otherwise she will be excessively and unnecessarily worried.

Remember, cancer is basically a "sore." As it grows it begins oozing a little fluid and then a little blood. Then, as time passes—perhaps weeks and months—that sore begins oozing more and more blood. This pattern of bleeding is quite different from the sporadic episodes of bleeding that almost all women occasionally have (see Q. 791). The real key, though, is whether or not abnormal uterine bleeding is persisting.

If a woman is over forty and her uterine bleeding persists almost daily for more than three months, she should see a doctor and expect that diagnostic tests will be done. Most doctors feel that a woman does not even need to see a doctor until the bleeding has lasted three months or unless there is some aspect of the problem that really worries her. If a woman is under forty years of age, it is unlikely that uterine cancer is the cause of her bleeding. Therefore, there is less urgency in diagnosing the cause of her bleeding, but neither she nor her doctor should delay diagnosis and treatment for too many months.

Types of bleeding that indicate the need for a D&C, classified by ages, are the following.

*Before menopause (younger than the age of forty).* Bleeding between periods that persists month after month usually needs to be evaluated by D&C. Most of the time the doctor will find that the woman is not ovulating regularly. This type of bleeding is not dangerous and is not caused by cancer.

There are some conditions, however, that can increase your chance of having a uterine problem earlier than the age of forty. For example, if you are twenty-five to fifty pounds overweight, you are three times as likely to develop cancer of the uterus as other women; and if you are fifty pounds overweight, you are nine times as likely to develop cancer of the uterus as an average-weight woman; if you are a diabetic, you are more likely to develop cancer of the uterus; and, if you have had infrequent menstrual periods for many years, you are more likely to develop endometrial cancer. If you fit into one of these categories, you should be sure your doctor knows it; and if you are having abnormal bleeding, you might suggest to him or her to consider a D&C at an earlier age than might otherwise be done.

*Bleeding over the age of forty.* If you have an episode of bleeding between periods and start having regular periods again after a month or so, you do not need a D&C. If, however, you start having bleeding between periods that persists for more than three months, you need a D&C. Also, if you start spotting between periods, excluding just after or just before a period, and this spotting continues for three or four months, you need a D&C.

*After the menopause.* Any unexplained bleeding after the menopause requires a D&C. **This is an absolute rule** and you and your doctor should never violate it unless the bleeding is from the vulva or from the vaginal walls. Even then most gynecologists will suggest going ahead with a D&C except where they can actually see the bleeding coming from a scratched or scraped place on the vulva or vagina.

Nothing in life is perfect, and this includes a D&C. A study done in 1979 showed that only 75 percent of D&Cs were accurate in showing cancer. This means that, even if the doctor had done a D&C and found no irregularities, if you continue bleeding you probably need to have another D&C (or office curettage) done. If the doctor feels a D&C does not need to be repeated, you will be told that, but remember that if the doctor suggests another D&C because you are continuing to bleed, it is a reasonable suggestion.

Although a D&C is inconvenient and somewhat expensive for a patient, it is a safe procedure and is an invaluable test providing vital information for a woman.

**796** **After a D&C done for bleeding, my doctor said that I had endometrial hyperplasia. What is this, and what should be done?**

Hyperplasia merely means overgrowth of the tissue of the lining of the uterus. Hyperplasia of the endometrium can be broken down into four different groups.

*Hyperplasia.* In this condition, the lining of the uterus is simply overgrown, but has no precancerous cells. A woman having this change of her uterine lining should be cautious. She should be given hormones that will absolutely regulate her if she has irregular periods. This treatment can cause hyperplasia to revert to normal. A woman with hyperplasia should have another endometrial biopsy or D&C done after a few months to make sure that her uterine lining is not becoming more abnormal. There is an increased chance of developing cancer of the uterus during the next ten years if she has hyperplasia of the endometrium. If her cycles cannot be regulated or the follow-up testing of the lining of the uterus continues to show hyperplasia and the woman has had all the family that she wants, it would probably be best for her to have a hysterectomy.

*Adenomatous hyperplasia.* This abnormal form of hyperplasia has no cancer cells present, but about 25 percent of women who develop it will have cancer of the uterus sometime in the next ten years. In spite of this a woman does not need to have a hysterectomy immediately. She should make sure that she has absolutely regular menstrual periods and should be tested again in a few months to see if the cells are continuing to be abnormal. If they are or she cannot regulate her periods, she should go ahead with a hysterectomy if she has had all the family she wants.

*Atypical endometrial hyperplasia.* With this more severely abnormal form of uterine hyperplasia, about 80 percent of women will develop cancer of the lining of the uterus at some time during the following ten years if not treated. A woman ordinarily needs to have a hysterectomy if this condition exists.

*Severely atypical endometrial hyperplasia.* This abnormality is considered to be cancer, but it is confined to the surface of the uterine lining. All women with this problem will have continued change in the uterine lining progressing to actual invasive cancer (cancer growing down into the tissues of the body) unless they have a hysterectomy.

Although treatment with hormones will usually cause the tissues of the uterine lining to revert to normal, in the atypical and severely atypical stages of hyperplasia it is generally best not to try this unless there is some specific reason to do so. The treatment involved is the use of Provera or birth-control pills and repeated uterine scraping for testing on a long-term basis. You and your doctor can discuss this and decide what is the best treatment in your situation.

distinctly different types of cancer and are treated in almost totally different ways. (See Q. 757–760.)

Once endometrial cancer is diagnosed, the condition is "staged" to classify the extent of the cancer in the body. The different stages of endometrial cancer are:

*Stage I-A.* The size of the uterus from the opening of the cervix to the top of the inside (measured at D&C) is eight centimeters, about three and a half inches, or less. Uterine size is important because the more a uterine cancer has grown, the larger the uterus will be.

*Stage I-B.* The size of the uterus is greater than eight centimeters.

*Stage II.* The cancer has grown from inside the uterus down into (but not outside) the cervix. The doctor finds this extension of the growth by scraping the inside of the cervix at the time of the D&C. This cervical scraping is included as part of a D&C done to diagnose possible endometrial cancer.

*Stage III.* The cancer has grown out of the uterus into other areas of the pelvis, such as into the ovaries or down into the vagina (but not outside the pelvis).

*Stage IV.* The cancer has grown into the rectum, or bladder, or outside the pelvis into other parts of the body.

---

**797** **If cancer of the uterus is diagnosed, what procedure is followed?**

First let me state that "cancer of the uterus" or "uterine cancer" is a term that gynecologists use to refer to cancer of the lining of the uterus. This is actually cancer of the endometrium. If a patient has cancer of the cervix, that is referred to as cervical cancer, not uterine cancer, even though the cervix is part of the uterus. These are two

**798** **How significant is the type of cell that makes up the cancer?**

All cancer cells are not the same; some grow faster than others. "Grading" a cancer means classifying the aggressiveness of the cells that make up the cancer. The grade is assigned by the pathologist who studies the cancer cells from the uterus.

The following simple grading system is used by doctors.

*Grade I:* The architectural pattern of the growth is primarily glandular. This is a "better" tumor than the next two grades.

*Grade II:* The architectural pattern is a mixture of glandular and solid type cells.

*Grade III:* The architectural pattern is primarily solid.

## 799 What things besides stage and grade affect the way endometrial cancer will act in my body?

There are several things that affect the way the tumor will act in your body.

*Depth of the cancer.* The less deeply the cancer has grown into the wall of your uterus, the better off you are. However, the only way this can be determined is with a hysterectomy. If X-ray or radium treatment is necessary before a hysterectomy, the pathologist often cannot tell how deeply the cancer had grown into the wall of your uterus before such treatment.

*The location of the cancer.* If the cancer started and is growing in the upper part of your uterus, you are better off than if it started or is growing in the lower part of your uterus.

*Cancer cells in abdominal fluids.* If the cancer cells have broken loose and are floating freely in the fluid in your abdominal cavity, you are not as well off as if that fluid contained no cancer cells. The doctor can determine this only at the time of the hysterectomy.

*Lymph nodes.* If the lymph nodes inside your abdomen at the time of the hysterectomy are free of cancer, you are better off than if they have cancer in them.

*Age.* The younger you are when you are found to have cancer of the uterus, the better off you are.

*The type of cancer cell.* You are better off if you have a cancer that is adeno-acanthoma or adenocarcinoma. A cancer cell that is adenosquamous cancer, clear-cell cancer, squamous-cell cancer, or papillary adenocarcinoma is more aggressive and more likely to recur after treatment.

## 800 How are these different stages of cancer treated?

Each of the stages of cancer calls for medical care tailored to that specific stage.

*Stage I, Grade I.* This type of cancer of the uterus which has not invaded the wall of the uterus very deeply, usually can be totally cured by simple hysterectomy. If, however, the cancer is low in the uterus and involves some of the cervix, or if the grade of tumor is more aggressive, or if another complicating factor exists, radiation treatment must be included with the hysterectomy, either before or after—or a radical hysterectomy must be done.

*Stage II.* The treatment for this type of cancer can be either a radical hysterectomy or hysterectomy and radiation. The choice depends on which one your doctor feels will give you the best chance of a complete cure.

*Stage III.* When cancer has grown outside the uterus, the treatment depends on the location of the cancer. If it has gone into the ovaries the best treatment may be surgery first; a decision for or against radiation can be made after the surgery has been completed. If the cancer has spread to the vagina or to the supporting structures of the uterus, radiation is usually given first and then, if possible, a hysterectomy is done.

*Stage IV.* When the cancer has grown into the rectum or bladder or other areas of the body, individualized treatment is necessary. Treatment depends on what kind of tumor is present and where it has spread. Ordinarily treatment will be primarily with radiation and with chemotherapy.

## 801  Which chemotherapy is useful for cancer of the uterus?

Chemotherapy is usually begun when all the cancer cannot be removed at surgery or when the doctor thinks that cancer may still be present in the body after treatment. These drugs will also be given when a woman has seemed to be free of cancer, but it shows up again in her body several months or years later.

Ordinarily the treatment is with progesterone in high doses. Drugs such as Megase, Depo-Provera, or Delalutin are all progesterone preparations sometimes used to treat cancer of the uterus that persists or that recurs after initial treatment.

The patients who respond best to this type of treatment are those who are not elderly, who have had long periods of time from their initial treatment until a recurrent episode of cancer, whose recurrence of cancer was not in the pelvis, and whose grade of cancer was not very aggressive. Half of the patients who have this type of recurrence of cancer will have good response to therapy, many of them going several years without having further trouble with their cancer.

Progesterone drug treatment does not cause one's hair to fall out and does not have many of the toxic effects of other types of chemotherapeutic agents. In addition, progesterone preparations almost never cause

nausea. Unfortunately they rarely produce a complete cure from the cancer.

## 802  What if the progesterone treatment stops working? Is other chemotherapy recommended?

If the progesterone treatment does not work, other chemotherapy is called for. This is such an intricate and specialized field that we now have doctors, called oncologists, who are experts in the use of these drugs.

If you have a cancer that is not responding to other treatments, or if your doctor suggests that you start on some type of chemotherapy, I would encourage you to ask for a referral to an oncologist for consultation and treatment. If your doctor tells you that you have cancer growing but does not refer you to an oncologist, I encourage you to see one any way, at least for a second opinion.

Many people are afraid to talk to a doctor about chemotherapy, but such a consultation is often useful. If you have a cancer that has come back or one that was not initially removed completely, it is certainly worthwhile to talk to a chemotherapist about his or her recommendation for treatment of your problem. Although you don't have to do what is suggested, you will at least know what your options are.

## Problems of the Fallopian Tubes

A woman's fallopian tubes, or oviducts, are about three to four inches long. They are attached to the uterus at one end and have a delicate, flowerlike opening on the other end that takes in the eggs from the ovaries. These tubes (which look a lot like and are about the same size as relaxed, medium-sized earthworms) have the same delicate, peritoneal lining that covers all the organs inside the abdomen. They have two layers of muscle and are lined on the inside by a soft, delicate pink lining (mucosa).

The inside surface of the fallopian tube is made up of different cell types. Some of these secrete mucus. Others are specialized, with hairlike projections that produce a synchronous sweeping motion, which is responsible for propelling the egg down the fallopian tube and eventually into the uterus. The inside diameter of the fallopian tubes varies from one-twenty-fifth to one-sixth of an inch.

When we look at the function of the fallopian tubes, we understand to some extent how truly complex they are. A fallopian tube is capable of transporting sperm and ovum in opposite directions at different times during the menstrual cycle. How this feat is accomplished is unclear. The fallopian tube is responsible for moving the egg from ovary to uterus, but the sperm must come from an opposite direction—through the uterus into the tube—for fertilization to take place.

The fallopian tube provides the perfect environment for fertilization. For example, concentrations of bicarbonate and potassium are greater in oviductal fluid than in the body's plasma; these are just two examples of the multitude of beneficial environmental factors provided by the tube for successful fertilization.

Once the egg is fertilized, the fallopian tube continues to "handle it with care." The egg must stay in the fallopian tube for three days before it is delivered into the uterus, allowing time for it to grow and mature enough to survive in the uterine cavity as a pregnancy. If the fallopian tube passes the embryo into the uterus too early, neither the embryo nor the lining of the uterus would be ready for implantation and pregnancy could not occur.

It is not known exactly how the fallopian tube keeps the egg from passing on through. This is obviously another of the complex

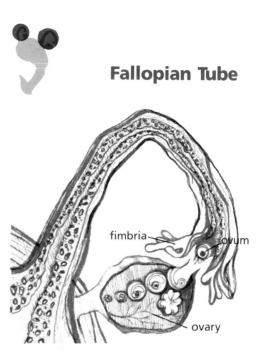

## Fallopian Tube

fimbria — ovum

ovary

mysteries of the human body that God designed in a special way.

Those of us who deal with problems of infertility feel that increasing knowledge of the function of the fallopian tubes will help us understand many cases of unexplained infertility, and application of the knowledge gained will probably enable doctors who do microsurgical fallopian-tube repairs to do them in an even more effective way.

The only function of the fallopian tubes is to enable a woman to become pregnant, and except in the rare case of malignancy or growths any surgery performed on the tubes is to help either increase fertility or produce sterility. No change results in a woman's body with fallopian-tube surgery (other than the desired effects of fertility or sterility), nor does removal of the tubes produce any generalized effect. Hormones from the ovaries do not travel the fallopian tube route into the uterus. The ovary introduces its hormones into the blood stream which carries the hormones via the heart back into the uterus, fallopian tubes, and other pelvic structures. Neither tying nor cutting the fallopian tubes affects the function of the remainder of the pelvic organs.

**803** **Since the fallopian tubes are important to my becoming pregnant, is there anything I can do to keep them healthy?**

There are three primary precautions to insure good fallopian tube health.

*Don't have intercourse with anyone who can give you an infection.* Gonorrhea and chlamydia are the infections most commonly associated with fallopian tube scarring, but other sexually transmitted diseases (STD) can also cause infection of the tubes. (See chapter 13.)

Even if a man has not had intercourse with anyone else for two or three years, he can still have and pass germs to you that can cause you to develop infection in your fallopian tubes and uterus. Such infections can cause sterility. In spite of modern antibiotics and microsurgical techniques to open scarred tubes, pregnancy may be impossible after such episodes of pelvic infection.

Obviously, the best way to avoid this type of infection is for you and your husband to have intercourse only with each other. God's injunction for marital fidelity is for the partners' own health and happiness.

If you enter marriage with someone who has had intercourse before, you could contract an infection from him. Whether or not one of you thinks there is an STD organism present, if either has had previous intercourse both should be checked and, if necessary, treated by a physician. Some STD organisms cannot be detected by a physician, but as you and your husband live together your bodies will tend to fight off any germs the two of you may have, or you can be treated if there are signs of infection. After a while the two of you as a couple will be free of such problems, except, perhaps,

occasional herpes infections or from scars left from previous infections.

*Don't use an IUD (intra-uterine contraceptive device) until you have had all the children that you want.* IUDs can cause an infection of the fallopian tubes that can leave them obstructed or unable to function adequately. Many people think that the Dalkon Shield is the only IUD that causes an infection in the female organs, but this is not true. Any IUD can cause pelvic infection; the Dalkon Shield just happened to be the most popular IUD when physicians noticed that IUDs could cause pelvic infection. And it did cause a higher rate of infections than other IUDs. Even the newest IUDs should not be used if you want a future pregnancy.

*Don't get your tubes tied until you know that you will not be interested in getting pregnant in the future.* A sterilization procedure is done to make you permanently sterile; it is not designed to be reversed. Even though most physicians warn patients that sterilization is permanent, many patients come back wanting their sterilization reversed. (See Q. 812, 813, 925–929.)

**804** **What is the result of infections in the fallopian tubes? What should a woman do if she suspects such an infection?**

Infections of the fallopian tubes are normally associated with infections of both the uterus and the ovaries. Such infection (called pelvic inflammatory disease or PID) can cause ulceration of the inside lining of the fallopian tube. Scarring can develop. The fallopian tubes can become completely blocked, and the delicate fimbriated ends of the tubes can become completely closed and destroyed. If the tubes are completely closed they may fill with fluid and become quite distended, swelling to several inches in diameter. If both of a woman's tubes are damaged and closed in this fashion, she obviously would be sterile.

Even if the tubes are not completely closed, scarred areas of the lining of the tube may have destroyed the tubes' hair cells (ciliated cells). In that case there is no current of fluid to bring the egg down the tube. This can result in infertility or, if such an egg was fertilized, the embryo might fail to pass through the tube, resulting in a tubal ectopic pregnancy.

One episode of infection by a sexually transmitted organism does not usually cause sterility, but if the infection flares up several times, a woman can become totally sterile.

If a woman has been exposed by intercourse to germs that might cause a pelvic infection and she starts developing pelvic pain and fever, she should see a doctor immediately for antibiotic therapy. The doctor will first need to make sure that she does not have appendicitis, a tubal pregnancy, an ovarian cyst, or some other medical problem.

PID (pelvic inflammatory disease) is discussed more extensively in chapter 13, especially Q. 1155, 1164–1172.

## 805 Can the fallopian tubes become infected with tuberculosis?

Yes. Approximately 10 percent of patients who have active tuberculosis of their lungs (not just a TB skin test that has become positive) will also develop tuberculosis of their pelvic structures. Tuberculosis was on the decline in the United States and had actually become uncommon, but with increased immigration during the past few years the number of cases of tuberculosis in our country has risen.

Tuberculosis in the pelvis seems to occur because the tubercular organism from the lungs is carried into the pelvis by the blood. Tuberculosis can cause infertility. If tuberculosis has developed in a woman's pelvis, she must be treated with adequate antibiotics to preserve the pelvic structures. If tuberculosis of the pelvis becomes too extensive, the patient will need both hysterectomy and antibiotic treatment.

For a more extensive discussion of this problem, review Q. 219–222.

## 806 What is a tubal, or ectopic, pregnancy?

An ectopic pregnancy occurs when the fertilized egg is implanted in the fallopian tubes instead of in the uterus. As the fallopian tube is not distensible enough to allow the development of a normal pregnancy, the tube eventually ruptures, causing internal bleeding, possible shock, and even death. Approximately 2 or 3 percent of all maternal deaths caused by pregnancy in the United States are the result of tubal ectopic pregnancy.

Ectopic pregnancies are becoming more common because of the increased number of women whose fallopian tubes are scarred as a result of infections, IUDs, and fertility surgery. Such scarring can "catch" a fertilized egg, causing it to start growing in the tube.

## 807 What are the symptoms of an ectopic pregnancy?

A doctor and a patient suspect a tubal ectopic pregnancy if the following symptoms exist.

*A missed period.* A woman may be pregnant any time she misses a period. It may be a normal uterine pregnancy or an ectopic pregnancy. If the next two signs occur, the pregnancy indicated by the missed period may be a tubal pregnancy.

*Bleeding from the uterus.* If after the last period was missed and before the next period is due a woman begins having abnormal bleeding, an ectopic pregnancy may be suspected. This bleeding may be heavy but is usually light; it may be continuous or intermittent. Such bleeding can be a sign of a miscarriage, but if there is also pain in the pelvis, the possibility of an ectopic pregnancy is even stronger. Occasionally a woman with a tubal pregnancy will not have uterine bleeding.

**Pain in the pelvis.** Patients who have a tubal ectopic pregnancy usually have discomfort, such as sharp pains or aching in the low abdomen. Frequently women are able to identify the exact time that the pain started, such as when they were cooking a certain meal or when they were having intercourse.

If you are pregnant and have noticed any of these signs, be sure to let your doctor know so he or she can evaluate you for a tubal pregnancy. Tubal pregnancies are discussed in greater detail in Q. 344–350.

## 808 Are there abnormalities of the fallopian tubes that are not due to infection?

Yes. These noninfectious abnormalities include *salpingitis isthmica nodosa,* various tumors and cysts, and cancer of the fallopian tubes. All of these problems are extremely rare.

## 809 What is *salpingitis isthmica nodosa?*

This disease is so uncommon that it does not even have a common name. It is a problem involving nodular thickening of the fallopian tubes. These thickenings, when viewed under the microscope, are small cavities in the wall of the tube communicating with the central canal of the fallopian tube. It is felt, therefore, that the problem is caused when the tubal lining bulges out through the muscular layer and proliferates

to form the glandlike appearance of these nodules.

Although this condition is not dangerous and does not lead to malignancy, its most bothersome aspect is that it can cause infertility. If this problem is found and a woman is trying to become pregnant, a doctor can cut out the areas of the fallopian tubes that are involved and sew the ends of the tubes back together. Surgery of this type must be done with microsurgical technique to have the best chance of success. Fortunately only the inner half of a fallopian tube is usually involved in this process, so the outer part and the ends of the tubes with the delicate fimbria that are so important to egg intake can be left intact. (See Q. 924.)

## 810 Which tumors and cysts can occur on the fallopian tubes?

"Hydatid cysts of Morgagni" can occur. These cysts are normally only one-quarter to one-half an inch in diameter and are found near the open end of the fallopian tube. Apparently they are structures that would have become part of the tubes that carry sperm if the person had developed as a male. Instead they exist in the female as small grapelike structures attached near the end of the fallopian tubes. These cysts are present in at least two-thirds of the women who have surgery—they are not an abnormality.

Occasionally one of these growths may be several inches in diameter. When it is discovered, a doctor would not know it is a simple hydatid cyst and would probably need to operate to determine exactly what it is. Any time a woman has a mass two to three inches in diameter in her pelvis that does not go away in a few weeks, she needs to have surgery.

Other growths of the fallopian tubes may occur. Tumors of the fallopian tubes include fibroid tumors (just like fibroids of the uterus), hemangiomas (tumors of the blood vessels), and dermoids (tumors that seem to develop from primitive cells in the body that are capable of producing various types of tissue in one tumor—thyroid, fat cells, and oil glands). See the discussion of ovarian dermoids in Q. 830 since dermoids occur in ovaries much more commonly than in the tubes.

## 811 Can cancer of the fallopian tube occur?

Yes, but cancer of the fallopian tube is the rarest cancer of a woman's female organs. It accounts for only 0.5 percent of all the cancers of the female organs. Only about five hundred cases of this type of cancer have been reported in medical literature.

With this type of cancer a woman would normally see the doctor because of abdominal enlargement, low abdominal pain, and abnormal bleeding. Occasionally a woman with this type of cancer will have a fairly heavy discharge of watery blood because of the development of bloody fluid in the tube. This fluid is discharged through the uterus and vagina.

The doctor's exam would show a mass in the pelvis, and finding such a mass and the uterine bleeding would necessitate a D&C to check for cancer. Then an abdominal operation would be performed to remove the mass. During the surgery the doctor would find the fallopian-tube cancer.

Normally a doctor will suspect ovarian cancer in a woman with a pelvic mass, since it is so much more common than cancer of the fallopian tubes. It does not make any difference if the doctor does not definitely determine which type of cancer is present before surgery. The surgery is the same if it is an ovarian cancer or a tubal cancer: removal of the uterus, tubes, and ovaries. After the hysterectomy, unlike the treatment of

ovarian cancer, X-ray therapy would probably be necessary.

If the cancer is a "carcinoma," the cure rate can be as high as 50 percent if the growth is fairly small; if the growth is a "sarcoma," the cure rate is much lower. Fortunately sarcoma is even more rare than carcinoma; only thirty cases of fallopian-tube sarcoma have ever been reported in the world.

## 812 Is tubal ligation for sterilization a recommended operation?

If a woman knows for sure that she never wants to become pregnant again, a tubal ligation is a good operation (see Q. 1104). If there is any doubt, perhaps another method of birth control should be used.

Doctors have argued back and forth through the years about whether or not a tubal ligation will cause a woman to have problems with her uterus and ovaries later on. Some doctors say that a woman is more likely to end up having a hysterectomy later on and that she will be more likely to have growths on her ovaries if she has had her tubes tied. Statistics, however, have not shown any increased chance of either one of these problems after a tubal ligation. As a matter of fact, recent statistics have shown that sterilization definitely has no effect on the future health or function of a woman's body. It appears to be true that the tubes serve no other function than to facilitate pregnancy.

A woman who has a tubal ligation should realize that, even though her tubes are tied, she can still become pregnant. The chance is remote, varying from one in five hundred to one in two or three thousand. It does not matter whether the tubes are burned and cut, have an elastic band applied, have a clip put on them, or whether they are tied and cut; there is always a remote chance of pregnancy in the future. However, since the chance of subsequent pregnancy is so small, I advise my patients not to worry but to enjoy their newfound freedom.

Women can have their tubes tied either immediately after delivery (postpartum sterilization) or at some other time. Patients who choose to have a tubal ligation immediately after delivery must realize that a baby can be born looking totally normal but develop fatal complications the next day, or during the next few days, weeks, or months. A woman should not have her tubes tied if she would want another baby if something happened to this one. If you think that you would want another child if your newborn died, then you should wait to have your tubes tied until some later date.

A tubal ligation done at some time other than immediately after delivery is called an interval sterilization. It can normally be done on an outpatient basis and normally a laparoscopy sterilization or a mini-lap sterilization procedure is used (see Q. 1106–1109). If your doctor says that he or she needs to make a large incision and keep you in the hospital for two or three days in order to perform the surgery, the doctor is not doing one of these simpler procedures and probably has not learned how. I think it would be wise for you to find a doctor who can do a mini-lap or laparoscopy sterilization. This necessitates a much smaller incision, meaning less danger to your body and a shorter recovery time. (See Q. 1099–1118.)

Most patients have the idea that a fallopian tube extends from the uterus like a finger from a hand; if it is cut off, it will just fall away and die. This is not true. The fallopian tube is attached to and supported by a thin sheet of tissue through which blood vessels and nerves come up to the tube along its entire length. If the tube is cut in its midportion, the outer half of the tube still has an adequate blood supply and is still present in the body. This explains why doctors are able to cut the scarred portion of the tube ends away and sew the tubal segments back to-

gether in patients who want to have a sterilization reversed. (See illustration on p. 591.)

---

**813** **Is reversal of a sterilization possible?**

Yes. Such an operation is often possible for both men and women. (See Q. 925–929.) Most women are surprised to learn that this procedure has been available for years. I did my first successful tubal repair in 1971. Since then the techniques that I and other microsurgeons use have improved dramatically.

If your fallopian tubes have not been terribly damaged by the sterilization technique used and you and your husband are otherwise normally fertile, there is a 75 percent chance of your getting pregnant after having the reversal surgery done. In stating this high success rate I am assuming that your doctor would use microsurgical techniques.

But this means that 25 percent of women who have had a tubal sterilization will not be able to become pregnant later, even with surgical reversal of the original procedure. The only help available to these women is the "in vitro" (test tube) fertilization process. Fortunately centers that can do in vitro fertilization are growing in number around the country.

The operation to repair fallopian tubes is much more involved than the original sterilization. It requires a major abdominal incision, because the doctor must do the procedure meticulously and carefully, using the microscope. Those of us who do these procedures find that it can take from two to four hours for the repair. Three to five days' hospitalization is required, with a three- to five-week recuperation period afterward. The cost, including the surgeon's fee, normally is in the thousands of dollars.

I always counsel my patients who want reversal of their sterilization to approach the surgery with the attitude that since they cannot get pregnant the way they are, they might as well give it a try. If they do become pregnant, that's great! If they don't, at least they have done all they could and will have no regrets later on.

## Problems of the Ovaries

The human ovary is another of God's miracles. Its complexity is seen in its anatomy, its function, and its effect on a woman's menstrual cycle and on her total life process. Most women rarely think about the significance of their ovaries, although these organs are responsible for major changes in her life: the development of breasts, her menstrual periods, and her ability to conceive. The normal function of the ovaries can be seen in the regularity of a woman's menstrual cycle, a process which continues until the "death" of the ovaries at menopause, determined by the ovaries' internal time clock. God has beautifully orchestrated this process, and when a woman realizes this it can make her appreciate God's greatness even more.

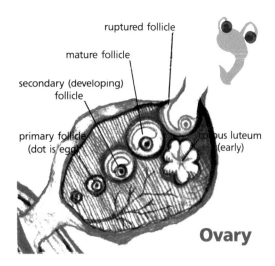

ruptured follicle
mature follicle
secondary (developing) follicle
primary follicle (dot is egg)
corpus luteum (early)

**Ovary**

envelope (the cortex) inside of which is a core (the medulla). The ovary is much like a golf ball in that it is white, its surface is irregular, and it has an outer covering and an inner core.

The outer covering of the ovary contains the egg cells, and all the activity responsible for the production of an egg each month is in that layer. The inner core of the ovary is primarily supportive. It contains blood and lymph vessels and connective tissue.

In chapters 1 and 2, we discussed the ovaries at length. For an in-depth understanding of the ovary's development and function, you might want to review those chapters.

---

## 814 What is special about the anatomy of the ovary?

The ovary is suspended on ligaments that extend from the uterus to the side of the pelvis (utero-ovarian ligaments and infundibulopelvic ligaments). These ligaments are capable of "moving" the ovary, making it more accessible to the fallopian tube for egg pickup. During pregnancy these ligaments are able to stretch dramatically, lifting the ovaries as the uterus enlarges.

The ovary is about one and a half inches in diameter and is made up of an external

## 815 What causes the ovaries to cease functioning and start the menopause process?

Menopause begins when all the eggs of the ovary have deteriorated or been ovulated. Since a woman's estrogen comes from the follicles surrounding the eggs, when there are no more eggs there is no more estrogen. Why most women have lost all their eggs at about the same time of life is unknown, but it occurs in a fairly consistent time range and is set by a woman's genes. The average age for menopause is from forty-eight to fifty-three. Many women, of course, start menopause five years before that and many five years after, and a few women develop menopause even outside these limits.

The whole subject of menopause is discussed more extensively in chapter 5.

## 816 What can I do to make sure my ovaries stay healthy?

There are only three things that a woman can do to help keep her ovaries healthy.

*Pelvic examination.* From the time a woman becomes sexually active, or reaches the age of twenty to twenty-five, she should have an annual pelvic examination. The doctor can determine whether or not there is an enlargement of the ovary during such an examination. If an enlargement of the ovary of two inches (five centimeters) or.more is found, the doctor will want to evaluate it carefully. An enlargement of that size may indicate a growth on the ovary.

Abnormal uterine bleeding indicates a need for a pelvic examination to check the ovaries along with other pelvic organs. An ovarian growth can cause a change in menstrual bleeding or cause bleeding between periods.

A woman who has pelvic pain should be examined. Such pain may indicate a growth on the ovary. An ovary with a growth on it can twist on its supporting ligaments, cut off its own blood supply, and become tender. An examination by a physician would determine whether or not this condition is present.

*Avoid infections of the ovary.* Any process that causes infection or scarring of the fallopian tubes can also affect the ovaries. Therefore, sexually transmitted diseases can cause infections that might involve the ovary, producing abscesses that require surgical removal of the ovary, and even of the uterus, tubes, and ovaries. A less-severe infection can cause chronic pain and scarring

and adhesions of the ovary to surrounding tissues, making it less able to produce a pregnancy. Even in this condition, however, the ovary will continue to produce the estrogen that the body of a reproductive age woman needs. In addition, IUDs can be the source of infection that not only involves the tubes but also affects the ovaries in such a way as to cause adhesions, scarring, pain, and decreased fertility.

*Do not have unnecessary ovarian surgery.* Even in this advanced medical age, many patients are subjected to unnecessary ovarian surgery. The most common reason for this is the presence of an ovarian cyst. Although cysts are often a part of the normal function of the body, this fact is sometimes misunderstood by both patients and physicians. Ovarian cysts are one of the most common sources of unnecessary surgery done by poorly trained or unscrupulous physicians.

## 817 How are ovarian cysts "normal"?

Each month the ovary forms a follicle around an egg. At the time of ovulation, this follicle breaks open and releases that egg. This follicle is a cyst, and it can be felt by a doctor during a pelvic examination if that exam is done just before ovulation. Normally such cysts will be two to three centimeters, or about an inch, in diameter. They are normal and occur every month and should cause neither you nor your doctor any concern.

Occasionally a follicle cyst can fail to break open at ovulation time. It then absorbs more fluid into itself and becomes larger. Such a cyst can sometimes be mildly painful. This enlargement can be felt by a doctor doing a pelvic exam.

## 818 When a follicle cyst enlarges, what should be done?

If your doctor tells you that you have an ovarian cyst and that you need surgery "now," you should get a second opinion from another doctor, and that doctor should be a gynecologist. Exceptions to this would be:

If you are through menopause. A doctor should not be able to feel a woman's ovary if she is postmenopausal. If the ovary can be felt at all it probably has a growth. You definitely need surgery if your doctor tells you that the ovary is enlarged or seems to have a cyst.

If the ovary seems "unusual" in some way to the doctor: unusually tender, unusually hard, unusually big (larger than three inches).

If you know your doctor well enough to be confident that he or she is well trained and will not recommend unnecessary surgery.

A good doctor can safely recommend conservative therapy rather than turning immediately to surgery if your ovary is only about two inches in diameter or smaller. My routine is to put a patient on three weeks of birth-control pills, starting the pills on the fifth day of the next period that comes up, and then examine her just before she finishes that three weeks' supply of the pills.

Birth-control pills "de-activate" the ovaries, allowing the fluid in a simple follicle cyst to absorb away. The ovary will usually return to normal size with just three weeks of birth-control pills.

I usually prescribe Enovid-E in this situation. Although this is a higher-dose birth-control pill than some, it is effective in suppressing the ovaries. The small-dose birth-control pills are more likely to fail in this respect.

If you cannot take birth-control pills, your doctor can watch the cyst for three or four months to see if the ovary will absorb the fluid out of the cyst on its own.

If the cyst goes away, either with birth-control pills or after three or four months of observation, you have a normal ovary. You have no increased risk of developing cancer, and you can think of that ovarian cyst as a normal part of the function of your body. You

will also have avoided ovarian surgery that could have caused scarring of your ovaries and possibly decreased your fertility in the future.

---

## 819 What if the cyst does not go away?

If your doctor has said that the cyst is five centimeters (two inches) or larger, or if it is smaller than that but does not go away under either of the conditions listed above, surgery is necessary. Unfortunately a doctor cannot tell by looking at a cyst whether or not it is a true growth, a malignancy, or a simple follicle cyst. Because of this a laparoscopy is usually not adequate for evaluating an ovarian growth. It is generally necessary to have a major incision made in your abdomen so that the doctor can remove the growth. This can usually be done with the side-to-side, bikini-type incision, about six inches long, in your low abdomen along the top of your pubic hairline.

Surgery is not done to get rid of a simple cyst, which is normal for the ovary. It is done because a cyst that does not go away is probably an ovarian growth; and growths on the ovary have a 2–3 percent chance of being cancer.

If you have an ovarian enlargement that is smaller than five centimeters but does not get smaller over a period of several months, you probably need to have surgery. When this situation exists, there is usually something wrong with the ovary. It is often a growth.

If you have any reason to question the competence of your physician, consult another doctor. If you have been going to a general practitioner or a general surgeon, I suggest you transfer to a gynecologist before you have any surgery on your ovaries. Because of their training and experience, gynecologists are better able to tell you what might be going on with your ovary and if you actually need surgery. They are much more able to do such surgery without endangering your future fertility. (See Q. 824.)

## 820 Is laparoscopy of no value in evaluating ovarian enlargement?

Any good gynecologist will occasionally use the laparoscope to look at an ovary that has stayed enlarged. But as stated in question 819, if your ovary is five centimeters or larger, the growth usually needs to be removed, not just looked at or biopsied.

If your ovary is smaller than five centimeters but is still staying enlarged, the doctor may want to look at it with a laparoscope. Such an enlargement can be due to endometriosis, or it can just be scarring or adhesions in the area of the ovary that does not involve the ovary at all. It could, of course, be a tumor.

The problem with laparoscopy for ovarian growths is that the laparoscope cannot look into the ovary to see what is causing it to be enlarged. If something abnormal is found, the surgery that can be done at laparoscopy is limited. The doctor can put a needle into the ovarian enlargement to see if there is fluid present (aspiration). If there is, the fluid will be sent to the pathologist for examination. The doctor can sometimes biopsy an ovarian cyst to make sure it is just a cyst and not a tumor. The problem with this is that if a tumor or cancer is present, it would be best for the growth to be taken out intact and not broken open by a biopsy first. Biopsying can allow leakage of the material from the growth, and if that material were cancerous, that would not be good.

However, with the laparoscope the doctor will occasionally be able to tell that the enlargement of the ovary is not significant. This would prevent a more major operation.

## 821 Will sonograms (ultrasound studies) or X-rays tell if surgery is needed for a pelvic mass?

Sonograms and X-rays can sometimes tell if a growth or cyst is present in a woman's pelvis. There are some special situations in which they might be ordered, but usually the doctor's pelvic exam is more accurate than an ultrasound or X-ray of the pelvis in determining what is happening or what needs to be done. Once the doctor has found a pelvic growth, X-rays and ultrasounds can help determine what it is.

## 822 What type of major surgery is necessary if I have a growth on my ovary?

First, let me state that while a growth on a woman's ovary is most likely not malignant, the only way she can know for sure is with surgery.

This type of surgery requires an abdominal incision, probably bikini-type about six inches long, done under general anesthesia or occasionally spinal or epidural anesthesia. During the surgery, the doctor can do one of three different types of operations on the ovary:

*Shelling the growth from the ovary.* A growth may be taken out of an ovary in much the same way an avocado pit comes out of an avocado, especially if it is a dermoid cyst. Such a growth is not totally "free," but with careful dissection it can be removed, leaving most of the ovarian tissue still intact. With very small sutures the doctor can sew the ovarian edges back together so that no raw surfaces are left along the edge to adhere to the surrounding tissues, causing adhesions that might later cause fertility problems or pain.

*Removal of the entire ovary.* If the growth has destroyed most of the normal ovarian tissue, it cannot be separated from that tissue. In this case the doctor will probably remove the entire ovary. This is a simple operation most of the time; the doctor merely clamps the base of the ovary, cuts it away, and sutures the tissue from which the ovary came so that it does not bleed.

*Removal of both ovaries, tubes, and the uterus.* (See Q. 825.)

---

## 823 What is the recovery from ovarian surgery like?

A four- or five-day hospitalization is usual after such surgery. I then advise my patients to have someone else do their cooking and housekeeping for the first two weeks they are at home. If they do this, they will be less likely to be tired later on. After three to four weeks, most women can return to normal activity.

---

## 824 Why do you recommend that a gynecologist do ovarian surgery?

Surgery on the ovary done in the old-fashioned way is just about the easiest abdominal surgery a doctor can do, and all doctors who do abdominal surgery think they can operate on ovaries as well as anyone else. Most general practitioners and general surgeons, however, are unaware that 75 percent of women who have surgery on their ovaries will end up with adhesions and scarring that can cause either pain or infertility later on. In addition, many of these doctors are not aware that many ovarian growths can be "shelled out" of the ovaries, leaving them normal in both hormone and egg production. For example, I know of a sad case in which a teenager had dermoid cysts on both ovaries. Although dermoid cysts are the kind that are most easily shelled out of an ovary, the general surgeon who discovered the growths removed both the girl's ovaries, leaving her sterile and without natural hormones for the rest of her life.

My suggestions are these:

Permit only a gynecologist to operate on your ovaries, and then only a gynecologist whom you feel will be gentle and careful in doing the surgery.

If you are below the age of forty, encourage your doctor to shell out the growth if possible. Shelling out a growth of an ovary takes more time than removing the ovary, but you never know when your other ovary might require removal. It is best to keep your ovaries, if you can, up to the age of forty. (See the next question regarding the reason that removal of the ovaries may be wise at this age.)

---

## 825 I have a growth on my ovary, and my doctor says that he will probably do a hysterectomy and remove both ovaries during surgery. Is this necessary?

If you are going to have surgery for an ovarian growth, removal of the uterus, the tubes, and both ovaries is a good idea if the following circumstances exist:

You do not want more children.

You don't want to have further trouble with ovarian growths or take the chance of having ovarian cancer in the future.

You are over forty or forty-five and do not mind taking a hormone pill every day starting now.

You would definitely need to take hormones until about the age of fifty if you had your ovaries removed before your menopause. If you did not do this, your chance of developing osteoporosis later on would be very high.

Having your ovaries removed at forty would make you different from other women, as far as hormones are concerned, but only until the age of menopause. At menopause there is no difference in a woman who has had her ovaries removed (surgical menopause) and a woman whose ovaries stop working on their own (natural menopause). If you have your ovaries removed at forty and you take estrogen and progesterone by mouth, you can be just like women who still have their ovaries. Then at the age of menopause (from about forty-eight to fifty-five) both you and they will have to decide if you want to continue taking hormones for the rest of your life as is now recommended by most gynecologists. (See Q. 265–280.)

You do not have to take hormones for the rest of your life if you have both ovaries removed, but there is good rationale for the three points mentioned above. If you have a growth in one ovary, there is about a 15-percent chance that a similar growth might develop on the other ovary. If you have had all the children you want and are nearing menopause anyway, you may as well go ahead and have both your ovaries removed to avoid the possibility of another ovarian growth. Having both ovaries out would, of course, eliminate the possibility of ever developing ovarian cancer.

A doctor who is going to remove both ovaries would almost always recommend removal of a woman's uterus and tubes too; unless she was young and wanted to keep her uterus, hoping that one of the new infertility techniques would allow her to be the recipient of an embryo from another woman.

If a woman has both ovaries removed, most of the time she will immediately start taking hormones. If she has her uterus removed, she can take her hormones without ever again having vaginal bleeding. Of course, if the uterus is removed, that eliminates any future chance of a woman developing cervical or uterine cancer. A woman feels no worse during the hospital stay if she has only her ovaries removed or has ovaries, tubes, and uterus removed.

When I talk to patients who are forty or over about this procedure, I give them the choice of removal of the uterus, tubes, and ovaries or surgery only on the affected ovary. Recovery from either surgery is essentially the same. Some women are quite glad to be finished with having menstrual periods and free of any chance of ever having an ovarian, uterine, or cervical growth. Others are quite adamant in wanting only the ovary with the growth taken out. Leaving one ovary does not increase the chance of uterine cancer developing later.

Most thoughtful gynecologists are not absolutely sure how to advise a patient who is around forty or forty-five years old. I have changed my recommendations back and forth through my years in practice. I now feel that if my wife had an ovarian tumor and was forty years old or older and we did not want any more children—and she did not have any big emotional problem with having her uterus, tubes, and ovaries removed—I would want her to do just that.

I have seen many women develop ovarian cancer later in life after having ovarian surgery when they were in their forties without having both ovaries removed. They and their families could have been saved lots of agony if both ovaries had been removed.

I am not implying, however, that a woman who has had cysts, growths, or surgery on her ovaries has a greater chance of developing ovarian cancer in the future. She does not.

Since it is now felt that almost all women need to take estrogen continuously from menopause on, removing the ovaries at the age of forty to forty-five only means that a woman would need to take oral hormones a few years longer. This same reasoning also applies to almost any surgery done through an abdominal incision on the pelvic organs in women over forty. (See Q. 159–173.)

---

## 826 If 95 percent of ovarian growths are not malignant and are not cysts, what are they?

Let me clarify that statement: 95 percent of ovarian growths are not malignant for women below the age of forty-five. If a woman is above that age and has a growth on her ovary, there is a 33-percent chance of malignancy.

The ovary can produce more than twenty different varieties of ovarian tumors, including both nonmalignant and malignant tumors. A woman's ovarian growth may be absolutely benign (nonmalignant), it can have borderline malignancy, or it can be overtly cancerous. In addition, a growth that a woman has on her ovary may have no capacity for producing hormones. On the other hand, some growths may produce hormones in such quantities that a woman's body will undergo dramatic changes, such as increased hair growth, baldness, and an enlarged clitoris. Both benign and malignant ovarian growths can be hormone-producing tumors.

For the purpose of clarity, nonmalignant ovarian tumors will be divided into two groups: those that do not produce hormones and those that do. I will primarily point out the facts that make them different from other tumors. For an in-depth discussion, you would need to see a medical textbook. Most doctors are quite willing for a patient to sit in their waiting room and read from one of their textbooks.

## 827 Which nonmalignant tumors do not produce hormones?

There are five benign tumors that do not normally produce hormones. I say "normally" because any tumor of the ovary can irritate it, causing it to produce increased amounts of hormones. These increased hormone levels can make a woman have irregular or abnormal periods. Those five tumors are: serous and mucinous cystadenomas, dermoid cysts (teratomas), fibromas, Brenner's tumors, and endometriosis.

## 828 Are serous and mucinous cystadenomas dangerous?

Yes, because if a mucinous cystadenoma is allowed to remain in the abdomen, it can rupture. If this happens portions of the growth can begin growing on other organs in the abdomen, producing mucus in the abdominal cavity. Although this is not a malignancy, it is difficult for a gynecologist to remove all of the mucus-producing tissue from the abdominal cavity. Even after surgery for removal of this material, it is common for women to continue to produce this mucus material, resulting in abdominal fullness, discomfort, adhesions, and other medical problems. The medical term for this unusual condition is "pseudomyxoma peritonei." This condition can cause death, and is rare. I have never treated a woman for it.

The primary problem with cystadenomas of the ovary is that they can be malignant. If a woman has an enlargement of the ovary and that enlargement is due to this type of tumor, it must be removed to prevent serious complications.

## 829 How are cystadenomas treated?

Removing a cystadenoma of the ovary almost always means removal of the entire ovary. Occasionally, if a cystadenoma is quite small, it can be cut out of the ovary. This type of tumor does not develop a capsule from which it can be shelled.

If a cystadenoma is found in one ovary, there is a 10-to-15-percent chance it will also be present in the opposite ovary. Although this is not a reason for both ovaries to be removed in a young woman, a woman in her forties would probably be best treated by removing both ovaries, the tubes, and the uterus. (See Q. 825.)

## 830 What are dermoid cysts?

Dermoid cysts (benign cystic teratomas) make up 30 percent of all nonmalignant tumors of the ovary. They occur most often during the reproductive years, though they have been found in newborn babies and in women after menopause.

A dermoid cyst, or a teratoma, is a tumor of the egg cells of the ovary. An egg cell will occasionally begin growing without fertilization. A fertilized egg, of course, has the potential of developing into a human being, but a tumor growing from an unfertilized egg has the capability of developing any of the tissues that make up a human body. A dermoid cyst, therefore, will typically contain hair, teeth, oil and sweat glands, cartilage, and other body tissues.

Because of the presence of these various tissues, a doctor may be able to diagnose a dermoid by taking an X-ray of a woman's abdomen. For some reason dermoids often have teeth growing in them, and these teeth seen on an X-ray can be the tip-off of a dermoid's presence.

This type of tumor can normally be shelled out of an ovary and the ovary closed with fine sutures, allowing resumption of normal ovarian function. Because dermoids often occur in the reproductive years, a gynecologist must do this procedure carefully so that fertility remains intact.

There are important reasons why dermoids should be removed. First, about 2 percent of them can be malignant. Second, a dermoid could rupture, spilling its contents into the abdomen. Also, any tumor in an ovary can interfere with regular ovulation and can affect otherwise normal fertility. Finally, since any of the body's tissues can be present in a dermoid, there can occasionally be enough active thyroid tissue to cause a woman to be hyperthyroid. This condition is called struma ovarii and is unusual.

When a dermoid is present in one ovary, there will also be one in the other ovary about 12 percent of the time.

## 831  What are fibromas?

A fibroma of the ovary is a tumor made up of fibrous connective tissue. This solid, firm tumor does not become malignant, but if neglected, it can get quite large.

A woman having a fibroma will occasionally also have fluid in the chest cavity around the lungs and excessive fluid in the abdominal cavity. This condition is called Meig's Syndrome. Removal of the fibroma causes this fluid accumulation to go away spontaneously. Removal of the fibroma usually requires removal of the entire ovary because the fibroma often causes the ovarian tissue to disintegrate completely.

When a fibroma is present in an ovary, there will also be a fibroma in the other ovary approximately 25 percent of the time.

## 832  What are Brenner's tumors?

Brenner's tumors, so named because of the doctor who described them in 1907, interest physicians because they are not sure from which cell in the ovary they arise. Part of the tissue of a Brenner's tumor is fibrous connective tissue, but there are also cells present which are similar to the surface cells of the ovary.

Most Brenner's tumors are benign, which is fortunate as they can occur in young women. Because they rarely occur in both ovaries and are rarely malignant, simple removal of the affected ovary seems to be adequate treatment in a young woman, but the entire ovary must be removed. If a woman does not want any more children, the best treatment is removal of the uterus and both ovaries and tubes, because this eliminates most of the tissues to which the tumor would spread in its early stages.

## 833  Can I have endometriosis of the ovary?

If endometriosis is present in the substance of the ovary, it is called an endometrioma. A doctor cannot determine without surgery if an enlargement of an ovary is due to endometriosis, although a laparoscopy may be sufficient to tell that endometriosis is present. When the doctor does look into a woman's pelvis and finds an endometrioma, he or she will almost always find implants of endometriosis in other areas of the pelvis. (See Q. 174–179, 953–960.)

## 834 Which nonmalignant ovarian tumors do produce hormones?

There are two, both of which are discussed in the following questions: granulosa-theca cell tumors, and tumors that produce male hormones.

## 835 What are granulosa-theca cell tumors?

This tumor of the ovary, which produces female hormones, can occur and has been observed in young girls at birth and also in women well past menopause. About 50 percent are found in women after the menopause and 5 percent in children before they start their puberty.

Because these tumors produce increased amounts of female hormones, they can do unusual things to the female in whom they are growing. In prepubertal females they can cause premature puberty, including the development of breasts, genital hair, menstrual periods, and shortness of stature. If a woman develops one of these tumors during her reproductive years, it can cause her to have irregular periods, or even a lack of periods. If a tumor of this type occurs after the menopause, it can cause a woman to resume bleeding from the uterus and to have sensitive, enlarging breasts.

Another unusual characteristic of this tumor is that it can occasionally produce malelike hormones that can cause a woman to have increased hair growth, decreased breast size, and other symptoms of male hormones in her body. Additionally, these tumors can rupture, bleed into the abdomen, and cause severe abdominal pain, necessitating emergency surgery.

Only about 5 percent of these tumors occur on both sides. Approximately 3 percent of them are malignant.

Treatment for a young woman, if the tumor is not malignant, is removal of the entire ovary. If the woman is older and has had all the children she wants, the best treatment is removal of the uterus, tubes, and ovaries.

## 836 Which tumors can produce male hormones?

Tumors that produce male hormones are unusual, and in my entire experience as a gynecologist, I have seen only one. The outstanding characteristic of these tumors, which have strange names such as gynandroblastoma, Sertoli-Leydig cell tumor, and lipid cell tumor, is that the male hormones they produce will cause significant changes in a woman's body. A woman may stop having menstrual periods and develop a beard, acne, baldness, deepening voice, and an enlarged clitoris.

These tumors ordinarily do not occur in both ovaries. If a person is young, removal of a single ovary is probably adequate. Because these tumors can be malignant, however, if a woman has had all the children she wants or is age forty or older and wants to have both ovaries removed, she should have that done.

## 837 If a growth in my ovary is (premalignant) "borderline malignant," what should I do?

During recent years doctors have come to realize that they cannot tell whether or not some tumors will "act" malignant, or in other words, will spread. They call these tumors "borderline malignant." As many as 20 percent of ovarian tumors may fall into this category, and many young women will have such tumors.

If women with borderline malignancy of an ovarian tumor have the affected ovary removed, they will usually not develop any spread of that tumor to other parts of their body. It is impossible to know for sure what will happen because the uterus and other ovary could already contain some malignant cells. A woman who has had all the children she wants should probably have her ovaries, tubes, and uterus removed. If it is important to her to maintain fertility, she can have only the affected ovary removed, as long as she has more frequent examinations than she would have had otherwise and understands that she is taking some risk.

### 838 Are there any techniques available for early detection of ovarian cancer?

No, there are not. This is one of the reasons that cancer of the ovary is a frustrating problem for both patients and doctors. There is no way to detect it early, and even if there were an early-detection technique, five thousand women would have to be screened by that technique in order to find one woman who had cancer of the ovary. Because of the problem of early detection, a woman often does not even know that she has an ovarian cancer until it has progressed fairly far. When a diagnosis of cancer of the ovary is made, 75 percent of the time it will have already spread out of the pelvic structures into other parts of her body.

There are four suggestions that doctors give.

If your ovary is enlarged and does not shrink, have surgery done to evaluate it.

If abdominal discomfort is present—including such things as distension, mild pain,

unusual indigestion—have a pelvic examination. It is not adequate for a doctor to merely feel your abdomen; he or she must do a pelvic exam to evaluate your pelvis adequately. Persistent vague symptoms of abdominal discomfort can be signs of an ovarian cancer.

If a tumor develops in one ovary, if you have completed your family and if you are age forty or older, let the doctor remove both ovaries and the uterus.

If you are having a hysterectomy for some other reason and are forty years or older, have the doctor remove your ovaries too. If you do not want both ovaries removed, at least have one removed. The less ovarian tissue there is in your body, the less likely you are to develop cancer of the ovaries during the next part of your life.

### 839 Why be so aggressive about preventing ovarian cancer?

About 2 percent of all women develop ovarian cancer. In 75 percent of these women the cancer will have already spread out of their pelvic structures into other parts of the body by the time it is found. Because of this, ovarian cancer is the leading cause of death from cancer of the female organs.

The death rate from cancer of the ovary is now equal to that of uterine cancer and cervical cancer combined. Even though far fewer patients actually develop cancer of the ovary than develop cancer of the uterus and cervix, the cure rate for cervical and uterine cancers is better because they can be detected earlier than ovarian cancer.

### 840 What will be done if my doctor suspects before surgery is done that I have cancer of the ovary?

Your doctor will order a complete blood count. If you are anemic, a blood transfusion may be necessary so you will have plenty of blood during surgery. The doctor will probably order kidney and colon X-rays to be sure that these organs are not involved in the cancerous process. Occasionally a doctor may want a CT scan, a sophisticated X-ray that shows a picture of a slice through the body (a cross section), instead of the usual X-ray view which is taken much like you would take a picture with a camera, or an ultrasound examination of your abdomen. These procedures provide some additional information about the location of any tumor tissue. Normally, though, these are not necessary.

Your doctor will discuss with you the fact that if cancer is present, the incision will need to be from your pubic bone straight up to your umbilicus and then around your umbilicus on up for another three or four inches. A large incision is necessary for a complete evaluation of the abdomen, to see whether or not the tumor has spread from the ovary, and to allow removal of as much cancer as possible.

You will need to prepare yourself for this type of surgery by being in as healthy a state of mind and body as you can be. The operation can take from three to five hours, because the doctor will want to be especially careful and thorough when doing the surgery.

---

### 841 What is done during surgery for ovarian cancer?

After the incision is made, the first thing the doctor will do is irrigate various parts of your pelvis with salt water (saline) and retrieve the fluid to check for free cancer cells in your abdomen. A pathologist will check the fluid.

Next, the doctor will look and feel all through your abdomen, including the under surface of your diaphragm and over your kidneys, as well as the apron of fat (the omentum) that hangs from your colon and stomach. He or she will look around your pelvic structures carefully.

The purpose of this careful examination is to determine first, if cancer is present, and second, how far the cancer has gone. Finally, the goal of this surgery is to remove as much of the cancer as possible. Unless your abdominal cavity is examined carefully, the doctor will not know what percentage of the cancer he or she has been able to remove. Remember, any chemotherapy treatment success is partially based on the amount of cancer left in your abdomen at the completion of surgery.

---

### 842 What surgical procedures will the doctor perform if I do have ovarian cancer?

If you still want to have children, if your cancer is totally contained inside the ovary, and if it is a fairly nonaggressive type of cancer, the doctor may remove only the ovary where the cancer is growing. In every other situation the doctor will remove your uterus, tubes, and ovaries.

The gynecologist will normally remove the omentum and any cancer implants found growing anywhere in your abdomen, as well as any lymph nodes that are enlarged, since they may contain cancer.

Nodules of cancer can also grow on the intestines. If a large nodule cannot be cut off the surface of the intestines, a portion of the intestines may need to be cut out to remove the growth. Since ovarian cancer is usually a surface growth, this is not often necessary. In my years of practice, while doing an operation for ovarian cancer I have had to do only two intestinal resections and one colostomy. (A colostomy is a procedure which routes the colon to the outside through the abdominal wall instead of through the anus. Bowel movements, therefore, must come through the colostomy instead of through the anus. An intestinal resection means removing a segment of bowel, then sewing the ends back together.)

Once the doctor has removed as much of the tumor as is possible, you will be evaluated for the use of chemotherapy. The use of radiation (X-ray) treatment for cancer of the ovary is not often necessary because, in this case, it is ordinarily not as effective as chemotherapy and may produce complications. The exception to this is the treatment of a dysgerminoma. (See Q. 847.)

## 843 What is the outlook for patients with ovarian cancer?

Cancer of the ovary is so frightening that it is normal to feel scared if you have it. You are fortunate, however, to be living at this time, when treatment for ovarian cancer is much better than it once was. In past years doctors often opened patients up, biopsied the growth, and then closed the incision, telling the patient that the cancer was incurable. This was in earlier days when chemotherapy was not as good as it is now, when the best surgical procedures for ovarian cancer had not been determined, and when general surgeons often did this type of operation. Today most patients with ovarian cancer are operated on by a surgeon/gynecologist team or by a specialist in gynecologic cancer surgery. This insures expert surgery and an increased chance for cure.

## 844 Is chemotherapy effective for ovarian cancer?

There are several chemotherapy drugs that are used for treatment of ovarian cancer, and these drugs may be used alone or in combination with each other. The choice of drug therapy will, of course, be in the hands of a specialist who understands the use of these drugs, their benefits, their side effects, and how these relate to your condition.

In years past the outlook for patients with ovarian cancer was fairly hopeless, but with today's drugs and techniques, many patients treated with chemotherapy are free of ovarian cancer for many years, and some seem to be totally cured.

Many patients object to the idea of the use of chemotherapeutic drugs, and I can understand their feelings. For ovarian cancer, however, these drugs are useful. I strongly encourage my patients to take them in this situation. They are not pleasant drugs, of course, but you do not have to take them forever, and they give you a much greater chance of a cure or at least a longer life. Without them the cancer will almost always continue to grow, even after the best surgery.

## 845 What does "staging" mean in relation to ovarian cancer?

The "stage" of a cancer refers to how extensive it has become. It is a technical term, and there is a precise definition for each stage. The term *stage* does not refer to whether a patient is in the early or late stage of life. Staging a patient's cancer helps the doctor to define clearly how far along the person's cancer is. It is also useful when doctors with different treatment techniques compare notes in an effort to find the most effective method.

## 846 What are the different stages of ovarian cancer?

The stages of ovarian cancer are:

*Stage I:* The cancer is confined to the ovary; it has not spread.

*Stage II:* The cancer is confined to the pelvis. It may involve, in addition to the ovary or ovaries, a fallopian tube, the uterus, or some of the lining tissue of the pelvis (peritoneum).

*Stage III:* The cancer has grown outside the pelvis but is still inside the abdomen. It may involve lymph nodes in the abdomen or the lining of the intestines or other areas of the abdomen.

*Stage IV:* The cancer involves the liver or areas outside the abdomen, such as the lungs or lymph nodes in other parts of the body.

---

**847** **What chance of living do I have after my ovarian cancer is found and treated?**

Your chance of cure is based on the type of cancer you have and in what stage it is when the surgery is done.

*Type of cancer.* A few types of ovarian cancer have special characteristics that make chances for survival better. For instance, if a *"dysgerminoma,"* an ovarian cancer that occurs often in young women, has not spread outside of the ovary, removal of the ovary can cure the patient. If tumor tissue is later found elsewhere in the body, this recurrent cancer can be treated with X-ray therapy and often cured. In addition, some ovarian cancer is quite sensitive to chemotherapy. This type of therapy should definitely be tried in these cases.

*Grade of cancer.* The degree of malignancy of the cells is important. Aggressiveness of cancer cells varies from person to person, even when the same type of tumor is involved, but that aggressiveness (or nonaggressiveness) determines how quickly the cancer spreads and how much trouble it causes. For instance, if at surgery you have a cancer that is exactly as extensive as another woman's, yet your cancer is Grade I (a mildly aggressive cancer) but the other woman's cancer is Grade III (much more aggressive cancer), your chance of living for five years is three or four times greater than the other woman's.

*Amount of tumor left at first surgery.* In years past doctors opened patients up, found cancer, closed them back up, and told them they had an inoperable cancer and would die within a few months. Today this should almost never happen. If the cancer is removed so that there is no piece of cancer remaining in the body thicker than one-half inch, the chance of surviving for five years is greatly increased. The reason for this seems to be that if the cancer cannot be totally removed, the cancer that is left in a woman's abdomen can be penetrated by the chemotherapeutic drugs if it is a maximum thickness of one-half inch.

If you or a friend or relative has surgery done and the doctor merely closes you up, saying you are "inoperable," immediately call one of the phone numbers given at the end of this chapter. Get the name of a gynecological cancer specialist in your area and contact him or her. Don't give up. You may have months or years of useful life left if you are cared for properly.

*Woman's age.* The age at which a woman develops cancer is also significant. The younger a woman is when she develops cancer, the greater her chance of survival.

Because all of the above factors are important, it is almost impossible to predict an overall chance of survival from ovarian cancer. In general, however, the following survival rates are quoted by those who treat cancer of the ovary.

*Stage I:* About 50–60 percent of women will survive for five years.

*Stage II:* About 40–60 percent of women survive for five years.

*Stage III:* About 5 percent of women survive for five years.

*Stage IV:* About 3 percent of women survive for five years.

It is important to remember that these figures mean nothing except that the more extensive the ovarian cancer is, the less likely you are to live for five years. If you have a cancer that is a low-grade malignancy, such as Grade I or II, you are fairly young, and the doctor who operated on you did a thorough job of getting most of the cancer out, you have a much better chance of living for five years than a patient who is a great deal older, who has a Grade III or IV cancer, and in whom the doctor had to leave large pieces of the cancer behind at the time the surgery was done.

## 848 How will my doctor know if chemotherapy is successful?

In order to check the success of the treatment, additional surgery is necessary. This second operation, usually done a year after the initial surgery, is called a second-look operation. As it is a vital and significant step forward in the care of women who have ovarian cancer, it is most important that it be done.

This second-look operation is major surgery, of course. As large an incision will be made the second time as was made the first time. Biopsies will be taken from all areas of your abdomen. If there is cancer present anywhere in your abdomen, the doctor will try to cut all of it out, even if it requires taking out a part of the colon, the small intestines, or some other structure that can be removed at such surgery.

No one likes the idea of a second operation, but this type of surgery is extremely helpful in getting you well. In order to "qualify" for a second-look operation, patients must have no evidence of any cancer being present on abdominal or pelvic exam. In one sense, therefore, the fact that a patient needs a second look is an extremely good sign. However, it only means that there is no

cancer that can be felt in the pelvis or abdomen. This may mean that no cancer has grown back and that any cancer that was there after the first operation was killed by chemotherapy. Of course, it can also mean that cancer is still present but just cannot be felt.

## 849 I have ovarian cancer and I am scared. Can you help me?

The life of one of the most afflicted, troubled men who ever lived is chronicled in the Bible. His name is Job, and his wisdom is helpful to anyone facing the possibility of death:

> Man's days are determined;
> You have decreed the number of his months
> And have set limits he cannot exceed.
> (Job 14:5)

All of us should have the same attitude. Whether or not you have ovarian cancer, your attitude toward life and death can be, "I will not live on this earth forever; I will, however, live as long as God wants me to live. I may die tomorrow of a car wreck, next year of ovarian cancer, or when I am ninety-five of a heart attack, but whenever it is, God controls the time."

If you do have ovarian cancer, it should be encouraging to note that approximately 30 percent of women who have cancer of the ovary do not die as a result of that cancer; they die of other diseases and problems that ordinarily affect womankind. It seems best, therefore, for a woman to accept gratefully the days that God has given her.

It is absolutely vital for a woman to fight as hard as she can to overcome all the obstacles that life may present, including ovarian cancer. It is important to have surgery, take chemotherapy, and to have the second look operation, but all of this should be done without bitterness and anger. Becoming bitter and angry makes you unhappy and more uncomfortable and also makes those people around you unhappy, uncomfortable, and unsure of how to relate to you.

Talk freely with your physician about your chances for survival. It is important to ask what type of therapy is recommended and what side effects you might have. Many doctors are uncomfortable discussing these things so you may need to lead your doctor into telling you what you need to know.

I think the reason doctors are uncomfortable in discussing this subject with patients is that they feel it is their own failure if they cannot cure a patient. Because their own egos are involved, they find it more difficult to discuss with the patient what might happen if the cancer continues to grow.

Of course you want a doctor who believes he or she can cure you and who will not easily give up. But if your doctor cannot give you good emotional support, talk to your pastor, priest, or rabbi, or see a psychologist or psychiatrist. Such counseling can be of great help in hard times.

---

**850** **Where can I get more information about ovarian cancer?**

A toll-free number has been established by the National Cancer Institute. The number is easy to remember: 1-800-4-CANCER. If you call, you will be connected with the Cancer Information Service in your area which provides information and confidential answers to your personal questions about cancer.

Since this service was established in 1976, it has responded to more than two million inquiries from the general public. The response to these calls is confidential, and you will receive, if you wish, free publications on specific cancers and also on techniques for cancer prevention, cancer treatment, and for coping with cancer.

There are three offices that are not tied into the main number. These are:

| | |
|---|---|
| Washington, D.C. | 202-636-5700 |
| Alaska | 1-800-638-6070 |
| Hawaii | 808-524-1234. |

In addition, the public library will have books, magazines, and further information on cancer. There also is a new publication with information about cancer called *Cancer Update*. Order it from P.O. Box 55007, Sherman Oaks, California, 91413.

Finally, you might call a hospital that specializes in cancer and ask for the gynecology department. The cancer hotline can tell you how to reach the nearest cancer hospital in your area.

---

## Problems of the Breasts

The human breast is obviously important to human beings since we are classified as a species, along with other "animals" who nourish their young with milk, by the Latin word for breasts: *mammal*. Also, not long ago human breast milk was necessary for the continuation of the human race. Now, although mother's milk is still the best food for a baby, there are alternative methods of feeding our young. The breast is not exclusively nurture-related, however. In today's society, a woman's breasts have taken on a new significance in areas of psychological importance and social and sexual relationships.

Because of the importance of the breast in all these areas, there is a great deal of concern when something seems to be wrong with them. Parents are concerned if a daughter's breasts do not seem to be developing properly, and the girl herself is often concerned if her breast development does not equal that of her friends. Women and their husbands are extremely concerned about breast lumps. The specter of cancer, with its potential for causing the loss of a breast, always overshadows the finding of such lumps.

In the questions that follow, we will discuss various diseases of the breasts. Other aspects of the breast are discussed elsewhere in the book: In chapter 1 we discussed the basic anatomy of the breasts; in chapters 2 and 3 we discussed developmental abnormalities of the breast in baby, child, and adolescent; and in chapter 11 we will discuss the problem of galactorrhea (milky secretions from the breasts). Refer to those chapters and to the Index for further information.

## 851 If I develop a problem with my breasts, will my gynecologist treat it?

If the problem involves breast lumps or breast cancer, your gynecologist will probably refer you to a surgeon who will do a breast biopsy and/or breast surgery. This is because most gynecologists come from specialized educational programs that provide no training whatsoever in the treatment of breast growths and breast cancer.

Because you probably go to a gynecologist for your annual exam, however, he or she will most likely be the one you first see when you think something is wrong with your breasts. A gynecologist is usually the one who evaluates a breast problem and who will give you guidance as to what to do about it.

If your annual checkups are normally done by an internal-medicine specialist, a general practitioner, or a family practitioner, that doctor will offer the same help in evaluating the problem and will refer you to a general surgeon if the situation warrants.

The information we offer in this section is the type of information you would receive from a gynecologist; we will not attempt to delve in great detail into breast surgery or breast cancer.

The gynecologist's limitation in the care of your breasts does not mean he or she is unimportant in the care of your breasts. Gynecologists do more breast exams, in fact, than general surgeons do, because of the number of patients they see for annual examinations. And, because gynecologists are familiar with the administration of hormones, they are much more likely than a general surgeon to be able to help you avoid aggravating and recurring breast nodules by use of appropriate hormones. This alone may help avoid many biopsies that a general surgeon might otherwise need to do. In addition, a gynecologist will usually be more knowledgeable and understanding if you have a problem with breast pain and will often have suggestions for relieving such discomfort.

## 852 Is there anything I need to do between annual examinations to keep my breasts normal and healthy?

Yes. You should do regular breast self-examinations (BSE), since 90 percent of breast lumps are discovered by women themselves, using this technique. Remember, even though you may have very recently had a breast examination by your physician, you could have an early breast cancer growing in your breast right now. If you wait twelve months for another exam, that cancer could have grown to a dangerous stage before it is found.

Since you cannot go to your doctor often enough to feel safe about your breasts, you should do breast self-examinations once a month, right after your period. It is important to do the exam at that time, because then your breasts are the least swollen and knotty. If you have a breast nodule, your doctor may want you to check your breasts more often than once a month. Choose a special way to help you remember when to check your breasts. For example, check them on the fourth day of your menstrual period; if you are on birth-control pills, do a BSE on the day you take the first pill each month; or if you have had a hysterectomy or have gone through the menopause, check your breasts on the first day of the calendar month.

Many of my patients will not check their breasts each month. Some are afraid that they might find a lump others say they just forget. Both reasons, while understandable, are foolish. Failing to examine the breasts will not keep a breast lump from developing; it will only allow it to become dangerously far along before it is found.

If you cannot remember, or cannot make yourself do a BSE, have your husband do it! However, if he is going to have that responsibility, be sure he knows how to check the breasts thoroughly and objectively. (BSE is not the time for "fooling around"!)

You should continue to check your breasts even if you are pregnant or nursing. There have been many sad cases in which women found a breast lump during pregnancy or while nursing, but they or their physicians assumed those lumps were caused by the hormones of pregnancy or lactation, only to find out later that they had been neglecting a breast cancer.

Many women feel that they would not know a "significant" breast lump from an insignificant one. As one who has felt many breast cancers, I can say with conviction that if you feel a breast cancer in your breast, you will almost certainly know it. There is something "different" about the way it feels. Just do the exam. Don't worry about whether or not you would feel a breast cancer—you would.

Obviously all those who encourage you to do a regular BSE, such as your doctor and the American Cancer Society, know that you are not a professional "breast checker." In spite of that, we still encourage you to do

BSE because we know that if you have a breast cancer, you will detect it sooner than if you were not examining your breasts regularly. The only reason you say you do not think you would know a breast cancer if you felt one is that you have never felt one. Take my word for it: you would know!

---

## 853　How is a breast self-examination done?

I will describe the classic technique for BSE. You probably will need instruction about BSE before you can do it properly. (See p. 486.)

If you feel any lumps anywhere be sure to let your doctor know.

I find that many women will not do the entire BSE procedure. If you are one who absolutely will not do all of it, at least check your breasts in the shower with soapy fingers, or check them in bed, lying on your back.

In addition to the instructions on p. 486, it is a good idea to get your doctor to show you how to do a breast examination. I use a movie in my office that gives BSE instructions. In addition, I have plastic models of the female breast, complete with various-sized lumps, so that my patients can get an idea of what a breast lump feels like. Your doctor may have these instructional tools available. If so, take advantage of them. If not, encourage your doctor to get them.

---

## 854　Which symptoms might indicate breast problems?

There are several important danger signs that should be checked by your physician:

a lump in the breast or in the axilla (armpit)

discoloration of the skin of the breast

# Breast Self-examination

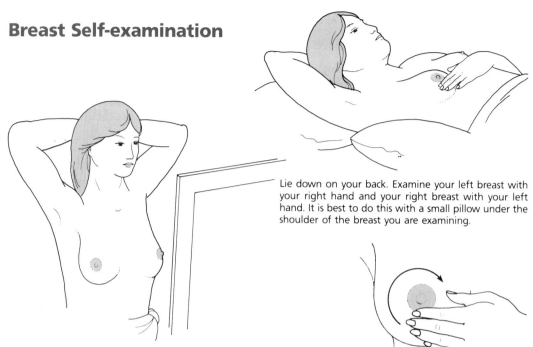

Lie down on your back. Examine your left breast with your right hand and your right breast with your left hand. It is best to do this with a small pillow under the shoulder of the breast you are examining.

Stand or sit in front of a mirror where you have good lighting. Place both hands on top of your head and pull your arms back. Observe your breasts carefully, looking for indentations of the skin (retraction), puckering, and any irregularities or thickening of the skin. Look at the nipples to be sure that they are the same as they were in previous months. Don't be surprised if your breasts are not the same size; no woman's breasts are exactly symmetrical.

Examine your breasts with your fingers together flat against your breast, with gentle but firm pressure. Work from the outside toward the nipple, or from the nipple out, in a circular, spiral pattern.

Also feel the area around the nipple. Squeeze the nipple gently to see if there is any discharge.

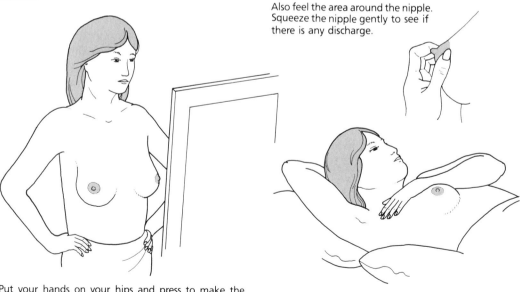

Put your hands on your hips and press to make the breasts "stand out." Then do the visual check again.

Feel up under your arm in your armpit (axilla).

bleeding or discharge from the nipple

lumpiness of the breasts that makes one breast look different from the other

dimpling of the skin of the breast

retraction of the nipple

prominent veins of the breast that have not been present before

thickening of breast skin

area of the breast that is hot or warmer than the rest of the breast or than the other breast

sore on the breast or nipple that does not heal

unusual pain in the breast

---

## 855 Is it normal to have painful breasts?

Yes, it can be quite normal to have painful breasts. Pain that fluctuates with the menstrual cycle is almost always due to normal changes in the body and not to breast disease.

Breasts are made up of cells that are sensitive to estrogen and progesterone. As the estrogen level increases during the menstrual cycle, and as progesterone adds to the increased stimulation of breast tissue, the breasts will become sensitive, especially during the days just before the menstrual period.

Some women have breasts that are unusually sensitive to these hormone fluctuations of the menstrual cycle. Their breasts can become so tender just before their periods start that they cannot sleep on their stomachs or hug their husbands. This is normal for them. The woman who has this type of pain does not need to worry, since it is not a sign of cancer or of any other disease process.

If the breasts hurt or if a lump hurts, the problem is usually not cancer. It is most likely due to normal hormonal changes of the breasts or it is fibrocystic disease. Cancer

is so slow in growing that it does not normally cause breast pain.

---

## 856 Can breast pain be due to an abnormality?

Yes, breast pain can be caused by several different problems.

*Fibrocystic disease.* Breast pain can be caused by this disease process. (See next question.)

*Pain due to nerves of the chest wall.* A woman who has had a neck injury can have resulting irritation of the nerves that go to the wall of the chest. Women may think the pain they are having is in their breast tissue, but an exam will show that it is actually in the wall of the chest.

*Pain from structures in the chest wall.* It is not uncommon for patients to have pain in a rib, or in cartilage between the rib and the breastbone, and assume it is breast pain. An examination will usually identify this pain across the wall of the chest. If one of the muscles of the chest wall or its attachment to the bone becomes irritated, pain can develop under the breast and seem to be breast pain. Careful examination usually identifies the source of such pain.

*Blood clot in a vein of the breast surface (Mandor's disease).* Occasionally a vein of the skin over the breast will become clotted, causing tenderness and pain. It takes careful examination by a physician to make this diagnosis. This condition is not dangerous, but it must not be confused with inflammatory cancer of the breast, which is an extremely malignant process.

---

## 857 What is fibrocystic disease of the breasts?

Fibrocystic disease is caused by an overreaction of the breast tissue to the normal female hormones. The cells of your breast tissue have estrogen receptors, and this is how your breasts "know" that estrogen is around. When the cells of your breasts sense the presence of estrogen, they thicken and grow. In fact, this is how your breasts develop in the first place.

A large number of women have breast tissue that overresponds to normal estrogen and progesterone production. Their breasts thicken up too much during the week or two before a period. Then during and after the period, when the hormone levels of the body decrease and the breasts lose the hormone stimulation, too many of the cells in the overstimulated breasts break down, filling the ducts of the breasts with excess cellular debris. All this material forms pockets of fluid which cause the pain and cysts of fibrocystic breast disease. Some degree of fibrocystic disease of the breasts occurs in 50 percent of women. Some authorities say that all women have some elements of fibrocystic change in their breasts! It is not truly a "disease," however—neither an infection caused by a germ nor a growth, such as a tumor. It is merely the interaction of a woman's hormones with her breast tissue.

---

**858** **What problems can fibrocystic breast disease cause?**

Fibrocystic disease can cause several problems.

*Pain.* The fluctuation of hormones in a woman's normal cycle cause fibrocystic breasts to swell and change more than they should, and these fibrocystic changes can cause pain. The pain from these changes normally increases during the premenstrual time and decreases after the period has ended. As stated previously, such pain is usually not a symptom of cancer because cancer is unlikely to put enough pressure on the breast tissue to cause pain, at least until it has been growing for a long time.

*Lumpiness.* Fibrocystic disease causes breasts to be lumpy. Many women think that breast tissue is merely fat and that any nodularity or firmness in their breasts is fibrocystic disease or a tumor. Normal breast tissue, however, is embedded in the fat of the breasts, and breast tissue itself is gland tissue and is firm, just as most other gland tissue of the human body is firm. A man's testicles are glands and demonstrate the naturally firm nature of gland tissue. The firm tissue you feel embedded in the fat of your breast is breast tissue. When you examine your breasts, it is not this firm, glandular tissue that is significant; rather it is change in that tissue that you are looking for.

Some nodularity of breast tissue is normal and to be expected with the monthly changes in the breasts. When you do a BSE you are looking for something different, for discrete firm or rubbery nodules or discrete cystic areas. I describe them to my patients as being separate, distinct areas not actually embedded in the surrounding tissue, something like a small peeled grape that moves easily.

When you are checking your breasts and find a nodule, it can be a fibroadenoma; it is more likely to be that than it is to be cancer. Breast nodules, or fibroadenomas, are a result of fibrocystic disease. These lumps are hard to diagnose, and since a doctor cannot tell whether a lump is a fibroadenoma or cancer, breast biopsies or other diagnostic tests are necessary. Fibroadenomas are present in both breasts in from 12 to 25 percent of women who develop them.

*Cancer.* Women who have true fibrocystic disease of the breasts (fibroadenomas proven by biopsy) or who have cysts large enough for fluid to be drawn out of them with a needle (aspiration) are more likely to have cancer of the breast than other women. The increased risk of cancer is about two or three times the average woman's risk.

---

**859** **What should I do if I find a lump in my breast?**

If you find a lump in your breast, make an appointment immediately to see a doctor for evaluation. There is no need to panic, however. If a breast cancer is present, it has already been growing for several years before it became large enough to feel. A few days' delay will not make any difference in your chance of recovery.

Allow yourself time to be sure you are seeing a good doctor. It is most important to see a doctor who will give you proper consultation and will give thorough consideration to your problem. This is far more important than for you to rush madly into a biopsy.

Most women see their gynecologist first. If your doctor agrees that what you are feeling is a definite lump or cyst, you will usually be referred to a good general surgeon. If your gynecologist thinks that what you are feeling is not a distinctly abnormal area, he or she will tell you so and may suggest that you do nothing now but return after one or two menstrual periods to see if the area has become less nodular. If in time the area becomes less noticeable, it is almost certainly not cancer but only a fibrocystic change. If your doctor is unsure about the nature of the irregular area, he or she may suggest diagnostic techniques to find out for sure. (See Q. 862–869.)

## 860 What will a doctor look for when checking a breast lump?

There are several things a doctor will look for when checking a breast lump:

***Changes in the skin or nipples.*** Changes of this type mean that a growth is more likely to be cancerous. They might include dimpling of the skin over the lump or discoloration, perhaps reddening, of the skin or nipple. Don't let an acne-type pimple on your breast or nipple scare you too badly, though; these are actually in the skin, not down in the breast tissue, and are almost always insignificant.

***An isolated lump.*** If your lump is isolated and not a part of a thickened area in the breast, it is slightly more likely to be cancer. A lump that is part of a group of other lumps, or part of a generally thickened area in the breast, is more likely fibrocystic disease.

***Attachment of the lump.*** If the lump seems attached to the skin or to the chest wall, it is more likely malignant. Benign lumps in the breast do not usually attach in this fashion.

***Hard consistency.*** If your lump is hard, it is more likely to be cancer than if it is soft and easily compressed.

## 861 Are there high-risk categories for breast cancer?

There are certain situations that make it more likely that you will develop breast cancer sometime in your life than the average person. These factors are not meant to scare you, but to help you be more careful. You can, of course, have all of these factors existing in your life and never develop cancer, but women with some of them need to watch their breasts more carefully, consult their doctors a little sooner, and have biopsies a little more often than other women. The higher-risk categories for breast cancer are:

*Being a woman.* Men do get breast cancer, but rarely; it occurs in less than 1 percent of the male population.

*Women over thirty-five.* If you are over thirty-five, you are more likely to develop breast cancer than those who are under that age. Less than 4 percent of breast cancer occurs in women under thirty-five.

*Family members with cancer.* If you have a family member who has had breast cancer (mother, sister, or aunt), you are two or three times more likely to develop breast cancer than the average woman.

*Previous breast cancer.* If you have had breast cancer already, you are more likely to develop breast cancer in the remaining breast than the average woman.

*National origin.* If you are Jewish, you are more likely to develop breast cancer than if you are not.

*Menstrual cycle record.* If you started menstrual periods before the age of twelve or began menopause after the age of fifty, you are more likely to develop breast cancer.

*Childbirth record.* If you did not have your first child until after you were thirty years of age or if you have never had a child, you are more likely to develop breast cancer than a woman who had her first child before she was thirty years old.

*Alcohol consumption.* If you drink alcohol daily, whether it is wine, beer, or hard liquor, you are more likely to develop breast cancer than if you do not consume alcohol that often.

*Weight.* If you are 10 percent above the average weight for your height and age, you are more likely to develop breast cancer.

*Fibrocystic disease.* If you have fibrocystic disease of the breasts, you are more likely to develop breast cancer.

*Diet.* Recent studies have indicated that women who eat the typical American diet, which is high in meat and fat and low in fiber, have an increased risk of breast cancer.

---

**862** **If I have a suspicious lump, are there diagnostic procedures and tests that can be done after the physical examination?**

Yes, there are several tests that can be administered to help evaluate the breasts.

These are discussed in the next seven questions. Although these tests are good and certainly have their place, if your doctor feels that a breast lump should be biopsied, you should have it done. There is no test of the breasts, other than biopsy, that can tell with total accuracy whether or not a malignancy is present.

I had a patient several years ago who had a hard nodule that I was quite concerned about. I referred her to a surgeon. Instead of going to the surgeon, however, she had a mammogram, or X-ray of the breast. Since the mammogram did not show signs of cancer, this woman did not go to the surgeon for several months, and then not until her arm had already begun swelling as a result of her cancer spreading to the lymph nodes under her arm.

*Remember:* Tests are useful, but if a doctor feels that you need a breast biopsy, have it done. Almost all persistent lumps need to be biopsied.

---

**863** **If a biopsy is the only truly accurate method of diagnosis for breast lumps, what is the value of the other tests?**

Occasionally tests can indicate the presence of cancer when you and your doctor do not otherwise suspect the possibility of cancer. For instance, 45 percent of the breast cancers that are found by mammograms are so small that they cannot be found on examination by you or your doctor. If a breast cancer is found by mammogram before it can be felt on exam, a woman has an 80-95-percent chance of being totally cured. If, however, her cancer is not found until it can be felt by examination, she has a 50-70-percent chance of cure.

If a woman has routine mammograms, they can show a breast cancer two years before it would grow large enough for her to feel on breast self-examination. Obviously,

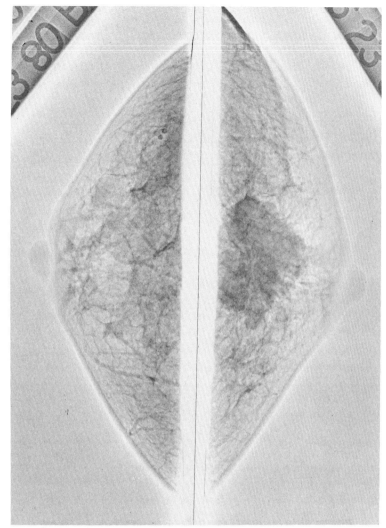

Reproduction of a mammogram. The darkened area on the right breast is suspicious and, until proven otherwise, is presumed to be cancerous.

therefore, if your cancer is found before it is large enough for you to feel it, your chance of cure is excellent. Tests for breast cancer are a great help.

## 864   What is a mammogram?

A mammogram is simply an X-ray of the breasts. The examination itself is called mammography. The purpose of this X-ray, as

with any X-ray, is to find abnormalities inside the body. The Xerox Corporation has refined the procedure for X-ray of the breasts, using a technique they developed called Xero-radiograph, or Xerograms. This is the technique most often used in the United States for mammography.

The procedure is simple and for most women free of pain. Some women dislike the fact that they must undress to the waist for the exam, and other women find that the pressure of the instrument against their breasts is uncomfortable. It is necessary, however, that the breasts be compressed during the procedure to reduce the thickness of the tissues being X-rayed. Thinner tissues allow a better X-ray picture.

## 865 What problems make a mammogram necessary?

Mammograms should be done in the following situations.

- Women of any age who have such irregular, lumpy, firm, or enlarged breasts that an adequate breast examination is impossible should have a mammogram done on a regular basis. They should, however, continue doing their own BSE. Even though it is difficult to do on certain types of breasts, BSE is still a vitally important examination.
- Patients who have suspicious breast symptoms, such as a lump, nipple discharge, bleeding from the nipple, severe pain, or persistent redness of the skin of the breasts need to have a mammogram done.
- Patients who have no symptoms or problems but who are in high-risk categories (see Q. 861, 866, 867), need more frequent mammograms on a schedule recommended by their physicians.

## 866 Who should have routine mammograms, and how often should they be done?

The American Cancer Society and the American College of Radiology make the following recommendations for routine mammograms on patients who are having no problems.

Women should have an initial screen or baseline mammogram at the age of thirty-five. After the age of forty, women should have a mammogram every one or two years until age fifty. The frequency is based on the incidence of breast cancer in their families. From the age of fifty on, an annual mammogram should be done.

## 867 Why should I have a routine mammogram if I do not feel a lump and am having no other breast problem?

A breast cancer exists in the breast tissues for many months before it grows large enough to be felt by you or your doctor. If you are having routine mammograms, a breast cancer can be detected two years before you could find it on breast self-examination. At this stage you have an 80-95-percent chance of complete cure with good treatment. Not only is the prospect of cure exciting, but the peace of mind that comes with knowing that you have little chance of having recurrent cancer is wonderful.

The American Cancer Society has good reasons for mammograms done according to the above schedule.

Deaths due to breast cancer can be decreased by 40 percent in women who are over fifty years old who have mammograms done yearly. Newer techniques have decreased radiation exposure from mammograms by two-thirds in recent years, making it a safer procedure than it was in the past. (See next question.) In addition, the accuracy of mammograms has increased, making it a more reliable procedure.

## 868 Are mammograms dangerous?

The American Cancer Society and the American College of Radiology recommend that mammography machines expose a woman to no more than one rad of radiation for an entire mammogram study. This is an extremely small amount of radiation. A study showed that the average radiation given even as long ago as 1977 was from 0.1 to 0.7 rads, well below the danger level that the American Cancer Society set. Since doses this low are being routinely used by radiologists, there seems to be no risk to you from yearly mammograms. Not a single case of breast cancer has ever been found to be due to mammograms, and the benefits of finding early breast cancers far outweigh any risk that might be associated with mammograms.

Much of the fear associated with mammograms resulted from a 1972 report from the National Academy of Sciences, widely publicized by syndicated newspaper columnist Jack Anderson. This report had a devastating impact on mammography. The fear that cancer is caused by mammograms still lingers in the minds of many people because of this.

The 1972 study that Anderson reported on was prepared from information that is not applicable to the mammograms that are done with today's newer techniques. I hope that you will erase all fear of mammograms from your mind and will adhere absolutely to the mammogram schedule advocated by the American Cancer Society and the American College of Radiology. (See Q. 866.) Dr. D. M. Eddy in 1980 showed that mammograms can save the lives of 500 out of every million women studied each year. With today's more sensitive studies, the lives of even more women are being saved.

---

## 869 What other screening tests of the breasts are done?

There are presently three other screening tests. These are sometimes done routinely and sometimes done only when breast problems are found.

*Thermography.* The American College of Radiology expressed its opinion of thermography in a strongly worded policy statement issued at the Radiologic Society of North America in Chicago in 1983, and reported in *Journal of the American Medical Association* (February 10, 1984, Vol. 251, No. 6): "Thermography, a direct method of measuring skin temperature, either as discrete values or in the form of visual image, is ineffective for detecting clinically occult breast cancer and should not be used as an indicator for biopsy."

This is a very strong statement. Let me try to clarify the place of thermography in detection of breast cancer. Thermography is useful only in helping a doctor make a *final* decision about a patient's breast abnormality. Even then it is useful only if a doctor is familiar with thermography's limitations and pitfalls. Thermography can only augment, never replace, mammography. It is absolutely wrong for any doctor to suggest that a patient have a thermogram *instead of* a mammogram.

Any breast area that is abnormal enough for a competent doctor to recommend biopsy needs to be biopsied regardless of thermograms, mammograms, or any other testing procedure. The danger of thermography is that it may give a false sense of security, convincing a doctor and a patient to forego a breast biopsy until too late.

In the past few years there has been a great emotional enthusiasm for the use of thermography. There is even an American Thermographic Society. The instrument used is small enough to fit into a physician's office; many doctors have bought these instruments. Because of their financial investment in them and their emotional commitment to them, these doctors continue to do thermograms on their patients as screening procedures. It now seems quite clear, from excellent studies, that this is not legitimate. Thermograms have very little usefulness in breast evaluation.

*Ultrasound of the breasts.* An ultrasound machine sends out sound waves and receives them back with an echo-receiving device, "drawing a picture" on a screen of the image that is received. This is a safe procedure, and there is no X-ray-type radiation involved. Although this technique can sometimes detect breast cancer, it is not as reliable as mammograms or translumination of the breasts with light. In the future ultrasound may be capable of more accurate diagnosis of breast lumps.

*Translumination of the breasts with light.* This new, exciting technique has some fancy names, such as "computerized multispectral translumination" and "light scanning." It, too, involves no X-ray-type radiation, and it is not painful. The technique merely involves the projection of light into the breast, with visualization of the diffusion of the light through the breast by a computerized system that ultimately projects an image on a TV screen. Several studies have shown that this technique is as accurate as mammography.

*Nuclear magnetic resonance.* Known as NMR this is the most advanced CT scan technique to date. It is available in relatively few centers in the United States at this time, however. Doctors who have access to one of these instruments have found it to be surprisingly successful in evaluation of breast nodules. NMR has not been in such use long enough for its role in breast evaluation to be adequately determined, but it may, in time, be found to be very useful. It is an expensive procedure, costing three hundred to five hundred dollars per exam, and is probably best suited to patients for whom mammography is not satisfactory and who are at high risk for developing cancer of the breasts.

No presently available technique will detect every breast cancer, and using more than one technique for evaluation of the breasts will significantly decrease the percentage of cancers that escape detection. If there were no money or time factor involved, it would seem best for a patient to have both a mammogram and a light scan done according to the schedule that the American Cancer Society and American Radiologic Society recommend for routine evaluation by mammogram. If you can get these two tests done each time you have a routine breast evaluation, I suggest that you go ahead and have both of them. If you do not have the money or the time, then it seems best to have mammograms done on the schedule recommended by the American Cancer Society.

---

**870** **In what situations would translumination be advisable over mammography?**

There are some cases when translumination is advisable.

> For the patient who absolutely refuses any X-rays, this technique will provide some degree of evaluation without the use of X-rays.

> Similarly, if for some reason a patient must have frequent examinations of the breasts by other than BSE or a physician, this technique can be used as often as necessary, even every month, with no X-ray exposure.

> Even though a mammogram delivers little X-ray-type radiation, women who are younger than thirty-five and who have breast lumps that need diagnosis might benefit from the use of light imaging rather than from mammograms, to reduce the total X-ray exposure over so many years.

> Some breasts are so dense (radiographically dense breasts) that a mammogram is not as reliable as desired. Light imaging is useful in these cases. If a mammogram is questionable, a light image might help in deciding whether or not a biopsy is necessary.

> Finally, after a patient has had augmentation mammoplasty (breast implants), a

mastectomy (removal of the breast), or breast biopsies, light translumination can be used along with mammograms to help evaluate her breasts accurately.

## 871 What is aspiration of a breast lump?

Aspiration is an essentially painless procedure in which a doctor inserts a needle into a breast lump in an attempt to draw off the fluid. If there is fluid and if it is clear, you can be assured that it is highly unlikely that you have a breast cancer. Furthermore, if there is no residual mass left in the breast after aspiration, and the fluid is either clear or cloudy, it is almost certain that you do not have breast cancer. It is important, however, that you have follow-up examinations done as your doctor instructs and that you also continue to do your own monthly breast examination.

If the fluid that is aspirated is bloody, or if the mass does not go away after aspiration, the doctor will probably recommend a mammography and an excisional biopsy. You should follow this recommendation.

## 872 Should I have a breast biopsy even if a mammogram is normal?

Neither mammograms, light studies, nor any other tests are absolutely accurate. If you have a breast lump, even if the mammogram is negative, and your doctor recommends a breast biopsy, you should have it done. The mammogram before a biopsy will not only give the doctor more information about the possibility of breast cancer, it will also help determine if you have a suspicious area in the opposite breast that you cannot feel and that also needs to be biopsied.

## 873 What is involved in breast biopsy?

A breast biopsy is ordinarily a simple procedure. It is normally done through a small incision. More and more surgeons are doing such biopsies in an outpatient setting, although your doctor may not have access to such an operating situation and may need to admit you to the hospital.

The surgeon injects a local anesthetic, or an anesthesiologist gives you general anesthetic. A small incision is then made, and through it the suspicious portion of the breast is removed. Stitches are used to stop bleeding and the incision is closed. Healing is usually complete within three weeks.

There are great advantages to having a breast biopsy. If a woman is worried that she has breast cancer, a breast biopsy can reassure her that she does not. If she does have cancer, the biopsy insures treatment as soon as possible, giving her the best chance of cure.

## 874 If the doctor does a breast biopsy and finds cancer, will my breast be removed while I am asleep?

Many breast biopsies are now done in an outpatient setting. A doctor will not do a breast removal or mastectomy in an outpatient surgical facility or in the office.

Studies have shown conclusively that when a cancer is present, a breast biopsy does not cause that cancer to spread, provided that the mastectomy is not delayed for more than two weeks. Therefore, breast biopsies are often done in an outpatient setting. This allows a patient to go home the day of her biopsy and wait the day or two it takes to get the report from the pathologist. Another advantage of this procedure is that it allows you time to compile information so that you can decide on either a lumpectomy or a mastectomy. (See Q. 878.)

Often, though, the most logical procedure

is for you to go to the hospital for your biopsy and have it done under general anesthesia. The pathologist can look at the tissue under the microscope while you are still asleep. This takes only a few minutes, and if the pathologist finds cancer, your surgeon can proceed with a mastectomy. In this way you get the entire procedure over at one time. You avoid having two operations (first a biopsy, then later a mastectomy) and you do not have the anxiety of waiting one or two days for the pathologist's report.

## 875 If a breast lump is not cancer, what else can it be?

Eight out of ten breast lumps are benign. Those nonmalignant breast lumps might be:

*Thickening or cysts.* Such thickening or cysts may be the result of fibrocystic disease of the breasts.

*Fibroadenomas of the breast.* This is usually a solitary mass in the breast, occurring in women between the ages of fifteen and thirty-nine. These lumps are usually easy to feel, are smooth and firm, and tend to move around when palpated. The problem is that a doctor cannot tell for sure by feel alone whether a lump is a simple fibroadenoma or an early breast cancer. A breast biopsy is almost always required to determine whether or not cancer is present. Mammography and light scanning can often help with the diagnosing.

*Intraductal papillomas.* This problem is caused by an overgrowth of normal duct lining. Papillomas can cause oozing of fluid, often bloody in nature. This, of course, scares a patient and concerns her doctor. The doctor's concern, however, is not to be too radical with a situation that is almost always nonmalignant. Mammograms help make sure there is no cancer present. Follow-up exams are recommended. Sometimes resection of a portion of the breast

from which the ducts come is necessary to stop the bleeding problem and to confirm that there is no malignancy present.

The doctor will often get a Pap smear of the fluid from the nipple for the pathologist to check for cancer cells. This is useful, but not totally reliable. If bleeding persists, your doctor will almost certainly want you to have a biopsy, even if the mammogram is normal.

## 876 Why do I hear so much about breast cancer?

You hear a lot about breast cancer because breast cancer is the most serious malignancy affecting women in the United States, and the entire world. In 1983, 34,000 American women died of breast cancer, a figure which represents 18 percent of all female deaths due to any type of cancer. One in eleven American women will have breast cancer in her lifetime. This risk is not only important for older women; breast cancer is the leading cause of all deaths in women between forty and forty-four years of age.

These statistics are not cited to scare you but to encourage you to do two things: be faithful about doing your breast self-examinations, and follow the American Cancer Society guidelines for mammography.

## 877 What surgical techniques are used to treat breast cancer?

Four techniques are used for the treatment of breast cancer.

*Radical mastectomy.* This procedure involves removing the entire breast, the underlying chest muscles (pectorals), and the lymph nodes under the arm. There are variations of this type of operation, but all of them are drastic, leaving the chest wall quite

# Types of Mastectomies

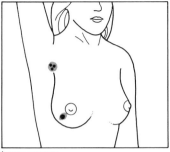

lumpectomy

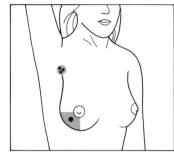

quadrectomy

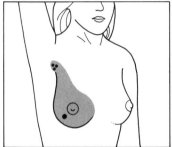

simple mastectomy

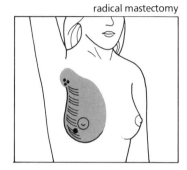

radical mastectomy

- ● tumor
- ▦ area removed
- ⁚• axillary nodes

disfigured. In addition, these procedures can restrict movement of the arm and cause edema, or swelling of the arm.

This procedure is not done routinely in this country anymore. About the only indication for its use is when the cancer has invaded the muscles under the breast. In this case, those pectoral muscles must be removed to get around the cancer. A second reason for this operation is if the patient and doctor do not have access to a treatment center that can give good radiation therapy. Then the patient and doctor must rely on surgery alone to cure the cancer.

*Simple (total) mastectomy.* This operation involves removal of the entire breast and the lymph nodes under the arm. The pectoral muscles are not removed. Because of this, disfigurement is not so drastic, swelling of the arm is uncommon, and arm move-

ment is not restricted at all. This is the operation most commonly used by United States surgeons now.

The only absolute reason for even simple mastectomy is if the tumor involves a third or more of the breast. If a breast cancer is this large, trying to cut the cancer out would leave the rest of the breast so deformed that it might as well be removed. Studies have shown, however, that the cure rate for simple mastectomy is no better than when only a part of the breast is removed and radiation therapy given. (See Q. 878.)

***Segmental resection of the breast and quadrant resection of the breast.*** These two operations involve cutting around the breast cancer widely, taking out as much as a fourth of the breast tissue. These operations are normally accompanied by a separate incision under the arm, through which the doctor removes the underarm lymph nodes. This gives some idea of how far the cancer has spread in the body and how likely is a cure, since the fewer involved lymph nodes under the arm, the more likely the cure. Radiation is used with these surgeries.

***Excision of the cancer lump itself (lumpectomy).*** It is possible for the doctor to merely cut the lump itself out of the breast, with no attempt to excise tissue around the cancer. A lumpectomy is normally done only when the breast cancer is early and small and always involves removal of axillary (underarm) nodes. Radiation therapy is also used and can cause complications such as swelling and stiffness of the breast and skin discoloration. (See Q. 878.)

While European physicians have embraced more limited surgery for breast cancer, most surgeons in the United States still do mastectomies for breast cancer. The motivation behind the American approach is good—it is felt that mastectomy is more likely to provide a cure—but several studies now indicate that other more limited techniques may produce as great a chance of cure as mastectomy.

Physicians who care for women realize that all women are very concerned about breast surgery. Therefore, various methods of treatment have been devised; these options have been used long enough now that the surgical management of breast cancer is no longer automatically a mastectomy but can be tailored to a woman's particular situation.

---

**878** **My doctor's standard operation is total removal of the breast for any breast cancer, and he will not consider more limited surgery. Where can I get more information?**

The National Cancer Institute has set up a hotline for cancer information. Through this hotline you can get information about all aspects of breast cancer: surgery, treatment, and prevention.

The telephone number for the cancer hotline is 1-800-4-CANCER. There are three offices in the United States that are not tied into this number. They are:

| | |
|---|---|
| Washington, D.C. | 202-636-5700 |
| Alaska | 800-638-6070 |
| Hawaii | 808-524-1234 |

Controversy is presently (1985) raging among surgeons over the wisdom of a woman with a small breast cancer having a lumpectomy and radiation instead of a mastectomy. The report of a significant ten-year well-designed study by Bernard Fisher, M.D., professor of surgery at the University of Pittsburgh School of Medicine, released in March 1985 showed that for small breast cancers (smaller than 1¾ inches across) lumpectomy plus radiation was as likely to cure the cancer as mastectomy. This study was conducted with the support of the National Cancer Institute and was called the National Surgical Adjuvant Breast Project (NSABP).

Such information can help a woman with breast cancer and her doctor decide which surgery is best for her. About 50 percent of women with breast cancer have tumors small enough for them to consider lumpectomy and radiation instead of mastectomy. This option rewards women for examining their breasts and finding a cancer early enough to take advantage of this procedure.

---

**879** **Is breast reconstruction a good idea after mastectomy?**

Because the emotional impact of breast surgery is so great, reconstructive surgery for the breast is a major breakthrough in the overall treatment of patients with breast cancer. A Gallup Poll revealed that 60 percent of women felt that their womanhood would be impaired if they had to have a breast removed, 18 percent felt that the loss of a breast would be more important to them than the loss of a limb, and 9 percent of women said they would "rather die" than have a breast removed! Obviously, then, a woman's breasts are a symbol of femininity and sexuality to her, and losing a breast can have significant psychological trauma.

Having a breast reconstructed can be an important step in adjusting to breast cancer for many women. Not only will a woman look and feel better and therefore be less self-conscious, but she will also be more comfortable.

In addition, if women do not fear the disfigurement of breast cancer so much because they know they can have a breast reconstruction, they will, hopefully, examine themselves more regularly, have necessary surgery done more quickly, and therefore have better survival statistics and less physical problems.

---

**880**  **If I know I am going to have a mastectomy, and I am considering breast reconstruction, should anything special be done in preparation for that?**

If you are going to have a mastectomy, it is important that you discuss with your surgeon the fact that you plan to have breast reconstruction done. Since increasingly more breast reconstruction is being done as a part of mastectomy surgery, your doctor will not be too surprised by your desire. The procedure would be carefully planned in advance as your surgeon, plastic surgeon, and possibly radiologist consult with each other. During the surgery, your surgeon would then make incisions in your breasts in the least visible areas, allowing the plastic surgeon, who would be on hand during the surgery to "take over" following the mastectomy and do the best possible reconstruction.

Plastic surgeons are able to construct breasts that are very acceptable cos-

metically, allowing a woman to dress as she did before surgery. When the surface skin and nipple are "salvaged," the result is completely lifelike; when skin must be grafted, as is necessary following radical mastectomies, and nipples "made from scratch"— using tissue from the inner thigh, the labia, and other parts of the body—the result is still quite acceptable. In both cases form and comfort, the two major considerations in most cases, are established.

Research has shown that breast reconstruction reduces a woman's anxiety about subsequent sexual relations. The same research indicates that women have less feeling of loss, less grief, and less depression following mastectomy if they have breast reconstruction done. Such surgery also seems to lessen the fear of recurrence of the cancer.

It is important to point out, however, that while mastectomy is emotionally traumatic, studies have shown that the severe trauma is fairly short-lived. Even without reconstruction, most women are able to accept the loss of a breast after a few months. Unfortunately, during the transition time, many women present a false attitude of casualness about their breast surgery. If you have had a mastectomy and you are hurting emotionally because of it, be sure to discuss this with your physician or have him or her refer you to a counselor with whom you can discuss and resolve your anxiety.

---

**881**  **I have breast pain, breast nodularity, and breast lumpiness that bother me a great deal. What should I do?**

There are many women who are continually bothered by breast pain and breast lumpiness. These women may or may not have had several breast biopsies (all benign) or are constantly under surveillance by their physicians for their lumps, with the warning that biopsies must be done if the lumps persist. Such lumps cause a great deal of worry and concern.

I strongly recommend that a woman who continues to have this problem do her best to get that discomfort ended so that she does not have to live under a cloud of worry about her breasts. Life is too short to worry all the time. There are several things that seem to be effective.

*Good breast support.* A woman who has breast pain should wear brassieres that give especially good support. For years I have recommended Pennyrich brassieres because they can be custom-fitted to a woman's particular needs. There are other brassieres that do just as good a job. Many women have found that if they wear a comfortable sleeping bra at night, they will have less breast pain.

*Restrict caffeine.* Caffeine contains the chemical methylxanthine (as do theophylline and theobromide, drugs for treating asthma and lung congestion). Although carefully controlled studies have not conclusively proven the effect of the caffeine-free (methylxanthine-free) diet on the breasts, some studies have indicated that 70 percent of women have less breast tenderness and less nodularity if they get off these products.

Eliminating caffeine from the diet means no coffee, tea, chocolate, or soft drinks containing caffeine. Fortunately each of those items is now manufactured "caffeine free." Caffeine is also an ingredient in many other regularly used products, including prescription drugs (Percodan, Soma Compound, Synalgos, Emprazil, Fiorinal, Migral, Cafergot, Empirin with Codeine, and Repan) and in numerous nonprescription drugs (Anacin, Sinarest, Stanback Analgesic Powders, Triaminicin, Vanquish, Anorexin, Bromo Seltzer, Cope, Dexatrim, Dristan, Empirin, Excedrin, Midol, and NoDoz). Check the labels to be sure the products and prescriptions you use do not contain caffeine

if you are trying to restrict or eliminate caffeine in your diet.

I encourage patients who have breast pain or fibrocystic disease to maintain a caffeine-free diet. Although there is a slightly increased chance of having breast cancer in women with fibrocystic disease, the main reason to cut out caffeine is not to prevent cancer but to lessen the problems of fibrocystic disease and the worry it produces. After getting off caffeine, it may take three or four months to detect any difference in the breast symptoms.

*Take vitamin E.* I have been telling patients for years about the use of vitamin E. I suggest they use up to one thousand international units per day. I know of no reliable study that "proves" a positive effect, but vitamin E has been widely recommended for this problem by competent physicians all over the country. They (and I) have found that it significantly helps many patients. Vitamin E used in this way is more than just taking a vitamin in the usual way. It is using a vitamin as a medicine. On this large dosage you may feel bloated, have oily skin, become irritable, and have other side effects. If you have such problems you would want to stop taking the drug.

*Birth-control pills.* Many studies now have shown that women who are on birth-control pills have less fibrocystic disease and fewer breast lumps, require fewer breast biopsies, and experience less breast pain. The studies suggest that you have to be on the pills for more than two years to have the greatest effects. The use of birth-control pills may be the best long-term treatment for this particular problem. If you can and want to take birth-control pills for your breast problem, I strongly suggest that you ask your doctor about using them. Recent studies even indicate that women who have been on birth-control pills for a few years have less chance of developing breast cancer in the future than women who have not taken birth-control pills.

*Danocrine (danazol).* This drug will stop breast pain and breast nodules in up to 80 percent of women who use it. This is probably the most underused technique for helping women with breast pain and nodularity. It works most of the time, and most women have no side effects from taking the drug. In my experience, general surgeons do not usually even mention this drug to their patients. I have many patients who have general surgeons following them for breast pain and nodules and who have had biopsies of these masses, and yet have never even heard that Danocrine might help them avoid this problem. I believe the reason general surgeons do not mention Danocrine is that they rarely use hormones in their practice and are not comfortable prescribing them. Gynecologists, who use and discuss hormones all the time, are more comfortable prescribing a drug like Danocrine.

Danocrine has been approved by the FDA for breast problems. A daily dose of from 400 to 600 mg for three months can stop a woman's problem for years. It can stop pain and make breast lumps go away, allowing a woman to avoid biopsies. Don't try to avoid this drug if you and your doctor think it can help you. I have never had a patient have a significant problem with it when she took it for only three months. (See Q. 176, 956 where we discuss the use of Danocrine for endometriosis to learn more about this drug.) Do not misunderstand: If you have a *specific* lump and your doctor recommends a biopsy, have it done. Then start on Danocrine to help avoid future lumps.

## 882 What is a subcutaneous mastectomy?

A subcutaneous mastectomy is surgery in which a woman's breast is hollowed out, leaving a skin sac with a nipple, into which a breast implant has been put. Subcutaneous mastectomies are recommended for women who have a high risk of developing breast cancer. Such people include women with a strong family history of breast cancer and those who have already had breast cancer in one breast. Subcutaneous mastectomies are also recommended for women who have continual major problems with fibrocystic disease.

Although this operation can eliminate these problems, it should not be entered into lightly. In the first place, subcutaneous mastectomy does not remove all risk of having breast cancer because some breast tissue is always left behind. Second, it is major surgery and can result in loss of the breasts completely. For example, a patient of mine had this procedure done and, as a result, developed infections under the skin of both breasts. She had to have the implants removed and subsequently had five more operations, which finally resulted in removal of both nipples and of some of the skin of both breasts.

The fact that such things can happen should not scare you away from surgery that you need, but it should warn you that having your breast hollowed out, and an implant put in to replace it, is not necessarily a simple and uncomplicated procedure. Choose your surgeon carefully; you want a doctor who will not only make wise recommendations but who will also do excellent surgery.

Do not confuse this surgery with the much simpler and far less dangerous "breast job" (augmentation mammoplasty) that many women have done by a plastic surgeon.

## 883 Can anything be done to prevent breast cancer?

The possibility of a link between diet and cancer is a much-debated and frequently discussed subject. While a correlation has not been definitely proven, there is enough evidence to strongly suggest a positive link in many cases. A National Cancer Institute study provides the following data, based on the dietary histories of 577 women (aged thirty to eighty), with breast malignancies, and of 826 disease-free women: the more frequent the consumption of beef and pork, the greater the risk; the more frequent the eating of sweet desserts, the greater the risk; and using butter at the table, and frying with butter or margarine as compared with vegetable oils, increases the risk.

Since these guidelines are conducive to overall good health anyway, with or without the cancer link, it makes sense to incorporate them into an "every day, for a lifetime" diet regime.

## An Afterword

It is evident from the material in this chapter that women do develop problems in their sexual and reproductive organs. I have seen many different responses from patients when I tell them they have a medical problem. Some women get mad; some are frightened. Others try to ignore the problem. These are normal responses. It is important, however, for a woman with a medical problem to overcome these initial reactions and resolve to do all she can to eliminate her problem. Fortunately, today women have access to medical care that was undreamed of a few years ago. Take advantage of these medical breakthroughs. There are medications available today, including certain hormone-type drugs, that can easily solve extremely difficult problems of the female sexual and reproductive organs.

The availability of modern-day medicines does not always mean that a woman can avoid a surgical procedure. However, problems that required major surgery in the past can now often be taken care of with minor surgery, such as laparoscopy or hysteroscopy. Even if a major operation is needed, such surgery is now safer than ever before. Women who do have major surgery today are usually released from the hospital after only a few days' stay.

If you have a problem, find a doctor who is medically expert, honest, and will communicate with you. Take advantage of the support of your family and friends. Then get the problem taken care of as soon as you reasonably can so that you can get past that hurdle in your life and get on with other things.

# 11

## Infertility

There is, I believe, no stronger stress in a couple's life than the continued absence of the child that they long to have. This chapter will be of vital importance to those couples whose fondest wish—the conception of a child—has, to this point, been denied.

A psychological evaluation of infertile couples released in 1985 showed that 50 percent of the women and 15 percent of the men felt their infertility was the most upsetting experience they had ever had.

The emotions stirred by childlessness run strong and deep. They always have. Hannah, mother of the biblical prophet Samuel, remained infertile year after year despite intense longing for a child. The anguish shared by Hannah and her husband, Elkanah, mirrors the heartache of thousands.

"Hannah," Elkanah entreats tenderly, "why are you weeping? Why don't you eat? Why are you downhearted? Don't I mean more to you than ten sons?" (1 Sam. 1:8). Poor Elkanah. He was only trying to help. In fact, he was hurting as much as she was.

Fortunately this particular story had a happy ending. Hannah steadfastly continued to approach God with her problem, going year after lonely year to the temple to pray for a child. Eventually God answered her prayer, blessing Hannah and Elkanah with a son.

Unfortunately not all infertility stories have the same happy ending. Not everyone who wants a child will have one. However, exciting new advances in the treatment of infertility make it possible for an ever-increasing number of infertile couples to achieve pregnancy.

I strongly encourage any infertile couple to pray, as did Hannah and Elkanah, asking God to grant the desire of their hearts for a child. In the final analysis, I believe that it is God who opens and closes the womb; it is God who makes the final decision about pregnancy.

True, a couple may not conceive, but then God's wisdom must be respected and trusted. He is to be praised no matter what—because every aspect of his plan for us is in our best interest.

God has made it possible for us to develop new understanding and treatment for the causes of infertility. Those with infertility problems have at their disposal some of the most modern and up-to-date medical care available in any field of medicine. All this technology gives you a fighting chance of achieving the pregnancy you so long for.

The encouraging fact for those of you who have not yet become pregnant is that every year new tests and treatments are being developed. The techniques of microsurgery have brought fertility to thousands of people during the past ten years; and the laser, bromocriptine, and in vitro fertilization (test-tube babies) bring realistic hope of fertility to thousands today.

This chapter contains a wealth of information for those couples who are infertile. There are also some important facts for those couples who are planning to delay starting their families for several years. A third group who will benefit from this chapter are those whose infertile friends and relatives have shared with them their anguish. The lives of this third group of people will be blessed by sharing with their childless loved ones information that may prove to be a solution to their infertility problem.

Those couples who seem to be infertile need first of all to know whether or not they are, in truth, infertile. Next they need to know what to do about it if they are infertile.

I urge you strongly not only to read the chapter but also to keep in mind that the sooner you get an infertility problem treated, and the more appropriate that treatment is, the more likely you are to have success: a healthy, normal baby!

The questions that follow are those that I am most frequently asked by infertile couples.

## 884 What does the word *infertility* mean?

Infertility refers to the condition of a couple who may be capable of producing an offspring but have not achieved pregnancy after trying for one year or more. A woman who habitually miscarries, failing to bring a baby to full term, is also considered to have a problem of infertility. (See Q. 324–336.)

## 885 What is the difference between "infertility" and "sterility"?

Sterility means that either the man or the woman is totally incapable of achieving pregnancy. For example, if a woman has had a hysterectomy, or has some major deformity or disorder of her female organs that prevents her from becoming pregnant, then she is truly sterile. A sterile man is one who has no sperm, who has had a vasectomy, or who has other complications that prevent the occurrence of fertilization.

## 886 How often is infertility a problem?

Infertility exists in about 10–15 percent of marriages. After attempting for one year to conceive, approximately 85 percent of couples will have achieved pregnancy. After eighteen months of attempted conception, that figure increases to approximately 90 percent. Those couples unable to achieve pregnancy after that length of time are considered to have an infertility problem.

## 887 When should I consult a doctor if I am unable to become pregnant?

If you are under thirty and have not become pregnant during eighteen months of trying, you should see a physician knowledgeable in infertility evaluation and treatment. If you are over thirty, I suggest that you see a doctor after only a year of trying to conceive. This is because infertility evaluation and the resulting treatments take time, and even more time is required to achieve pregnancy after the problem has been diagnosed and solved. It is particularly important that a woman over thirty not delay seeing a doctor if she suspects that there is a fertility problem.

## 888 Is there an age when fertility begins to lessen?

Until recently doctors assumed that a woman's fertility level remained relatively constant until she reached forty, at which point fertility began dropping off. A new study, however, indicates that fertility drops much sooner.

More tests will have to be conducted before doctors can feel totally confident about the results, but at this point it appears that there is a possible risk in postponing pregnancy much beyond the mid-thirties.

A study, done in France and reported in a 1984 issue of the *New England Journal of Medicine*, showed that a woman's fertility rate starts dropping from the age of thirty on. Up to age thirty a woman's chance of conceiving was reported by them to be 74 percent. The study further reported that women in the thirty-one to thirty-five age group had a fertility rate of 61 percent; those beyond age thirty-five had a fertility rate of 53 percent. These percentages are somewhat low for normal marriages. The study was based on women having artificial insemination. However, the reported decreased fertility rate that comes with age is a reality.

In addition, men's sperm counts are lower now than they were in the past. Doctors have been observing a gradual decline in sperm counts during the past thirty or forty years. In the early 1800s sperm counts were normally greater than eighty to a hundred million per cc of ejaculate. Now the average male's sperm count is in the range of forty million, and we consider twenty million to be normal.

It is interesting to note that men who have a sperm count of more than two hundred and fifty million have a higher incidence of infertility. Apparently there is something somewhat abnormal about counts that are so high.

Lowered sperm count may be due to pollutants in the atmosphere, to diet, or to general lack of exercise, or to excessive exercise. It may also mean that because people are delaying their attempts to get pregnant, when they finally come to see a doctor for an infertility problem, the male's sperm count has already dropped, since age can affect sperm production.

What I am saying is that delaying your family until you are older can make it more difficult to become pregnant, not just because of the female's lessened fertility, but also because the male is somewhat less fertile.

**889** **Are you saying that if I delay pregnancy until after I am thirty-five, I may have difficulty becoming pregnant?**

Yes. Women who put off their childbearing for their convenience, for their profession, or for other reasons run the increasing risk of not ever becoming pregnant. Although I do not recommend that a woman become pregnant when she does not want a baby, I do encourage patients to think carefully about their priorities. If they are delaying pregnancy for convenience or for a selfish motive, they may regret that decision in the future.

**890** **If there are, as people tell me, things I might do to stimulate a pregnancy—for example, "just relaxing," having sex only during ovulation, adopting a child—why do I need to see a doctor?**

First, all of those things are popular misconceptions. Many factors can cause infertility, and only a competent doctor can determine the source of your own or your husband's infertility.

One of the most popular myths concerning becoming pregnant is that "if you'll just relax and quit worrying about it, you will become pregnant." However, the *reason* you are not relaxed is that you are not getting pregnant: not the reverse! Several studies on this subject show that this type of tension does not inhibit fertility. It is normal for you to feel upset each month when you find out that you are not pregnant. This will rarely interfere with your chances of becoming pregnant.

There is an exception to this rule, however. Severe emotional and physical stress can cause ovulation to become erratic or to stop. If that occurs, naturally it will lessen your chance of becoming pregnant. If your periods are regular, however, there is no reason to "worry about worrying."

Another myth is that if you adopt a baby, you will become pregnant. In reality there is no increased chance of becoming pregnant after adopting. Researchers have compared childless infertile women with those who have given up hope of pregnancy and have adopted. The incidence of subsequent pregnancy is no greater in the adopting group.

The third myth concerning stimulating a pregnancy is that it is best to avoid having sex until ovulation occurs, so that the man can "save up" his sperm and have a higher sperm count.

Most urologists believe that this is not only not helpful, but that it may be harmful. When a male goes for several days without intercourse, the sperm start getting "old," resulting in lessened fertility. On the other hand, having sex four or more days in a row can also lessen the sperm count.

The best tactic for achieving pregnancy is to have intercourse three or four times a week, especially at ovulation time. One hint for being as fertile as possible is for the wife not to take aspirin-containing products and prostaglandin inhibitors during ovulation time.

Another myth concerns so-called fertility pills. These pills, such as Clomid, are used for a specific problem: to make a woman who is not ovulating establish regular ovulation. They are helpful only in such cases. They are not the miracle cure for all infertility problems, as some people seem to believe.

Other misconceptions about cures for infertility include undergoing a D&C or taking thyroid medication and/or hormones. One of these treatments may solve an existing infertility problem, but none of them is a universal solution to infertility. These procedures are effective for many patients, but they only treat specific problems.

## 891 What kind of physician should I see for an infertility problem?

You should go to a physician who is skilled in evaluating and treating infertility problems. Valuable time can be wasted seeing a doctor who is only mildly interested or slightly knowledgeable about treating infertility.

Some physicians have not developed expertise in handling infertility problems. Patients are occasionally just given a card on which to record their menstrual cycle. They are instructed to do this year after year, but are never offered any true fertility evaluation.

## 892 How can I know if a doctor is skilled in handling infertility and its treatment?

There are several things you can do.

Ask the doctor if he or she does much infertility work. If the doctor does only a small amount, you should probably find someone else to do your evaluation.

Ask your doctor if he or she does laparoscopies (examination of the female organs with a special instrument passed through the abdominal wall). If a woman does not become pregnant during the process of her initial infertility evaluation, the final test is often a laparoscopy. Any doctor who does not do laparoscopies is not ultimately competent to complete your fertility evaluation.

Call your local Planned Parenthood office and ask them for the names of doctors who specilize in infertility evaluations and treatment.

Contact the following groups:

**Resolve, Inc.** This national lay organization has compiled a good directory of infertility specialists.

**The American Fertility Society.** Most U.S. doctors interested in infertility are members.

**Young Couples International.** This new organization has a registry of doctors who provide infertility care.

Use your common sense. If your doctor does not appear organized, does not have a step-by-step plan for your evaluation, or is doing little to help you achieve pregnancy, you probably need to change doctors. Remember, if you have gone eighteen months without becoming pregnant, you have an infertility problem and need testing right now, not "next year."

## The Initial Infertility Evaluation

### 893 What can a physician do to help me with my infertility problem?

A competent physician in fertility evaluation procedures will provide accurate information about the causes and treatment of infertility, dispel any misinformation you may have on the topic, have an intelligent and systematic approach to your problem, be able to project how soon you should be able to get pregnant, assuming there is a solution or treatment for your problem, and be able to counsel you about adoption options if you decide to choose that means of having a child.

### 894 How can the physician discover the reasons for my own or my husband's infertility?

The doctor will attempt to uncover the reasons by doing a thorough evaluation of the reproductive tracts of both you and your husband. The investigation will also include obtaining a comprehensive medical history on both of you to ascertain if there is a general medical complication causing your infertility. Finally, the doctor will discuss your sexual activity to be certain that you are having proper frequency of intercourse and at the right time of the month.

During the first visit the medical history,

the sexual-habits evaluation, and a complete physical examination of the wife will usually be done. If no cause is found initially, the couple is scheduled for a second series of tests. Since infertility can be caused by either or both the husband and wife, it is essential that both undergo the standard tests. If, for example, the doctor finds a malfunction in the man's reproductive tract, clearing that up will not solve the couple's infertility if the woman has blocked tubes.

I want to emphasize that if you do not get off to a proper start with a doctor, chances are that you will not receive as efficient and comprehensive a workup as you need. If from the beginning the doctor does not obtain a good medical history or does not plan to test both you and your husband, I suggest that you not remain with that doctor.

### 895 How long does an infertility workup usually take?

The infertility evaluation can usually be completed in two to three months, but specific problems may involve an additional few months.

### 896 How much does infertility evaluation and treatment cost?

The cost depends heavily on how soon your problem is diagnosed and what treatments will be necessary to eliminate it. The costs will increase as more office visits, medication, surgical procedures, and tests are required.

In calculating costs, two factors are important considerations. First, insurance policies are now beginning to cover these procedures. Second, while this care can add up to a sizable amount of money, remember that adoping a child is also quite expensive. Adoptions usually cost from $5,000 to $20,000 per child (1985).

The following list gives the average cost for various tests and treatments for infertility in Austin in 1987:

- $150, initial office visit (consultation and examination)
- $200, initial lab studies
- $170, X-ray of uterus
- $75, Sims-Huhner test
- $45, office exam each month during use of Clomid
- $23, cost of the usual five Clomid pills each month
- $50, cost of an ultrasound study (three or four studies can be required each month)
- $75, intrauterine insemination, IUI, with washed sperm
- $2,500, cost of laparoscopy (doctor's fees, outpatient operating facility, laboratory fee)
- $7,000, cost of major surgery for scarred tubes or endometriosis
- $5,200 per month, in vitro fertilization
- $4,200, GIFT procedure

## 897 Should my husband accompany me on the first visit to the doctor?

Definitely. He should be involved with you during the entire process. Conceiving and raising a child should be a joint effort, and infertility is just as much his problem as yours.

The evaluation cannot take place without your husband's cooperation, since he is involved in not only the questioning and testing but possibly also in the treatment phases of the process. If your husband is present at the first interview, he will have a better understanding of the entire program. This should make him more supportive of your efforts to become pregnant.

Additionally, some of the procedures may require that you change your normal sexual routine. This will require his support and cooperation. His attitude is much more likely to be positive and helpful if he has been involved in this effort from the start.

Finally, if your husband has met your doctor, he will feel more comfortable about calling him or her if he has any questions.

## 898 What kind of advice might the physician give us on the first visit to his or her office?

After obtaining your history and doing an examination, the doctor will offer you some general advice to enhance your chances of conceiving. During the first visit, for instance, I make several suggestions.

If the man wears jockey-style underwear, I advise him to switch to boxer shorts. The reason for this is that the testicles need to be cooler than the rest of the body in order to achieve optimum sperm production. Testicles normally hang outside of and away from the body for that reason. Close-fitting underwear holds them much closer to the body than does a pair of boxer shorts.

I instruct women patients to begin taking their temperatures every morning with a basal thermometer. This thermometer is necessary because it detects a narrower range of temperature than a regular fever thermometer. The thermometer should be shaken down and put at bedside every night. First thing each morning the thermometer is put under the woman's tongue for five minutes before reading and recording the results. A temperature chart should be kept faithfully for three months and brought back on subsequent visits to the doctor. This chart presents a graphic demonstration to infertility patients of the timing of their ovulation. It shows whether or not they are ovulating and helps them to schedule intercourse accordingly. However, recent studies have shown that the ovulation time indicated by BBT charts can be wrong one-third of the time.

A very useful new technique allows a woman to check her urine for her body's pro-

# Sample Temperature Record

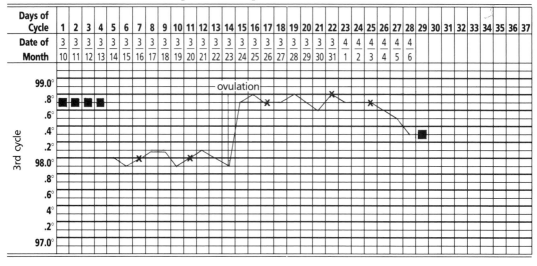

| Days of Cycle | 1 | 2 | 3 | 4 | 5 | 6 | 7 | 8 | 9 | 10 | 11 | 12 | 13 | 14 | 15 | 16 | 17 | 18 | 19 | 20 | 21 | 22 | 23 | 24 | 25 | 26 | 27 | 28 | 29 | 30 | 31 | 32 | 33 | 34 | 35 | 36 | 37 |
|---|---|---|---|---|---|---|---|---|---|---|---|---|---|---|---|---|---|---|---|---|---|---|---|---|---|---|---|---|---|---|---|---|---|---|---|---|---|
| Date of | 3 | 3 | 3 | 3 | 3 | 3 | 3 | 3 | 3 | 3 | 3 | 3 | 3 | 3 | 3 | 3 | 3 | 3 | 3 | 3 | 3 | 3 | 3 | 4 | 4 | 4 | 4 | 4 | 4 | | | | | | | | |
| Month | 10 | 11 | 12 | 13 | 14 | 15 | 16 | 17 | 18 | 19 | 20 | 21 | 22 | 23 | 24 | 25 | 26 | 27 | 28 | 29 | 30 | 31 | 1 | 2 | 3 | 4 | 5 | 6 | | | | | | | | | |

x—intercourse

■ menstration

## Instructions:

1. Immediately after waking in the morning and before arising, eating, drinking or smoking, place the thermometer under your tongue for at least five minutes. (Do this every morning except during menstruation.)
2. Record the reading on the graph by placing a dot at the proper location (be accurate). If intercourse has taken place during the previous twenty-four hours, cross the dot (X).
3. Insert the date at top of column in space provided for date of month.
4. Consider the first day of menstrual flow as the start of a cycle. It is not essential to record the temperature during menstruation. However, indicate menstruation with a ■ on the graph starting at extreme left under number one day of cycle. As flow diminishes resume temperature recordings.
5. Any obvious reasons for temperature variation such as an infection, insomnia, or indigestion should be noted on the graph above the reading for that day.
6. If you detect ovulation by a twinge of pain low on one side of the abdomen or by a few drops of vaginal bleeding about midcycle, indicate it on the graph.

duction of luteinizing hormone (LH). When the pituitary gland produces this hormone, it causes ovulation to occur thirty-eight hours later. This technique allows a couple to schedule intercourse or insemination much more reliably than with a BBT chart.

Next I recommend proper frequency and timing of intercourse. No matter how fertile you are, if your sexual timing or habits are wrong you will probably be slow to achieve pregnancy. For example, I have had as patients several couples who were having intercourse only once a month, and this only at random times. Having sex about three or four times a week, spread out over the week, seems to produce the greatest chance of pregnancy. This pattern is most important to follow around ovulation time.

Finally, I recommend that a woman remain in bed on her back, for at least thirty minutes after each act of intercourse during the ovulation period. (She should lie on her stomach if her uterus is tipped or retroverted.) This allows the semen to pool around the cervix and facilitates the sperm's access to the uterus.

---

## 899 Is there anything else my husband and I can do to improve our chances of conceiving?

Good general health and sound lifestyle habits can have a positive effect on a person's fertility. If the woman diets excessively, is extremely obese, or exercises too strenuously, the functions of the body are changed enough to prevent normal secretion of hormones and therefore a normal menstrual cycle.

I always advise my patients to avoid the following things while they are trying to get pregnant.

*Cigarette smoking.* Chemicals in cigarette smoke combine with red blood cells, preventing them from carrying a normal load of oxygen. This is one reason that smokers are less likely to gain weight. If body tissues are so starved for oxygen that they cannot grow properly, it is reasonable to assume that the reproductive system may not function properly either. Studies have conclusively shown a significantly decreased fertility in smokers.

Furthermore, once pregnancy occurs, it is imperative for the well-being of the child that the mother stop smoking. The best time to stop is before pregnancy occurs, especially if you have infertility problems.

*Alcohol.* Little is known about alcohol consumption and fertility, but we do know that a heavy drinker does not have normal body functions in many respects. Much more is known about alcohol used during pregnancy, and none of it is good. (See Q. 474, 475.) As with cigarettes, for the baby's health and your own, you need to stop alcohol intake, preferably before you get pregnant. This may help you to achieve pregnancy sooner. It is my recommendation that there be either no drinking or drinking only in highly controlled moderation (two to three drinks per month) for both the husband and wife who are trying to achieve pregnancy.

*Other drugs.* Even less is known about the effect of other drugs on fertility. Marijuana research suggests that this drug can affect the production of a normal egg, inhibit ovulation, and lower sperm count. When no longer used, there seems to be no effect of the drug on fertility later in life. Heroin, cocaine, barbiturates, and so on used excessively are known to cause malnutrition, poor health, irregular ovulation, and therefore some degree of infertility. Some tranquilizers can cause the cessation of periods and thus interfere with fertility.

A man's sperm production and sex drive may be affected by all these substances too. Cigarettes can have a significant effect on sperm production. I advise all the husbands in infertile couples to stop smoking. Alcohol can lead to impotence; marijuana can affect production of sperm; heroin, cocaine, and barbiturates can affect both libido (sex drive) and general health; and tranquilizers or anti-depressants reduce sperm production in animals and may do the same in men.

It is important to note that sperm production that begins "today" in a man's testicles does not appear in his ejaculate for about seventy-five days. Whatever he does today, therefore, will not affect his sperm count or his sperm fertility for seventy-five days. In addition, to improve his sperm he must start right now for sperm that will be ejaculated two-and-a-half months from now.

The maxim concerning infertility and the use of any drug is, "Don't use the drug." If you are going to the inconvenience and expense of diagnosing your infertility and having it treated, maximize your chances for pregnancy by stopping all drugs, including cigarettes and alcohol.

### 900 What reasons for infertility might the physician discover during the examination on the first visit?

The following abnormalities, each of which can interfere with fertility, are evaluated during the initial physical examination.

*Vaginitis.* If a vaginal infection is found it must be treated, as it can delay the occurrence of a pregnancy.

*Growths or abnormalities in the pelvis.* These may be fibroids of the uterus, ovarian tumors, or endometriosis. Additionally, if some congenital abnormalities are found on pelvic examination these must be evaluated and may need to be treated.

*Cervical stenosis.* This is a narrowing of the opening into the uterus. It can prevent or make it difficult for the sperm to gain access to the uterus. This condition is often due to an earlier abortion, cervical cautery or freezing, or a cervical conization (excision of cervical tissue).

*Unusually heavy or abnormal patterns of hair growth and/or moderate-to-severe acne.* These symptoms can be indicative of an excess production of male hormones (even in women) and may suggest the need for hormone studies. Such studies usually, however, prove to be normal.

*Physical abnormalities.* These can indicate abnormal growth patterns in the body that could be due to congenital problems such as chromosomal abnormalities. One of the most common of these is called Turner's syndrome or ovarian agenesis (see Q. 107), a problem that requires more extensive treatment and counseling than just dealing with infertility. However, these problems occur infrequently.

### 901 Which tests will the physician order for me and my husband following the first visit?

A fairly standard series of tests will be ordered. All of them are designed to evaluate the proper functioning of your body in general as well as of sexual organs and to identify problems that could be causing your infertility.

The common causes of infertility, such as a low sperm count, are first tested. The simplest, nonsurgical tests are also done first, followed by more involved tests and treatments until a cause is discovered and the proper therapy found. Often the problem can be cleared up quickly and easily, and pregnancy will occur without the need to proceed to the more advanced tests and procedures.

### 902 What initial tests are ordered for the man?

Most gynecologists working with infertility will order only a semen analysis.

If this test for sperm count and health and semen health is normal, the husband usually needs no further testing. It is wise, therefore, that this be one of the first tests ordered for any infertile couple.

*Sperm agglutination.* This test to make sure the female is not allergic to her husband's sperm varies in popularity. This is now felt to be a relatively rare fertility problem and one for which testing is not very reliable.

## 903 What tests would be ordered for the woman at the time of the first office visit?

A group of tests that any doctor would obtain during a thorough general checkup are also recommended for a woman with an infertility problem.

*Complete blood count.* This checks for anemia or a chronic blood problem that could affect both fertility and the health of the mother and the fetus.

*Complete urinalysis.* This checks for evidence of a chronic kidney disease, which could affect both fertility and a pregnancy.

*SMA 21.* This checks for any evidence of liver disease, gout, diabetes, kidney malfunction, and several other problems that can affect fertility in the female.

*T3 & T4 and/or a TSH test.* These check thyroid function. It is unusual for a thyroid problem to cause infertility, but it does occur and should be checked.

*Rubella titer test.* This tests resistance or lack of resistance to German measles (rubella) which, if contracted during pregnancy, may cause severe abnormalities in the baby. (See Q. 520–523.) If the test shows you have no resistance to rubella, immunization should be done and for the next three months you should use good contraception. You may continue testing during this time.

*TB skin test.* If a woman has had tuberculosis, it may have affected the female organs and caused infertility.

*Prolactin test.* The prolactin level needs to be checked because this hormone can indicate a small tumor in the pituitary that could be preventing pregnancy. Not all physicians do this routinely.

*Progesterone testing.* Some doctors like to have a blood test for progesterone. This is done a few days after ovulation and indicates that a woman's ovary did release an egg and then developed a corpus luteum that is producing progesterone, the hormone necessary for preparing the lining of the uterus for pregnancy.

## Further Steps in Infertility Evaluation

## 904 What is the next step in the infertility evaluation?

After the couple has had the first consultation and the above-mentioned testing, the doctor will review the results. Any indication of a problem should be clearly explained by the doctor so that the couple will understand exactly what is going on and what will happen next.

If no apparent cause for infertility was found during the first series of questions, tests, and examinations, a hysterosalpingogram and a Sims-Huhner test are scheduled for the woman.

## 905 What is a hysterosalpingogram (HSG)?

This X-ray test is used to view the inside of the uterus and fallopian tubes. It is a nonsurgical procedure. An X-ray dye is squirted through the cervix, up into the uterus, and through the fallopian tubes so that these organs may be X-rayed and any abnormality will be outlined.

The test can show several things: whether or not your uterus is formed normally; whether or not there is scarring inside your uterus from a previous miscarriage or an operation such as an abortion; and whether or not your tubes are open. While this X-ray is not foolproof, it does give doctors a fairly reliable picture of that area.

Since this procedure can cause cramping, I usually have patients come in for a paracervical block on their way to the X-ray clinic. The procedure takes only about twenty or thirty minutes, and is a very important part of an infertility evaluation.

---

### 906    What is the postcoital (Sims-Huhner) test?

While awaiting the hysterosalpingogram, or soon after, a postcoital or Sims-Huhner test (SHT) needs to be done. This test examines the cervical mucus and its reception of your husband's sperm.

Your husband's ejaculate (material that comes from his penis during intercourse) is mostly mucus. Once the ejaculate is in your vagina, the sperm swim out of it and into your cervical mucus. If your cervical mucus is not receptive to the sperm, it acts as a barrier to the sperm reaching the uterine cavity.

For the SHT, several scheduling considerations are necessary. First, intercourse must take place from two to six hours prior to the scheduled office visit set up for the SHT. Second, the office visit must be scheduled one or two days before ovulation.

During the procedure the doctor will take some of the mucus from the cervix, put it on a laboratory slide, and look at it under a microscope. There should be many active sperm, and these sperm should have good direction as they swim—as though they know where they're going.

This test produces a good indication of

## Hysterosalpingogram

dye outlines uterine cavity and channels in the fallopian tubes

dye spills from open tube

instrument inserted in cervix, using plunger, dye is released

Hysterosalpingogram (hystero-uterus; salpingo-fallopian; gram-picture)—an X-ray picture of uterus and tubes is obtained by injecting dye into the uterine cavity, filling the cavity so that the dye overflows into the fallopian tubes, and then taking an X-ray. This procedure can reveal many types of abnormalities.

the condition of the husband's sperm and the woman's cervical mucus. If the sperm are immobilized or killed, the mucus is "unhealthy and hostile," and the condition probably needs to be treated. (See Q. 916.)

Actually, some recent studies have shown that a "good" or "bad" SHT may not be as important as previously thought. In the studies, a laparoscopy done at the right time of the month and after intercourse showed that sperm had actually traveled up into the uterus and tubes in some women with "bad" SHTs, and no sperm had reached the uterus and tubes in some women with "good" SHTs. Conclusions on this particular problem, obviously, are currently ambiguous. Nevertheless, most doctors will try to get the cervical mucus healthy and receptive to sperm, or will try to bypass unhealthy cervical mucus with the new technique called intrauterine insemination with washed sperm. (See Q. 973, 974.)

# Laparoscopy

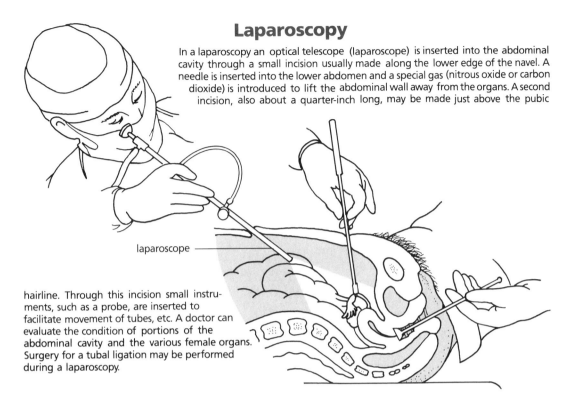

In a laparoscopy an optical telescope (laparoscope) is inserted into the abdominal cavity through a small incision usually made along the lower edge of the navel. A needle is inserted into the lower abdomen and a special gas (nitrous oxide or carbon dioxide) is introduced to lift the abdominal wall away from the organs. A second incision, also about a quarter-inch long, may be made just above the pubic

laparoscope

hairline. Through this incision small instruments, such as a probe, are inserted to facilitate movement of tubes, etc. A doctor can evaluate the condition of portions of the abdominal cavity and the various female organs. Surgery for a tubal ligation may be performed during a laparoscopy.

It is important to understand that a Sims-Huhner test is not a substitute for a sperm analysis. The SHT does not tell a great deal about your husband's sperm specimen. To determine whether or not he is fertile, the doctor must have your husband take a sperm specimen to the laboratory for a competent evaluation. Just because his sperm do get into your cervical mucus does not mean he is able to fertilize you. Having a Sims-Huhner test will not prevent pregnancy during the month it is performed.

When all the studies mentioned above have been done and any abnormalities have been corrected, if pregnancy still has not occurred a diagnostic laparoscopy needs to be done.

## 907   What is a laparoscopy?

This is a minor surgical procedure that can usually be done with general anesthesia on an outpatient basis. After the surgery one's activities are limited only by feelings of fatigue and weakness that accompany relatively minor surgery and general anesthesia. There is not a great deal of pain following the procedure.

A laparoscopy takes about thirty minutes, unless some other procedure (laser, surgery) is done at the same time. After you are put to sleep, the physician inserts a needle through the lower edge of your navel. Three quarts of carbon dioxide gas are allowed to flow through the needle into your abdominal cavity, blowing it up like a balloon.

Two incisions are made—one in the lower edge of the navel and another just above the pubic hairline. Neither incision is more than a quarter of an inch long.

Through the upper incision the doctor inserts a telescope with optics so refined that the interior of the abdomen can be seen as though one were looking directly at it. Through the lower incision the doctor inserts small instruments such as a long probe, or an instrument with delicate teeth to pick things up and move them around.

About half of the time the laparoscopy reveals some abnormality, such as endometriosis, adhesions, or congenital abnormalities. These abnormalities are often correctable. Occasionally, using the small instruments that are employed during the laparoscopy, adhesions can be cut, biopsies can be taken, and the laser can be used without making larger incisions. At other times the abnormalities are too major to be corrected through these small incisions, and a major operation must be done later.

Most doctors always arrange for a laparoscopy to be done after ovulation. They normally dilate the cervix and scrape some of the uterine lining out (D&C) at the time of the laparoscopy. The procedure likely would not remove a just-beginning pregnancy because the embryo is so small and the entire uterine lining is not curetted. To absolutely avoid the possibility, however, some doctors perform laparoscopies before ovulation occurs. The D&C is beneficial because it gives a sample of the lining of the uterus to send to the pathologist for evaluation. The lab report tells whether or not this lining is responding properly to the hormones from the ovary and from other glands in the body.

Recovery from a laparoscopy takes a few days. A patient should stay in bed the evening after her surgery, getting up only to use the bathroom. The next day she can get up and do anything she wants, but she may not feel like doing much.

There is some pain as a result of laparoscopy. A woman may have shoulder pain, which is referred pain from the diaphragm where gas bubbles are causing temporary irritation. She may also have incision pain, but it is not excruciating and lasts only two or three days. Most women can return to full activity in two to four days, although some will be groggy and tired from the anesthesia for up to two weeks.

## 908 Is the use of the laser through the laparoscope a useful procedure?

The use of the laser during laparoscopy is an exciting and truly revolutionary technique that can save many patients major surgery. If you are going to have a laparoscopy done, it would be ideal if you could have it performed by a physician who has the training and desire to use the laser if necessary. Of course, it is also necessary that the operating room have the laser equipment available to hook up to the laparoscope if it is needed.

With the laser hooked up to the laparoscope, the doctor can operate in your abdomen without having to make a large enough incision to get his or her hands inside. With laser laparoscopy a doctor can cut adhesions, cut fibroids off the uterus, vaporize endometriosis, open fallopian tubes, and destroy cystic structures. Of course, the laser cannot be used to do any of these things if they are too large or too extensive. It is not a panacea.

The wonderful thing about laparoscopy, however, is that it can often be used to remove a mild abnormality that may or may not be responsible for infertility. For instance, mild endometriosis can cause infertility, but because it is mild, a doctor never knows if it really is the endometriosis that is causing the infertility. Without the laser laparoscopic technique, a doctor cannot adequately treat even the mildest endometriosis without either three to six months of Danocrine therapy or major surgery. But the question in his or her mind is, "Is such mild endometriosis really the problem?" The laser used through the laparoscope can eliminate such endometriosis completely. This will often lead to pregnancy, but even if it does not, it will eliminate this mild endometriosis from consideration in the fertility evaluation and treatment.

## 909 Is a laparoscopy really necessary?

It is my opinion that no physician has done a complete infertility evaluation until a laparoscopy has been performed. D&C alone is not adequate, because it is the less important part of this procedure. If a doctor suggests a D&C for fertility testing, he or she is probably unfamiliar with the best techniques for the diagnosis and treatment of infertility. You should probably at least get a second opinion.

For example, I once had a patient whose previous physician, except for failing to do a laparoscopy, had done an adequate infertility evaluation. The X-ray of her uterus and tubes was normal. On the basis of the evaluation the woman had undergone treatment for approximately three years. Because she continued to be infertile, however, I did a diagnostic laparoscopy on her and found that both of her tubes were completely closed. The X-ray of her uterus erroneously had looked normal and the physician did not investigate further. She had wasted two or three years because her original doctor had not done a laparoscopy.

My suggestion concerning laparoscopy is this: first have all the preliminary tests done. If everything seems all right and you are under thirty years of age, wait six to twelve months to see if pregnancy will occur. If it does not, have a laparoscopy and D&C. However, if you are over thirty, or if some abnormality is detected that would be clarified by a laparoscopy, go ahead and have it done immediately.

Even though everything appears to be normal on all other exams and tests, the laparoscopy is necessary to insure that the tubes and the rest of the pelvis are normal.

Many other surgical and nonsurgical procedures can be done to treat or diagnose a particular problem, but the foregoing material covers most of the initial studies necessary for proper evaluation of infertility.

## Male Infertility Problems

## 910 When a cause for infertility is discovered, is it more often with the female or with the male?

Problems with the male organs cause infertility about 30 percent of the time, while female abnormalities are also responsible about 30 percent of the time. A combination of factors causes about 40 percent of the problems.

## 911 What will be done if a problem is discovered with the man?

A low sperm count, unhealthy sperm, or a congenital problem are major factors in the problems that can cause male infertility.

A urologist ordinarily treats a man with an infertility problem. Here I will give only a brief overview of male infertility. As previously stated, most gynecologists specializing in fertility care can order the preliminary semen tests. Further testing and treatment will require seeing a urologist.

Two things are important for a man to remember when collecting a sperm specimen for analysis.

Do not abstain from intercourse for over four or five days before collecting the specimen, because this can make the sperm count lower than it really is. Two or three days is okay, or just follow your normal frequency.

Do not collect the specimen following withdrawal during or after intercourse. This contaminates the specimen with vaginal secretions and also makes it possible to lose part of the specimen, making it appear as though you have a lower sperm count than you do.

If the sperm analysis shows the production of few or no sperm (a sperm count that is twenty million or higher per cc of semen is considered normal), several other tests will be performed. These include hormone tests to be sure no hormone problem exists; testicular biopsies to see if sperm can be produced; X-ray vasographies (injection of dye into the vas) to pinpoint the location of blocked sperm ducts; and testing the sperm to see if they will penetrate hamster eggs. This test gives a clue as to whether or not they can penetrate the wife's eggs.

Treating the male usually is much simpler than treating the female, primarily because there are fewer choices for treatment and the problem can be treated fairly easily or not at all.

An infection in the semen can be corrected, whether it is from prostatitis, seminal vasiculitis, or some other type of infection. If there is a varicocele, an accumulation of veins around the testicle, the urologist may want to operate to tie off the engorged veins. The rationale behind this surgery is that the enlarged veins keep the testicle warmer than it should be. Testicles produce the best sperm counts when they are cooler than the rest of the body. When the varicocele is tied off, the testicle (or testicles) gets cooler and starts producing better sperm. Because testicular cooling may improve semen quality, you may want to apply ice to the scrotum each evening or use THD (testicular hypothermia device, available from Repro-Med Systems, Inc., Box 191, Middletown, NY 10949) to provide cooling in a much more scientific way.

If a man does not have a varicocele but still has "bad" sperm, the doctor may try giving him Clomid or some other drug. Al-

though the results are often unsatisfactory, their use is worth a try.

If this does not work, intrauterine inseminations with washed sperm can be done. (See Q. 973, 974.) Or, if that fails, in vitro fertilization can be tried. (See Q. 975–986.) If none of these techniques works, insemination with another man's sperm can be done. This is called artificial insemination with donor sperm, or AID. (See Q. 967–972.)

If a man has had a vasectomy for sterilization, he can have that vasectomy reversed. A doctor who uses microsurgical technique can open the scrotum where the initial incision was made for the vasectomy. The scarred ends of the vas can be cut open and sewn back together so that sperm can once again flow through the reproductive tract. If the vasectomy was done recently, your husband has an excellent chance of producing normal sperm that can result in a normal pregnancy for you. If it has been several years since the vasectomy, he has less chance of producing healthy sperm. If it has been more than ten years since a vasectomy was done, your husband may have only a 10–20 percent chance of being able to produce healthy sperm after his vas are repaired. The only way to know whether or not an operation to repair the vas will work is to try it. If your husband decides not to have this operation, or if after a vasectomy reversal no pregnancy occurs, the only alternative for you to become pregnant is to have artificial insemination done using donor sperm. (See Q. 967.)

---

## The Scope of Female Abnormalities Affecting Fertility

---

**912** **Which structural abnormalities in a woman could be discovered in an initial physical examination?**

A thorough, competent infertility doctor will usually find a variety of these abnormalities at the initial exam. A detailed description of treatment for these conditions follows.

*Abnormal vagina.* A tough hymen can prevent proper penetration of the penis; a vaginal blockage can prevent deposition of the semen by the cervix, and a vaginal infection can produce short-term infertility. When it comes to vaginal infections, trichomonas vaginitis (see Q. 690) is the worst offender.

*Abnormal cervix.* Cervical problems can inhibit fertility through abnormal cervical mucus due to cervical infection, previous cervical surgery, inadequate hormone stimulation of the cervical mucus, or a woman being allergic to her husband's sperm. Cervical stenosis (tight cervix) and mycoplasma or chlamydia cervical infections can also affect fertility.

*Abnormal uterus or abnormal endometrium (uterine lining).* There are many problems involving the uterus that can prevent conception, including fibroid tumors and congenital abnormalities. The inside of the uterus is called the endometrial cavity, and the lining of the inside of the uterus is called the endometrium. There may be polyps projecting from the uterine wall, fibroid tumors distorting the uterus or its cavity, or an infection of the uterus. The endometrium reflects the function of the ovaries and other hormones in the body. If these hormones are functioning abnormally, the lining of the uterus will not undergo proper changes during the female monthly cycle and will therefore not be receptive to pregnancy.

*Abnormal fallopian tubes.* Problems of the tubes may result from previous infection that scarred or blocked them, a previous sterilization procedure, congenital abnormalities that caused distortion of the tubes, previous tubal pregnancies, or endometriosis.

*Abnormal ovaries.* The ovaries may not function properly because of endometriosis, scarring from previous infection, polycystic ovarian disease, or some abnormality of hormone production by the ovary.

*Abnormal hormone functioning.* Since hormones control ovulation, abnormal hormone function can cause infertility. The hypothalamus, located at the base of the brain, monitors the release of hormones. This gland is the master control gland for the female cycle. Its abnormal function can cause an irregular cycle or prevent ovulation. Abnormal function of the thyroid or adrenal glands can also prevent normal ovulation.

## Vaginal Abnormalities and Infertility

**913** **How is a blockage in the vagina from a tight hymen or from a septum treated?**

The procedures to surgically open a hard and resistant hymen or to correct an obstruction in the vagina are relatively easy. General anesthesia may be required, but only for a short time. Usually such problems would be corrected by conventional surgery: cutting across the abnormal tissues and suturing them in a more open configuration. The laser, an instrument that produces an intense light beam that can evaporate tissue with little damage, corrects the problem most easily, but lasers are not always available.

**914** **What about treating a vaginal infection?**

A vaginal infection can prevent pregnancy, so it should be eliminated immediately.

Flagyl will be given if the germ is found to be trichomonas. For a fungus infection a drug such as Monistat or Gyne Lotrimin may be given. (See Q. 689–695.)

## Cervical Abnormalities and Infertility

**915** **What can be done if there is an abnormality of the cervix?**

If a cervix just "looks" abnormal, with ridges or irregularity as is frequently the situation if you were exposed to DES in your mother's womb, nothing needs to be done, as that condition is probably not contributing to your infertility. If the cervical opening is too tight because you have had cautery, freezing, or a conization of your cervix, something may need to be done, such as a dilatation of the cervix (as in a D&C). This procedure would require anesthesia.

Occasionally the opening of the cervix may be so small that the doctor will be unable to find it; usually the result of having had a conization done in the past. If surgery is required to repair the cervix and a D&C is not possible, then the doctor makes an incision in the abdomen, splits the uterus from above, and probes down through the cervix into the vagina in order to redevelop a cervical opening.

**916** **How can an abnormality in the cervical mucus affect fertility?**

The cervix has an active role in the process of reproduction. At ovulation time it produces mucus made up of chains of macromolecules which arrange themselves into parallel "rods of mucus" several millimeters in length. This physical arrangement of the cervical mucus seems essential for successful transport of the sperm. The mucus also acts as a filter.

Cervical mucus is the vehicle through which the sperm swim into the uterus, but it prevents the passage of the semen or of your vaginal secretions into the uterus. Semen is mainly mucus, with the actual volume of sperm a mere dot of tissue.

Both before and after ovulation the cervical mucus forms a dense mesh that causes it to become sticky. This prevents the passage of sperm, germs, or anything else into the uterus.

**917** **What can be done if my cervical mucus is abnormal?**

You may have an obvious cervical infection called cervicitis, which should be treated with antibiotics by mouth, with a vaginal antibiotic cream, or by treatment of the cervix with laser or freezing.

Certain cervical infections may exist without any symptoms yet still produce infertility, for example, infections with mycoplasma or chlamydia organisms. Because cultures of these germs are not always reliable, I routinely treat all first-time infertility patients and their husbands with tetracycline for two weeks to rid them of such organisms. Incidentally, the husband is treated because he can have any germ in his urethra that his wife has in her vagina.

Of the women with poor Sims-Huhner tests, approximately two-thirds will have cervical mucus that is thick, yellow, and abnormal-looking. A daily dose of some type of oral estrogen can sometimes change the cervical mucus, allowing pregnancy to take place.

If the cervical mucus seems to be normal but your husband's sperm are immobile when the mucus is examined (though the sperm count is good), there may be a "hostile factor" in the cervix or a missing factor in your husband's semen.

Testing for this problem can be done by mixing a donor sperm specimen with your cervical mucus on a laboratory slide. At the same time your husband's sperm specimen will be mixed with another woman's cervical mucus to determine whether the problem is due to your mucus or to his sperm.

If the poor Sims-Huhner test is because your husband has a small amount of semen (less than two cc), or a low sperm count (less than twenty million per cc), try inseminations with his sperm. (See Q. 962.)

Another technique to try if your husband's sperm count is low is to have him withdraw after the first burst of ejaculate is released into your vagina. This is done because the first portion of your husband's ejaculate has the highest concentration of sperm. If he withdraws after that is released, the "good" portion is not diluted by the last part, which has few sperm present. Remember, however, if your husband has a sperm problem and has a varicocele, he should get the varicocele fixed.

If the cervix has an infection that cannot be cleared up with antibiotics, or the opening is small and will not stay open adequately, some type of surgical treatment may be necessary. Conizations of the cervix—cutting out and sewing up part of the cervix—have been done in the past for these conditions. More recently cryosurgery (freezing of the cervix) and laser conization have been popular.

Many gynecologists, myself included, now feel that the laser is the ideal method of treatment for this type of cervical problem. It results in little scar tissue and leaves a healthier cervix on healing.

After having gone through this description of the traditional approach to treating infertility due to cervical problems, I must admit that most of the time pregnancy does not occur. A relatively new technique called intrauterine insemination with washed sperm (IUI) helps but pregnancy rates have not been as high as most of us had hoped. When I have a patient with a cervical problem today, I will ordinarily treat her with IUI. (See Q. 973, 974.) If a woman has an acutely inflamed cervix, of course, antibiotics have to be used to clear it up. Some of the other traditional techniques to get the cervix healthy might be used, but I would be planning to try IUI as soon as conditions permit. If pregnancy does not occur after using IUI for up to nine months, the couple should consider using the GIFT procedure. (See Q. 979.)

## Uterine Abnormalities and Infertility

## 918 What if my doctor finds an abnormality of my uterus?

If there is something growing in your uterus that is large enough for your doctor to feel, it will almost always be a fibroid tumor—a knot of muscle growing in the wall of the uterus which almost never becomes cancerous, but can prevent pregnancy or cause miscarriages.

Even when your uterus is enlarged by fibroid tumors to the size of a five- or six-months pregnancy, such fibroids can usually be removed without a hysterectomy but infertility often results due to distortion of the uterus.

However, it is a lot easier for a doctor to do a hysterectomy than to cut out all those fibroids. If your doctor is going to operate on you for fibroids and you want to remain fertile, be sure that he or she is competent and enthusiastic about working with infertility patients and that you have clearly indicated that you do not choose to have a hysterectomy.

I have removed as many as twenty-six fibroids from one uterus. The woman from

# Hysteroscopy

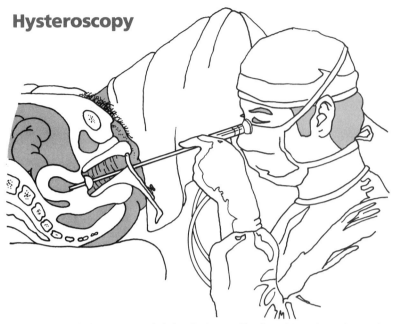

The insertion of a hysteroscope (a lighted telescopelike device) into the vagina and through the cervix allows evaluation of the uterine cavity.

whom I removed these fibroids had two subsequent pregnancies, after which I did a sterilization procedure because she did not want any more children.

An operation to remove fibroids requires an incision in the abdominal wall. If the inside cavity of the uterus is entered in the course of that surgery, it will later be necessary to have a cesarean section for delivery, assuming that pregnancy is achieved eventually.

**919** **What if an X-ray of my uterus by hysterosalpingogram shows scarring or polyps inside my uterus?**

If this happens a D&C and diagnostic laparoscopy should be done. Hysteroscopy, if available, might be useful as well.

If there is scarring in the uterus (synechiae), it needs to be evaluated by a D&C. When I do a D&C for this reason, I always do a laparoscopy at the same time. If a patient has had enough disease or trauma to her

uterus to cause scarring there, she may also have scarring of her tubes and ovaries.

When the X-ray shows abnormalities in the uterine cavity, it is most important that they be corrected. Scarring in the uterus can cause both infertility and miscarriage, and small polyps or growths inside the uterus seemingly act like an IUD (intrauterine contraceptive device) in preventing pregnancy. Therefore it is necessary that these abnormalities be removed.

An instrument called a hysteroscope should be used for problems of this type. This instrument is inserted through the cervix; it has a lens system with a fiber optic light (see glossary listing) that allows visualization of the interior of the uterus. With the hysteroscope, abnormalities inside the uterus can be seen. Small instruments are available for operations with the hysteroscope. Polyps can be removed, scars cut apart, and congenital abnormalities corrected, all without making an incision into the uterus.

Occasionally some of the abnormalities

seen on the X-ray of the uterine cavity cannot be operated on with a hysteroscope. In this situation the doctor must make an incision in your abdominal wall in order to cut the uterus open from above and take out the polyps or growths.

## 920 What if the hysterosalpingogram shows that I have been born with an abnormal uterus?

As a female baby develops inside the mother's uterus, the baby's own uterus is formed from two halves: one from the right and one from the left side of her body. Normally these meet in the middle, fuse, and then develop an opening in the middle which becomes the uterine cavity.

Occasionally the two halves of the uterus form on each side of the body but do not come together in the middle. Variations of this type of abnormality occur. They may range from a woman's having two vaginas lying side by side—with two cervixes and two halves of a uterus that function as two normal, separate uteri—to having only a small indentation in the top part of the uterus.

An abnormal uterus may or may not be a problem for you. If you have not had miscarriages and have had no trouble getting pregnant, you need not be worried if your doctor tells you that your uterus did not form properly.

Having two uteri (uterus didelphys) usually does not cause fertility problems. However, it can result in miscarriages or premature deliveries. When this is thought to be the problem, the two uterine bodies can be sewn together to form one cavity. This is done by making an incision in the abdominal wall, opening the two uterine bodies, and sewing them together.

A less severe form of abnormal uterine development is the septate uterus. The two halves of the uterus come together but do not fuse completely. As a result there is a wall either partial or complete, between the two halves of the uterus.

Any of these abnormal situations is compatible with totally normal reproductive capacity. In other words, you may be able to become pregnant normally and carry babies in a totally normal fashion. If you are having trouble becoming pregnant, you should have a complete evaluation for other possible problems of fertility before any type of surgery is done on your uterus. If everything else seems normal and the only abnormality is the uterine abnormality, then it is reasonable to have surgery to correct it.

I had as a patient a young woman who had become pregnant several years ago in one side of her double uterus. Her physician at the time told her that she should have an abortion, as she would surely miscarry or deliver prematurely. She took his advice and had the abortion.

After moving to our city she came to me and asked that I repair her uterus so that she could have a baby. I then had to tell this young woman that the abortion had been unnecessary and that her uterus did not need repairing, unless it was proven that she could not carry a pregnancy.

After the uterine cavity has been evaluated, the tissue that lines that cavity, the endometrium, should be evaluated. This is accomplished by an endometrial biopsy, as explained in the next question.

## 921 How is an endometrial biopsy done? Is it painful?

An endometrial biopsy is done in the doctor's office, usually without anesthesia. However, although the procedure is quickly accomplished, it is painful.

I have given patients nitrous oxide (as some dentists do) to relieve the pain. This has worked so well that I now recommend this technique for certain other simple-but-painful procedures that are done in the office.

An endometrial biopsy is done by inserting into the uterus a small, hollow, round tube with a sharp lip. As it is drawn back, some of the lining of the uterus is collected. This tissue is fixed on a slide and studied under the microscope by a pathologist.

Because this procedure hurts, I usually try to wait to do it until I do a laparoscopy. The D&C done at laparoscopy is, therefore, basically an endometrial biopsy.

## 922 What if an endometrial biopsy or D&C shows that the lining of my uterus is abnormal?

Endometrial biopsies are done primarily to be sure that the body is ovulating and producing normal hormones after ovulation, and that the uterus is being prepared by those hormones to receive and nurture a baby. If no ovulation is occurring, this will usually be proven by the results of the biopsy. A luteal phase defect is diagnosed in part with this same test. (See Q. 946, 947.)

Occasionally the endometrial biopsy done to check for hormone changes finds an infection. If the endometrium is infected, antibiotics may be prescribed. Another endometrial biopsy or a D&C may be done later to evaluate the effect of the treatment of the infection.

An infection inside the uterus could also involve the tubes and ovaries. This can be determined by performing a laparoscopy at the time a D&C is performed.

## Fallopian-Tube Abnormalities and Infertility

## 923 What if my physician finds that my fallopian tubes are abnormal and suspects that is causing my infertility? What produces such abnormalities and how can they be treated?

Several problems may cause the fallopian tubes to be abnormal. These problems comprise the most common cause of infertility, accounting for 35 percent of infertility in couples, and over 50 percent of female-related infertility.

*Sexually transmitted diseases (STD).* Gonorrhea and certain other infectious diseases (such as chlamydia) are spread by intercourse. Such infections are commonly called PID—pelvic inflammatory disease. These organisms can result in infections in the fallopian tubes that can cause them to close completely or become so scarred inside that an egg cannot pass through them. Occasionally an egg gets partially through the tube, where it becomes lodged and fertilized, resulting in an ectopic or "out of place" pregnancy.

To explain what is meant by adhesions and scarring of the tubes and other organs, I often use this example: If you scrape the sides of two of your fingers till they are quite raw and then bind them together for several weeks, they will grow together. Physicians would refer to the scar that held the fingers together as an "adhesion." This is what happens to the tubes, ovaries, intestines, and other organs inside the pelvis as a result of infection. They stick together, and the scars that hold them together and distort them are adhesions.

Infections from gonorrhea cause infertility in 11 percent of women with a first infection, 23 percent with the second infection, and 54 percent with three or more such infections. If the infectious organism is chlamydia, the percentages are even higher. (See Q. 1167.)

*Intrauterine devices.* Women who use IUDs run a greater than normal risk of pelvic infections (two to three times normal) and such infections usually occur during the first few months that an IUD is in place. Because of this increased risk of infection, I counsel women not to use IUDs unless they have had all the babies they want. If a woman has used an IUD she has doubled her chance of being infertile.

*Endometriosis.* Endometriosis can cause distortion and scarring of the fallopian tubes and the surgery that is done to remove endometriosis can also result in damaged fallopian tubes. Endometriosis is a fairly common cause of infertility, and infertility may be the only symptom of her endometriosis. (See Q. 953–960.)

*Elective abortion.* A small but significant percentage of women who have chosen to have abortions will have infertility problems later due to infections of the tubes as a result of those abortions.

*Previous pelvic surgery.* Any surgery done on the pelvic structures can result in scarring of the tubes and subsequent infertility. Since some pelvic surgery is unnecessary, my advice is that you not let a doctor operate on you, especially for an "ovarian cyst," unless you know it is absolutely necessary.

*Tubal (ectopic) pregnancy.* Tubal pregnancies are both a result of and a cause of scarred tubes. When a tube is scarred, it can trap a fertilized egg, causing an ectopic pregnancy. That pregnancy can then severely damage the tube, and subsequent surgery for the ectopic pregnancy can cause more tubal scarring.

*Appendicitis.* An infected or ruptured appendix can cause so much infection in the pelvis that it can result in a great deal of scarring of the female organs. I once had to

do a hysterectomy on an infertility patient who had contracted severe pelvic inflammation from her appendix.

*Voluntary sterilization.* "Band-Aid" sterilization has made female sterilization so acceptable and easy that many women are having it done. And, as the news of its successful reversibility spreads, more and more women are requesting a reversal of a previous sterilization. Surgical reversal of a tubal ligation can usually be done successfully but it does leave some scarring of the tubes. (See Q. 925–929, 1107, 1118.)

---

**924** What can be done if my fertility evaluation shows I have scarred or blocked fallopian tubes?

First, if the problem was discovered with a hysterosalpingogram, a laparoscopy needs to be done to determine the probable cause and the extent of the damage. If surgery is called for, the doctor should be able to give you a general idea of your chances of pregnancy if you elect to have such surgery. Remember that the choice is yours. Your health will not be damaged if the scars are left alone, but removal of them may increase the possibility of your achieving pregnancy.

If your tubes are blocked or there is a moderate amount of scarring, there is probably a 30-percent chance of pregnancy following surgery. One thing to remember is that after such surgery there is a greater than normal chance of your having an ectopic pregnancy. I still generally encourage patients to go ahead with surgery because, short of in vitro fertilization, it is the only chance they have of becoming pregnant.

If you choose to have the surgery, the physician should use a microsurgical technique. He or she will usually do the surgery through a six-inch "bikini" incision in your lower abdomen, made crossways just above your pubic hairline. Your surgeon should not only be familiar with microsurgery, but enthusiastic about the technique and willing to take the time required to use it correctly. Microsurgery is advantageous for many reasons.

*Gentleness.* Obviously, gentleness is important in handling delicate tissue; microsurgery involves the use of small instruments and small sutures.

*Irrigation.* Prolonged exposure of tissue to drying can cause further adhesion formation. Therefore the doctor will constantly moisten the tissues with a saline solution during the surgery.

*Control of bleeding.* Blood on tissue can cause adhesions to develop more easily. The careful use of sutures, cautery, and the laser (when available) to control bleeding is an essential part of microsurgery.

*Covering of raw surfaces.* The tissue (peritoneum) that normally covers the organs in the abdomen can be pulled over raw places, decreasing the chance of adhesion formation.

*Magnification.* Magnification can be achieved with the use of magnifying glasses (called loupes) or with the use of operating microscopes. These devices make it possible to use smaller sutures and smaller instruments during the surgery. Because of the tubes' delicate anatomy, this is especially important if they must be worked on.

Once these microsurgical techniques are used to excise adhesions and scars and separate adhesions that hold the tubes and ovaries together, your doctor will close the incision. You will stay in the hospital about four or five days after the day of surgery.

Your physician may administer injections of antibiotics to prevent infection and cortisonelike drugs to prevent scar formation. The latter drug often produces temporary euphoria. You may feel better than you thought you would following surgery, but after you get home you may experience a few days of depression.

Although you may feel fine within a few weeks, it may take your pelvic tissues a long time to become normal enough to produce a pregnancy, especially the tissues of the delicate inner lining of the tube. I tell patients I have operated on that they will probably not become pregnant for a year, and possibly longer. If pregnancy does not occur after one or two years, further evaluation and treatment may be necessary. Ultimately, in vitro fertilization or adoption may be the only options available for obtaining a child.

The statistics of 30-percent chance of pregnancy following surgery apply when the problem of infertility is due to fairly serious pelvic adhesions, but the chances are better with less severe adhesions.

---

**925** **What if I have had a previous sterilization and now want to get pregnant?**

A sterilization can usually be reversed. (See Q. 813.) Occasionally, though, a sterilization reversal cannot be accomplished. Some sterilization techniques almost totally destroy the fallopian tube, making it unlikely that a tubal reversal could be done.

Back in 1971 and 1972, when doctors began doing "Band-Aid" sterilizations, the tubes would often be burned in two places. This is essentially doing to a tube what you do to a piece of bacon when you fry it. If your sterilization was done in this fashion, you probably do not have enough tube left for your physician to repair.

If, however, your sterilization was done with the coagulation (electrical burn) technique in only one area of the tube, you may have enough tube left to repair.

If you had a Fallope Ring or a Hulka Clip, or some other method of sterilization in which cautery was not used, you have a greater chance of pregnancy following the repair of your tubes.

**926 How does the doctor determine whether or not my sterilization is reversible?**

Your doctor would probably order a hysterosalpingogram. If this X-ray showed that some open tube was protruding from the uterus, and if your doctor felt that the technique used to do your sterilization probably did not destroy too much of your fallopian tubes, he or she might suggest that you go ahead with the major repair surgery.

Most of the time, there is enough tube on at least one side to repair adequately. Occasionally, however, the doctor will find that both tubes have been too severely damaged by the sterilization to be repaired. In this case the operation would be unsuccessful. The doctor could, of course, make sure at the time of this operation that your ovaries were in proper position for your having in vitro fertilization done later if you desired it.

If there is some question in the doctor's mind, after the initial evaluation, that your tubes might have been too damaged by your sterilization procedure to be repaired, he or she will probably want to do an evaluating or diagnostic laparoscopy before performing the more major operation. This allows him or her to determine if there is enough tube left for the repair to give you a reasonable chance of subsequently getting pregnant.

It is important to realize that having your tubes tied did not change your body's function in any way and getting your tubes put back together will not either. For instance, PMS will not get better and periods will not be more regular.

**927 What happens after the doctor determines the condition of my tubes?**

Once the doctor has evaluated your condition and your husband's sperm and has determined that there are no other fertility problems, then you would be scheduled for surgery to reverse the sterilization surgery.

This operation involves a large incision in your abdomen. When your abdomen is open, the doctor can directly examine your tubes to determine whether or not he or she can proceed with the surgery. The doctor will then position the tubes so that they are visible through the operating microscope (or through the loupes), cut off the scarred stumps of the tubes, cauterize bleeders, and sew the two tube openings together with very fine suture. The suture used is smaller than a human hair and difficult to see with the unaided eye. Many physicians, including myself, like to use the laser to cut the scarred tubes. It not only cuts precisely, but it seals blood vessels as it cuts, which is good microsurgical technique. This also shortens operating time.

**928 What are the success rates for sterilization reversal procedures?**

Subsequent pregnancy rates are about 75 percent. This means, of course, that about 25 percent of the women who go through all this surgery will still not become pregnant. However, the women who do have this surgery can feel satisfied that they have done everything they could, short of in vitro fertilization, to achieve pregnancy. They will have no regrets later in life because they will know that they tried.

**929 Are there any complications following sterilization reversal?**

There is one possible problem other than the complications common to any surgery. After having this type of surgery, there is an increased chance of having a tubal pregnancy. This is disappointing, of course, especially if only one tube could be repaired during surgery and the tubal pregnancy destroys that one tube.

## Ovarian Abnormalities and Infertility

**930** What can be wrong with my ovaries that prevents me from getting pregnant?

The primary job of the ovaries is to put out an egg every month in a process called ovulation. If ovulation does not occur at all, you cannot get pregnant. If ovulation is irregular, you may not be able to become pregnant, or it may take months or years for you to become pregnant. The main ovarian problem associated with poor ovulation is polycystic ovarian disease (PCOD), sometimes called the Stein-Leventhal syndrome. It is for this problem that fertility pills such as Clomid are often used. (See Q. 931.)

The secondary job of the ovaries is to produce hormones in adequate amounts and with proper timing. If the ovary does not produce hormones in this way, pregnancy will not occur or will be much delayed. One form of this problem is called luteal phase defect. This is sometimes treated with Clomid, but other treatments are also used.

Occasionally the ovaries do not work well because they are enmeshed in scars that resulted from infection or surgery. This can interfere with the egg getting out of the ovary and can cause the ovary to become so irritated that it forms cysts and releases the egg irregularly or produces hormones erratically. The major treatment is to cut the bonds that are interfering with ovarian function. As the fallopian tubes are almost always involved when such scars and adhesions are present, this form of surgery is

the same as that used to repair the fallopian tubes. (See Q. 924.)

**931** My doctor said I might have polycystic ovarian disease. What is this, and how is it treated?

Polycystic ovarian disease (PCOD) is an abnormality of the ovaries that produces irregular periods and infertility. Although there are numerous other causes of irregular periods, if you have had irregular periods since puberty it is likely that you have this disease.

Other common symptoms of PCOD are obesity and a tendency to be more hairy than your blood relatives. Although these two characteristics are not always present in PCOD cases, when they do occur the odds are ten to one that you have PCOD.

Since PCOD is a dominantly inherited disorder, a woman with several relatives who also have irregular periods and excess hair growth has an even greater likelihood of having the disease. Another sign of possible PCOD is enlarged ovaries.

PCOD seems to stem from a lack of normal enzyme production by the ovaries, which causes them to produce more male hormones and less female hormones. The ovary does produce some male hormones normally. More than 85 percent of women who have PCOD have elevated levels of one or both of the male hormones—androstenedione or testosterone.

Because of the ovaries' failure to ovulate and the overproduction of male hormones, the pituitary produces too much luteinizing hormone (LH), the hormone that makes the ovary release its ripened egg, but only a normal or slightly below normal amount of follicle-stimulating hormone (FSH). This is an attempt to make the ovary release its eggs.

PCOD can be treated with medication. Before treatment, tests should be done to make sure the symptoms are not caused by abnormality of the adrenal glands, the pituitary, or the thyroid, although your doctor may have already tested you for such problems with earlier blood tests.

---

**932** My doctor said Clomid or Serophene is used to treat PCOD. What are these drugs and what do they do?

Clomid and Serophene are actually the same drug: clomiphene. This drug causes a woman to ovulate 80 percent of the time and to become pregnant 50 percent of the time. This is why the drug is known as "the fertility pill."

Clomiphene was first studied in 1960 as a possible contraceptive aid. Surprisingly during this research it was found to induce fertility.

The chemical structure of clomiphene is similar to estrogenic substances. Scientists think that the hypothalamus, the large control gland at the base of the brain, regards clomiphene as the body's own estrogen. Once the clomiphene is taken in by the hypothalamus, the hypothalamus cannot measure the true amount of estrogen in the body's circulation and perceives it to be low. This causes the hypothalamus to signal the pituitary to stimulate the ovaries, which makes them ovulate.

In addition to inducing ovulation, the use of clomiphene often creates regular twenty-eight- or twenty-nine-day menstrual cycles, with ovulation on day fourteen or fifteen. This cycle makes it "easier" for pregnancy to occur. With regular periods intercourse can be more accurately timed to coincide with ovulation, and the endometrial lining is developed in the most normal fashion for reception of a fertilized ovum.

The ultimate goal of using clomiphene is pregnancy, and it has truly been a miracle

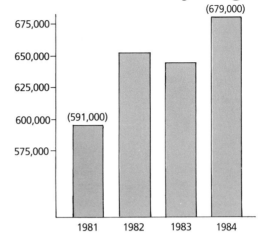

**Number of Prescriptions Written for Fertility Drugs**

drug in helping thousands of otherwise infertile women achieve pregnancy.

---

**933** Are any side effects or multiple births connected with the use of clomiphene?

Yes, there are some side effects, but these are generally unimportant and not too bothersome.

About 10 percent of women taking clomiphene will have hot flashes similar to those experienced in menopause, although it does not cause menopause to start. Occasionally there is some abdominal swelling and bloating (5 percent experience this). There will sometimes be breast discomfort (2 percent), nausea and vomiting (about 2 percent), visual symptoms, such as bright spots of light (1.5 percent), headaches (about 1.5 percent), and dryness or partial loss of hair (about 1.5 percent). The cause of these symptoms is generally unknown, but in all cases the symptoms disappear when the medicine is no longer needed, leaving no permanent effects. Occasionally a patient will feel some discomfort in her ovaries as they enlarge in response to the clomiphene.

If you should develop one or more ovarian cysts while taking clomiphene and continue to take it, the ovary can become huge: as big as a softball or even bigger. This can cause pain and can also cause the release of more than one egg, which increases the possibility of a multiple pregnancy. This is the primary reason for a monthly check by the doctor before prescribing more clomiphene.

In summary, the drug seems to cause almost no health hazards, and its side effects seem to be limited only to the month in which it is taken.

Although there is an increased chance (about 8 percent) of having a multiple birth, most of these are twins. I have only had one patient get pregnant with triplets due to clomiphene, and none have had more than triplets. However, as of this writing there have been one sextuplet birth and three quintuplet births reported in the world among women who took clomiphene.

The miscarriage rate for clomiphene users is only 20 percent, which is the same rate as in normal pregnancies.

---

### 934 Is there an increased risk of having an abnormal baby while using clomiphene?

Most studies show that there is a slightly increased risk of abnormalities in pregnancies produced by clomiphene. The increased risk is so small, however, that experts conclude that the benefits definitely outweigh the risks. Most researchers believe that the increased risk of having an abnormal baby is due to the already existing subfertility (decreased fertility) of the couple who must use clomiphene to achieve pregnancy rather than to the clomiphene itself.

---

### 935 How is clomiphene taken?

Patients are given a prescription for five clomiphene tablets, and each clomiphene tablet contains 50 mg of clomiphene citrate. One tablet is taken each day for five consecutive days, starting on the third to fifth day of the menstrual cycle. The cycle is always counted with the first day of the menstrual period being "day one."

Women taking clomiphene must be examined by their physician each month during the menstrual period, although there are a few fertility specialists who feel comfortable about not examining their patients each month. Most patients will ovulate with the first dose of clomiphene citrate. If they do not ovulate after two or three months, the dosage may be increased to two clomiphene tablets per day for five days, or even up to four or five clomiphene tablets per day for each of those days. Also, ovulation can sometimes be induced by taking clomiphene for a total of eight days rather than five.

Patients on clomiphene should keep a daily temperature chart every month to determine when they ovulate. This is done by using a basal body thermometer. If no period comes and the temperature did not go up about the fifteenth day, ovulation did not occur. However, if the temperature went up at ovulation time (and stays up) and no period comes, you are probably pregnant. By the way, this is almost as good an indication of pregnancy as a pregnancy test.

---

### 936 How often does ovulation occur while using clomiphene, and how often does pregnancy follow the use of clomiphene?

About 80–90 percent of women taking clomiphene will ovulate. Of these, 50 percent achieve pregnancy. Some of these women will have been treated with clomiphene without having a complete fertility evaluation. A complete workup is essential if a comprehensive and effective treatment program is to continue.

## 937 What if I still don't have regular periods after taking clomiphene for several months?

Human chorionic gonadotrophin (HCG) can be given as a single shot in the muscle on day fourteen or fifteen of your cycle. Normally you will ovulate thirty-eight hours later. When HCG is used, you should have intercourse the day of the shot and on each of the next two days.

Human chorionic gonadotrophin is a hormone which is extracted from the urine of pregnant women or from the placentas that result from normal births. HCG is structurally and biologically similar to luteinizing hormone (LH), the hormone produced by the pituitary that "kicks" the ovary and makes it release its egg. A woman who is not ovulating properly may have poor production of LH from her pituitary and the HCG shot takes the place of the LH that the body should be producing.

Doctors will sometimes want patients who are not responding readily to clomiphene, and who thus need HCG, to have an ultrasound examination of their ovaries done just before and just after ovulation. The ultrasound machine can show if follicles are developing on the ovary and when they are releasing the egg. This helps both the doctor and patient know if and when ovulation is occurring. HCG is a very safe drug. I have never had a patient with an allergic reaction to it, and it does not increase a woman's chance of having twins or triplets.

## 938 Is there any other treatment to try if ovulation does not occur when using clomiphene or human chorionic gonadotrophin, or if I still have not become pregnant after using clomiphene for a long time?

If ovulation is not occurring at all or is irregular, or if prolonged use of clomiphene has not resulted in pregnancy, the next treatment might be with Pergonal.

If you are not ovulating because the pituitary is not producing enough follicle-stimulating hormone (FSH), the only known way to increase your FSH level is by using Pergonal. This drug is being used more and more with fertility patients, but its use is complicated and expensive.

Pergonal contains a hormone called human menopausal gonadotrophin (HMG), so called because it is extracted from the urine of women who have gone through menopause. Pergonal stimulates the ovaries of an infertile woman in the same way the hormone it contains "tries" to stimulate the ovaries of a postmenopausal woman.

Menopause occurs because the ovaries have come to the end of their life span. They "die" and stop producing estrogen. The pituitary gland, however, remains alive and well. When it perceives that the ovaries are not producing estrogen any more, it works overtime trying to force the ovaries back into production. In its attempt to do this, the pituitary produces more and more follicle-stimulating hormone (FSH), the hormone that causes the ovary to increase its production of estrogen and to mature an egg.

Because of this increased production of FSH, the excess spills into the urine from the blood stream of postmenopausal women. It becomes possible, therefore, to extract FSH from the urine of postmenopausal women and administer it to infertility patients.

## 939 When is the use of Pergonal indicated?

There are four groups of women who need Pergonal.

*Women whose pituitary glands are not producing follicle-stimulating hormone (FSH) and thus are not ovulating.* Problems that can cause this to happen include growths or diseases that destroy all or part of the pituitary, thus keeping it from producing enough hormone. Surgical removal of the pituitary would also place a woman in this category.

*Women whose pituitaries are producing FSH, but who are still not ovulating.* Most of these women are having irregular periods and have polycystic ovarian disease (PCOD). They should try clomiphene first, but if several monthly courses of clomiphene do not cause ovulation, Pergonal can be tried.

*Patients who have had a tumor (adenoma) in the pituitary.* If these patients do not start ovulating after their pituitary tumor is treated, they need Pergonal.

*Women who have abnormal cervical mucus.* If a woman's infertility seems to be due to a cervical mucus abnormality and other methods of treatment have been unsuccessful, Pergonal might be tried. Pergonal almost always causes the cervix to produce exceedingly abundant and healthy cervical mucus. This is an aggressive treatment for this problem, but it often results in pregnancy. (See Q. 917.)

## 940 How is Pergonal taken?

Injections of Pergonal are given in increasing amounts daily, starting soon after a menstrual period begins, until tests shows the ovary is ready to ovulate. At this point a shot of human chorionic gonadotrophin (HCG) is given, and the couple has intercourse the day of the shot and then daily until the temperature goes up, usually two more days.

To determine the amount of Pergonal to give, the doctor will usually want to measure both the amount of estrogen in the woman's blood and the size of the egg-containing follicles on her ovaries. The latter is done with an ultrasound (sonogram) machine. These tests are usually done daily from about day seven until the follicles are large enough to have a mature egg. The size

of the follicles on the ovaries is important because, when the ovaries are ready to release an egg, the ovarian follicles containing the eggs will each be about two-thirds inch in diameter. When the ovary with its cysts is "ready," the HCG injection is given, making the ovary release its egg(s).

An alternative program using both Clomid and Pergonal is also available and is less expensive.

## 941 What are the results of using Pergonal?

If patients are properly selected (those who actually have a chance to get pregnant with Pergonal), up to 75 percent will conceive. However, a slightly higher-than-normal number of these pregnancies end with miscarriage (28 percent), so only about half of the treated patients will carry a baby to term. Don't be too discouraged by this. If you are able to get pregnant once, you probably can again.

## 942 What about complications with Pergonal?

You may have read in the newspaper that Pergonal is the fertility drug that can cause women to have five, six, or seven babies at a time. Because Pergonal is being used to push the ovaries hard, they sometimes are overstimulated. This can have its most dramatic effect in producing a pregnancy with twins, triplets, quadruplets, or more. This happens 20 percent of the time. (About 15 percent are twins; 5 percent are more than twins.)

Another complication is that the ovaries can become much larger than was meant to happen. This "hyperstimulation" occurs less frequently than it did in the past because physicians have learned how to use the drug more precisely. When hyperstimulation does happen, the ovaries can become as large as volleyballs and cause pain and dehydration. An occasional death has even been reported.

Treatment with Pergonal is not simple. It requires a great deal of time, dedication, and money. It also requires being able to get to the doctor almost daily during the first half of the cycle.

---

### 943  When should Pergonal not be used?

Pergonal should not be used if the woman is postmenopausal, either because of premature menopause or because of regular menopause that occurred at the normal age. In menopause the FSH level in the blood is already high, and more FSH, given as Pergonal, will not help.

In addition, Pergonal should not be used until other fertility problems have been proven to be absent by a complete evaluation.

---

### 944  What can be done if I ovulated with clomiphene and Pergonal but still did not get pregnant?

After using Clomid and then Pergonal without a pregnancy, a wedge resection of the ovaries can be considered. Drs. Stein and Leventhal, early leaders in fertility treatment, discovered that after they removed part of the ovaries of women with polycystic ovarian disease (PCOD), the women would develop regular periods. Up to 95 percent of their patients ovulated after such surgery.

By cutting out part of the ovaries there is

## Ovarian Wedge Resection

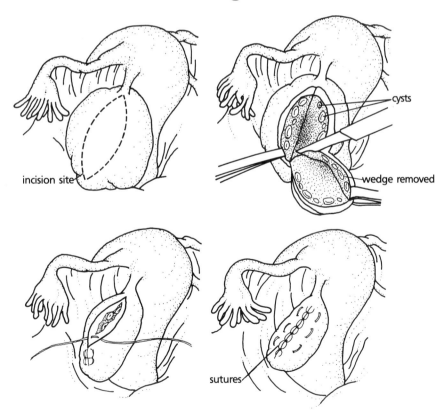

incision site

cysts

wedge removed

sutures

less hormone secreted from them. The control glands (pituitary and hypothalamus) then react by putting out more stimulating hormones to make the ovaries work harder. It is this increase in follicle stimulating hormone (FSH) and luteinizing hormone (LH) from the pituitary that drives an ovary to begin putting out eggs each month.

## 945 How is such ovarian surgery done? Is it dangerous?

After making an incision in the abdomen, the doctor cuts an "orange slice" portion out of each ovary. After the segment of ovarian tissue is cut from each ovary (up to one-third to one-half of the ovary may be removed), the ovary is reclosed. As mentioned in the previous question, this procedure is called a wedge resection of the ovary.

As to danger involved, there are risks connected to any surgery, of course. The primary danger with this operation is that it is so simple to do that any physician who does surgery can do it. Do not let a physician make the decision to do this procedure on you unless you know that he or she is competent in the area of fertility treatment, that it is a "last resort," and that it will be done with the microsurgical technique described in Q. 924.

The next greatest danger from this surgery is that it can produce adhesions, or scar tissue, around the ovaries and tubes. Studies show that up to 50 percent of women develop scarring and adhesions from this operation.

It is extremely important that the surgery be done by a gynecologist who has expertise in fertility and in this particular procedure. The ovary must be closed delicately and carefully, with very small sutures, so that there is absolutely no bleeding from the ovaries at the conclusion of the operation. This helps prevent scarring.

There are other techniques practiced by gynecologists interested in fertility surgery that can be employed to help decrease adhesions. These include keeping tissues moist, using Ringer's lactate instead of saline during the operation, and putting Hyskon (a substance that decreases the possibility of the tissues sticking together) into the pelvis after the operation and before closure of the abdomen.

Most women who are infertile because they are not ovulating can be made to ovulate with one of the medications we have discussed. It is a rare patient who needs ovarian surgery for this purpose.

## 946 My doctor has said that I have a "bad luteal phase." What does that mean?

The medical term usually used for this is "inadequate luteal phase." At ovulation, the ovary forms a corpus luteum, which then produces a hormone called progesterone. The normal production of progesterone results in changes in the inner uterine lining that will cause a menstrual period to start fourteen days after ovulation if no pregnancy has occurred.

If the progesterone production is normal and the lining of the uterus is properly developed in anticipation of pregnancy, then pregnancy can occur. If the production of progesterone from the ovary is insufficient, the luteal phase is inadequate. This problem apparently stems from a lack in the corpus luteum of the cells that produce progesterone. In this situation there is nothing wrong with the lining of the uterus itself, other than the fact that it has been poorly prepared for pregnancy.

## 947 How is an inadequate luteal phase diagnosed?

There are three diagnostic methods in practice now. Luteal phase inadequacy is often

# Hormone Levels During Menstrual Cycle

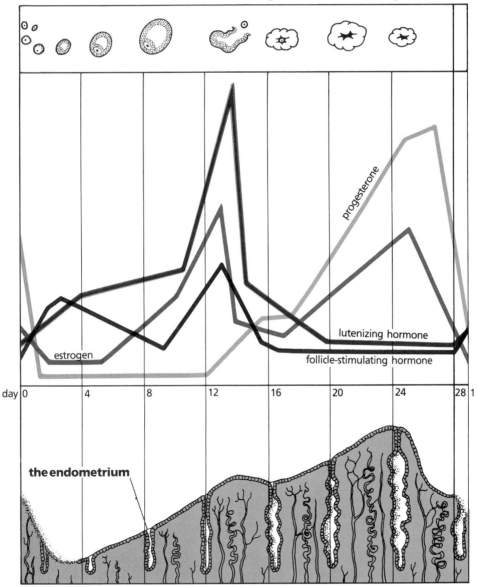

day 0     4     8     12     16     20     24     28 1

progesterone

lutenizing hormone

follicle-stimulating hormone

estrogen

the endometrium

diagnosed by the doctor after study of a woman's basal temperature chart. If her period starts ten days or less after ovulation, she probably has an inadequate luteal phase. If her temperature rises slowly or goes up and down during the time after ovulation, this can also indicate an inadequate luteal phase.

Inadequate luteal phase may also be diagnosed by having a laboratory blood test, which measures the amount of progesterone in the blood. This must be done daily for three or four days after ovulation. One problem with this is that doing it for only one month is not enough; it must be done for several months to reach a conclusive diagnosis. This is expensive, inconvenient, and primarily a research tool.

A third method of diagnosing an inadequate luteal phase is an endometrial biopsy. (See Q. 921, 922.) The lining of the uterus undergoes precise changes every day of a woman's cycle from ovulation until menstruation starts, usually on the twenty-eighth day. The lining has a corresponding precise appearance on each particular day after ovulation. If biopsy of a uterus is done on day twenty-three as determined by a temperature chart, but the tissue appears to be characteristic of day twenty-seven, there is an inadequate luteal phase. If the two are not within two days of each other, a luteal phase defect probably exists.

## 948 Since an endometrial biopsy is done after ovulation, will it cause me to have an abortion if I am already pregnant?

There are good studies that show that an endometrial biopsy usually does not interfere with early pregnancy, but this is always a possibility.

A great deal of information is gained from an endometrial biopsy done after ovulation that cannot be obtained any other way. Since it is usually performed on women who are infertile, there are few who would unknowingly be pregnant. Of these few who might be pregnant, the biopsy would have a slight chance of ending their pregnancy. Because the chance of hurting an early pregnancy is so slight, and the information gained is so helpful, almost all infertility specialists feel the procedure is necessary in certain situations. A couple may wish to use

contraceptives the month a biopsy is going to be done.

## 949 How is an inadequate luteal phase treated?

There are several different treatments. The most common is the use of clomiphene. Vaginal suppositories, which are inserted into the vagina if the body's temperature goes up at ovulation, may be prescribed. Some investigators have reported as much as 50–60 percent pregnancy rates in patients treated this way.

The disadvantage to using the progesterone suppositories is that they are expensive and messy. In addition, this medication may be difficult to obtain.

Other methods of treatment have not been used as widely and are not at this point felt to be as reliable as the suppositories. These include the use of bromocriptine (Parlodel), HCG, and Pergonal (See Q. 937, 938).

## 950 Are there other causes and treatments for irregular ovulation?

Yes. If the body is secreting too much prolactin, menstrual cycles become irregular and the breasts begin secreting fluid. The condition can become severe enough that a woman will not be having any menstrual periods (amenorrhea) and will be secreting a great deal of fluid from her breasts (galactorrhea). Parlodel (bromocriptine) is a drug that will usually decrease the amount of prolactin and enable ovulation to occur normally.

Prolactin is secreted from the pituitary gland, a small gland at the base of the brain. If the gland becomes overactive, it will release too much prolactin. Sometimes this occurs if there is a small tumor (pituitary adenoma) present in the pituitary gland.

Pituitary adenomas are the most common tumors in the human body, present in

# Endometrial Biopsy

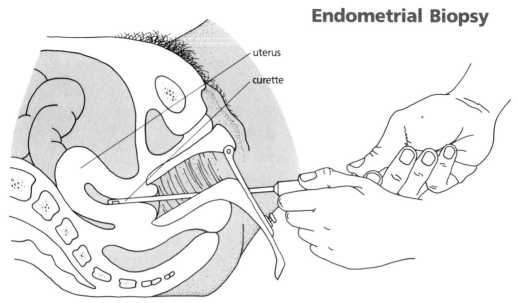

When an endometrial biopsy is performed, a small piece of tissue is scraped from the lining of the uterus and removed for miscroscopic evaluation.

30 percent of all people. Most of these are small and do not cause any problem. Until 1969, when a blood test was developed to find elevated levels of prolactin, there was not even a reasonable way to know that they existed.

If a blood test shows a high prolactin level, a second test, a CT scan (computer X-ray of tissue inside the body) of the pituitary, is needed to see if a tumor is present. If the CT scan shows that there is no tumor, the patient probably only has an overactive pituitary gland. In that situation, treatment with Parlodel usually (in 90 percent of the women) halts the excess production of prolactin, stops the breast secretions, allows normal periods to begin, and, for many, pregnancy occurs.

If the CT scan indicates a tumor, treatment is usually necessary, whether or not a woman is attempting to become pregnant. It can follow one of two directions. If the tumor is small, treating it with Parlodel is often successful. But if these tumors are large or do not respond to medication with Parlodel, surgical removal is usually necessary. Decisions concerning these problems and any surgery involved require consultation with specialists in endocrinology and neurosurgery.

Although high prolactin levels are not a common cause of infertility, most infertility specialists occasionally have a patient with this problem. I routinely do a prolactin level test on all infertility patients. Abnormal periods are a definite indication for such a test.

---

## 951 How is Parlodel taken, and are there any side effects?

Ordinarily Parlodel is taken in a dose of 2.5 mg, twice a day. This dose may be increased by your doctor if it seems necessary.

Occasionally women taking Parlodel may experience nausea, vomiting, diarrhea, or even faintness. These symptoms are usually of short duration, especially if the initial dose is only a small fraction of what is eventually used every day. The drug does not seem to cause severe reactions and has not been shown to cause any congenital abnormalities in children of women who take the drug. Of course, as soon as a woman knows that she is pregnant she should stop taking it.

## 952 Is Parlodel ever indicated if the prolactin level is normal?

For some infertility patients who have tried other treatments and have not become pregnant, a doctor will occasionally order Parlodel "empirically." This means that the drug is given even though there is no clear indication for its use. Physicians are finding that women sometimes become pregnant after they are started on Parlodel, even though they have tried unsuccessfully to achieve pregnancy for a long time. Parlodel is not a magic solution to infertility, but it can be tried.

## Endometriosis and Infertility

## 953 What is endometriosis, and how does it cause infertility?

Endometriosis is probably the most common cause of infertility in women over the age of twenty-five. It affects an estimated 25 percent of women over twenty-five, and it causes infertility in 25–30 percent of all women who cannot get pregnant. Fortunately it is usually treatable and is not difficult to diagnose.

Endometriosis is tissue like that which lines the inside of the uterus (the endometrium) that began growing in the wrong place in your body. During each menstrual period it is normal for some menstrual flow

to back up through the tubes and into the abdomen. This fluid contains live endometrial cells that will, in some women, attach and start growing where they do not belong: behind or in front of the uterus, on the ovaries or tubes, or on the intestines. This is endometriosis.

A problem then results because this tissue still acts as if it were inside your uterus and still responds to the same hormones as before. The tissue thickens up in response to the female hormones prior to ovulation. Then at menstruation time the tissue breaks down, producing bloody material just like the uterus does each month.

Bloody material released from endometrial tissue outside the uterus obviously cannot get back through the tubes and out the vagina. Instead it forms pockets of blood wherever it is growing. The irritation of this blood causes scarring to develop. This scar tissue damages the female organs and can even become severe enough to make a hysterectomy necessary.

Endometriosis can cause the buildup of enough scar tissue to create a blockage in the fallopian tubes and can scar ovaries and tubes so that it is difficult for the egg to get from the ovary to the tube, or envelope the ovaries so that an egg cannot get out.

Also, endometriosis apparently is the source of excessive production of hormones called prostaglandins. These prostaglandins may be released into the peritoneal fluid that bathes the internal organs and cause spasms of the uterus and tubes, inhibiting their ability to transport the egg properly. Prostaglandins can even affect the ovaries' ability to produce normal hormones or to release the egg normally. This may be how even mild endometriosis causes infertility.

## 954 How is endometriosis diagnosed?

A doctor usually discovers endometriosis when he or she does a fertility evaluation, but the only way the doctor can know conclusively that endometriosis is present is to do a laparoscopy.

I would strongly urge you not to let a doctor treat you for endometriosis based merely on what is found on an office pelvic exam, because the doctor's conclusions may be inaccurate.

I well remember a young woman I planned to operate on for bad menstrual cramps. I was going to cut the presacral nerve to stop her cramping. During a physical examination preceding that surgery, I felt nodules in her pelvis; I was certain that when I operated on her I would find that she had endometriosis. However, when I operated I was quite surprised. There was no endometriosis.

My point is that laparoscopy is essential to the diagnosis of endometriosis, so do not be treated without it.

---

## 955 Are there symptoms of endometriosis that I might notice myself?

Endometriosis sometimes, but not always, causes:

pain with menstrual periods

deep pain with intercourse

pain with bowel movements

pain in the center part of the lower abdomen

painful urination

blood in the urine and/or stools

spotting prior to periods

heavy periods

infertility

In the early stages and occasionally even with extensive endometriosis you may not have any of these problems. Endometriosis usually does not develop quickly, and it may take years to become widespread and for the condition and symptoms to worsen. If you know you have endometriosis and are interested in becoming pregnant in the future, you should be under the care of a doctor well versed in the care of endometriosis. The greatest risk is that you never know at what stage it will affect your fertility. You also never know when it will progress to the point that you can no longer have "fertility surgery" and will need a hysterectomy.

---

## 956 How is endometriosis treated?

For infertility patients treatment consists of either surgical removal of the endometriosis or the use of a drug called danazol (Danocrine). Because endometriosis can cause sterility, it is important that treatment not be withheld, particularly if you are over thirty years of age. If you are over thirty or are in a hurry to become pregnant, I recommend surgery over danazol because it is a more expedient and conclusive treatment.

If Danocrine is used, patients usually need to take it for six months to clear up the problem. Your chance of pregnancy after taking this drug is about the same as having surgery (75 percent in mild or moderate cases and up to 40 percent in more severe conditions). After taking danazol for six months, you may have to attempt pregnancy for a year before you could know whether your infertility had been reversed. If you did not become pregnant, you would need surgery. In this case you would have wasted more than a year of time. Younger patients have the luxury of all this time; older patients may not.

Before major surgery or danazol is considered, a laparoscopy is done to determine conclusively the presence of the disease. During the laparoscopy, if only minimal or moderate endometriosis is present, it can sometimes be cauterized or treated with laser. (See Q. 908.)

If your doctor finds endometriosis that cannot be treated with laser laparoscopy, he or she may want to go ahead with major surgery, but this should be done only if you agreed to this prior to the laparoscopy. I usually do a laparoscopy in an outpatient operating facility. A few days later, when the patient is feeling alert and well, I meet with her and her husband in my office. At that point we discuss the laparoscopy results, the treatment called for, and the chances of fertility resulting from that treatment. I prefer this to proceeding with major surgery immediately after laparoscopy, since the patient is still asleep and cannot participate in decisions about her therapy.

If you choose to have your endometriosis treated surgically, be sure that it is done by a doctor skilled in fertility surgery. It is much easier to do a hysterectomy than carefully excising endometriosis so that a patient's fertility is restored. Some general surgeons are especially prone to do hysterectomies. So are some gynecologists who are not interested in spending the tedious time it takes to cut out or laser each little spot of endometriosis. Be sure you have a competent and willing gynecologist and that you do not give permission for a hysterectomy to be done at that point: unless your doctor explains beforehand why it will probably be necessary.

## 957 How is endometriosis treated surgically?

The operation requires an incision like that used for a hysterectomy (either "bikini" or up-and-down). Time in the hospital after surgery is usually four to six days, followed by a two-week recovery period at home.

The concept behind such surgery is fairly simple, but the surgery is not. The doctor cuts out, or vaporizes with the laser, every bit of endometriosis to be found. If it requires cutting an ovary open, the gynecologist does that. If he or she can leave one ovary and tube fairly normal, the other ovary and tube may be taken out if they are badly scarred.

Also, if the uterus is retroverted or leaning back, the surgeon suspends it (sews it forward). The laser may be employed to remove hard-to-reach areas of endometriosis.

If the doctor is of my school of thought, he or she will also do a presacral neurectomy. This involves cutting the network of nerves from the uterus, tubes, and ovaries, hoping to further relieve any residual spasm of the uterus or tubes and make it easier for the egg to get down the tube. Cutting these nerve fibers can also help alleviate the cramps that so often accompany endometriosis, but it does not affect sexual responsiveness or feeling. If you become pregnant after a presacral neurectomy, however, you will usually not feel labor pains as strongly as normal.

It is sometimes necessary to remove part of the colon or part of the bladder in order to get all the endometriosis. This in no way affects your ability to urinate or have bowel movements after recovery from the surgery. The idea is to remove every spot of severe endometriosis present.

## 958 How effective is this surgery?

The chance of pregnancy following this type of surgery depends on how advanced and extensive the endometriosis was. If it was not too bad, there is a 75-percent chance of getting pregnant. If, however, the endometriosis was fairly severe, the chances decrease to 40 percent or less.

The severity of endometriosis is classified from Stage I to Stage IV. If your doctor finds that you have endometriosis, you should ask what stage your disease is in. This will help you understand your situation and more intelligently participate in treatment decisions.

## 959 Can endometriosis keep coming back?

Doctors can never be sure that all endometriosis has been removed. Some can be left in areas of scar tissue, and there can be microscopic implants that are impossible to see at surgery. There is always, therefore, the possibility of endometriosis growing back. Approximately 13 percent of patients who have had surgery for endometriosis will require a second surgery. Only a small percentage will require a third operation.

When a patient has had endometriosis surgery and still does not become pregnant, a repeat laparoscopy should be done to see if she has recurrent endometriosis. A laser laparoscope might then be used to get rid of any endometriosis still present.

## 960 Can endometriosis occur in the uterus itself?

Yes, it can. When endometriosis exists in the muscular wall of the uterus, it is called adenomyosis. When that occurs, it is as though the lining of the uterus has developed roots that have gotten cut off from the surface endometriosis. These areas of endometriosis then grow, bleed, and form a scar in the wall of the uterus. This causes the uterus to be irritable, resulting in infertility.

Unfortunately the diagnosis for adenomyosis is difficult and not reliable. However, the following pattern often suggests the presence of the disease. An infertile patient, who has been totally "worked up," including laparoscopy, and treated for whatever problems were found, still does not become pregnant. Months later, at a second laparoscopy, there is some suggestion that her uterus is more boggy and vascular, perhaps slightly larger than a normal uterus. Only then is adenomyosis suspected.

The only treatment for this disease for the woman trying to achieve pregnancy is

danazol, given in a dosage of 200 mg, three or four times a day for three to six months. If adenomyosis was actually the cause of her infertility, the woman may then be able to achieve pregnancy following the treatment.

## 961 If all the preceding avenues of evaluation and treatment are exhausted, what means remain for having a child?

There are three topics yet to be covered in this chapter. All of them are pertinent to our discussion of infertility and all are of interest to those couples who want to pursue every means available to have a child.

These three topics are artificial insemination (by husband and donor sperm), in vitro fertilization (test-tube babies), and adoption.

## Artificial Insemination

## 962 What is artificial insemination?

Artificial insemination involves the injection of sperm into the vagina or uterus by artificial means rather than by normal intercourse. There are three types of artificial insemination: AIH, insemination with the husband's semen, AID, insemination with a donor's semen; and IUI, insemination with semen (either husband's or donor's) that has been "washed" so that sperm can be put directly into the uterus (intrauterine insemination). (See Q. 973.)

The technique of insemination by AID or AIH is simple. The man collects the semen by masturbating into a clean container which does not need to be sterile. The specimen is brought to the doctor's office for insertion into the woman's vagina. If AID is

## Artificial Insemination

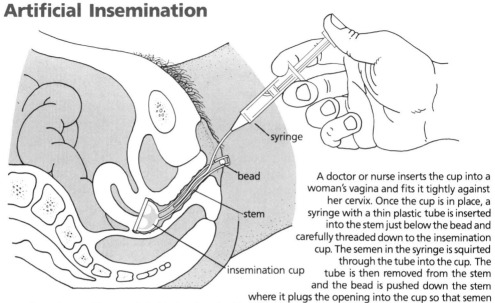

syringe

bead

stem

insemination cup

A doctor or nurse inserts the cup into a woman's vagina and fits it tightly against her cervix. Once the cup is in place, a syringe with a thin plastic tube is inserted into the stem just below the bead and carefully threaded down to the insemination cup. The semen in the syringe is squirted through the tube into the cup. The tube is then removed from the stem and the bead is pushed down the stem where it plugs the opening into the cup so that semen cannot escape from the cup. The stem is twisted and pushed back into the vagina. The sperm swim out of the semen and into the woman's cervical mucus as would occur with normal intercourse. After approximately four hours, the woman herself removes the cup.

used, the specimen is from an anonymous donor or through a sperm bank.

The doctor places a special plastic cup, with a tube on one side, over the cervix. The collected semen is squirted through the tube and into the cup. A small plastic bead is used to plug the tube to keep the semen from escaping.

The cervical cup keeps the semen at the cervical opening and allows the sperm to swim into the cervical mucus and then into the uterus. Inseminations can be done without the cup, but most doctors prefer to use it.

Though insemination is a simple procedure, it will help very little if other causes for infertility exist. For this reason all other factors should be ruled out first.

---

**963** **For what reason is artificial insemination with the husband's semen used.**

The most common reason for trying AIH is that the husband has a low sperm count,

although intrauterine insemination seems to be replacing AIH for this problem, because IUI is much more effective. (See Q. 973.)

AIH is helpful in other situations too. Some men, for example, are unable to develop or maintain an erection, or a man may have an abnormal opening in his penis which causes the semen to exit at the base of the penis. Other men have had a prostate operation which causes the semen to squirt back into the bladder upon ejaculation instead of out of the penis. In situations like these, AIH enables the doctor to place the semen in the vagina so that conception may take place.

In the case of the last example, semen is obtained by inserting a catheter through the man's penis into his bladder to recover the semen after he masturbates. Another technique is for the man, after masturbation, to strain down as with urination and at the same time push on his low abdomen with his fingers in order to "push" the semen out of the bladder. Before masturbating for either of these techniques the man must empty his bladder of urine. Intrauterine insemination (IUI) will probably prove to be more effective than AIH in this situation.

If the husband's sperm count is low, the doctor will probably instruct your husband to collect only the first part of his ejaculate for either AIH or IUI, because the first part of the ejaculate usually contains the greatest concentration of sperm.

Occasionally, however, the last part of the ejaculate will contain more sperm. Through tests done on the sperm, a doctor can determine which portion of the ejaculate is best in an individual case.

## 964    How effective is AIH?

Results with this technique are variable. Some people report as high as a 20 percent pregnancy rate with AIH, obviously a fairly low percentage. If the husband's sperm are poor, there ordinarily is a better chance for pregnancy to occur if his sperm problem can be corrected, or if intrauterine insemination is used, rather than using his sperm for AIH.

There is no "magic" with AIH. The husband usually would deliver the sperm to your cervix a lot better the natural way, through intercourse. This is one of the reasons why IUI is rapidly replacing AIH.

## 965    Wouldn't it be better if the doctor squirted some of the semen directly into the uterus rather than into my vagina?

This would seem like a good idea, but what your husband passes when he ejaculates is mostly mucus. When all the sperm from his ejaculate are concentrated, they amount to no more than just a small pellet of tissue. If the ejaculate were drawn into a syringe and squirted into your uterus, most of what would go into the uterus would be mucus.

Furthermore, this mucus can cause a reaction in the uterus that can produce terrible cramps, or in some cases a generalized body response, including feeling ill and fainting.

In the past, doctors would try putting a small amount of semen into the uterus at the time of insemination in an attempt to bypass bad cervical mucus. Again, because of the problems with the injection of semen into the uterus, including the low pregnancy rate, intrauterine insemination has been recently developed as a more effective technique. (See Q. 973.)

## 966    Why can't my husband's sperm be concentrated by freezing many of his specimens and then taking the live sperm from them?

This technique has been tried and has not been useful. When a specimen with low sperm count is frozen, many of the already-limited number of sperm are killed, thus making it impractical to improve chances of pregnancy.

## 967    When is artificial insemination with donor sperm used?

Donor insemination (AID) is useful if a husband has no sperm, because of birth defect, disease, injury, or previous sterilization; if he has an extremely low sperm count; if he has a genetic disease he does not want to pass on to a child; or if insemination or intercourse with his "abnormal" sperm do not result in pregnancy.

In addition, if a woman has Rh-negative blood which has resulted in previous stillbirths, she could be inseminated by an Rh-negative donor, thus bypassing the Rh problem. This is rarely necessary today because of the use of Rho-Gam. (See Q. 536.)

## 968 What are some of the objections to the use of (AID)?

There are negative arguments to having artificial insemination using donor sperm (AID). Many religious faiths oppose this type of conception.

Many husbands feel that having their wives inseminated by another man's sperm is a reflection on their own virility, or they do not like the idea of their wives being pregnant "by another man." Some people will not consider AID because they feel it is "unnatural."

Many couples are now rejecting AID because of the fear of transmitting the AIDS virus from donor to patient. The technique for freezing semen, holding it for six months, and then testing the donor again for AIDS before using the semen has decreased the possibility of AIDS transmission via AID. But this technique is not completely reliable and therefore I have stopped doing donor inseminations in my office. Another infection is also of great concern: cytomegalo virus (CMV) that can cause a baby to be badly deformed when it is born.

I believe that no couple should consider donor insemination unless both parties feel totally confident that it is what they want.

## 969 For what reasons do you consider AID a good idea?

Without AID many couples would not be able to have a baby. Second, if AID is used to achieve pregnancy, as opposed to adoption, the baby gets at least half of its genetic make-up from one of the parents. Third, many women seem to prefer carrying and delivering their own babies.

## 970 Does AID always work?

No. Donor inseminations produce pregnancies in only about 70 percent of the women on whom they are used. Those who are under the age of thirty are a little more likely to achieve pregnancy by inseminations (about 75 percent) and women who are over the age of thirty are a little less likely to become pregnant with AID (50–60 percent.)

## 971 Do all doctors do inseminations using donors?

No. Many physicians are now greatly concerned about passing AIDS or other infections to their patients. Even with extreme care, this is a real possibility. In addition, enlisting a large enough group of men to obtain a choice of donors for patients is a time-consuming task. While frozen semen from a commercial sperm bank can be used, this requires that a doctor have a liquid nitrogen tank in which to keep the frozen semen after it arrives in the office. This is not only a lot of trouble but is moderately expensive. Also, many doctors find the frozen semen produces pregnancies less often than fresh semen.

An AID program requires a doctor who is willing to take the time to pick and choose among men who are eligible sperm donors to make sure that the donors are men who are considerate, thoughtful, reliable, in good health, and without history of genetic disease, or it requires a doctor who will go to the trouble and expense of handling frozen semen.

## 972 Are there legal problems with AID?

The legal status of donor inseminations has not been totally settled by the courts. It is agreed that a husband who consents to his wife's being inseminated by a donor is legally that child's father from then on. Currently, the legal problems resulting from the transmission of viruses and diseases via AID have not been addressed.

## 973 What is intrauterine insemination, and why is it used?

Intrauterine insemination (IUI) is a relatively new technique for the treatment of infertility. This procedure involves the insertion of washed sperm (from husband or donor) directly into a woman's uterus. How likely it is that a woman will become pregnant with this technique is not yet known, but many women who had not conceived with other procedures have become pregnant with IUI. Although there may be other reasons found for the use of IUI in the future, many physicians now are trying IUI for the following problems.

Husband has a low sperm count, poor sperm motility, small volume of semen, excessive volume of semen, or semen that is too sticky.

Wife has cervical mucus in which sperm are not surviving: "bad" Sims-Huhner test. (See Q. 906, 917.)

Pregnancy is not resulting when there is no obvious cause for infertility, or when the cause for infertility seems to be corrected but pregnancy does not occur, as when a woman is taking clomiphene and having regular ovulation but without subsequent pregnancy.

Husband has retrograde ejaculation. (See Q. 963.)

## 974 How is IUI done?

The semen is allowed to liquefy or is drawn back and forth through a needle to make it liquefy.

The semen is then mixed in a test tube with some tissue culture media, a liquid that is normally used to grow human or animal tissues in the laboratory. This fluid is spun on a centrifuge. Since the sperm are heavier than the other contents of this mixture, they go to the bottom of the tube. The fluid on top of the sperm is suctioned off and discarded, and more tissue culture fluid is put on top of the sperm. The contents are mixed up again and the process repeated.

A small amount of tissue culture media is then added to the now well-washed sperm, and the tube is shaken.

This solution, which now contains all the sperm, is gently squirted directly into the woman's uterus. The uterus does not react to the tissue-culture media and washed-sperm mixture in the negative way it reacts to semen, although some women will have mild cramping with IUI.

I normally do this procedure two times each month, as close to the time of ovulation as possible. The actual insemination is a simple procedure, both for the doctor and for the patient. It usually causes no more discomfort than a regular pelvic exam, although it does take time to allow for washing of the sperm.

Positive aspects of the procedure, other than the fact that it does not hurt, are that as far as we can tell now there are few complications, and patients for whom there was "nothing left to try" are now getting pregnant using IUI.

## In Vitro Fertilization

## 975 What about test-tube babies?

In vitro fertilization–embryo replacement (IVF-ER) is the procedure of last resort for certain infertile couples. There are good reasons for this being a final choice. A major reason is that in spite of intense and time-consuming medical therapy, the pregnancy rate is fairly low: about 25 percent.

Another negative factor associated with in vitro fertilization is the expense. It costs several thousand dollars a month for the procedure, and medical insurance usually pays only a part of the bill.

Additionally, the procedure requires injections, blood tests, ultrasounds, and a laparoscopy every month. In spite of all this, IVF-ER is now a standard technique for the treatment of infertility. I believe every woman who is not getting pregnant by using other techniques and whose problem might respond to IVF-ER should consider taking advantage of this procedure.

## 976    How is in vitro fertilization accomplished?

The procedure is theoretically fairly simple. It has been found that a woman who has IVF done is more likely to become pregnant if she can have three embryos put into her uterus with IVF-ER. Normally a woman's ovaries produce only one egg a month. To make her ovaries develop more than one egg in a given month, an IVF patient receives Pergonal or a combination of clomiphene and Pergonal, starting soon after her period begins. These drugs are given daily until the ovaries contain two, three, or more healthy appearing follicles (cysts).

When the follicles have developed properly, as measured by repeated ultrasound observations and repeated blood estrogen tests, each one of them usually contains a healthy egg. When these eggs seem to be at maturity and just before the body ovulates on its own, a laparoscopy is done. At laparoscopy the doctor inserts a needle into each follicle separately, applies suction, and draws the follicular fluid with its egg out of the ovary and into a separate container for each egg.

After a period of time varying from a few minutes to a few hours, a solution containing sperm is placed with each egg in its dish. Fertilization occurs in those dishes. The doctors can tell the next morning if the eggs have been fertilized.

After the embryos (the eggs that are fertilized) have grown for two or three days, they are drawn into a thin plastic tube. A speculum is put in the woman's vagina, just as with a pelvic exam, and the tube with the embryos is painlessly inserted through the cervix into the uterus. The embryos are gently pushed into the cavity of the uterus.

If the embryos stay in the uterus and continue their growth, pregnancy is established and nine months later a baby (or babies) is born. Even though more than one embryo

## In Vitro Fertilization and Embryo Transfer

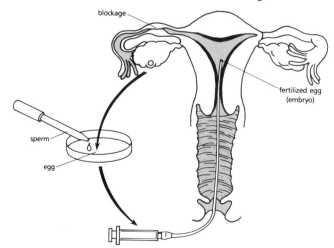

# Development of Egg in the Uterus

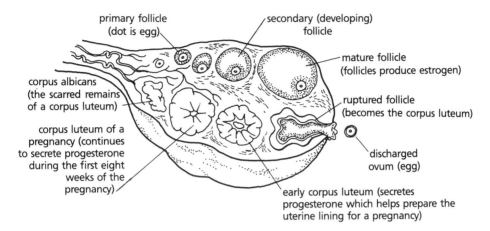

primary follicle (dot is egg)

secondary (developing) follicle

mature follicle (follicles produce estrogen)

corpus albicans (the scarred remains of a corpus luteum)

ruptured follicle (becomes the corpus luteum)

corpus luteum of a pregnancy (continues to secrete progesterone during the first eight weeks of the pregnancy)

discharged ovum (egg)

early corpus luteum (secretes progesterone which helps prepare the uterine lining for a pregnancy)

may be placed in the uterus, all of them do not usually survive.

If pregnancy does not occur, and it does only about 25 percent of the time even when living embryos are put back into the uterus, the woman can repeat the process. Because of the expense and anxiety associated with the procedure, most couples wait a few months before trying again. They can, however, try as many times as they want to.

---

## 977 When should in vitro fertilization be considered?

There are several problems of infertility for which in vitro fertilization is especially useful. It can be used if a woman's fallopian tubes are irrevocably blocked or destroyed. If the tubes are simply blocked, a greater chance of pregnancy might be obtained by her undergoing microsurgery to open them than by her having in vitro fertilization. However, a woman who has had surgery done to open her tubes but has not become pregnant would be a candidate for having in vitro fertilization.

Other situations that might warrant this procedure are unsuccessfully treated endometriosis, infertility of unknown cause, or infertility due to a husband's poor sperm count since his few sperm can be put directly on the eggs.

For in vitro fertilization to be possible using the technique generally followed at this time, the ovaries must be visible at laparoscopy. This is necessary because the follicles that develop the eggs must be seen in order for the doctor to insert a needle into a follicle to draw out an egg.

A technique in which a needle is inserted through the abdominal skin or through the vagina into the follicles, using ultrasound guidance, may make it possible to retrieve eggs from ovaries so encased in scar that they cannot be seen at laparoscopy. Eventually this procedure could become more commonly used than the laparoscopy technique because it is less complicated and less expensive.

A couple should not consider in vitro fertilization unless both are enthusiastically in favor of it, since the emotional and financial drain is great.

---

## 978 What objections are there to the use of in vitro fertilization?

Many objections have been voiced against

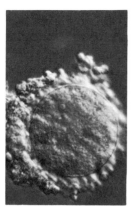
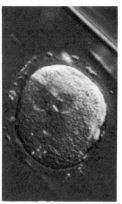
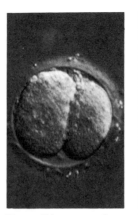
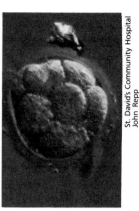

Immature egg, as viewed through microscope

Egg in pronuclear stage (soon after fertilization)

Two-cell human embryo, about twenty-four hours after fertilization

Eight-cell human embryo, about thirty-six to forty hours after fertilization, ready for transfer to uterus

so-called test tube babies. Some of these are based on personal feelings that the procedure is "unnatural" or on religious beliefs ("men playing God"). Other people are afraid, and rightly so, that in vitro fertilization in the wrong hands might be used in an unethical fashion (selective breeding or unwarranted destruction of embryos).

I feel that there are many technical procedures that humans c n use either maliciously or beneficially, and this particular procedure is in that category. It is obvious that this technique can be mishandled and misused, but it also offers the wonderful benefit of pregnancy to women who do not otherwise have a chance of achieving pregnancy.

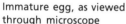

**979** What techniques, other than the traditional in vitro fertilization procedures, are being developed and used to achieve pregnancy?

Three methods of achieving pregnancy that go beyond the regular IVF techniques are:

*Frozen embryos.* Unused embryos are frozen and "banked" for use in subsequent months if pregnancy is not achieved initially.

*Embryo transfers.* Embryos conceived in one woman are "washed out" of her uterus and transplanted into the uterus of an infertile woman.

*Surrogate mothers.* A woman will contract with a couple to bear and deliver their child, which is conceived either by embryo transfer from the woman or by insemination of the surrogate's egg with the man's sperm.

*GIFT procedure.* A recent adaption of IVF is a procedure called gamete intrafallopian transfer (GIFT). This procedure, in most programs, is limited to women with one or two normal fallopian tubes. GIFT is done exactly like IVF through the point at which the eggs have been removed from the woman's ovaries. Instead of being allowed to wake from anesthesia at this point, however, the woman is kept asleep for a short additional time. While she remains on the operating table, eggs and sperm are drawn into a thin plastic tube. This tube is brought into the operating room and inserted through the incision made for the needle that was used to retrieve the eggs. The tip of this plastic tube is threaded into one of the fallopian tubes and eggs and sperm are squirted into the fallopian tube. The procedure is repeated with the other fallopian tube. The instruments are removed and the incision is closed. The woman is allowed to wake up and go home, hopefully to become pregnant. No other treatment is necessary, except perhaps the use of progesterone shots or progesterone vaginal suppositories until she knows whether or not she is pregnant. With GIFT, pregnancy occurs spontaneously in the woman's fallopian tube, the place where pregnancy normally occurs. The embryos then pass into the uterus where in the normal fashion they either become a growing pregnancy or pass on out as a very early miscarriage. Preliminary studies indicate a 30-percent pregnancy rate with this procedure. It is somewhat less expensive and less time-consuming than IVF.

## 980  How are frozen embryos used?

During the in vitro fertilization procedure, it is often possible to grow more than three embryos. In our in vitro fertilization program we often have six or more embryos develop from a woman's eggs. Although a woman has a greater chance of achieving pregnancy when three or four embryos are put back in her uterus, the chances do not increase if more than four embryos are transferred.

It seems reasonable to freeze the extra embryos so that if the woman does not get pregnant with the initial IVF, the extra embryos can be thawed and transferred back into her uterus at the appropriate time for pregnancy the next month. This would allow the woman to have two (or perhaps more) embryo transfers into her uterus with only one laparoscopy procedure to secure the eggs.

## 981  What problems are associated with the transfer of frozen embryos?

There is a major technical problem with this procedure today. In spite of the fact that several centers around the world are attempting this procedure and actually transferring frozen embryos back into women, only a few pregnancies have occurred. No doubt this problem will be solved in the future.

Another problem involved is a moral one. The availability of this procedure raises moral dilemmas of deciding what to do with the extra embryos if pregnancy is achieved on the first attempt, or if the embryos are not needed because of ill health or death of the mother. A widely publicized example of this situation is the Australian couple who died before their frozen embryos were used. The American Fertility Society presently recommends that frozen embryo procedures be restricted to research programs.

## 982  What is an embryo transfer?

The term *embryo transfer* describes the moving of a live embryo from the uterus of one woman to that of another. In 1984 this technique was used to produce several pregnancies in infertile women. Steps in the procedure are:

A fertile woman (the egg donor) is inseminated with the semen of an infertile woman's husband.

After five days, the inseminated woman's uterus is flushed out daily for three days, or until an embryo is found.

If and when an embryo is flushed out, it is transferred to the uterus of the infertile wife, who then carries the pregnancy produced by the other woman's egg and her husband's sperm.

## 983  What problems are associated with the embryo transfer technique?

A major moral problem with this procedure arises when the fertile woman (egg donor) becomes pregnant from the insemination and the embryo does not flush out. She must decide to have an abortion or continue the pregnancy. The corporation (Fertility and Genetics Research, Inc.) which applied for a patent on this procedure requires their egg donors to agree to have an abortion if the embryo does not flush out. The term *menstrual extraction* used in their publications and newspaper interviews is merely an early abortion.

An additional problem with embryo transfer is that the flushing itself can kill an embryo.

## 984 What is a surrogate mother?

A surrogate mother, one who carries and delivers a child for someone else, has been used in these situations.

If a wife has no uterus, tubes, or ovaries, she cannot become pregnant. Her husband's sperm can be used to impregnate a woman who will carry the child. When the baby is born, the couple adopts the baby from the surrogate mother.

If a women has no uterus but does have ovaries, her eggs can be collected by the in vitro fertilization procedure and fertilized by her husband's sperm. The embryos that result can be transferred to a woman who is able to carry the pregnancy. After the child is delivered, the surrogate mother releases it, through adoption, to its "real" parents.

## 985 What problems may result from using surrogate mothers?

A major problem that may develop from the use of a surrogate mother is the possibility that she could become pregnant by her own husband or another man. In 1984 a widely publicized situation occurred when the surrogate mother delivered a child with congenital abnormalities. Subsequent testing proved that it was her husband's child and not that of the couple who had hired her to be a surrogate mother.

Another problem that may surface with surrogate pregnancy is that by the time a woman has carried a child to term and given birth, she has usually developed an emotional bond with that child. A recent widely publicized court case graphically demonstrated the problems caused by the emotional ties of a mother to the baby she has been carrying.

## 986 How do you feel about the use of these three techniques to achieve pregnancy?

It is my personal commitment to do all I can, within my ethical and moral limits, to aid infertile couples in achieving pregnancy. In the process I remind myself and the couple that there is a higher goal in life—the dignity of the individual, the preservation of the family as a unit ordained by God, and the maintainance of healthy relationships between the members in those families. Regardless of the intensity of their desire to have a child, I believe infertile couples must not and should not be coerced into using any technique they cannot wholeheartedly accept. Nor should a doctor engage in procedures which violate his or her ethical or moral beliefs.

## Adoption

## 987 Do some couples who come to you with a fertility problem decide to forego infertility evaluation and treatment and try to adopt a child?

Yes. I believe no one should go through infertility evaluation and treatment who does not want to.

Many couples do not want to expend the time and money, or go through the frustration and inconvenience, involved in the evaluation. For those couples adoption is the answer to their childlessness, unless they find themselves achieving pregnancy before the adoption process is complete.

## 988 How long should we persist in infertility treatment before we "give up" and consider adoption?

My general recommendation is this: after you have had a full evaluation and have had a year of treatment without becoming pregnant, you should consider starting the adoption process.

I encourage you to continue trying to become pregnant, however, because the adoption process often requires two or more years of waiting before a child actually arrives in your home. It is possible that during this time you could become pregnant.

Adoption agencies generally do not mind if you continue your attempts to become pregnant while working with them on an adoption. If you become pregnant, you can always cancel the adoption process.

Trying to adopt a child has an additional advantage if you have been unsuccessfully trying to become pregnant for quite some time. It can be a pressure-relief valve for you and your husband, even while you continue your infertility treatments, because you will know that one way or the other, at the end of two years, you should have your new baby.

A doctor can be of great help, not only in working out a plan for your infertility evaluation and treatment, but also helping with the adoption process. The three of you should keep talking as you proceed through every step of the fertility evaluation and as you consider adoption.

## 989 We don't want to adopt a baby. Is that abnormal?

It is quite normal not to want to adopt a baby, and many couples feel this way. Just as no couple should undergo an infertility workup unless they want to, no one should adopt a child who does not want to.

If you feel that you cannot, without reservation, accept an adopted child as your own, it would be foolish to adopt. It would not be good for you or the child and might result in more anguish than being childless. I also believe, for the same reason, that one mate should not push the other into adopting if he or she has any reservations.

## 990 How do we begin the adoption process?

It is best to contact adoption agencies in your area, but not necessarily in your local community. Most agencies have a waiting period before they will even take an application.

You should find out which agencies have specific rules about age, religion, race, and so on that would prevent your getting a baby from them.

It is often helpful to communicate regularly with an agency, so that they know you are sincerely interested in adopting. Call them, write them, and have your doctor write them. Don't be overbearing, insistent, or impatient. Gentleness and persistence are essential. Perhaps it would encourage you to know that most of my infertility patients who do not become pregnant are eventually able to adopt a baby.

## 991 How much does an adoption cost?

The cost of adopting a baby varies, but it can range from $5,000 to $20,000.

## 992 Is it possible to adopt a baby through a doctor or lawyer?

When adoptions are carried out through an agency, there is little risk of you ever being forced to return the baby to the natural mother. Although a judge cannot usually reverse the adoption except on certain specific grounds, such as the biologic mother having given up the child because of fraud or coercion, it can happen.

About 75 percent of adoptions are conducted through agencies. This is primarily because most pregnant women will go to an adoption agency, rather than to a doctor or a lawyer, when they want to give up their baby. Also, private adoptions are illegal in some states and limited in others.

If you are unable to get a baby through an agency, however, you might try the private route.

---

## 993 What about adopting foreign, minority, impaired, or older children?

These are specialized situations, each entailing specific problems.

Foreign adoptions are possible, but they involve many delays and obstacles. There are American agencies that specialize in foreign adoptions. You can get their names and addresses by writing the Children's Bureau of the United States Department of Health & Human Services, P.O. Box 1182, Washington, D.C. 20013. One organization specializing in foreign adoptions is Los Ninos (1106 Radam Circle, Austin, Texas 78745; phone (512) 443-2833).

If you are interested in adopting minority, biracial, impaired, or older children, you might contact orphanages in your area or your local child-and-family service organization.

One word of advice: be sure to get adequate counsel about problems you might face in the future as a result of such an adoption. By the way, all states except Hawaii have subsidy programs for parents who adopt hard-to-place children.

---

## 994 Is it possible for me to breast-feed an adopted baby?

It is possible! In fact, 50 percent of women can, at least partially, nurse their adopted babies. Before they receive their adopted baby, however, they need to get their breasts started producing milk. One technique is as follows: a woman starts taking 25 mg of chlorpromazine three times a day and vigorously stimulates her nipples about every one to three hours. She needs to do this for several weeks before the baby arrives.

Obviously a woman who does this must be dedicated to it, and know that 50 percent of the time all her dedication is not going to produce milk. Even when it does, the mother will usually not produce enough milk to provide all the nutrition a baby needs. Most of the time a mother must give her baby supplemental feedings or find a wet nurse: another woman whose milk production is still present after having had her own child. The LaLeche League, International (9616 Minneapolis Ave., Franklin Park, Illinois 60131; Phone: 312-455-7730) can be of great help and encouragement in this endeavor.

---

## Emotional Support for the Infertile Couple

---

## 995 Why are my husband's and my own emotions running so out of hand as we consider and work on our infertility?

As stated in the introduction to this chapter, I believe that few stronger stresses come into a marriage than the continued absence of a longed-for child.

Often a couple with an infertility problem needs counsel. If you and your husband are frustrated, tell your doctor. If it seems wise he or she will help you find a counselor who will be able to help you. Counselors have a good success rate in helping people who basically have everything together but are grappling with a single problem.

The biggest danger is for you or your husband to deny that you are upset by your current problem. Every couple who confronts a period of infertility is upset to some degree. Infertility wends its way into every part of your life: your schedule, your intimacy with each other, your finances, your comfort, and your social life.

It is normal for you to "hate" Mother's Day and your cousin who just told you she was pregnant, and to resent it when your friends ask when you are going to "decide" to have a baby.

All this is normal. The danger lies in denying these emotions. Talk about your feelings with your doctor, your pastor, a close friend, and see a psychologist or psychiatrist when the pressures are too heavy.

**996** **Are there organizations that might give me emotional support during this time of infertility?**

There are several. One is an extremely warm and helpful Christian group that publishes a newsletter. They can be reached at the following address:

Stepping Stones
2900 N. Rock Rd.
Wichita, KS 67226

Resolve, Inc. is a lay organization with many chapters throughout the United States. The national office is very helpful in providing information about infertility.

Resolve, Inc.
P.O. Box 474
Belmont, MA 02178-0474
(617) 643-2424

Another organization is in the Los Angeles area. It provides counseling, referral, and support:

Infertility Resources, Inc.
527 Eighteenth Street
Santa Monica, CA 90402

This group has a catalog of sympathy and announcement cards for miscarriages and stillbirths, booklets to help siblings and grandparents deal with their feelings, booklets on what family and friends can do, scrapbooks to preserve memories of a lost baby, and burial cradles for miscarried babies. Their newsletter includes articles, letters, and stories for those who have lost babies and lists current services offered (referrals to support groups, funeral directors, speakers, pen pals, literature, helpline, and telephone volunteers).

Loving Arms
1415 East Wayzata Blvd.
Suite 22
Wayzata, MN 55391

A national organization of physicians interested in fertility problems includes both gynecologists and urologists, and it is a good source for names of physicians with this interest:

American Fertility Society
1608 13th Avenue, South, Suite 101
Birmingham, AL 35205

This newly formed organization has a very informative newsletter and a registry of physicians that provide infertility care:

Young Couples International
216 Calhoon St.
Charleston, SC 29401

**997** **Are there periodicals that are helpful to infertile couples?**

Yes. Currently there are at least three newsletters, published by Stepping Stones, Young Couples International, and Resolve, Inc. The addresses for these organizations are given in Q. 996.

**998** **What is the future of infertility treatment?**

The possibilities in the area of infertility are barely tapped. I have been telling patients for a long time that there are hundreds of things controlling fertility that we don't even know exist and therefore cannot begin to treat.

## An Afterword

We are learning more about infertility all the time. The use of the laser in infertility surgery, in vitro fertilization, greater knowledge about the hormones controlling reproduction—all these are exciting advances, and they herald real hope for infertility patients in the future.

The fact that these techniques are possible does not eliminate the validity of the feelings and emotions that are a part of life itself. Human beings are not meant to go through life as pawns of science, and the ultimate goal of life is not achievement of pregnancy and parenthood.

As future procedures for the solution of infertility come along, it is most important to evaluate them carefully before accepting or becoming involved with them.

# 12

# Birth Control—Temporary and Permanent

The same Bible that tells us in Psalm 127 that children are a gift from God (Ps. 127:3) also speaks of the responsibilities of parenting:

If anyone does not provide for his relatives, and especially for his own family, he has disowned the faith and is worse than an unbeliever (1 Tim. 5:8, RSV).

It is pleasant to have children (most of the time!), and there are many rewards in seeing them grow and mature and become individuals in their own right. With every privilege, however, comes responsibility, and there is an enormous responsibility in having children. A husband and wife must be willing and able to care for the children that they decide to have.

There are many factors to be considered in family planning. During a time when husband and wife are extremely busy, it may be best for them to delay pregnancy. If a husband and wife need time to get their own relationship straightened out, it is often best to postpone temporarily the extra stress of a newborn child. Economic factors influence almost every couple that is thinking about getting pregnant. There may be numerous other factors for prospective parents to consider as they plan their family, but often the final decision about when to have, or when not to have a child is as much emotional as intellectual.

Contraception allows a husband and wife to plan for the children they want to have. It allows having the "right" number of children and permits them to time the arrival of those children so that the family is well prepared for them.

Contraception is a double-edged sword, however. It can allow the delay of a family until it is no longer possible for the couple to conceive. It can also make it convenient for a couple to delay starting a family until they eventually feel too old to do so, thus cheating themselves out of one of the most significant blessings life has to offer.

Because there are such effective methods of contraception available, I feel that it is vital that couples be educated about them. Since God has given us minds capable of reason, with proper thought we can decide how to use our sexuality, how to use contraception, and how to plan our families.

Each of us should let God work in our minds and actions, so that the ultimate result is God's will for us as individuals and as families.

## Choosing a Birth-Control Method

### 999 What is the common goal of all methods of contraception?

The goal of contraceptives is to keep the sperm from meeting and fertilizing the egg. Birth-control pills, for instance, accomplish this by preventing the ovary from releasing an egg; vasectomies serve the same purpose by preventing a man's sperm from passing out of his testicles into his ejaculate.

Since the definition of contraception found in Webster's New Collegiate Dictionary is "voluntary prevention of conception or impregnation," we will not and should not discuss abortion as a technique for contraception. If an unwanted pregnancy oc-

curs, contraception either failed or was not used. When pregnancy occurs, a totally different set of considerations is called for. (See Q. 223–236.)

### 1000 What should be considered when a couple is deciding on a birth-control method?

Many things must be considered in choosing a method of birth control, some of which are:

*Family size.* A couple must decide how many children they want and when they want to have them. There are many factors to be considered, such as the importance of not delaying pregnancy until a couple has become too old to want children or has developed a fertility problem; the importance of being off birth-control pills for three

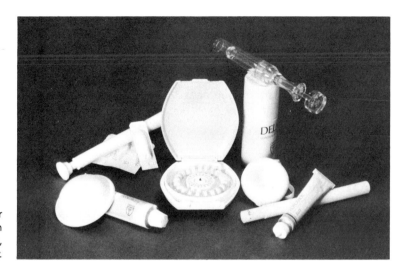

Birth-control devices for women: diaphragm (with jelly), suppository, pills, foam, sponge, and jelly.

months before pregnancy is attempted; and the fact that it may take a fertile, normal couple up to a year of trying to achieve pregnancy.

*Mutual acceptability.* A couple is best served by a method of birth control that suits both of them. Some women feel fine on birth-control pills and can take them; others do not feel well when they take birth-control pills and should not take them. Some men do not mind using condoms (rubbers), but other men hate them.

*Spontaneous and carefree sex life.* A contraceptive should serve the same role in a couple's sexual relationship that an appropriate backdrop serves in a play. It should be in the background to enhance what is going on but should not interfere with or overpower the action. A contraceptive foam, for instance, should be inserted in the vagina no more than half an hour before intercourse and is most effective if inserted at least fifteen minutes before intercourse. Some couples are able to use foam under these conditions without it interfering with their spontaneity. Others find that these requirements totally interrupt their foreplay and their spontaneity.

*Freedom from worry.* A couple's contraceptive method should allow freedom from worry about physical damage or health problems as well as freedom from anxiety about an unwanted pregnancy. For example, many women can use an IUD (intra-uterine contraceptive device) without worrying about the possibility of it making them sterile. Other women worry so much about the IUD causing damage that they cannot enjoy its use. Some couples can use condoms alone for contraception, even with the accompanying 20 percent pregnancy rate, because these couples are not seriously worried about the possibility of getting pregnant.

---

**1001** **How important is it that contraception be a mutual decision between husband and wife?**

It is enormously important. Communication is one of the vital necessities of a marriage, and mutual agreement in the area of sexual activity and contraception is essential to a deep and sensitive understanding between husband and wife.

Discussion about contraception should begin as part of a premarital examination for the woman, and the couple should have an open discussion with the physician about sexual relations and contraception. But even more important is the couple's discussion about contraception after leaving the physician's office. Any couple planning marriage should read the material in this chapter before seeing their doctor, so that they can ask better-informed questions and arrive more quickly and knowledgeably at a decision about contraception.

## 1002 Since there are so many reliable contraceptive techniques presently available, why are there so many unplanned pregnancies?

To avoid pregnancy it is absolutely necessary that an effective birth-control method be used and that it be used correctly. Many pregnancies occur because of careless use of contraceptive techniques. There are other reasons, however.

*Failure of a reliable contraceptive used correctly.* Although rare, failures of even the best birth-control methods can happen. Pregnancies have occurred in women using all forms of birth control, from condoms to the Pill.

*Using a "less-effective" contraceptive technique.* Some devices have a higher pregnancy risk. Condoms, for example, have a higher "failure" rate than birth-control pills! Be sure you are aware of the risks of pregnancy with the technique you use.

*No contraceptive used.* Any time a couple has intercourse and one of them is not absolutely sterile, pregnancy can occur. This applies to "sentimentalists" who do not want to stop sex play in order to use their contraceptive properly; couples who rely on the rhythm method; couples who lack the discipline necessary to use birth control correctly; couples who dislike the contraceptive technique they are using; and women who are in their forties or early fifties who have irregular periods and think that they are menopausal and cannot become pregnant.

*Desire for pregnancy.* I have had many patients who became pregnant while they were using a generally reliable contraceptive technique. Some of these patients admit that they or their partner, deep down, really wanted to get pregnant and were careless about using their contraceptive.

## 1003 Why are there so many different kinds of contraception?

There are many contraceptive techniques because there is no one perfect method. Some people do well with one type of contraception, and others do well with another. You must find the method that is best for you. Your doctor can help you do this, as can the information in this chapter.

If you are using a contraceptive method with which you are dissatisfied, switch to another one. If you do not like the technique you are using, you will probably not use it as regularly as you should, increasing your chance of an unplanned pregnancy.

Couples today are fortunate in that they live in an age when there are several effective methods of birth control. In addition, a number of new methods of birth control are being studied and perfected. (See Q. 1127.)

## 1004 Isn't sterilization the best method of birth control?

Sterilization is the most effective birth-control method, except for abstinence and hysterectomy, but sterilization is only for people who absolutely never want another child. I cannot overemphasize that fact. Almost every week a patient comes to my office because she wants a sterilization reversed.

Surgery to reverse a sterilization can be done. But no matter how expertly done, 25 percent of women having tubal reversal surgery will still not be able to get pregnant. These women can then undergo in vitro fertilization, but this is an even more expensive and time-consuming process. (See Q. 925–929, 975–978.)

The only time to consider sterilization is when you know beyond a shadow of a doubt that no matter what happens in the future—divorce, remarriage, death of a child, whatever—you will absolutely not want to be pregnant again, or that because of a health problem you should not become pregnant again.

The birth-control methods we will survey in the next few questions are techniques that will prevent pregnancy now but still give you the option of becoming pregnant later. A detailed discussion on each technique will be presented elsewhere in this chapter. You should use one of these methods until you are certain that you want to be sterile for the rest of your life, then have a sterilization if you like.

## 1005 Aren't pills, IUDs, and sterilization procedures dangerous?

There are risks involved with almost everything, and birth control is no exception. No known contraceptive has a death rate as high as that of pregnancy, however. Although the death rate from either pregnancy or birth control is relatively low, one estimate is that the death rate from pregnancy is over five times greater than the death rate traceable to the use of birth-control pills.

For example, IUDs usually do not cause any generalized health problem, but they can cause infection in a woman's pelvic organs that can result in infertility or sterility. Use of an IUD increases the risk of infertility by 50 percent.

Sterilization carries some risk, but in this case the risk is over in one fell swoop. After the surgery, which always carries some risk, a patient does not need to worry at all about any dangers relating to contraception.

The point is that if a woman gets pregnant, there is a potential health risk from that pregnancy that is statistically higher than the risk of any birth-control method she might use.

## 1006 What birth-control method do you recommend to your patients?

I do not push my patients into using one particular contraceptive method; I give them information on various methods, discuss the pregnancy rates and health risks involved, and then try to help them decide what is best for them. I usually give my patients the following information.

The best contraceptive method is the birth-control pill. If you can take the Pill, it is the method I recommend. You have the lowest chance of pregnancy occurring with it, and it is reversible. There is a lower chance of uterine or ovarian cancer later on in life in women who have used oral contraceptives for a few years than in women who have not. Finally, women on birth-control pills have fewer breast lumps than women not on the Pill. Newer research is indicating that women who have used birth-control pills for a period of a few years at some time in their life may even develop less breast cancer than women who have never used oral contraceptives.

The IUD is an effective contraceptive technique, but you should use an IUD only if you never plan to get pregnant again but do not want sterilization. There will be a small but significant number of women who will develop sterilizing infection and scarring of their tubes from an IUD. Because of this I think it is best that you not consider using an IUD unless you are fairly sure that you do not want any more children. The chance of being made sterile by an IUD is only 3–5 percent, so most women are still quite fertile even if they have used an IUD several years. The drawback is that you may never know if something has happened to affect your fertility, and you may later decide that you do want more children.

The only other reliable methods of birth control, in my opinion, are "barrier" methods, such as suppositories, foam, sponges, diaphragms or condoms. These methods, used alone, carry a pregnancy rate of about 20 percent. This percentage includes everyone, even those people who are not disciplined enough to use their contraception all the time or who forget to use it. The women most likely to be "safe" using a barrier method of contraception are those who will be well-disciplined in its use and who will also use an additional barrier method during the fertile week of ovulation.

Rhythm, withdrawal, douching, and all the variations of these techniques have a high pregnancy rate. They should not be used unless the couple is aware that an unplanned pregnancy is a strong possibility.

The silicone-plug technique, which involves "plugging" the fallopian tubes, is still basically a research procedure. Too few people have had silicone plugs removed to determine if pregnancy is possible after their use. This is probably because once a woman has gone through the expense and discomfort of having the plugs put in, she is unlikely to ever want to have them taken out and have to go through it all over again! (See Q. 1092–1098.)

## Birth-Control Pills

### 1007  How do birth-control pills work?

Birth-control pills contain synthetic estrogen and progesterone that produce an artificial menstrual cycle in your body. They do this by "putting to sleep" your own ova-

ries and your normal hormone system. Because your ovaries are, in effect, asleep, they do not release any eggs and you cannot get pregnant. With no egg to fertilize, the sperm merely swim into your body, die after several hours, are then absorbed by your body as small packages of protein, or they are passed out of your uterus and vagina with other secretions.

The Pill has other effects on a woman's body that increase its potency. It affects the passage of an egg through the fallopian tubes; it changes the lining of the uterus making it unreceptive to a fertilized egg; and it makes the cervical mucus more difficult for the sperm to penetrate.

### 1008  How are birth-control pills used?

When you begin taking birth-control pills, you should decide what time of day you would most easily remember to take them. It does not matter whether it is morning, noon, or at bedtime. You should take your pill within two hours of the same time every day for maintenance of the best hormone level in your body. Many women like to take their oral contraceptive at bedtime to avoid any sick feeling or nausea that the pills might produce.

Oral contraceptives are available in two different types of packages—twenty-one day and twenty-eight day.

*Twenty-one-day packages.* The twenty-one-day pill packages provide a pill a day for twenty-one days. After you finish this package, you then take no pills for seven days. You are protected from pregnancy all month long, even during the seven days that you are taking no pills.

To begin the twenty-one-day package the first time, start the pills on the fifth day of a period. "Day one" is the first day of a period, not counting the day or two of slight spotting that precedes the period for some women. Once you start the pills, take one a day for twenty-one days (three weeks). Then stop the pills for seven days and start a new package.

For example, if your present period started on Sunday, you would count Sunday as day one of your period and start your pills on Thursday. You would then take the pills daily for three weeks, stop for seven days, and then start a new package. Following this schedule you will always take your last pill on a Wednesday and start the next package on a Thursday, one week later.

You will almost always have your period the week you take no pills. Your period will usually start a couple of days after you stop taking the pills, and it may or may not stop by the time you start your next package of pills.

If you prefer, you can arrange your schedule of pill intake so that your period always comes during the week, avoiding having a period on the weekend. Merely delay starting your next package of pills until the next Sunday, or start them a few days early so that the starting day is on a Sunday.

*Twenty-eight-day packages.* The twenty-eight-day packages contain the same type and same number of hormone pills as the twenty-one-day packages, but the twenty-eight-day packages also contain seven "sugar pills" (nonhormone) to be taken at the end of the hormone-pills schedule. The reason for this type of packaging is to help you remember when to start and stop the hormone pills each month. The nonhormone pills are merely a mechanism for timing.

All twenty-eight-day packages instruct you to start the first pill on a Sunday. Therefore, the first month you take them, you should begin the pills on the Sunday after your period begins. If your period begins on a Saturday, then begin your pills the next day. If your period begins on a Sunday, start your pills that evening. If your period begins on Monday or any other day of the week, start your pills on the next Sunday. The sugar pills

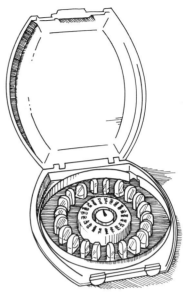

21-day package of oral contraceptives

in the package are the seven pills at the end that are a different color. While you are taking these pills your period will start, because they contain no hormones.

Do not skip any days between the end of one twenty-eight-day package and the beginning of the next.

*The preceding information was adapted with permission from a patient-information booklet written by my associate, Jo Bess Hammer, M.D.*

If you have recently given birth, you can start oral contraceptives between the third

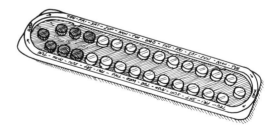

28-day package of oral contraceptives

and sixth weeks after delivery. If you are breast-feeding, however, or if there is any possibility that you might be pregnant again, you must not take birth-control pills.

As soon as you start taking the pills, you are probably protected from getting pregnant. If you switch to a different brand of pill, you are probably safe as soon as you start that pill. I say "probably" because there are some physicians who feel that there is a slightly higher chance of pregnancy occurring when a woman first starts oral contraceptives or when she changes to a different brand of pill. If you want to be the most safe from pregnancy, use a contraceptive foam or condom for the first ten days you are on a new pill. Another technique that provides reliable safety from the first day is to take your first pill on day one of your period the month you start your new pills. This is not only safe but also eliminates the need to use a barrier form of protection.

## 1009 How long can I take birth-control pills?

Extensive research has shown that women may use an oral contraceptive for as many years as they want to without any permanent change to their reproductive and hormone systems. Except for the week off each month, the pills do not have to be discontinued until age thirty-five. Women who smoke must stop taking the Pill at the age of thirty-five; and some physicians also advise even nonsmokers to stop oral contraceptives at the age of thirty-five. In the package insert that comes with the pills, the FDA suggests forty years of age as the cut-off time for taking the Pill for nonsmokers and thirty-five as the cut-off for smokers.

## 1010 What should I do if I miss a pill?

Don't panic! If you miss a pill, just take an extra one the next day. If you miss two pills, take an extra pill a day for two days. It is unlikely that you will become pregnant if you do this, but if you absolutely do not want to risk pregnancy, it would probably be best for you to use a barrier contraceptive, such as a vaginal foam or condoms, with intercourse for the next ten days. With the higher-dose pills that were used in the past this was not so critical, but with the lower dosage now in use missing a pill is more likely to allow a breakthrough ovulation and pregnancy. Remember, the pregnancy rate with birth-control pills is low, but the women who are more likely to become pregnant are those who take their pills erratically.

Missing pills, by the way, will not damage your body at all.

## 1011 I have had bleeding during the twenty-one days that I take my pills. Is something wrong? What should I do?

One of the most common problems with birth-control pills is breakthrough bleeding. This is bleeding during the twenty-one days a woman is taking her hormone-containing pills. This is almost never a sign of a medical problem, nor is it in any way harmful for a woman's body. Some women bleed while taking oral contraceptives because the small amount of hormones contained in birth-control pills cannot keep their uterine lining from shedding. This does not increase the chance of pregnancy.

Of course, if bleeding persists it could be due to a medical problem, such as a tumor or a pregnancy. Therefore, if bleeding persists for more than two months, call your physician.

There are basically three methods of treatment of breakthrough bleeding.

Change to another brand of birth-control pill. Your doctor will help you decide if this is wise to do and will prescribe an alternate brand.

Add an ethinyl estradiol 0.02-mg tablet, a form of estrogen, to your hormone intake each day. Increasing the amount of estrogen in your body will usually build up the uterine lining enough to stop breakthrough bleeding. You would, of course, need your doctor's advice and a prescription for this hormone.

Double up on your birth-control pills. This is a good, simple technique. You already have the pills and do not need to call your doctor to do it, although you may want to check. Just take an extra pill a day, out of an extra package, until the bleeding stops. Then take an extra pill for an additional three to four days. After that, drop back to one pill a day.

If you allow the bleeding to persist, you may start having cramping and heavier bleeding than you normally have with a period. When breakthrough bleeding gets this heavy, it may take several days to get the bleeding stopped when you finally do change your hormone dosage. If you start treatment for the breakthrough bleeding and you come to the end of your package before the bleeding stops, stop the pills, go one week without them, then start a new package of pills at the regular time. Remember, it is normal to bleed at the "wrong time" during the first one or two months you are on a new pill. Don't worry about this, but if it bothers you follow one of the suggestions given to control it. If you have breakthrough bleeding after the first two months, it is best to follow one of the suggestions given to stop it.

---

**1012**  **I have bad cramps when I have breakthrough bleeding during the time I am taking the twenty-one pills. Is this normal?**

Yes. Many women have worse cramps when they have breakthrough bleeding than they normally would have with their periods when they are not on the Pill.

This increased cramping is probably normal. If it is too severe, however, call your doctor. It is possible for a woman on oral contraceptives to become pregnant and to have either a miscarriage or a tubal pregnancy.

---

**1013**  **If I do not bleed during my week off the pills, does that mean I'm pregnant?**

Probably not. Some women have no bleeding at all during the week they are off their pills. In this situation your doctor will often suggest that you get a serum pregnancy test, because taking birth-control pills while pregnant may result in congenital abnormalities of the baby. Because of this it is always best to have either a period or a negative blood pregnancy test before resuming the oral contraceptives. If you do not have a period after you stop your pills, and you do not want to have a serum (blood) pregnancy test, use barrier contraceptives—contraceptive foam and condoms or a diaphragm—until you have a period and can resume taking the pills.

If this happens with a particular brand of pills more than two times, ask your doctor about switching you to a different brand of oral contraceptive.

---

**1014**  **What are the chances of pregnancy occurring while taking the Pill?**

The risk of pregnancy is extremely low. Of two hundred women who use the Pill for one year, only one will become pregnant. This is almost 100-percent effective, a higher contraceptive rate than any other reversible method of contraception available today.

If you take certain drugs while you are on the Pill, you should use additional contraceptives during the cycle you usually take pills, or increase the strength of your oral contraceptive to a 50-mg pill. These drugs decrease the effectiveness of birth-control pills:

Anticonvulsants
    pheyntoin
    primidon
    barbiturates: (phenobarbital)
    carbanazephina (Tegretal)

Antibiotics
    ampicillin
    rifampin
    tetracyclines (the small dosage most people use to treat acne does not decrease the potency of birth-control pills)

## 1015 Which women cannot use birth-control pills?

Women should not use oral contraceptives if they:

are over forty

are over thirty-five and smoke

are pregnant

have had breast cancer (unless they have physician approval)

have liver damage or liver disease

have (or might have) cancer of the uterus

have blood clots in their legs

have had a stroke

have hypertension (except by approval of their physician)

have severe headaches or seizures

are diabetics. Diabetics are more likely to develop hardening of the arteries, strokes, and other blood vessel prob-

lems—problems that can be aggravated by birth-control pills.

have high cholesterol levels. These women are at a greater risk for developing heart attacks and other blood-vessel problems.

## 1016 Will birth-control pills prevent future pregnancies when they are discontinued?

No. Reliable studies have shown that birth-control pills do not affect a woman's future fertility. For a few months after discontinuing oral contraceptives, a woman's periods may be somewhat irregular, which can prevent pregnancy initially. After a few months fertility is as normal as though she had never taken birth-control pills. This does not mean that a woman may not have trouble getting pregnant or may not have a miscarriage later. However, those things are possibilities for any woman, whether or not she has been on birth-control pills.

## 1017 Are there detrimental side effects of birth-control pills?

With the modern lower dose oral contraceptives, women have fewer side effects than they did with earlier pills. However, side effects may still occur. For example, a woman may feel tired, bloated, headachy, or irritable; she may gain weight; she may have a decreased desire for intercourse; she may develop tenderness of her breasts; she may be nauseated or have vomiting; and she may have spotting or bleeding at times other than during her menstrual period.

Liver tumors (hepatomas) are more likely to occur in women who take birth-control pills, but they are extremely rare. I have never seen a patient with this type of tumor. Some studies suggest that birth-control pills may be related to cancer of the breast, but other research has shown that there is no significant relationship between the two. As a matter of fact, the most recent studies indicate that women who have taken the Pill for several years have a decreased chance of developing breast cancer later on in life.

Women on oral contraceptives do tend to have an increased risk of cervical cancer. Since cervical cancer is related to sexual activity, however, most researchers feel that the increased risk of cancer of the cervix in women on birth-control pills is caused by increased sexual exposure. (See Q. 1145.)

---

**1018** **Why shouldn't women who are over thirty-five, and/or who smoke, take birth-control pills?**

Simply stated, it is too risky. Women who are over thirty-five and on birth-control pills have a slightly greater risk of developing problems with circulation through their blood vessels. Smoking greatly magnifies that risk. All studies on this subject prove that this is true. The typical warning printed on the insert that comes with each package of birth-control pills says:

---

WARNING

Cigarette smoking increases the risk of serious cardiovascular side effects from oral contraceptive use. The risk increases with age and with heavy smoking (15 or more cigarettes a day) and is quite marked in women over thirty-five years of age. Women who use oral contraceptives should be strongly advised not to smoke.

---

An example of the kind of studies that led to this warning is one done by Drs. Shapiro, Slone, Rosenberg, Kaufman, Stolley, and Mittinen, which was reported in the 1979 volume of the *Lancet Medical Journal.* Their

research showed that the risk of heart attack for a woman who smokes more than forty-five cigarettes a day increases almost tenfold: from the normal factor of 4.5 for a woman on birth-control pills to a factor of 40. Their studies also clearly showed that women over thirty-five, the age at which the risk of heart attack begins increasing in the population anyway, were more likely to be the victims of such problems.

If a woman is a heavy smoker, almost all authorities feel that some method of contraception other than birth-control pills would be safer for her. If a woman is over thirty-five and is a smoker, she must not use oral contraceptives.

---

**1019** **How does the fatality rate of oral contraceptive users compare to that of users of other methods of contraceptives or to those who use no contraception?**

Women who use birth-control pills are physically safer statistically than women who use no method of contraception. Some reliable recent studies have also shown that there is no difference in the death rates for non-smoking oral contraceptive users under the age of thirty-five and those who use other methods of contraception. See the accompanying chart for more information.

The reasons for these two findings are as follows.

Women who use no contraception can become pregnant, and pregnancy can cause a higher rate of clots in blood vessels, complications such as surgery and infections, and even a greater chance of death than for women who use birth-control pills.

Although a woman using a barrier method of birth control (such as diaphragm, condom, or foam) is less likely to get pregnant than if she were using no contraception, there are still enough pregnancies with com-

| Method | Annual Pregnancy Rate per 100 couples using a specific contraceptive method | Cost per Year | Annual Mortality Rate per 100,000 women using a specific contraceptive method (from method, complications, or unintended pregnancy) Age | | |
| | | | 15–24 | 25–34 | 35–44 |
|---|---|---|---|---|---|
| No method | 60–80 | — | 7.2 | 12.0 | 27.0 |
| Condom | 10 | $30 | 1.4 | 0.4 | 0.4 |
| Withdrawal (coitus interruptus) | 23 | — | 2.0 | 1.6 | 3.2 |
| Spermicides (jellies, foams, creams, suppositories) | 18 | $50 (foam) | 1.6 | 1.2 | 2.5 |
| Sponge | 9–15 | $100 | 1.6 | 1.2 | 2.5 |
| Diaphragm with spermicides (includes doctor's visit) | 19 | $50 (foam) $160 (diaphragm) | 1.6 | 1.2 | 2.5 |
| NFP—(natural family planning—periodic abstinence) | 24 | — | 2.0 | 1.6 | 3.2 |
| IUD | 5 | $131 (first year) | 1.2 | 1.3 | 2.0 |
| Birth-control pill | 2.4 | $172 (incl. dr. visit) | 0.6* 3.0** | 1.6* 10.2** | 23.0* 84.5** |
| Vasectomy | less than 1 | $271 (one time) | rare | rare | rare |
| Tubal sterilization | less than 1 | $1180 (one time) | 4 per 100,000 procedures | | |

\* nonsmoker
\*\*smoker
The annual death rate per 100,000 women from auto accidents is 10.1 percent; from smoking-related lung cancer it is 23.7 percent.

plications to make the death rate as high as that of women taking oral contraceptives.

# 1020 Are there beneficial side effects from the use of birth-control pills?

Based on figures for the mid-1980s, taking oral contraceptives allows almost 60,000 American women annually to avoid hospitalization. The use of oral contraceptives is responsible for the hospitalization of about 9,000 women, but the hospitalization of the majority of these women could have been avoided if the women over age thirty-five had stopped using the Pill and if women had discontinued smoking while they used oral contraceptives.

Some of the other benefits of using birth-control pills include:

*Less chance of unwanted pregnancies.* A woman using oral contraceptives will rarely become pregnant unless she wants to and therefore lessens her risking the potential dangers associated with any pregnancy, including less chance of ectopic pregnancy.

*Insures routine check-ups.* Women cannot get birth-control pills unless they see a physician. This means that they will have such things as yearly Pap smears and breast exams. It also means that they will often get in the habit of the "annual exam" and will continue it even after stopping the use of the Pill. This one habit has probably saved far more women from cancer and other medical problems than all the problems the Pill has ever produced.

*Less menstrual cramping.* Birth-control pills may be the only method of helping a woman who suffers from severe cramps who has not been helped by any other medication.

*Lighter menstrual periods.* Birth-control pills usually make a woman bleed less with her periods. This is especially beneficial if a woman usually has extremely heavy periods.

*Less pelvic inflammatory disease (PID) from gonorrhea.* Women who are on birth-control pills are up to 50 percent less likely to get infections of the uterus and tubes from venereal disease. Those who do get such infections generally have milder infections than women who are not on the Pill. However, they are just as (or more) likely to get pelvic inflammatory disease from chlamydia. A chlamydia infection can be even more destructive to the female organs than gonorrhea, so a woman should not rely on oral contraceptives to protect her from sexually transmitted disease.

*Fewer breast lumps.* Statistics have shown that women on birth-control pills have only one-fourth to one-half as many breast lumps as women who are not on oral contraceptives. This means, of course, far less chance of needing (or having to worry about) breast biopsies.

*Less ovarian cancer.* Women who have used birth-control pills for a few years during their reproductive age have a significantly lower risk of developing cancer of the ovary in the future. These women have one-third less ovarian cancer than women who have never been on the Pill.

*Less uterine cancer.* Women who have been on oral contraceptives have a significantly decreased chance of later developing cancer of the endometrium (lining of the uterus) and are as much as two and a half times less likely to develop uterine cancer than women who have never been on birth-control pills.

*Less rheumatoid arthritis.* Some studies suggest that women who have taken birth-control pills may have half as much chance of developing rheumatoid arthritis in the future as women who have not been on the Pill. A recent study done at Mayo Clinic, however, suggests this may not be so.

*Fewer ovarian cysts.* Women on oral contraceptives will not develop the ovarian cysts that are a part of the body's attempt to produce eggs each month, because the body is not trying to produce eggs at all while the birth-control pill is used. The advantage of this is that it is much less likely that you would be told by your doctor that you have an enlarged ovary and that you need ovarian surgery. (See Q. 818.)

---

**1021** **How soon may I try to become pregnant after I stop taking birth-control pills?**

You should wait three months after stopping the pills before you try to become pregnant. Use foam, rubbers, or some similar technique during that three-month period. Studies have shown that if conception takes place during the first three months after oral contraceptives have been discontinued, there is a slightly greater chance of the baby having a congenital abnormality. The chance of that happening is extremely small; if you do get pregnant during that time, you do not really need to worry about your baby.

The major reason for waiting three months is that your body may take that long or even longer to start having regular periods. If you get pregnant before your periods are regular, you may not know for sure when you got pregnant or when you are due.

## The Intrauterine Contraceptive Device (IUD)

### 1022 What is an intrauterine contraceptive device, or IUD, and how does it work?

An IUD is a device that is inserted into a woman's uterus to prevent conception. Such devices can cause infection in a woman's uterus and/or fallopian tubes, resulting in infertility. Lawsuits have resulted in all but one U.S. manufacturer discontinuing production of IUDs. Only Progestasert (See Q. 1040.) is available today.

No one knows exactly how an IUD works. It seems fairly certain, however, that the IUD produces its contraceptive effect in several different ways. It causes changes in the enzymes inside the uterus, which makes it "hostile" to both sperm and eggs. It causes white blood cells to be drawn into the uterus. These white blood cells actually "eat up" the sperm and the eggs that get into the uterine cavity. Since an IUD causes more uterine contractions than would otherwise be normal, an egg may be flushed through the uterus before it can be fertilized. It is also possible that an already fertilized egg may be flushed out of the reproductive tract. (See the next question.)

Copper-wire-wrapped IUDs have additional contraceptive effects. The copper that is absorbed into the uterine fluid interferes with the development of the uterine lining, making it hostile to egg implantation. It also draws more white blood cells into the uter-ine cavity, making it even less receptive to sperm and eggs. Finally, it is toxic to sperm, affecting their ability to fertilize eggs, and it is undoubtedly hostile to eggs too.

### 1023 Can an egg become fertilized with an IUD in place?

Yes, it is possible for fertilization to take place, and some women are troubled by the possibility of an IUD "aborting" the implantation of such an egg. Because of the many other modes of action of the IUD, however, it is unlikely that fertilization occurs very often.

If the possibility of an IUD causing the loss of a fertilized egg bothers a woman, she certainly should not have an IUD inserted.

### 1024 How is an IUD inserted?

Before inserting an IUD, the doctor will talk with you and examine you to make sure that you can use an IUD and that you are not pregnant. Warn the doctor if you think there is any possibility of your being pregnant. Having an IUD inserted while you are pregnant could cause a serious uterine infection and an abortion.

After the examination the doctor will insert the IUD. First a speculum will be inserted into your vagina and the doctor will grasp the cervix with an instrument (a tenaculum) which will cause cramping. Then he or she will pass a probe into your uterus to check the direction and depth of your uterine cavity causing more cramping, and next will insert into your uterus a small plastic tube, smaller than a straw, which contains the IUD.

The IUD is pushed out of the tube into your uterus, where it pops open and into position. The tube is removed, leaving a string (attached to the IUD) dangling into your vagina. The doctor will cut the string to a length that will allow you to feel it, but not so long that it extends from your vagina.

# Intrauterine Contraceptive Devices (IUD)

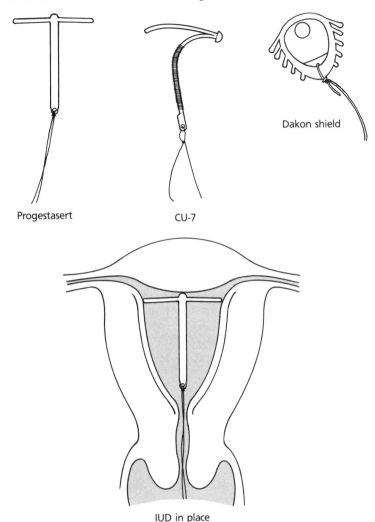

Progestasert

CU-7

Dakon shield

IUD in place

---

**1025**   **How can I tell if my IUD is staying in place?**

You should check for the IUD string by feeling inside your vagina before you have intercourse each time for the first month. An IUD is most likely to fall out during that time and it can fall out without your being aware of it, so be sure to check.

The doctor will want to see you again about a month after the IUD is inserted to check for any possible problem.

Sometimes, even several months later, the dangling IUD string will become a great deal longer. If this happens, it merely means that a small loop of the string was caught on the IUD as it was put in. It has now become unlooped, and the extra length allows the string to extend from the vagina. Do not pull it! Go to your doctor so that he or she can cut it shorter.

It is wise for you to check for the IUD string at least once a month, and the best time for this is right after a period. If you cannot feel the string, see your doctor. Otherwise you need to see the doctor only at the time of your annual exams, unless you develop any of the problems mentioned in the next several questions for which medical advice is suggested.

## 1026 What immediate effects can I expect after having an IUD put it?

Immediately after an IUD is inserted, you may have some cramping and some spotting of blood. This cramping and spotting can continue as long as you have the IUD in, but this is unusual. (See Q. 1030, 1031.) Most of the time a woman will stop having cramps and spotting after a few hours or days. It is quite common, however, for a woman's period to be heavier while she has an IUD, and it is also normal to have increased cramping with periods as long as the IUD is in place.

Your husband may be able to feel the IUD string during intercourse, but it probably will not bother him. If it does, your doctor may need to cut a bit more off the string.

## 1027 How effective is an IUD?

Studies show that of one hundred women who use an IUD for a whole year, only one or two will become pregnant during that year. These statistics show that the IUD is an effective method of birth control.

## 1028 How does an IUD affect fertility?

Infections of the pelvic organs (pelvic inflammatory disease, or PID) occur more often in women who use IUDs than in women who do not. When an infection occurs, the tubes can be scarred so abnormally that they cannot carry an egg into the uterus, producing infertility or absolute sterility. The risk of infection is three to five times greater for women who use an IUD. If a woman has had a PID, she is even more likely to develop infection again if she has an IUD put in.

It is possible for a woman who has an IUD to develop an ectopic (tubal) pregnancy, just as she could have a normal pregnancy. The progesterone-containing-type of IUD seems to cause more ectopic pregnancies than the other IUDs.

## 1029 What other problems may result from IUD use?

The primary undesirable side effect of the IUD is infection, but there are other problems, which are discussed in the next eight questions:

bleeding and spotting

pain

IUD falling out

IUD turning

IUD perforating the uterus

IUD becoming imbedded in the wall of the uterus

difficult removal of IUD

actinomycosis infection

## 1030 What should I do if my IUD causes spotting or bleeding?

A woman can start bleeding the moment she has an IUD put in and continue to have it as long as the IUD is present. This is not the norm nor is it dangerous, but most women will not tolerate such bleeding.

It is more likely that spotting and bleeding will occur intermittently. It is normal for a woman to start spotting or bleeding a year or two after insertion of the IUD. Such bleeding is usually due to the IUD, and removal of the IUD usually stops the bleeding.

This bleeding is not dangerous unless it becomes very heavy and persists for many weeks.

If a woman is forty or over, spotting or bleeding between periods may be an indication of cancer of the uterus. The IUD should be removed and a D&C or endometrial biopsy done to check for the possible presence of cancer. If you have such bleeding and are in this age group, check with your doctor promptly.

## 1031 Will an IUD cause pain?

It can. From the day an IUD is inserted, a woman could have pain from it. If this pain persists for several weeks, a woman usually has the IUD taken out by her doctor. I think this is wise, because such pain could indicate a low-grade infection of the uterus that could get worse.

It is common for a woman to have an IUD in place for a year or two and then start having pain. If the pain is a minor problem, it is fine to leave the IUD in place. If it becomes more constant and more severe, the IUD should definitely be removed.

If you develop pain while wearing an IUD, see your gynecologist first. When I insert an IUD I warn patients that they could have pain anywhere from the lower chest to their mid-thighs from the IUD! Gynecologists have learned that IUD pain can be felt anywhere in the central part of a woman's body. I cannot overemphasize this. I have had patients who went to doctors other than gynecologists and who even had surgery for pain, only to find out later that all the pain was caused by their IUD. If there is any question about whether or not pain is due to an IUD, I encourage you to get it taken out to see if the pain goes away.

## 1032 What if my IUD falls out?

I tell every patient in whom I insert an IUD to check the string before each act of inter-

course during the first month and then once a month after that. I do this because it is quite possible for an IUD to fall out without the woman knowing it. Most of the time, however, a woman will feel cramping if the IUD is working its way out.

If you think you are losing or have lost your IUD, you should see your doctor. If the string is not present, the doctor can determine whether or not the IUD is still in the uterus by two methods: either by putting a probe inside your uterus in an attempt to detect a "clinking" of the probe against the metal of a copper IUD, or by ordering an X-ray or an ultrasound scan. An X-ray will show whether or not an IUD is present. An X-ray is limited in that it will not show whether the IUD is in your uterus, but it will almost always show if an IUD is present somewhere in your abdomen. An ultrasound scan can show whether or not an IUD is in your uterus, but will occasionally miss an IUD if it is present in a woman's abdomen but not in her uterus. Therefore a doctor will occasionally need to order both an ultrasound and an X-ray to locate a lost IUD.

If your IUD has fallen out, you can have another one inserted. About 50 percent of women will be able to retain a second IUD even though the first one fell out.

## 1033 Can my IUD still be in place even if I can't feel the string?

Yes, it can. If the IUD turns in its position, it can pull the string up inside the uterus. In this case you will not be able to feel the string, nor would your doctor be able to see it.

If you have "lost your string," it is important to have an X-ray or ultrasound to see if the IUD is present, as mentioned in the previous question. This not only shows the presence of the IUD, but it makes sure the IUD has not perforated the uterus and lodged somewhere else in your body. (See next question.)

## 1034 What is the possibility that my IUD will perforate, or poke through, the wall of my uterus?

Less than 1 percent of women who have IUDs have the IUD perforate the uterus. If this does happen, it almost always occurs at the time of insertion when, as the doctor pushes the IUD into the uterus, it is pushed through the wall of the uterus.

If this happens, or if at some later point in time an X-ray shows your IUD to be lodged outside your uterus, the doctor can do a laparoscopy. (See Q. 907.) Normally with this procedure the doctor can find the IUD and pull it out of your abdomen without making a larger incision. If not, a larger abdominal incision will be necessary in order to remove the IUD.

It is important that you have the IUD removed if it has perforated the uterus.

## 1035 Can an IUD become imbedded in the wall of the uterus?

Yes, but if this happened you would not know it until the doctor tried to remove the IUD. If it had become stuck in the muscular wall of the uterus, the doctor would often not be able to get it out and would probably break the string trying to remove it. In this situation the doctor would have to admit you to an operating room for a D&C to remove the IUD.

## 1036 How is an IUD removed?

Most of the time removing an IUD is a simple process. The doctor merely grabs the string and pulls.

It is fairly common, however, for the

string not to be visible when you want your IUD removed. If the string cannot be seen, the doctor will probably have to use an "IUD hook," a device which has a slit in its tip just the right size for grasping an IUD. Once he or she has located the IUD, the doctor attempts to "hook" the IUD so that it can be pulled out.

Most of the time a doctor can remove an IUD in this fashion. If not, the doctor may have to dilate the cervix and use a larger instrument to remove the IUD. This would necessitate hospitalization and general anesthesia and would, essentially, be a D&C. (See Q. 788.)

## 1037 What is actinomycosis infection?

*Actinomyces* is a fungus organism that can begin growing inside a woman's uterus because of the presence of an IUD. This fungus infection can cause sterility and/or necessitate a hysterectomy because of pelvic abscess formation. Actinomycosis infections usually occur when an IUD has been left in a woman's uterus for many years.

When you have an IUD in place and a Pap smear shows the presence of actinomycosis, the IUD should be removed. After two or three months, when the body has had time to rid itself of this fungus, another IUD may be inserted.

## 1038 What are the advantages of using an IUD?

The primary advantage of an IUD is that a woman can have an effective contraceptive device without doing anything more than going to the doctor once a year (unless there is a problem). She does not need to take a pill and she does not need to use any device or medication just before intercourse.

Another good thing about the IUD is that there is usually no immediate harmful effect if a woman delays changing her IUD. (See next question.)

---

## 1039 Is it necessary to have an IUD changed or removed if I am not having any problems?

Most companies that make copper IUDs recommend that they be replaced every three years. The World Health Organization and other international groups that use these devices, have found that there is only a very slightly increased chance of pregnancy if a woman keeps her IUD in place for four years.

I now tell patients that they can keep an IUD in for four years, as long as they realize that there might be a slightly increased risk of pregnancy during the fourth year. Most choose to change their IUD after three years, but if they are a few months late getting in to have it changed, they do not have to worry about any increased risk of pregnancy.

---

## 1040 Which IUD is best?

When they were available, most physicians suggested a copper-wire wrapped plastic IUD. The copper IUD seems better than the all-plastic IUD for several reasons:

*Less menstrual blood loss.* This is probably because the copper IUD is smaller and therefore less irritating to the uterine lining.

*Better tolerance by women who have had fewer children.* Women who have had no children, or only one child, tolerate the smaller, copper IUDs better than the larger, all-plastic IUDs.

*Fewer IUDs will be lost.* The copper IUD stays in the uterus better than the plastic IUDs. Again, this is because of its smaller size and shape.

*Can be accepted by a smaller cervix.* Because the copper IUD is smaller, it can be inserted through a cervix that has a small

opening. The all-plastic IUDs require a larger cervical opening.

Other than the fact that it is the only IUD available, the main advantage of the Progestasert is that it significantly reduces the volume of menstrual blood loss with each period, which means it may be best for a woman who has heavy menstrual periods. One disadvantage, however, is that a woman will have a longer period and often have spotting during the month just before and after a menstrual period. In addition, this device must be removed and replaced every twelve months, and the chance of ectopic pregnancies is greater in women who use the Progestasert. Because of the disadvantages I do not use this device except when patients specifically ask me to.

---

## 1041 Which women cannot use an IUD?

Several conditions indicate that a woman should not use an IUD:

pregnancy

infections in the uterus, tubes, or ovaries (now or recently)

deformities of the uterus

abnormal uterine bleeding

pelvic cancer

abnormalities of the blood-clotting system (free bleeding)

severe cramping with menstrual periods. Women with this condition may not be able to tolerate an IUD but may try one if they wish.

possible future desire for pregnancy. Women who have no alternative birth-control option may feel that they have no choice but to use an IUD, but they must realize there is a risk of becoming sterile from the IUD.

## The Diaphragm for Contraception

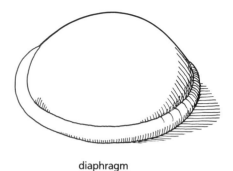

diaphragm

### 1042 What is a diaphragm?

A diaphragm is a dome-shaped rubber cap with a flexible spring rim. (See illustration.) It is approximately three inches in diameter.

Actually, a diaphragm should be called the diaphragm-plus-jelly contraceptive, because the diaphragm itself does not produce any significant contraceptive effect. The diaphragm merely holds the contraceptive jelly against the cervix; it is the jelly that kills the sperm. If only the contraceptive jelly is put into the vagina, the jelly will "glob up" into one corner of the vagina, making it relatively ineffective as a contraceptive.

Since the diaphragm does not completely seal off your upper vagina, sperm can swim around the edges of it. When they do this, they are killed by the contraceptive jelly. Even if you have a small hole in your diaphragm, any sperm that swim through the hole are usually killed by the jelly held in position by the diaphragm.

### 1043 How is a diaphragm obtained?

A doctor must prescribe and fit a woman's diaphragm. A set of fitting rings will be inserted into your vagina one at a time until one is found that fits. A diaphragm should be comfortable, and it should fill the area from the back of your vagina to your pubic bone.

Occasionally patients find that the size that seems best to the doctor is not the one that is most comfortable to them. When this happens the doctor will usually give them a size smaller or larger to meet their individual comfort needs. As long as the diaphragm stays in place during intercourse, it does not really matter that the size be absolutely precise.

One of the most important aspects of getting a diaphragm is remembering to purchase the jelly to use with it. Contraceptive foam, by the way, should not be substituted for the jelly; pregnancy would be much more likely to occur.

### 1044 How is a diaphragm inserted?

It is most important that your doctor, or the nurse, explain carefully how the diaphragm should be used. Basic instructions include the following.

Hold the diaphragm by the rim, with the cup facing up. Spread about a three-inch strip of jelly on the soft, central part of the cup. Use a little jelly around the rim so that it will slide into your vagina smoothly.

Mash the edges of the diaphragm together to make it long and thin, so that you can insert it into your vagina. Most women find it easier to insert a diaphragm when they are standing on one foot with the other foot up on the bed or the commode. The first few times you do this you may find it easier to lie on your back with your legs pulled up and apart. You can get your fingers deeper into your vagina that way.

In putting the diaphragm in place, you should insert the back edge of the diaphragm behind your cervix and the front edge up under your pubic bone. You should then be able to feel your cervix through the soft, central part of the diaphragm. Your cervix feels much like the end of your nose.

Some women prefer using a diaphragm inserter. This is a plastic stick with blunt hooks on it. The diaphragm is stretched out on it, inserted into the vagina, and then slipped off the inserter. Further positioning is the same as when no inserter is used. This device can be obtained at your pharmacy.

## 1045　When should a diaphragm be inserted, and when should it be removed?

You should insert your diaphragm no more than one to two hours before intercourse. The jelly will lose some of its potency and will tend to drain out of the vagina if you wait longer than that. Most women put their diaphragms in before they start sexual play, but some couples prefer putting in the diaphragm together as part of their foreplay. As soon as the diaphragm is in place, it is safe to have intercourse.

You should leave the diaphragm in place for six to eight hours after intercourse so that all the sperm deposited at intercourse will be dead by the time the diaphragm is removed.

## 1046　Is it safe to have intercourse more than once with one diaphragm insertion?

It is best for you to put an application of contraceptive foam in your vagina on top of the diaphragm if you repeat intercourse after more than an hour or two. Or your husband can wear a condom as an alternative to using the foam.

## 1047　How is a diaphragm removed?

To remove your diaphragm, simply put your finger up behind your pubic bone, hook the edge of the diaphragm, and pull it out. If you cannot get it out the first time you use it, don't panic. Simply go to your doctor and let the doctor or nurse help you. Don't start digging around for it because you can scratch yourself and cause bleeding.

It will probably not hurt your body if you forget your diaphragm and leave it in your vagina for several days. I had a patient a few years ago who forgot to take her diaphragm out after intercourse and didn't find it for several months! Menstrual flow goes right around the edges of a diaphragm. However, since toxic shock has occurred in women who use the diaphragm, it should not be kept in for more than twenty-four hours.

## 1048　What effects does a diaphragm have on intercourse?

Most women cannot feel the diaphragm at all when it is properly fitted, just as most women cannot feel the presence of a tampon. A man will usually feel a difference since his penis makes contact with the rubber of the diaphragm. This is not normally a problem.

## 1049　What is the chance of pregnancy with a diaphragm?

Statistics show that the chance of pregnancy with a diaphragm is in the range of four to twenty per hundred women in a year. If a woman uses a diaphragm carefully, she probably has no more than a 4-percent chance of pregnancy; if she is careless and intermittently forgets to use her diaphragm, she has a 20-percent chance of pregnancy. Many women have used the diaphragm for many years with no pregnancies resulting. From the turn of the century until the mid-1960s, the diaphragm was the mainstay of birth-control methods.

I suggest to patients that they use their diaphragms every time they have intercourse, except while they are actually bleeding from their menstrual period. Around the time of ovulation, I suggest that they put a plunger of contraceptive foam in on top of the diaphragm (or have their husband use a condom) in addition to using the diaphragm with its jelly. They should do this three or four days before ovulation and three or four days after ovulation. (Ovulation usually occurs fourteen days before the next period is going to start.) If a woman's periods are irregular she should use double protection all month long. In my years of practice, only one or two patients correctly using a diaphragm became pregnant. If you would rather not use this extra contraceptive technique at the time of ovulation, you and your husband can accomplish the same goal by abstaining from intercourse during this time.

---

## 1050 Are there women who should not, or cannot, use the diaphragm?

There are several factors to be considered when deciding whether or not to use a diaphragm for contraception.

*Lack of discipline.* If you know that you are not disciplined enough to use a diaphragm, or your husband is not patient enough to wait for you to put it in after sexual advances have been started, don't fool yourself. Use some other method of birth control.

*Discomfort.* Some women find a diaphragm uncomfortable. If changing diaphragm sizes does not solve the problem, choose another method.

*Dislike of the mess.* The contraceptive jelly used with a diaphragm causes a little more mess than some of the other birth-control methods. Some couples find this helpful because of the extra lubrication; other couples can't stand it. If you or your husband do not like the mess, don't use the diaphragm method.

*Dislike of the odor.* Some women and some husbands find the odor of contraceptive jelly offensive. If you or your husband feel this way, switch to a different technique, or try a different type of jelly.

*Irritation.* Some women experience irritation from contraceptive jelly. I have not had a patient with a true allergy to such medications, but I have had many patients who were irritated (or whose husbands were irritated) by the contraceptive jelly. If this is a problem for you and changing to a different jelly does not help, don't use a diaphragm.

*Fear of pregnancy.* The diaphragm is not the most effective method of contraception. If you feel you absolutely must not get pregnant, do not use a diaphragm for protection. You will be constantly worried about pregnancy and this will affect sexual relations with your husband. Choose another method.

*Urinary-tract infections.* Use of the diaphragm can cause some women to develop bladder infections. Apparently the pressure of the diaphragm on the bladder is the cause of this. If you continually have urinary-tract infections of your bladder or kidney, be sure your doctor knows you use a diaphragm. Even if the doctor doubts that there is an association, you might stop using the diaphragm and see if there is any improvement. Be sure to use an alternate form of contraception during that time.

*Effect on fertility.* There are no effects on future fertility with the use of the diaphragm. And recent research has also shown that there is no harmful effect on babies conceived while a couple is using a diaphragm and jelly.

---

## 1051 Are there any disadvantages to the diaphragm?

Pregnancy is the primary disadvantage! When you use the diaphragm, you must consider the "risks" of using it as equivalent to the risks of being pregnant, including the medical complications that can accompany any pregnancy. Of course, when a couple wants to have a baby, they find the risks that can accompany pregnancy acceptable.

A minor disadvantage of the diaphragm is that it must be refitted if you have had a baby, if you have gained or lost more than twenty pounds, or if your diaphragm becomes uncomfortable.

With diaphragm use there seems to be increased chance of developing urinary tract infections. Occasionally toxic shock syndrome has been associated with the use of a diaphragm. In that situation, a doctor would recommend discontinuing the use of a diaphragm.

## 1052 What are the advantages of the diaphragm?

There are several advantages to using a diaphragm.

Except for the risks listed in Q. 1051, a diaphragm is completely safe.

A diaphragm is used only during intercourse. It therefore does not affect a woman's body at any other time.

If you have intercourse during your menstrual period, there is less mess because the diaphragm will hold the menstrual blood.

With diaphragm use, as with other "barrier" contraceptive techniques, there appears to be a decreased chance of acquiring a sexually transmitted disease. The contraceptive jelly not only kills sperm, it also kills some germs.

## 1053 Does a diaphragm require any special care?

Yes. After removing the diaphragm from your vagina, you should wash it with soap and water, rinse it well, dry it off, and place it back in its container. A light dusting of corn starch may be used. Avoid the use of talc which may contain irritants. Air and light can cause the rubber of a diaphragm to become brittle. A diaphragm is usable as long as the rubber is soft and pliable and it does not have holes in it. Diaphragms often last for many years.

## Contraceptive Foam

## 1054 What is contraceptive foam?

Contraceptive foam is a "barrier" type of contraceptive, which means that it kills sperm before they can get into the cervix. The foam coats the cervix and vagina, killing sperm that come in contact with it.

When the medication is taken out of its container into the vaginal applicator, it foams up. The advantage of foam is that it spreads out in the vagina and covers the cervix effectively. A contraceptive jelly will not spread as effectively as foam and will accumulate in one part of the vagina, failing to block the access of sperm to the cervix.

## 1055 How is contraceptive foam used?

After the medication is put in the applicator, the applicator is inserted into the vagina and the medication ejected into the vaginal canal. Ideally this should be done at least ten or fifteen minutes before intercourse so that the foam can spread around in the vagina.

However, the foam should not be put into the vagina more than thirty minutes before intercourse because it can begin draining out and have less contraceptive effect.

Most women do not feel the need for douching after using the foam. The medication seems to absorb into the body after intercourse and does not produce as much of a mess in the vulvar area as contraceptive jelly does.

## 1056 Does contraceptive foam produce any undesirable effects on intercourse?

Yes, there are a few drawbacks to the use of this method of contraception, which may bother some couples.

A couple often must stop sex play in order to insert the foam into the vagina.

The foam is messy, and some couples do not like that.

An additional plunger of foam must be inserted into the vagina before repeating intercourse.

## 1057 What is the chance of pregnancy when using contraceptive foam?

The chance of pregnancy is considered to be greater than that with the diaphragm or the condom. About ten to twenty pregnancies per hundred women can be expected to occur each year.

In order to minimize the risk, my advice to a couple who use foam for contraception is that they use it every time they have intercourse except during the bleeding of a menstrual period. In addition, during the week around the time of ovulation, the man should use a rubber or the woman a diaphragm. If a couple really wants to be sure that the woman does not get pregnant, they should use a condom plus foam or a diaphragm plus foam every time they have intercourse.

## 1058 Are there women who cannot use the foam?

There are three groups of women who might find another birth-control method more acceptable.

Women who are sensitive to the foam should not use it. I normally recommend Delfen Vaginal Foam. Some women (and men) find this irritating. If you find it so, try a different brand.

Couples who are not disciplined enough to use the foam regularly, especially those who will not stop and insert it after foreplay has started.

Women who feel they absolutely must not get pregnant because foam is not a totally reliable contraceptive, even when properly used.

## 1059 Are there effects on future fertility or on a pregnancy conceived during use of the foam?

The foam does not affect subsequent fertility and a woman can become pregnant immediately if she stops using the foam. Recent studies have shown no relationship between abnormalities in babies and the use of foam, even if pregnancy occurred during the use of contraceptive foam.

## 1060 What are the disadvantages to using contraceptive foam?

The following might be considered disadvantages:

high pregnancy rate

may be irritating

requires discipline

many people dislike the "mess"

### 1061 What are the advantages of contraceptive foam?

The real advantage of the contraceptive foam is that it can be conveniently available at bedside and can be inserted immediately. This allows great spontaneity of intercourse with a fair degree of contraception.

In addition, it seems to decrease the chance of contracting sexually transmitted disease; the foam not only kills sperm, it also kills germs. If your sexual partner might have such a disease, you are less likely to get it from him if you are using foam.

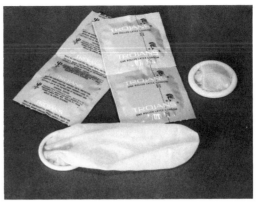

A condom, or rubber

## Condoms

### 1062 What are condoms, or rubbers?

A rubber (condom) is a contraceptive device used by a man; it fits onto his erect penis tightly enough to stay in place during intercourse, keeping the semen from getting into a woman's vagina. If a rubber has a hole in it or if it breaks during intercourse, the possibility of pregnancy is as great as if no contraception had been used.

Direct from the package, a rubber looks much like a miniature diaphragm; when unrolled it looks like a wiener-shaped balloon.

### 1063 How is a condom used?

A condom can be put on the erect penis immediately before intercourse. It is important, however, that a couple realizes that a man's penis may ooze a little semen before ejaculation, and that even small amounts of sperm deposited at the vaginal opening can result in a pregnancy. Therefore, it is extremely important that the husband's erect penis make no contact with the opening of the vagina without having the condom on.

### 1064 What effects does a condom have on intercourse?

Many women do not mind their husband using a condom, but most men do not like them because they lessen sensation during intercourse. Some condoms are available, made of a thinner material than rubber. They allow the man greater sensation. These are, of course, more expensive.

### 1065 What is the risk of pregnancy with a condom?

The chance of pregnancy with a condom is between ten and twenty per hundred women per year. The higher rates are for those couples who do not use the condoms as carefully as they should.

If a couple wants to use condoms as their primary contraceptive, I suggest they use them with every act of intercourse except during the actual bleeding of a period. In addition, during the week around ovulation, they should use a plunger of foam or a diaphragm along with the rubber. If a couple wants to be the most safe, they will use condoms and foam every time they have intercourse.

## 1066 Does a condom have a risk for subsequent fertility?

No, it is possible to achieve pregnancy with the next act of intercourse if no condom is used.

## 1067 What are the disadvantages to using condoms?

There are several undesirable side effects of condom use.

*Irritation.* Irritation of genital tissues may be a problem. If a couple finds a condom irritating, a different brand of condom may solve the problem.

*Effects on spontaneity.* A man must wait until he has an erection before he can put on the condom. Many people do not like this interference with their spontaneity.

*Lessened sensation.* Men often do not have adequate sensation with a condom. They often describe it as feeling like taking a shower while wearing a raincoat!

*Semen leak.* If a man and wife enjoy lying together after intercourse, the man's penis becomes flaccid. This allows the condom to leak semen that could cause a woman to become pregnant. It is important that once intercourse is over, the man withdraw to prevent the condom from leaking its contents into the vagina.

## 1068 What are the advantages to condom use?

The condom is immediately usable. It can be kept in the bedside table, in a suitcase, or in a purse or wallet. If a woman is planning to get up immediately after intercourse and does not want to have semen dripping from her vagina, she may want her husband to use a condom for that particular episode of intercourse.

In addition, the condom not only captures the sperm that comes from a man, it also catches his secretions if he has a sexually transmitted disease. Withdrawal immediately after intercourse is necessary for this to have any prophylactic effect against STD.

## 1069 What should be done if a condom breaks?

When a condom is put on, a half-inch of space should be left between the end of the penis and the end of the condom. This allows space for the ejaculate when it leaves the penis. A condom properly used is less likely to break.

If the condom breaks or if the man does not withdraw immediately, insert a plunger of foam into the vagina to try to kill any sperm that might have escaped. This will decrease the possibility of pregnancy from such an incident but will not totally prevent any chance of pregnancy.

## The Contraceptive Sponge

## 1070 What is a contraceptive sponge?

This contraceptive is just what its name implies: a sponge used as a contraceptive device. Strangely, the first birth-control method in recorded history was a sponge (used by women of ancient Egypt). And the "newest" nonexperimental contraceptive method (at the time of this writing) is a sponge.

While the ancient contraceptive sponge was simply an animal sponge, the modern sponge is made of a soft polyurethane material. It is approximately two inches in diameter and is impregnated with a contraceptive chemical that kills sperm on contact. (See illustration.)

The contraceptive sponge works in several ways, but primarily by releasing its chemical into the vaginal secretions. This chemical then kills any sperm that get into the vagina. The sponge does not act only as a barrier or as a spermicide; it also absorbs, traps, and kills sperm *before* they can reach the cervix. Because the sponge allows, in a sense, a time-release of the chemical, it can be put into the vagina many hours before intercourse and still be effective.

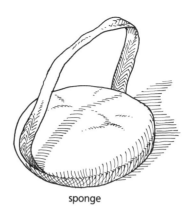

sponge

### 1071 How is the contraceptive sponge used?

The contraceptive sponge is moistened with water and folded enough to allow insertion into the vagina. It is put in so that the flat ribbon on the back serves as a handle for removal. The sponge can be worn for up to thirty hours but it must stay in place for at least six hours after intercourse to be effective. If you are going to leave it in for thirty hours, the last time you would want to have intercourse using that particular sponge should be no later than twenty-four hours after insertion.

### 1072 Does the sponge have any effect on intercourse?

Some women do not like the "full" feeling that the sponge produces, and some men do not like the feeling of the sponge in a woman's vagina. Other than this, the sponge really does not affect intercourse.

### 1073 What is the chance of pregnancy with a contraceptive sponge?

Of one hundred women who use the sponge for a year, about ten will get pregnant.

In order to minimize the risk, I advise patients to use the sponge just as they would a diaphragm or rubber. They should have the sponge in place every time they have intercourse except during the actual menstrual bleeding. During the week of ovulation they should use a condom along with the sponge.

### 1074 Who cannot use the sponge?

A woman who is sensitive to the chemical in the sponge cannot use it. Only about 2–3 percent of women develop an irritation from the sponge.

### 1075 What are the effects of the sponge on future fertility?

There are no effects on fertility from the use of the sponge.

### 1076 What are the disadvantages of using the contraceptive sponge?

Irritation from the chemicals and the risk of pregnancy are the most common drawbacks. In addition, some women have difficulty removing the sponge. Occasionally it will turn while it is in the vagina so that the handle is not in the right place. This is not dangerous. A woman merely needs to squat and bear down as though she were trying to have a bowel movement. This pushes the sponge down toward the vaginal opening so that she can flip it around, grab the loop, and pull it out. If this is not possible, the woman can go to her physician and have the sponge removed.

There is one extremely rare but possible side effect: the possibility of toxic shock. There have been a few sponge users who have developed toxic shock syndrome. The number, however, is extremely small when compared with the total number of women who have used the sponge. There is, in fact, a suggestion that the sponge may actually protect against this disease by killing the Staphylococcus aureus germs that cause toxic shock. Only time and future research will tell which is right.

## 1077 What are the advantages of sponge use?

The primary advantage of the sponge is that it can be inserted, left in place, and "forgotten" for a period of up to twenty-four hours before intercourse. Another advantage is that there appears to be a decreased chance of contracting a sexually transmitted disease, because the chemicals in the sponge not only kill sperm but also kill germs.

## Contraceptive Suppositories, Cervical Caps, and Injections

## 1078 What are contraceptive vaginal suppositories?

Contraceptive vaginal suppositories came on the market with great fanfare several years ago. They were touted as being the ultimate contraceptive, but they have not worked out that way. The primary problem with this method of birth control is a pregnancy rate that is about 10–20 percent per year, no better than the contraceptive foam.

The discussion in this chapter concerning the use of contraceptive foam applies almost word for word to the use of the suppositories. (See Q. 1054–1061.) If a woman prefers the suppository to the foam, she should use it instead of the foam. She should not use the suppository as her only contraceptive device, unless she does not mind getting pregnant.

If the suppository is used, it should be inserted with every act of intercourse except during actual menstrual flow. To increase its effectiveness a rubber, diaphragm, or contraceptive foam should be used with it during the week of ovulation.

## 1079 If I become pregnant while using a sponge, foam, or jelly, will this have any effect on my baby?

Studies to this point have indicated that there is no harm to babies whose mothers conceived while using these contraceptives.

## 1080 What is a cervical cap?

The cervical cap is a miniature diaphragm that fits over a woman's cervix, much like a condom fits on a man's penis. It simply acts as a barrier to the sperm getting into the cervix.

At present the FDA has restricted the use of the cervical cap to clinics or individual physicians who are complying with the research protocol. A list of the current cap providers can be obtained from the National Women's Health Network in Washington, D.C.

The cap has not been used widely in this

country. I have had few patients in my years of practice who have tried one. Its lack of popularity is probably related to the problems with the technique itself, the difficulty of finding a doctor who fits caps, and to its presently being an experimental technique.

To use a cervical cap, a woman must be able to feel her cervix, fit the cap onto her cervix, and be confident that it will stay there. A woman who cannot reach her cervix or cannot get the cap to stay on her cervix obviously cannot use it.

Those who advocate the cap feel that its primary advantage is that it can be left in place for from three to seven days and requires no extra contraceptive medication or device. They also say that since the cap is smaller, it interferes less with the sensation of intercourse than a diaphragm or contraceptive medication and will produce less pressure on a woman's urethra or bladder than a diaphragm.

My opinion is that the cap will never become a popular technique, primarily because of the difficulty most women have in locating their cervix. In addition, worry about whether or not the cervical cap is staying in place would keep most women from being comfortable with its use.

---

## 1081  What about contraceptive shots?

If a woman is given an injection of 150 mg of Depo-Provera, a long-acting progesterone, she will not become pregnant for three months. Studies have shown that the pregnancy rates with Depo-Provera are similar to the pregnancy rates with birth-control pills.

There are several problems with using Depo-Provera for contraception.

It has not been fully approved by the FDA. Except in unusual circumstances, your doctor cannot suggest it to you nor prescribe it for contraception. In 1984 it was approved for use in Great Britain.

Women who have had a shot of Depo-Provera may be unable to get pregnant for a much longer time than three months. Occasionally a woman will not resume her periods for as long as a year after a Depo-Provera injection. If a woman has plans for pregnancy in the next few years, she should absolutely not consider Depo-Provera as a contraceptive.

Women who receive Depo-Provera may have spotting or bleeding all the time or they may have no periods at all for many months.

Once Depo-Provera is injected into a woman's body, there is no way to remove it. She must allow her body to complete the absorption of the drug before its effect will be gone.

---

## Natural Family Planning

---

## 1082  Is natural family planning, the "rhythm method," effective for birth control?

The term *natural family planning* is now used instead of the "rhythm method" because this method of contraception employs the same techniques that are useful for becoming pregnant. Natural family planning implies control over both when one becomes pregnant and when one will not.

The first warning I give couples using this technique is that it does not work well if a woman's menstrual periods are irregular. For this purpose, I apply the word *irregularity* to anyone whose periods vary by more than one week from month to month.

With natural family planning, couples refrain from intercourse when they think an egg has recently been released, or is about to be released, by the woman's body. If there is no egg free in the body, there can be no pregnancy. The goal of this technique therefore, is for the couple to learn how to know when ovulation occurs so that no intercourse takes place around that time.

A key issue in the use of natural family planning is that only a small percent of women are absolutely regular in their menstrual cycles. A couple must therefore not have intercourse within two days of any predicted ovulation time.

A final factor to consider is that a woman who is normally quite regular can suddenly ovulate early or late in her cycle. A woman who uses natural family planning as a contraceptive can become pregnant if she has such an untimely ovulation.

The essence of this technique is that a couple must be able to predict when the wife is going to ovulate. If such prediction is not possible, then the technique will not work.

## 1083   How is natural family planning used?

A couple may use several different techniques to determine when the woman is ovulating. They can use one or all three of these to help them decide when it is safe to have intercourse.

*Recording the menstrual cycle.* With this method a woman records on a calendar when her periods come. Over a span of several months she can determine how regular they are. Many women are surprised when they actually record the occurrence of their periods as they often find that their cycles are much different (more regular or more irregular) from what they had thought.

*Basal body temperature.* This technique involves the purchase of a basal body thermometer (available at most pharmacies) and the use of that thermometer every morning. A woman shakes down the thermometer, puts it at her bedside, and, when she awakens in the morning, takes her temperature for five minutes and records it on the chart. A Basal Body Temperature Chart makes it much easier to keep a temperature record. These charts can be obtained from your physician or pharmacist. (See Q. 898 and accompanying illustration.)

About halfway through her cycle, a woman will notice a rise in her temperature. This happens when one ovary puts out progesterone at ovulation time. The body's response to this progesterone production is an elevation in temperature, which occurs just after ovulation.

*Evaluation of cervical mucus.* A woman can insert her fingers in her vagina, and with her second and third fingers gather some of the mucus coming from her cervix. By learning what her mucus looks like over a period of two or three months, a woman can learn to determine what type of mucus she puts out at the time of ovulation. Normally, just before and at ovulation time the cervical mucus will be much more abundant, much more watery and clear, and much more "stretchable" than at other times during the menstrual cycle.

*Pain with ovulation.* Many women feel low abdominal pain at the time of ovulation. Some women do not notice it, but many women who have not noticed it before will be aware of it when they are watching for it. This discomfort, caused by the egg coming out of the ovary, is called *mittelschmerz,* or "mid-pain."

*Cervical dilatation.* When a woman is checking her cervical mucus, she can also feel the cervical opening. This opening dilates from the end of the menstruation up to the time of ovulation and then contracts down again. A woman can feel this change and record it on her chart along with her temperatures and cervical mucus changes.

*Other symptoms.* There are a couple of other less common symptoms of ovulation. These can be slight spotting of blood at midcycle and/or breast discomfort, often a prickling or tingling sensation.

By observing the changes that occur in her body on a month-to-month basis, a woman can determine fairly accurately when she ovulates. Thereafter, by avoiding intercourse for two days before any possible early ovulation and for two days after any possible late ovulation, she can usually avoid pregnancy.

## 1084 What effect does family planning have on a sexual relationship?

Natural family planning can have a good effect in that both the husband and the wife are cooperating in family planning. It can have a deleterious effect in that there is a period of time each month during which they must not have intercourse if they want to avoid pregnancy. This discipline is more difficult for some couples than for others.

## 1085 What are the chances of pregnancy with natural family planning?

Studies have shown that a couple's chance of pregnancy varies greatly. The couples most likely to achieve pregnancy are those who do not have good instruction in the technique of natural family planning or who do not have the discipline to abide by it, or whose female partner does not have totally regular periods. Of these couples, as many as twenty or thirty out of every hundred conceive over a period of one year's time.

## 1086 Who should not rely on natural family planning as a method of birth control?

There are several contraindications to the use of natural family planning. First of all,

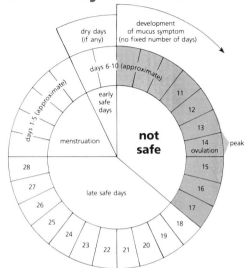

**Chart for Identifying "Safe" Days for Intercourse**

women who feel they absolutely must not get pregnant would be best served by another method of birth control.

In addition, those couples who do not have the discipline to abstain from intercourse at a specific time each month should not use natural family planning.

Finally, women who have irregular menstrual periods should not use this technique because they cannot determine when ovulation will occur. This includes women who produce poor cervical mucus, who have no symptoms of ovulation, and whose temperature charts are not easily interpreted, since they would find this technique extremely difficult to use.

## 1087 What are the effects of natural family planning on subsequent fertility?

The effects of natural family planning on future fertility are great! Not only does a couple do nothing that would interfere with future fertility, they also learn a great deal about the woman's fertile time. When they do want to have a baby, they may be much more capable of achieving pregnancy.

## 1088 Where can I obtain further information on natural family planning?

Ingrid Trobisch's book, *The Joy of Being a Woman* (Harper & Row), has an excellent description of natural family planning (pp. 33ff). In addition, The Natural Family Planning Federation of America, Inc., Suite A, 1221 Massachusetts Avenue, N.W., Washington, D.C. 20005, can provide information.

## Alternative Methods of Contraception

## 1089 What are "counterfeit" contraceptive techniques?

There are procedures many couples think of as contraception that are totally "counterfeit." Such techniques are totally ineffective, and if a couple continues to practice them pregnancy will often result. If a couple who uses one of these techniques has not conceived, it is only because they simply do not achieve pregnancy easily. Any healthy, normal, fertile couple who uses these techniques will be expectant parents sooner or later—and probably sooner.

These are ineffective contraception techniques.

*Douching.* Douching does not protect against pregnancy. Many sperm are in the cervical mucus within seconds of intercourse. Douching cannot wash this sperm-laden mucus out of the cervix. Pregnancy can certainly occur.

*Withdrawal (coitus interruptus).* This term refers to a man's withdrawing his penis from a woman's vagina before he ejaculates. This is not a good contraceptive technique, since some semen is released before ejaculation and this material—even at the entrance of a woman's vagina—can cause her to become pregnant.

An additional problem with this is that a man must maintain excellent control. His penis must be totally outside of his wife's vagina, and directed away from her vulva, before he ejaculates. Obviously a big minus to this technique is that intercourse is interrupted by a sudden separation just at the point of maximum pleasure.

*Plastic or other material used as a condom.* These materials (sandwich bags, plastic wrap) were not made for this purpose. The activity of intercourse can break them or they can leak, allowing conception to occur.

*Feminine hygiene materials.* None of the products sold for "feminine hygiene" (douches, deodorants, or other similar products) is effective for contraception.

*Breast-feeding.* Women often do not ovulate during the months they breast-feed, but a woman can start ovulating during this time. Remember, a woman ovulates before she has a period. She cannot wait, therefore, for a period to occur before she begins using contraceptives. She may have already ovulated and become pregnant, without having a period since her baby's delivery.

*No orgasm.* An orgasm is not necessary for pregnancy to occur. Women become pregnant with or without orgasm.

*Intercourse during a menstrual period.* I have implied several times in this chapter that a woman will not get pregnant during her menstrual period. In order to be absolutely correct, however, I must say that although I have never known a woman who conceived during her period, such a thing is possible. This is such a genuinely rare occurrence that I still say it is safe to have unprotected intercourse during a menstrual period. If you want to be absolutely, 100 percent sure you do not get pregnant, however, it is best to use contraception even during your menstrual flow.

## 1090 What about the morning-after pill—is there an effective one?

Gynecologists are frequently asked to supply a pill to use the morning after unprotected intercourse. These pills usually consist of an estrogen-type substance. Such medication taken the day after intercourse has been found to prevent conception most of the time. Recently, a combination of an estrogen and a progesterone, identical to that found in an Ovral birth-control pill and taken two times twelve hours apart, has sometimes been found to work as a morning-after pill if started within seventy-two hours of intercourse. Since no morning-after pill works every time (studies indicate it fails about 20 percent of the time), most doctors stopped providing them. They were concerned that such medications taken at such an early time in a pregnancy could damage the child. DES was commonly used as a morning-after pill until it was found that DES caused abnormalities in children born to mothers who had taken it during pregnancy. Although DES is a synthetic estrogen, its bad record made all estrogen administration suspect during pregnancy.

## 1091 Is abstinence a viable contraceptive method?

Abstinence is the only method of contraception, except for hysterectomy, that is 100 percent effective. It is not, however, one of the more popular methods of birth control, nor is it a healthy one for married couples. For those who are not married, abstinence has other great advantages. (See Q. 1145.)

## 1092 What are "silicone plugs"?

Silicone plugs are used to "plug up" the fallopian tubes, preventing the passage of an egg into the uterus and possibly preventing the sperm swimming up the fallopian tube to meet the egg.

When this technique was first introduced, it was seen as a permanent contraceptive, but one which might possibly be reversible.

With this technique both fallopian tubes are plugged by pushing silicone rubber, in liquid form, into the tube. A small bead of silicone forms inside the uterus, and from it a small thread of silicone leads to another bead at the other end of the fallopian tube. The two beads on either end keep the thread of silicone in place in the tube, effectively plugging it. The plug conforms to the inside space of the fallopian tube as the material hardens, blocking it without distorting it or sticking to the tissues.

The procedure is franchised but has not yet been approved by the FDA for general use. At this time it is considered a research technique, and its use is limited to clinics or individual physicians who are complying with research protocol.

## 1093 How are silicone plugs put in?

For insertion of the silicone plugs, a woman is first given a paracervical block, an injection of local anesthetic at the upper end of the vagina on either side of the cervix. This injection numbs the uterus so that manipulation can be done without significant pain.

The doctor dilates the woman's cervix enough to allow a hysteroscope (a small viewing instrument) through her cervix and into her uterus, so that the inside of the uterus can be seen. After locating the openings of the fallopian tubes, the doctor holds a hollow instrument against one of those openings and then forces the liquid silicone into the fallopian tube, where it quickly hardens into a plug. When this process has been repeated on the other side, X-rays are taken to prove that the plugs are in place. If they are, the procedure is over.

About 25 percent of the time the doctor will not succeed in plugging the tubes on the first try, in which case the procedure is repeated. A doctor will be unable to plug the tubes in about 10 percent of women, even after a second try.

## 1094  Are there side effects to the silicone plugs?

Complications from the effects of the silicone plugs have been minor. Pelvic pain has been reported; doctors have perforated the uterus in an attempt to do the procedure; and some women have irregularity of their menstrual periods as a result of having silicone plugs in their tubes. Generally, however, women who have these plugs do not have any problems. Currently, some patients have had plugs in place for over ten years.

## 1095  What is the chance of pregnancy with a silicone plug?

There have been a few pregnancies in women who have had the silicone plugs inserted. In one study, 338 women had the procedure attempted, 309 had proper plug formation from the procedure, and of these women only 3 became pregnant.

## 1096  Who cannot use the silicone plug technique for contraception?

Some women should not use this method of birth control.

Women who have, or have recently had, infections in their uterus or tubes.

Women with a great deal of scarring in the pelvis, which makes the uterus too immobile for the procedure.

Women in whom the doctor cannot find the opening of the fallopian tube when he or she checks the uterus with the hysteroscope.

Women with malignancy of any of the pelvic organs.

Women who have not completed their families—because the plugs may produce some degree of infertility.

## 1097  What are the advantages of the silicone plug?

The silicone plug is good for several reasons.

It does not require an incision for insertion.

It is an office procedure done under local anesthesia.

It is probably less damaging to the fallopian tube than the usual sterilization procedure done with surgery.

It can be removed or can stay in place permanently.

After the initial insertion, a couple does not have to bother with any other form of contraception.

## 1098 Are there any disadvantages to the silicone plugs?

Yes, there are many disadvantages to using the plugs.

*Still considered experimental.* Insertion of the plugs is classified as an experimental procedure. This means it is not a completely evaluated technique.

*Pain.* Even with the use of a paracervical block, insertion of the plugs is a painful procedure, though not usually intolerable.

*Difficult or impossible insertion.* A doctor will be unable to insert the plugs in 10 percent of women who undergo the procedure. It is frustrating to travel to a specific location for the procedure, go through the entire process, and not have the plugs successfully inserted.

*Limited availability.* Because it is still experimental, the procedure is available in only a limited number of locations in the United States.

*Pregnancy.* No birth-control method is 100-percent effective; this one is no exception.

*Losing the plug.* Aproximately 11 women of the group of 309 mentioned earlier had the plugs fall out.

*Infertility.* Very few pregnancies have occurred in women who have had their plugs removed. The plugs may produce some degree of infertility.

The disadvantages outweigh the advantages of this procedure in the opinion of most physicians. Few physicians think the silicone plugs will ever become popular.

## Sterilization

## 1099 What is sterilization?

A sterilization procedure is an operation done on a person's reproductive organs to make pregnancy impossible.

Such a procedure can be a great asset to a couple's sexual relationship. After sterilization they can have intercourse without fear of pregnancy and yet without the bother of birth-control pills, foam, rubbers, or diaphragms. Many women even find that their sexual responsiveness improves after sterilization.

## 1100 What are the methods of sterilization?

The methods of sterilization are:

*Tubal sterilization.* A woman may have surgery on her tubes so that an egg from her ovary and sperm are unable to make contact.

*Vasectomy.* A man may have the vas tied off, which prevents the sperm produced in his testicles from getting into the upper part of his body and eventually being ejaculated during intercourse.

*Hysterectomy.* Removal of a woman's uterus is a very effective contraceptive technique. Hysterectomy is the only absolutely 100-percent effective sterilization procedure, except for removal of a woman's ovaries, removal of a man's testicles, or abstinence. If a woman has "female problems" and is considering hysterectomy anyway, the desire not to have more children can be the deciding factor in choosing to proceed with a hysterectomy.

## 1101 When should I consider sterilization as a means of birth control?

First, you may have a medical problem, such as heart disease or severe diabetes which makes it dangerous for you to become pregnant. You, your husband, and your doctor would come to a joint conclusion to avoid pregnancy if these circumstances exist. Fortunately these life-threatening emergencies are rare.

Secondly, you and/or your husband may

have a problem with your genes that dramatically increases the possibility of having an abnormal child. Before having a sterilization for this reason, seek out expert genetic counseling.

Finally, you and your husband may have firmly decided that under no circumstances do you want more children.

You will probably know when you have come to the time in life when you are ready for sterilization. It is much like the decision to get married; it is both intellectual and emotional. Women who have not gotten married often ask how you know when you have met the right man, and the answer is, "You just know!" Sterilization is the same type of situation. All the intellectual facts may add up, but you should not have a sterilization done before you are emotionally ready.

Weigh your decision to have a sterilization carefully. Although sterilization reversal surgery can be performed, it is not always effective. For example, 20–25 percent of women who have had a tubal ligation reversed still do not get pregnant, and the longer a man has had his vas tied off, the less likely he is to have a successful reversal.

---

## 1102 What are some situations that could lead me to have a sterilization done now that I might regret later?

Some of them are:

*Dislike of other birth-control methods.* Occasionally a woman will want sterilization because she does not like using other methods of contraception. Sterilization, however, should be done because a woman never wants another child, not because she dislikes her present method of birth control. Compared to the devastation that comes into a woman's life when she realizes after sterilization that she wants another child, a little inconvenience with a birth-control method seems unimportant.

*Pursuing a career.* Many women begin the pursuit of a career believing that it is their only calling in life. There may be nothing wrong with feeling this way, but there is the possibility of a change of mind or lifestyle later on. If a woman has been sterilized while "pursuing a career," she may never be able to have a child if she changes her mind in the future.

*Youth.* I have seen many women in their early twenties who, after having had a child or two, had a sterilization performed. Unfortunately, many times such women have been divorced or widowed and remarried or have lost a child and wanted to have more children. These women often admit that they were too young and immature to have made the previous decision.

Statistics show that people who have a sterilization when they are below the age of thirty are more likely to want that sterilization reversed later. If you are in this age group and are considering sterilization, be cautious as you make the final decision to have the procedure performed. If you have any doubts about it, don't have it done.

*Fear of pregnancy.* Many people let fear of pregnancy frighten them into having a sterilization done. Sterilization, however, should be based on the decision never to have more children, not just on fear of becoming pregnant. Reliable birth-control methods are available that prevent pregnancy and at the same time allow normal fertility when discontinued.

*Emotional upheaval.* Many women have a sterilization done during a time of upheaval in their lives. Such women often decide as soon as one or two years later to have the sterilization reversed. I strongly encourage a woman not to have a sterilization done if she is in the middle of emotional trauma.

---

## 1103 Who should be sterilized, me or my husband?

Perhaps it is because I am a gynecologist that I tend to feel that it is best for the woman to

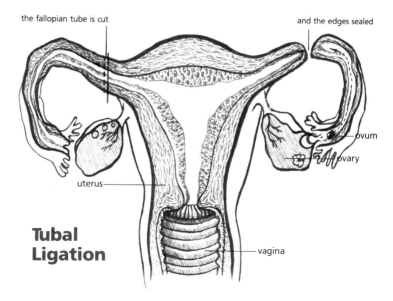

the fallopian tube is cut

and the edges sealed

ovum

ovary

uterus

**Tubal Ligation**

vagina

have the sterilization. She is the one whose body bears the risks inherent in pregnancy. If she is sterilized, she no longer has to worry about the risk, even if she loses her husband by divorce or death and remarries. If the husband is the one who has the sterilization and the woman enters into a new marriage, she must again consider what she wants to do about her fertility. While considering that she might become pregnant.

Most studies show that a vasectomy is more likely to fail than a tubal ligation. About one in a hundred men produce an accidental pregnancy after having been sterilized, whereas after a tubal ligation only about one in five hundred women will become pregnant.

## 1104   What is tubal sterilization?

Tubal sterilization, or tubal ligation, is now the most common method of sterilization for women in the United States. It is a procedure done to block the fallopian tubes so that an egg cannot pass through them to be fertilized. If the tubes are closed, a woman cannot get pregnant. (See Q. 1114, 1115.)

There are many different ways to have a

tubal ligation done, but all of them require some type of surgery. The next few questions discuss techniques for accomplishing tubal sterilization.

## 1105   What is an interval sterilization and how is it done?

An interval sterilization is one performed at some time other than immediately following a delivery. It is usually done through an abdominal incision.

When I entered practice, the only reliable way to perform a sterilization procedure on a woman was through a large abdominal incision. Since this was a major operation, it was not often done. Vasectomy was so much easier that most couples who wanted sterilization chose that route.

These days the abdominal incision method is outdated and unnecessary. If your doctor says he or she must make a larger than one inch abdominal incision to sterilize you, I suggest that you find a doctor who will do either a minilaparotomy or laparoscopy sterilization, as described in the next four questions.

## 1106 How is a laparoscopy sterilization done? Why is it called Band-Aid surgery?

Laparoscopy sterilization is the most commonly used technique for sterilizing women today. It is performed by using a special viewing instrument (laparoscope) inserted into the abdomen. It is not major surgery, and the patient can usually go home from the hospital the same day the surgery is performed. The procedure can be done with a local anesthetic, but general anesthesia is normally used.

Laparoscopy is sometimes called Band-Aid surgery, because the incisions required can be covered by a Band-Aid.

To do this surgery, the doctor dilates the cervix and inserts an instrument into the uterus to lift it to be able to reach under the uterus to get to the tubes. A small needle is inserted just under the umbilicus (navel), through which two or three quarts of carbon dioxide gas are allowed to flow into the abdomen. This lifts the wall of the abdomen off the intestines, so the operating instruments can be safely inserted into the abdominal cavity.

Most doctors use the "double puncture" technique, which requires two incisions. One is made just above the pubic hair line (about one-third inch long), and the other is made just under the navel (about a half inch long). After the laparoscope is inserted through the higher incision, it is used to observe the pelvic structures. Operating instruments, which are used to work on the tubes, are inserted through the lower incision. (See Q. 907.)

After the tubes have been blocked by cautery, clip, or band (see the following question), the instruments are removed, the gas is allowed to escape, and the incisions are closed.

I normally scrape the lining of the uterus at this time (a D&C) and send a sample to a pathologist. Since the cervix is already di-

## Skin Incisions for Laparoscopy Sterilization

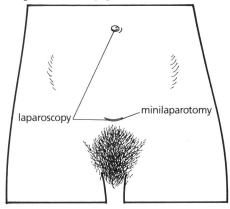

lated and the instrument is already in the uterus, it is a convenient time to test for premalignant or malignant tissue in the uterus. If the tissue is normal, the woman could feel confident that any uterine bleeding she had during the next year or two was not caused by cancer, because cancer does not develop that fast. Many doctors do not do this D&C. They feel that the cost of the tissue examination by the pathologist is not worth it, since the tissue will be normal for most women. However, most physicians do not charge extra if they do this type of D&C.

You may resume having intercourse without worrying about a possible pregnancy as soon as it is comfortable for you to do so.

## 1107 How are the tubes blocked during a laparoscopy?

There are three techniques that are used to block the fallopian tubes during a sterilization procedure.

*Cautery.* Cauterization is done to keep the tubes from bleeding when they are cut. After this electrocoagulation has been completed, each tube is cut through where the burn was made, usually about a third of the way from the uterus to the end of the tube.

*Hulka clips.* These are small clips with a copper spring. They are placed over the middle part of the tube and closed. Pressure keeps the blood flow from going through the part of the tube inside the clip. That part of the tube dies, separating the tubes into two sections.

*Falope rings:* A Falope ring is a rubber-band-shaped piece of silicone that is put around a "knuckled-up" portion of the tube. Such a ring is so tight that it cuts off the blood supply, causing the part of the tube it encircles to die thus dividing the tube.

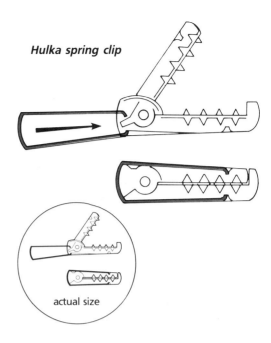

**Hulka spring clip**

actual size

### 1108 What is a minilaparotomy and how is it done?

A minilaparotomy is a sterilization procedure done without a telescopic instrument such as is used for laparoscopy. Only one incision is made for minilap sterilization, and it is a larger incision than that which is necessary for the laparoscopy techniques.

For this procedure the doctor makes a small incision just above the pubis and using a special instrument inserted into the uterus, pushes the uterus up against the wall of the abdomen just under the incision. With small instruments the doctor reaches into the incision, pulls the fallopian tubes up through the hole, and then ties and cuts them. This procedure usually is done under general anesthesia, though it is possible to do it with a local.

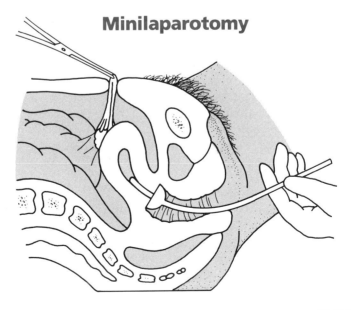

## Minilaparotomy

## 1109 What is the recovery from a laparoscopy or a minilaparotomy like?

Normally you will be able to go home the afternoon of the day you have the surgery performed. You should be on a liquid diet that evening and have someone stay with you through the evening and night. That night you should get up only to go to the bathroom. Getting up too often can cause small, residual bubbles of air or carbon dioxide gas to rise up under your diaphragm and cause pain that you would feel in your shoulders. This is called referred pain; it comes from the diaphragm, but is felt in the shoulders. Even if you stay down as you are supposed to, you may experience some shoulder pains, but this is normal.

Your doctor will probably have given you prescriptions for pain and for nausea, which often occurs after general anesthesia. The pain pills can be helpful for the discomfort from the incisions, the shoulder pain, or for the uterine cramping that occasionally occurs after this operation.

It is normal to have a little oozing of blood from the incisions, and it is also normal to bleed from the vagina for as long as a week or two after the procedure.

Starting the day after surgery, you can do whatever you feel like doing, though some women do not feel like doing much. I have had patients ranging from one extreme to the other. One patient went to a party the night of her surgery, but several did not feel well for two weeks after surgery. These latter women were not hurting; they were merely tired and sleepy from the anesthesia.

The average patient who has surgery on Friday afternoon will feel like going back to work on Monday. She may tire after a half-day and go home, and possibly do the same on Tuesday, but by Wednesday she will feel like working a full day.

It is fine to shower or bathe the day after surgery, but I advise patients to wait one week before they resume intercourse, douching, or the use of tampons.

Some patients feel bloated the first few days after this surgery. This is because the intestines do not handle food as efficiently for a few days after surgery as they did before, not because any carbon dioxide gas is still present. All carbon dioxide is absorbed out of the abdomen in only a few hours.

Bruising is common around the incisions. It can extend all the way from the navel to the pubic area, out to the side of the abdomen, and even to the flanks. Some of this bruising is due to the instruments being pushed through the wall of the abdomen, and some caused by the doctor grasping the skin of the abdomen to lift it up so that instruments can be inserted.

Normally the incisions cause little pain, but it is common to have a slight infection of the incisions. If you notice a little redness and pus oozing out of one or both of your incisions, apply warm, wet towels to the area as frequently as you can. If the area seems to be getting more and more inflamed and tender, call your doctor, who will probably prescribe an antibiotic.

## 1110 How is a vaginal tubal ligation— colpotomy—done?

Years ago doctors did sterilizations through the vagina. This required general anesthesia and an incision in the upper vagina, right behind the cervix. The doctor would pull the fallopian tubes down far enough to tie and cut them. The procedure allowed a woman to have a sterilization done without a larger incision in the abdomen.

However, this was not a reliable method of sterilization. The doctor was often unable to find both fallopian tubes after making the colpotomy incision and ended up having to make a large abdominal incision to complete the procedure. There was a greater chance of infection with vaginal surgery, because the vagina cannot be made as clean for surgery as can the skin of the abdomen.

If you can find a doctor who does laparoscopy, I urge you to do so. A vaginal tubal ligation should be considered only if it is impossible for you to have a laparoscopy.

---

**1111** **What is a postpartum sterilization?**

A postpartum sterilization is one that is done immediately after delivery of a baby, or the next day or two. If you are pregnant and know for sure that this baby is the last one you want to have, it is convenient and sensible to have the sterilization done immediately after the delivery.

The only warning I give my patients considering this procedure is that the most risky time in a human's life is the first twenty-four hours after birth. A baby can be born looking totally normal and die within that first day because of some major congenital abnormality which was impossible to detect at birth. This happens rarely, but if you feel that you would want another child if your newborn were to die, I recommend that you delay sterilization until at least the next day—or, perhaps more wisely, for about six months. I have seen similar problems occur when husbands have had vasectomies while their wives were pregnant with what they have decided would be their last child. If your husband is considering having a vasectomy done while you are pregnant, be sure that you and he have discussed the possibility of losing your child, either before or after delivery.

Postpartum sterilization can be done following either a normal vaginal delivery or a cesarean section.

*After normal vaginal delivery.* Immediately after delivery, the uterus is still quite large. The top of it is usually at the level of the naval, making the fallopian tubes, which are attached to the top of the uterus, easily accessible through a small incision under the navel. The doctor merely makes a single incision, reaches in first to one side and then the other, picking up each fallopian tube separately and pulling it through the incision so it can be tied and cut. The small incision is then closed with sutures.

A woman who has had a vaginal delivery and then a tubal ligation may want to stay in the hospital an extra day because of the discomfort of the sterilization, but this is not usually necessary. There is little risk in having this type of sterilization done; I have not had patients have any problems with it other than minor wound infections.

After a tubal ligation, a woman may do anything she would have otherwise done, including nurse her baby. There is no limitation, either in the hospital or after she goes home, that would not have been placed on her by normal recovery from delivery.

*After cesarean section.* This is the easiest of all sterilizations to do. After the doctor has sewn up the uterus, he or she merely reaches over, lifts each tube with a clamp, ties it with a suture, and cuts away the part of the tube that has been tied off. After tying the tubes, the cesarean-section surgery is completed as would normally be done. After this surgery a woman may have mild discomfort in her sides, but this is generally not nearly as uncomfortable as the C-section itself.

---

**1112** **After a sterilization procedure has been performed, what happens to the eggs a woman produces and to any sperm that enter her cervix?**

Both the egg and the sperm die inside the woman's body. The egg usually dies within twenty-four hours after ovulation, and most sperm will be dead within two or three days after entering the woman's body. After they die these cells are absorbed into the body, representing no more than a little added protein. There are millions of cells in a person's body that die and are absorbed and replaced every day. The absorption of dead egg and sperm cells is no different and does not hurt a woman's body.

## 1113 Is it harmful to my body in any way to have a sterilization done?

A sterilization procedure does not damage or change a woman's body in any way except to make it sterile. There is no increase in disorders of the female organs, nor any increase in psychiatric problems in women who have had sterilization done.

There are some gynecologists who tell patients that a sterilization will increase their chance of having cysts on their ovaries, menstrual abnormalities, depression, and other physical and emotional problems. Careful studies have proven that women who have been sterilized are at no greater risk from these problems than those who have not been sterilized.

Apparently what happens is that women who have had sterilization use that surgery as a point of reference. They say, for example, "Before I had my sterilization, I did not have abnormal periods." Women who have not been sterilized do not have that point to refer to and therefore have nothing to blame their abnormal periods or ovarian cysts on.

The Oxford Family Planning Study in Great Britain, which included 17,000 women who were observed for up to nine years after their sterilizations, showed that there was no increased chance of abnormality. This particular study showed, as other studies have done, that both women who have had sterilizations and women who have not had them have the same chance of being admitted later to a hospital for D&C or for hysterectomy.

## 1114 What is the chance of pregnancy after sterilization?

The pregnancy rate after a sterilization procedure is from one in five hundred to one in a thousand, but other studies show a rate of only one in three thousand patients. These rates apply to any of the sterilization techniques we have discussed.

There are some studies that indicate that a sterilization done right after delivery has a higher chance of pregnancy (one in five hundred) than a sterilization done with coagulation and cutting (one in two or three thousand). Other research, however, shows that a postpartum sterilization is just as successful as any interval sterilization.

I do many sterilization procedures every year, and I have had only one subsequent pregnancy occur; a tubal pregnancy in a woman who had had a laparoscopy sterilization several years earlier. I can reassure you that if you have had sterilization surgery by a competent surgeon you do not need to worry about whether or not you are going to get pregnant. Enjoy the freedom of your sterilization, and do not fret about the possibility of pregnancy. It is very unlikely.

## 1115 How can a pregnancy occur after both tubes have been blocked?

It is possible for a woman to have a pregnancy in her fallopian tube at the time of her sterilization. Even though the sterilization was done properly, such a pregnancy could pass on into the uterus and continue growing as a normal pregnancy or could be caught in the fallopian tube and become an ectopic pregnancy. Because of this a sterilization should be done in the first few days after a menstrual period, to make sure you are not pregnant at the time of the operation, unless you know for sure that you could not be pregnant because of some other reason.

It is also possible, though highly improbable, for a pregnancy to occur because of the body's ability to make its tubular structures "grow open" again. An example of this recuperative power is shown when your skin is cut. The body grows blood vessels (tubular structures) that cross the incision, reestablishing blood flow. In a like manner, when the tubes have been blocked the body tries to open them up again and is occasionally successful. The cut ends of the tubes do not actually grow back together. The stump of the tube attached to the uterus grows open, and an egg could be swept down that short piece of tube into the uterus. Because of the female body's tremendous drive toward pregnancy, it is surprising that more women do not become pregnant after sterilizations.

Another reason for pregnancy after a sterilization procedure is that the tubes were not adequately blocked by the operation. Normally it is fairly easy to see the fallopian tubes but if there are adhesions or scarring, it can be difficult to identify and reach the tubes. This increases the chance of pregnancy after such a procedure.

It might seem that doctors could X-ray the tubes after sterilization to be sure they are closed, but this is not a good idea. The pressure of pushing the dye through the uterus and into the tubes can blow the tubes open, making it more likely that a pregnancy would occur after the X-ray. In addition, since it may take the body several years to "grow a tube open" an X-ray today does not necessarily mean that your tubes will not open up next year.

---

## 1116 Is a sterilization procedure dangerous for a woman?

Any surgical procedure carries risks. Before any type of surgery, a patient should be told of the potential dangers that can accompany the operation. This is not just because lawyers advise doctors and hospitals to do this, but because a patient has a right to know that surgery does carry risks.

Just as there are always risks associated with surgery, there are potential problems associated with a sterilization procedure, including:

Damage to your intestines, which could necessitate a colostomy.

Bleeding into your abdomen, which could require a large incision so the doctor could locate the bleeding vessel and suture it. The bleeding could also lead to needing a blood transfusion, which could result in your developing hepatitis or AIDS.

Infection in your abdomen, which could cause a life-threatening abscess that could make a hysterectomy mandatory.

Death from complications of either the anesthetic or the surgery.

These dangers could scare a woman if she did not realize that not being sterilized, and then using a less reliable method of birth control, exposes her to the dangers of pregnancy!

There is no free ride. There is a risk to using other methods of birth control because of the possibility of becoming pregnant, and there is risk for the older women to continue to use birth-control pills because of her chance of developing blood clots. There is a risk to sterilization. What these risks amount to, therefore, is that a woman must decide which procedure is best for her circumstances at her specific period of life.

Statistics show that you are no more likely to die from having a sterilization procedure done than you are from riding in an automobile. Furthermore, although statistics show that four out of a hundred thousand women who have a sterilization procedure will die as a result of it, about nineteen out of a hundred thousand pregnant women will die because of the complications of pregnancy. The risk of a sterilization is lower than the risk for pregnancy and also lower than risking prolonged use of birth-control pills.

## 1117 What might indicate problems after a sterilization procedure?

The signs and symptoms you should watch for and immediately report to your doctor are:

Severe pain in your abdomen, especially if your pain increases in intensity.

Fever over one hundred degrees.

Heavy vaginal bleeding, heavier than a normal period.

## 1118 Can a sterilization be reversed?

Even though most people have been warned to be sure they never want another child before they have a sterilization, many people change their minds about having another child a few years later. Several situations are often associated with a woman's desire to be pregnant again.

*New marriage partner.* About 80 percent of women who want sterilization reversals want them for this reason.

*Death of an infant or child.* This accounts for about 20 percent of women who want reversals.

*Desire for more children.* This represents quite a small percent, unless there has been a change in marital partner after divorce or death of a spouse.

*Change in sexual responsiveness or emotional feelings after sterilization.* A very small percent of women will feel that they are not as responsive sexually or that they are in some way different emotionally after a sterilization. Psychological or psychiatric counseling would more likely solve such problems than would fallopian-tube repair.

While repair of the tubes can be done, it requires a major operation and an expense of between five and eight thousand dollars. Then, after all that, there is no guarantee that a pregnancy will result. Only 75 percent of women become pregnant after their tubes are repaired. Thus 25 percent will still not

become pregnant. The only hope for these women to achieve pregnancy is through in vitro fertilization. (See Q. 975–978.)

If a woman's sterilization resulted in destruction of most of her fallopian tubes or destruction of the outer (fimbriated) ends of the tubes, it will be difficult, or even impossible, for a gynecologic microsurgeon to do a tubal repair that will allow the woman a very good chance of pregnancy.

The most successful fallopian-tube repairs are those in which the fimbriated outer ends of the tubes and most of both tubes are still intact. If at least two and a half to three inches of tube are left after the repair has been completed, the chances of pregnancy are increased. In addition, the microsurgical technique for tube repair is most important. The pregnancy rates after repair are much higher if your doctor uses these techniques. (See Q. 924–929.)

## 1119 Are hysterectomies ever done as a means of sterilization?

I do not recommend having a hysterectomy primarily for sterilization purposes. Hysterectomies are often done, however, when a woman wants a problem with her uterus solved and also wants sterilization. Therefore, if you are having heavy periods, bad cramps, pelvic heaviness, or any other problem with your female organs, and you also want to be sterilized, a hysterectomy may be a good approach because it can serve both purposes. If a woman has no problem with her female organs, a laparoscopy sterilization is much easier and safer than a hysterectomy.

Your doctor should explain the choices you have for your care and let you make the decision. You may absolutely not want a hysterectomy, even if you do have heavy periods or other female organ problems. You may be so troubled by problems with your uterine function and so ready to be sterilized, that you would find a vaginal hysterectomy a good solution. (See Q. 663–677.)

If you decide to have a hysterectomy for this combination of reasons, I encourage you to have it done by an expert gynecologist who is familiar with doing vaginal surgery. A vaginal hysterectomy is one of the safest major operations done on women and also one of the most comfortable major operations for many women. Many of my patients who have had vaginal hysterectomies report that they had little discomfort during the recovery period from their operation, if no vaginal repairs were necessary.

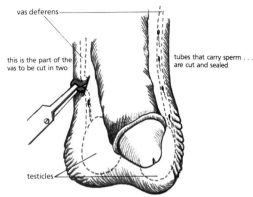

vas deferens

this is the part of the vas to be cut in two

tubes that carry sperm . . . are cut and sealed

testicles

## Vasectomy

---

## 1120  What is a vasectomy?

A vasectomy is a surgical procedure that makes a male sterile. It is a fairly simple operation, and it is almost always done with a local anesthetic. It is a simple procedure. A urologist or a general surgeon usually does this type of surgery.

The procedure involves an incision on the undersurface of both sides of the scrotum, about an inch to an inch and a half long. After locating the vasa (the tubes that carry the sperm from the testicles to the internal sexual organs) the doctor ties them off, cutting part of them away. The doctor may cauterize the vasa, put clips on them, or fold the ends back and tie them away from each other. No matter which technique is used, the procedure is still relatively simple.

After a vasectomy a man usually needs to rest for an hour or two and take it easy at home for the rest of the day. He should avoid hard or strenuous exercise for two or three days and should wear some support for his scrotum. Pain pills may be taken as needed. Discomfort ranges from mild to moderately severe, but almost all discomfort should have disappeared after seven or eight days.

A man may have intercourse as soon after a vasectomy as he feels comfortable doing so, but he should use some method of con-

traception until an examination of his semen shows that there are no sperm present. This may take two or three months.

If a man develops swelling and redness of his scrotum after the vasectomy, he should call his doctor immediately, especially if he begins running a fever.

---

## 1121  What complications can result from a vasectomy?

Several complications can occur.

***Formation of a hematoma.*** A hematoma is an accumulation of blood. A small blood vessel can continue to bleed after the operation, filling the tissues with blood. A doctor sometimes needs to drain a hematoma but may decide to leave it alone and let the body absorb the blood. Good scrotal support is important in this situation.

***Infection.*** Any site of the body that has been operated on can become infected. It is unusual for this to happen after a vasectomy, but if a man begins having swelling, heat, and tenderness of the tissues, infection is probably present. He needs to notify his doctor immediately.

***Epididymitis.*** This irritation of the collecting ducts of the testicle (epididymis) results from engorgement by the sperm that are still being produced by the testicle. This can occur up to several months after a vasectomy. Scrotal support and heat usually solve the problem.

**Granuloma.** There may be an accumulation of sperm, white blood cells, and other cells in the scrotum. This is called a granuloma and is a result of sperm leaking into the tissues surrounding the area of the vasectomy. Granulomas are not dangerous, but they may occasionally cause severe pain. One of the main problems associated with granulomas is that they can make successful reversal of a vasectomy impossible.

## 1122 How effective is a vasectomy at preventing pregnancy?

It is estimated that there is a failure rate with vasectomy ranging from about one in a hundred to one in five hundred men. Although the success rate with older vasectomy techniques is not quite as good as that for sterilization done on a woman, it is still an effective method of sterilization. Newer techniques (cautery seems safest) have significantly increased the success rate. If a couple chooses this method of sterilization, they should not worry about this extremely low chance of pregnancy. Instead they should enjoy the freedom from worry that sterility affords.

## 1123 Is it possible to reverse a vasectomy?

A vasectomy reversal can be successfully performed on most men, and subsequent pregnancy rates are as high as 80 percent. This requires an incision in the same area in which the original incision was made. The doctor must find the two ends of the vas, cut off the scar, and sew them back together. This is best accomplished by a urologist who is experienced in microsurgery.

The chance of fertility after a vasectomy repair is determined by three things: the surgeon should be an accomplished microsurgeon, enough vas to repair must be left,

and the last is the length of time from the vasectomy to the attempt at reversal—the shorter, the better.

If a couple desires pregnancy, and it has been less than twenty years since a man's sterilization, the vasectomy should be reversed to see if a successful pregnancy can be achieved. If it cannot, the only chance of achieving pregnancy is with insemination with donor sperm. (See Q. 962, 965, 967–972.)

## 1124 Are there any emotional or hormonal effects on men who have vasectomies?

Studies of men who have had vasectomies generally reveal that from 10–20 percent of them say that their sexual performance is improved after sterilization. This is probably due to the fact that they no longer have to worry about causing a pregnancy. Studies have also shown that there is no decrease in testosterone (male hormone) level.

Some men, however, feel that they cannot perform as well sexually after a vasectomy as they did before, but this is purely an emotional response to vasectomy. Generally, a man who has this problem is one who already had some psychological or emotional problem that the vasectomy merely brought to light.

## 1125 Are men who have had vasectomies more likely to develop atherosclerosis than men who have not?

Atherosclerosis, or hardening of the arteries, can lead to heart attacks. Several years ago, studies of monkeys who had vasectomies showed that they developed atherosclerosis more often than monkeys who had not had vasectomies. There is considerable variation, however, in the response to vasectomy by the bodies of different animal species.

The National Institute of Health, in response to these studies on monkeys, reported findings of their studies on men who had had vasectomies to the American Public Health Association annual meeting in Dallas in 1983. Based on their study of approximately twenty thousand men in four cities, they found no increased instance of heart attack or heart disease among men who had vasectomies.

**1126** **Do the sperm antibodies that men develop after having a vasectomy hurt their bodies?**

When a vasectomy has been done, the sperm which are still produced by testicles cannot get out of the testicles. They tend to invade the walls of the tubes in which they are trapped, producing a physiological antibody response to the sperm. In 1968, a doctor thought he found some relationship between vasectomy and ill health in a few men. His study generated several comprehensive, long-term, well-controlled medical studies that have since shown that there is no increased risk of ill health for men who had vasectomies. I feel that the evidence is quite clear that a vasectomy causes no increased risk to a man's health.

## Experimental Contraceptive Methods

**1127** **What new contraceptive techniques are being developed and studied?**

The *Dallas Times Herald* headlined a recent article, "Research Labs Are Pregnant With Ideas for Contraceptives." This is true.

There are many new contraceptive techniques being studied all over the world, since the "perfect" contraceptive method has not yet been found. However, it is unlikely that a single contraceptive technique, perfect for everybody, will ever be found.

Several contraceptives for men are being studied.

*Gossypol*. This chemical, an extract of the cotton plant, was discovered in the People's Republic of China. Taken daily it has been shown to produce an antifertility rate of 99 percent, which it accomplishes by decreasing the sperm count.

*LHRH*. Luteinizing hormone-releasing hormone is necessary for the proper function of the reproductive system of a human. It has been discovered, however, that if excessive doses of LHRH are given to the man, the reproductive system will "shut off," stopping the production of sperm.

*Hormone cream*. Researchers are studying a hormone cream, composed of estrogen and testosterone, which is absorbed into a man's body when rubbed on his chest or abdomen. This absorption seems to change the normal hormone function of the man's body so that sperm are not produced, yet it does not affect his sexual function or health.

Several contraceptives for women are also being studied.

*Hormone implants*. Pellets containing progesterone, called Norplant, are available. Using a local anesthetic these pellets are inserted just under the skin through a small incision, usually made in a woman's lower abdomen. The progesterone is absorbed into the body, where it acts much like birth-control pills. Since the pellets do not contain estrogen, they do not produce the problems of abnormal blood clotting as estrogens can. These implants can be left in place for up to five or six years and can be removed when a woman wants to become pregnant.

*Vaginal rings*. Rings, similar to the outer part of a diaphragm, and impregnated with long-acting progesterone, can allow the slow release of progesterone hormones into the body. Such hormonal absorption in the vagina thickens the cervical mucus, making it impenetrable by sperm. These rings can be impregnated with both estrogen and progesterone, both of which are in birth-control pills.

*Blockage of the fallopian tubes through the cervix.* Techniques are being studied for blocking the fallopian tubes by instilling different materials through the vagina and the cervix. Chemicals have been developed that, when pushed through the cervix into the fallopian tubes, scar the tubes enough to produce sterility.

*Vaccine.* Researchers are working on anti-pregnancy vaccines for both females and males. Testing on humans has not yet been started. This technique is probably years away from being perfected.

## An Afterword

Good contraceptive techniques are one of the miracles of modern medicine. There can be a real pitfall in all this manipulation, however. We can become so accustomed to having total control over everything in our lives that we become disoriented, upset, and angry when our planning goes awry. An unplanned pregnancy can lead to such a distorted statement as that written by a well-known professor and chairman of a major department of obstetrics and gynecology: "Unwanted pregnancy is a disease that should be treated as such."

That well-motivated physician, like many others in our society, seems to forget that it is God, ultimately, who "opens and closes" the womb. If we have done our best to avoid pregnancy and it still occurs, we need to view it as an unplanned blessing and expect a special gift from God in this "accident."

Most gynecologists, including myself, have seen couples who panicked over an unplanned pregnancy and rushed into an ill-thought-out abortion, only to come back a year or so later, unable to achieve pregnancy. Such couples often suffer an agony of self-incrimination for having destroyed a life and, in the process, having possibly destroyed their fertility. These people could have avoided all this heartache by accepting their surprise pregnancy as a blessing from God.

However, contraceptive techniques do provide great freedom from unwanted pregnancy and can be a boon to both mankind in general and to individual couples in particular.

# 13

# Sexually Transmitted Disease

Sexually transmitted disease (STD) is a nasty, convulsively grow-ing, worldwide epidemic. Its most likely potential victims seem to be blissfully unaware that they can get STD.

> It was the age of overindulgence. It was the age for tolerance of anything in anybody. It was the age of fear of imposing one's own social values on someone else. It was the age of the trivialization of sex. It was the age of anti-celibacy. It was the age when early teenage sex was commonplace. It was the age when homosexuality came out of the closet and became almost acceptable to those who once found it intolerable. It was the age of easy, irresponsible oversex, abortion on demand, chlamydia, and genital herpes. It was the age of AIDS.
>
> Not since syphilis among the Spanish, plague among the French, tuberculosis among the Eskimos, and smallpox among the Amer-ican Indians has there been the threat of such a scourge. Yet, the acquired immunodeficiency syndrome (AIDS) is different from any disease previously seen.
>
> From the introduction to an editorial in the *Journal of the American Medical Association*, June 21, 1985, by Dixie E. Snider, Jr., M.D. titled "The Age of AIDS: A Great Time for Defensive Living."

AIDS is not the only STD that medical experts are concerned about. The Centers for Disease Control and the Federal Health Resources and Services Administration recently declared war on the twenty known STDs infecting and ravaging the lives of Americans. Look at the statistics: 1 in 4 Americans will acquire STD at sometime in their life if they are now between the age of 15 and 55. Twenty-seven thousand new cases of STD occur every day in the United States.

Except for AIDS, STD is usually only a minor problem in men, especially if treated early. Almost all the severe complications of STD are experienced by women. James O. Mason, the director at the Center for Disease Control in Atlanta, recently said, "Sometimes I wonder why the female population doesn't stand up and scream about this."

A woman can have intercourse with a man who has not had intercourse with anyone else for years and still get STD from him. She too can carry STD for years and pass it on in the same way.

The most common preventable cause of infertility in the United States is infection of (with resultant scarring) the female organs, often caused by a usually curable sexually transmitted disease.

Precancerous and cancerous growths of the vulva, vagina, and cervix have increased alarmingly in numbers in the past few years. Research indicates that these conditions are almost always caused by a sexually transmitted factor, the human papillomavirus, the same virus that causes venereal warts.

In the following questions we will discuss some general facts relating to STDs as well as the most common forms of such diseases. There are a number of rarely occurring STDs which will be mentioned only briefly.

## General Facts About STD

### 1128 What is sexually transmitted disease?

Sexually transmitted disease, or STD, is a term that is used now for what was called venereal disease a few years ago. Because of the changed sexual mores of our society, these diseases are now the most common infectious diseases in the United States, except for colds and flu.

STD infections are passed from one person to another by intimate contact. This contact may involve the sex organs, the mouth, or the rectum. The delicate lining of these three areas, plus their warmth and moisture, allow the growth of the organisms that produce sexually transmitted disease. Because these germs require this type of environment, they are passed almost exclusively by intercourse and other intimate contact between two individuals.

### 1129 Who can get sexually transmitted disease?

The person who contracts a sexually transmitted disease is usually someone who had intercourse with another person who has such a germ. If you have intercourse with only your husband or wife, and he or she has never had intercourse with anyone else and never does so in the future, you are absolutely safe so far as sexually transmitted disease is concerned. The only exceptions are extremely rare, such as developing STD from an injection or from a blood transfusion.

No matter what your age or your status in society, you can catch one of these diseases if you violate the above rule even one time. Gonorrhea is less likely to grow in girls before puberty or women after menopause, but it can. You can get STD from intercourse with a doctor, a lawyer, or an Indian chief! It is not confined to one group in society. As a matter of fact, a person can catch two different venereal diseases at one time, even syphilis and gonorrhea. And it does not matter how neat and clean you are, or whether or not you douche after intercourse; you can still be infected with a venereal disease.

---

**1130** **What are some of the myths about sexually transmitted disease?**

There are too many myths about STD to discuss here, but reading this entire chapter will correct most misconceptions about sexually transmitted disease. Some of the most "popular" myths are these.

*"Sexually transmitted disease can be caught in some way other than by intercourse."* STD is passed only by intimate contact. It is true that venereal warts can occasionally be passed from hand to hand, but almost all the other STD germs are passed only by intercourse. They cannot be caught by shaking hands; they are not picked up on towels, toilet seats, door knobs, or dishes; heavy lifting and masturbation do not cause STD.

*"Sexually transmitted disease can be caught by kissing."* Although this may happen, it is uncommon. Oral/genital sexual contact, of course, can pass STD, but mouth-to-mouth kissing rarely does.

*"All STD infections can be cured."* Herpes and AIDS are incurable, which proves that all sexually transmitted diseases cannot be cured. Even when the infectious organisms of certain other STDs are themselves killed, the scars they produce in a woman's body can be a lifelong problem. Studies have shown, for example, that 6 percent of women who have one gonorrhea infection will end up totally sterile.

*"Homosexuals do not get sexually transmitted disease."* This is untrue. Both homosexual men and women can have STD. The most notorious example of this at the present time is AIDS. For years it was said that homosexual women did not contract STD, but this has recently been proved incorrect.

---

**1131** **Can a man have a sexually transmitted disease without knowing it?**

Certainly. Either a man or a woman can have these germs present in their body without knowing it. For example, one-third of the people who are infected with herpes, and who pass it on to others, have never had a sore.

Although the percentages may be different, this principle holds true for almost all sexually transmitted disease.

---

**1132** **If a man knows he has a STD, will he tell me?**

It is quite likely that he will not. Since STD infection in a man is usually only a trivial problem, and since he would probably consider being denied intercourse with you a major problem, there is a great chance that he would not tell you if he has a sexually transmitted disease. This is, of course, self-ish and inexcusable but often characterizes the masculine sexual drive. He may be unaware of his infection. No matter how much you may wish this were not true, it is a fact of life. And the woman is the victim.

The basic principle to remember is this: if a woman has intercourse with a male who has ever had intercourse with anyone else, she can catch a sexually transmitted disease from him, whether or not he has any symptoms. If you ignore this warning, you may end up as the victim of STD. In the same way, you can pass on STD to someone else.

If you marry someone who has had intercourse in the past, whether with a girl friend or a former marriage partner, it is possible that he can pass sexual disease to you. As you live together during the ensuing years, however, your doctor can help you control or get rid of most of the infections that might have been a part of your bodies at the start of your marriage.

## 1133 How can I know if I have a sexually transmitted disease?

You cannot know for sure without seeing a physician. Although your body might show signs of sexually transmitted disease, STD is generally found when a woman who suspects the problem goes to a doctor for testing.

You should ask a physician to test you for STD in any of the following situations.

If you know or suspect that you have been exposed to a sexually transmitted disease.

If you have symptoms that suggest the possibility of a sexually transmitted disease.

If you are certain that you do have STD by the presence of warts, herpes ulcers, and so on.

## 1134 How will a doctor determine whether or not I have a STD?

There are several things a doctor can do to determine whether or not you have a sexually transmitted disease. The medical procedure depends on the symptoms.

*Growths.* The doctor will check any growths and, if necessary, excise a small piece of one (a biopsy) to send to a pathologist for diagnosis. This is common procedure with venereal warts although it is usually not necessary.

*Vaginal discharge.* The doctor will have a culture done on your vaginal secretions to see if gonorrhea or chlamydia organisms are present.

*Syphilis.* If any other STD is present, syphilis may be too. A blood test will determine this, but not until at least twelve weeks after exposure. This is not too late for safe treatment of the infection.

*Pelvic infection.* If you have signs of pelvic inflammatory disease (PID), the doctor will start you on intensive antibiotic treatment to kill the infection as quickly as possible. The sooner the infection is cleared, the greater the chance of preventing scars that might cause subsequent infertility.

*The ulcer of herpes.* If you have a tender spot that might be a herpes infection, the spot can be cultured for the herpes virus.

With a combination of diagnostic and therapeutic tools, the doctor can determine which type of infection you have and tell you what to do about it. It is important that you and the doctor continue testing until you are totally free of infection or until you have an established pattern for treatment that both of you find acceptable.

## 1135 If I have STD, should I tell my sex partner?

If you have a sexually transmitted disease, you should definitely tell anyone with whom you have sex. In this way the two of you can work out a technique of sexual activity, such as refraining from intercourse or having intercourse with condoms and contraceptive foam, that will prevent your giving the infection to him and then his passing it back to you after your infection is clear.

A startling chain of events can occur when people do not tell their partners that they might be infected. Public health workers have found as many as two hundred people infected by venereal disease from one person who either did not know or did not tell a sexual partner about a STD infection.

## 1136 Do I have to notify the health department if I have STD?

Your physician should notify your local health department if you have a reportable STD, and you should insist that this be done. Officials there will talk to you (confidentially, of course) to find out with whom you have had sexual contact, so that these people can be treated and the transmission of the venereal disease ended.

The sexually transmitted diseases which are reportable in most states are syphilis, gonorrhea, lymphogranuloma venerium, chancroid, and granuloma inguinale. There are a few states that now require reporting of only gonorrhea and syphilis. Public-health physicians feel that chlamydia and herpes reporting will be required in the next few years by many states. Reporting of AIDS is already required by many states, but not as a venereal disease.

## 1137 If I have a STD, will my doctor find it when I have my annual examination?

No. Just as you can have another infection in your body that you are unaware of, so your doctor can be unaware of your having STD. Unless the infection produces abnormal dis-charge or growths in your body, your doctor would not usually suspect that you are infected.

Do not expect your doctor to ask you if there is any possibility that you might be infected by STD when he or she sees you for an examination. A doctor will not ordinarily ask this if you seem normal on exam. This is not because of embarrassment; but because most patients feel that a doctor suspects there is something wrong if he or she asks about a specific problem. Most patients, therefore, would assume that something seen in the exam made the doctor suspicious of a STD.

That is one of the reasons I do not routinely ask my patients about STD. The other is that I do not want to imply in any way that I suspect them of activity that could make a sexually transmitted disease possible.

Obviously it is up to you to tell your doctor if you think you may have a sexually transmitted disease.

If you are married and suspect that your husband may have had an extramarital affair, tell your doctor. You can be tested for STD and either relieve your mind about being infected or be treated if necessary.

I have had patients come to me with this problem, saying that they were terribly uncomfortable about discussing it with me. This is certainly a valid feeling on the part of patients, but let me assure you that doctors do not feel awkward in this situation. Your physician sees and treats this type of problem every day in people just like you. You should not let your embarrassment keep you from getting help.

## Venereal Warts— Condyloma Acuminata

## 1138 What are venereal warts, and what causes them?

Although the warts of condyloma acuminata look and act like ordinary warts, they are termed "venereal" because of their location (on the parts of the body normally associated with sexual intercourse), and also because they are a different type of wart from that which occurs on other parts of the body. A person can acquire venereal warts without having sexual intercourse, in spite of the implications of the name. The virus that causes these warts can occasionally be present on other parts of the body, especially the fingers, and can be spread by touch. In an adolescent or mature woman, however, infection by condyloma acuminata, or venereal warts, is usually a result of sexual intercourse.

Condyloma infections have increased remarkably in the last few years. Statistics in Britain show that there has been a 10-percent increase in the number of venereal-wart infections each year for the past ten years. Although reporting of condyloma infections in the United States is not required, there is every reason to believe that their incidence is increasing just as fast here as it is in Britain.

The number of people in the United States who have been infected with venereal warts is probably three times as many as have been infected with herpes. As the number of sexual partners increases, so does the likelihood that a woman will have venereal warts and herpes, and a person with one of these problems will often also have the other.

### 1139 What are the symptoms of venereal wart infections?

A woman usually notices this type of infection as a small bump or several small bumps on her vulva, either on her labia between her anus and the lower part of her vagina or around her anus. As time goes by, there may be more and more growths in this area. The warts may grow together and increase in size, sometimes becoming as large as a fist,

or they may occasionally clear up spontaneously for no known reason.

Warts may, and often do, grow up into the vagina (they may even start in the vagina and grow down), and they may also grow on the cervix. Warts of this type, however, rarely grow outside the moist, warm genital area.

Venereal warts often cause a vaginal discharge, and warts on the vulva will occasionally become mildly infected and sore and will bleed if scratched or handled roughly.

### 1140 What causes venereal warts?

These warts are caused by one of several of a group of human viruses, called human papillomavirus. When a woman has had intercourse with someone who has a venereal wart infection, she will not grow warts immediately. The viruses must incubate in her body for from two to six months before they start growing. It is not known if the virus is contagious during this incubation time.

If your sexual partner has not had intercourse with anyone else for one to two years and has no visible venereal warts, it is unlikely that he or she can give you venereal warts.

### 1141 Are venereal warts dangerous?

Venereal warts of themselves are not dangerous, but many researchers feel that they can produce changes in your body that can eventually cause cancer. (See Q. 740, 747.)

Venereal warts, however, are a real nuisance. They are irritating, cause soreness and itching, bleed or cause vaginal discharge, and cause pain with intercourse. The most aggravating thing about them, however, is that they can grow back again and again.

If venereal warts do grow back, this does not mean that they are cancerous. If your doctor has any question about this, he or she can send a biopsy of one of them to the laboratory for diagnosis.

## 1142 How are venereal warts treated and cured?

If the warts are ulcerated or are unusually hard or abnormal, the first thing the doctor should do is send a biopsy to the lab. Once the doctor and you have been assured that the growths are venereal warts, there are several different methods of treatment.

*Treatment of other existing medical problems.* Certain conditions seem to aggravate venereal warts. Vaginal infection is a primary offender. If you have a vaginal infection (trichomonas or some other type), this should be treated first to decrease the amount of vulvar moisture, allowing greater success in treating the warts.

One condition that encourages the proliferation of venereal warts is having a partner with an uncircumcised penis, since a man who has a foreskin often has warts under it, especially if he practices poor personal hygiene. Other contributing factors are pregnancy, taking birth-control pills, a faulty immune system (such as in a person who has had a kidney transplant and is on drugs for that), or diabetes. Patients who have one of these conditions will occasionally find their warts more easily controlled when the associated condition is eliminated or carefully controlled.

*Podophyllum.* A mixture of 10–25 percent of podophyllum in tincture of benzoin can be dabbed on each wart. If a woman's skin becomes severely irritated, she should wash this off, but I have found that women who have the worst reaction to podophyllum are more likely to have all their warts disappear with one or two applications than women who have almost no irritation from its use. Theoretically, the absorption of podophyllum by a wart causes the cells of the wart to stop growing and to die. This

may happen with some warts but not with others.

The doctor will usually have a patient return for treatment each week until her warts are gone. If they are not gone after two to four treatments, most doctors will then use another method of treatment.

Only a small amount of podophyllum is usually used in the vagina or on the cervix because of the danger of absorption, making a woman sick. It must not be used in pregnancy because of the possibility of absorption of the chemical into the mother's body, with resulting damage to the fetus. One of the following techniques is used if a patient has extensive vaginal or cervical warts or is pregnant.

*Laser.* The laser can be used to evaporate warts. This can be done with a local anesthetic or with general anesthesia in an outpatient operating room if there is a large number of condyloma. If a patient has venereal warts that are not clearing up after four treatments with podophyllum or with any other technique, I strongly advise her to see a doctor who uses the laser. Statistics show that warts respond better to laser than to any other method of treatment.

Since use of the laser is expensive, even those doctors who use the laser will usually try podophyllum first. If the warts do not respond to that treatment, the doctor will then suggest use of the laser, which is quite safe, even during pregnancy.

*Trichloracetic acid (Nevitol).* This acid can be applied to warts on the vulva, in the vagina, and on the cervix. Sometimes it is effective and sometimes it is not. If it does not work after two or three applications, the laser or one of the following methods should be tried.

*Freezing.* A "freezing," or cryotherapy, machine can be used to freeze warts. A local anesthetic will be administered for warts on the vulva, but warts in the vagina can usually be frozen without anesthetic. I have not found cryotherapy very useful for warts, because each wart must be frozen separately down to its base. Although some doctors use this technique with some success, I prefer the laser.

*Cautery.* Using a local anesthetic, your doctor can burn off, or cauterize, warts. This is a good treatment, especially if you have only a few warts. If you have many, the laser works better and will leave you much less sore from the treatment. The problem with cautery is that it will also burn normal skin around and under the warts, causing soreness and scar.

*5-Fluorouracil.* This drug, which is used in cancer chemotherapy, can be mixed in a cream base for use in the vagina or on the skin. It can be useful for warts, but it will almost always cause a great deal of vulvar irritation. If your doctor wants to prescribe this for you, it is fine to use and may work, but you should expect considerable vulvar irritation while using it. Some protection from the irritation may be obtained by covering the wart-free portions of your vulva with a heavy coat of Vaseline.

*Vaccine.* A few research centers have prepared individual vaccines from a woman's own warts. Reports indicate a long-term success rate for some of the people so vaccinated, but this is still in the research stage and not readily available for everyone. If you continue to have warts month after month and the laser or other techniques are not successful, you may want to contact a doctor who has an interest in this technique. One such doctor is L. Charles Powell, M.D., at the University of Texas Medical Branch in Galveston, Texas.

*Surgery.* Occasionally, whether you have only one persistent wart or several large ones, surgery will be necessary. Local anesthetic may be used, but usually general anesthesia is necessary. Surgery of this type can involve a combination of cautery, laser, and cutting of the warts.

## 1143 Are venereal warts dangerous during pregnancy or harmful to the fetus or newborn baby?

If the warts have grown so large that they block the birth canal, a cesarean section will be necessary. If you are pregnant and your warts are growing rapidly, the laser may be useful. *Do not let a doctor use podophyllum on you.* Occasionally the warts grow so fast during pregnancy that cesarean section is the only method for delivery.

Many doctors now believe that a baby born to a woman with venereal warts in her birth canal has a greater chance for developing vocal-cord papillomas (warts) in the first six to eight months. Since 60 percent of babies with these papillomas have been born to mothers with venereal warts, if you have such warts when you deliver your baby, it is probably best to have the baby examined by an ear, nose, and throat specialist about six months after delivery to make sure there are no polyps present. If your baby develops hoarseness, chronic cough, and has trouble making sounds, he or she should definitely be examined for polyps by such a specialist.

Incidentally, the virus that causes venereal warts cannot get inside the uterus and does not cause infections of the baby during pregnancy. (See Q. 424.)

## 1144 How can I keep from spreading venereal warts or getting them in the first place?

If you have had venereal warts and while you are being treated for them, you and your partner should use contraceptive foam and a condom every time you have intercourse. The rubbers keep you from spreading the virus back and forth to each other by preventing skin-to-skin contact with each other. Contraceptive foam has been found to kill germs. Therefore, if some of your secretions should touch your partner in spite of the rubber, the foam would tend to protect you. You should continue doing this for several months after you and your partner are free of warts, to make sure that the infection is not being passed back and forth.

If you have never had these warts, it would be best for you to use foam and a rubber when you have intercourse with anyone who has had intercourse with anyone else in the last six months. Although it is possible that one of you could still be carrying the virus after six months, this is unlikely. If one or the other of you has intercourse again with anyone else, you should start using the foam and condoms for another six months' incubation period.

This may seem like a lot of trouble, but most doctors who treat this problem have had many patients come back again and again for treatment of warts that would not go away. Anything you can do to lessen the chance of getting venereal warts or having them recur, is probably worth it. Prior to my use of the laser, one of my patients had warts continuously for over two years in spite of multiple treatment sessions. She still had them when she moved out of town after that two-year period. I have had two pregnant patients with vulvar warts that were as big as my fist (and that *is* big). All this is not only financially expensive; it is also emotionally costly. The experience of having venereal warts that will not clear up is frustrating. Using the foam and rubbers as prophylaxis against any STD will save you money, worry, and trouble later on.

One further word on the subject of venereal warts: once you have them, you should definitely have a Pap smear done every year. Most medical investigators think that most women who develop precancerous or cancerous cells of the cervix, as shown by an abnormal Pap smear, develop them as a result of a previous venereal-wart virus infection. This does not mean that you will inevitably develop precancerous cervical cells, but it does mean that the risk factor increases for you. Having a Pap smear every year will catch these changes if they occur, so that they can be treated before they become malignant.

---

**1145** **How are abnormal Pap smears associated with sexually transmitted disease?**

All abnormal Pap smears are not STD-related. Irritation and infection of the cervix from trauma or surgery or from diaphragm or tampon use are not intercourse-related and are not associated with venereal disease. An abnormal Pap smear caused by precancerous or cancerous cells (cervical dysplasia or neoplasia) almost never occurs in women who have not had intercourse. If a husband and wife have never had intercourse with anyone else, she will have only a small chance of developing cancerous or precancerous cervical cells.

The more sexual partners either member of a couple has had, the more likely is the woman to develop precancerous or cancerous cells of her cervix. For instance, if your husband dies and you remarry, you have an increased risk of developing precancerous cells on your cervix. The agent that causes precancerous cervical cells may have been passed to your new husband by his former wife, who may have had intercourse with someone when she was only a teenager.

The agent that seems to be most suspicious today as the cause of precancerous and cancerous cells of the cervix, the vagina, and the vulva is the same papillomavirus that causes venereal warts. This is not confirmed, but most researchers today think that if this virus is not the only cause of such changes on a woman's cervix, it is at least the major cause. (See Q. 747.)

There are some startling illustrations of the relationship between sexual activity and abnormal Pap smears. Some men cause every woman with whom they have sexual intercourse to develop a precancerous-type abnormal Pap smear. The second wives of men whose first wives died of cervical cancer are more likely to develop precancerous Pap smears than second wives of men whose first wives died of some other cause. This would seem to indicate that some men carry a cancer-producing factor in their bodies. We now know it is probably the papillomavirus.

Perhaps you are one of the many who read these facts who has had intercourse with someone other than your own mate, or you know that your spouse has had intercourse with someone else. What is done, is done; what is important now is that you have a Pap smear taken every year. Cervical cancer develops slowly, usually over a period of from one to seven years. Before the actual development of the cancer, abnormal changes can be detected in a Pap smear. The goal of a Pap smear is not to detect cancer but to detect *pre*cancerous cells before they turn into cancer.

If a Pap smear indicates that a woman has developed some abnormal cells, a colposcopy can be done and biopsies of her cervix taken. If this shows no malignancy, the precancerous cervical cells can be treated. (See Q. 741–756.)

Papillomavirus also seems to be the cause of the alarming increase in precancerous and cancerous growths on the vulva of women in our society, especially in younger women. (See Q. 669–673.)

Although chapter 10 contains a more complete discussion of diagnosis and treatment of disorders of the reproductive organs, the reason for mentioning them here is to be complete and to emphasize the fact that no discussion of STD *is* complete if it has only the tired, worn-out but still-true warnings about "gonorrhea and syphilis."

## Herpes

**1146** What should I know about herpes?

There is not only a lack of information on this subject, but there is a wealth of *mis*information. We know that 23 percent of sexually active Americans have been infected with this common sexually transmitted disease.

A person's primary, or first, herpes infection usually follows a general pattern of development. Tingling, itching, and burning of an area of the vulva (between the lower vagina and the anus, or around the anus) are usually the first symptoms of herpes infection in a woman. After two or three days that area will become red and form one or more fluid-filled blisters that rupture over a one- or two-day period, leaving small ulcers at the site of the infection. These ulcers can be extremely painful and tender to touch. They can be so painful, in fact, as to make intercourse impossible and occasionally so severe that urination cannot be tolerated.

Almost all people will have enlarged lymph nodes in their groin with their first herpes infection. They will also develop aching muscles, fever, nausea, and headache.

About 10 percent of herpes victims end up being admitted to the hospital with a first infection because of the pain or the inability to urinate.

These primary lesions usually last two to four weeks from start to total healing.

**1147** Can I have herpes more than once?

About 50 percent of patients who have had a primary herpes infection will have a recurrence within six months. This is not a new infection but merely an outbreak of the original herpes. Precisely because secondary infections can develop and there is no medication to prevent such infections, herpes is considered "incurable."

Secondary episodes of herpes are often triggered by emotional events, menstrual periods, intercourse, or trauma to the vulvar area. As the years go by patients will have fewer and fewer secondary lesions until, finally, many people will have no secondary lesions at all. Some people, however, will continue to have secondary herpes outbreaks for years.

Secondary outbreaks of herpes are almost never as uncomfortable as the first episode. Normally with secondary lesions the area becomes slightly red and forms the little fluid-filled blisters that break, leaving small, tender ulcers that clear up within a week or two.

If you have had a primary infection with herpes and do not develop any secondary infections, you have probably developed an immunity to herpes. If this is true, you would most likely not be able to get herpes again, even if you had sexual contact with someone with the disease. This has not been absolutely proven, but it is probably true.

---

**1148**  **What organism causes herpes?**

Genital herpes is usually caused by a virus called herpes simplex type II, which is almost always passed by sexual contact. Fever blisters are usually caused by herpes simplex type I, a virus usually caught in childhood.

In the past few years, research has shown that infections by these two viruses are not nearly so distinct and separate as once had been thought. About 15–20 percent of infections of the female genitalia are caused by herpes type I, and many of the so-called fever blisters that women have are caused by herpes type II.

If a woman is pregnant it makes no difference which type herpes she has, since ei-

ther type of virus can cause the same dangerous infection in the body.

---

**1149**  **How dangerous is herpes during pregnancy?**

If a baby is delivered through the birth canal while a woman has an active herpes sore, whether caused by herpes type I or type II, the herpes virus can get into the baby's body and infect the child. This infection in a baby is much different than it is in an adult. Herpes normally spreads all through the baby's body, and there is the possibility that the baby will die from the infection.

The actual incidence of passing herpes to a baby, however, is small. In Austin, Texas, for example, a city of about 500,000 people, a local neonatalist recently said that he could document less than twenty cases of suspected infant herpes infections in the history of the city.

Passing herpes to your baby can almost always be prevented merely by having a cesarean section instead of a vaginal delivery if you have a herpes sore or have had one within the month prior to delivery. (See Q. 425.)

---

**1150**  **What percent of herpes-infected babies die or are damaged?**

Studies indicate that from 70–100 percent of babies who actually contract a herpes infection as they are born to a mother who has herpes will die or have severe neurological damage as a result of the infection. From 30–75 percent of babies who develop this type of herpes infections are born to mothers who have no history of having had herpes infections, and did not even know they were carrying the virus in their bodies.

## 1151 How is herpes treated?

No virus infection, including herpes, is curable, because viruses do not respond to antibiotics as do pneumonia, gonorrhea, and other bacterial infections. A number of treatments have been tried for herpes, but only one has been found useful: a drug called Zovirax (acyclovir). When a patient uses this drug in capsule, injection, or ointment form with the first infection, it decreases the severity and duration of that infection and diminishes the possibility of a secondary outbreak.

If Zovirax is used with a secondary infection on a regular basis, it shortens the healing time for even these sores.

The injectible form of Zovirax can be used only in the veins and is best reserved for those with a severe primary herpes attack, infants with herpes infections, or herpes patients who have poor immune systems (those who have received transplant organs or who are on drugs to suppress their immune systems).

The ointment form of Zovirax may be used for any herpes outbreak. It speeds healing and decreases pain but to be effective it must be applied every three hours day and night until the sores have healed.

If victims are being bothered by recurrences of sores more than once a month, they may find that taking the capsule form of Zovirax daily either stops the sores from developing or decreases their frequency. At the present time the drug manufacturer cautions that the oral form should not be taken for more than a six-month period.

Do not fall into the trap of spending large amounts of money on so-called herpes cures. You are no more likely to find a herpes cure than you are to find a cure for the common cold, but you will probably spend a lot of money in a useless search.

A herpes vaccine has been developed, but it has not been thoroughly tested. By the time this book is published, it may be available.

## 1152 What should I do when I have active herpes sores?

There are some techniques that will help any herpes infection be more comfortable. They will not cure it, but they will make the infection more tolerable.

Wash the sores with soap and water.

Use a hair dryer to dry the area.

Do not wear tight clothes or nylon underwear. (Use cotton.)

Keep the area dry.

Use pain pills, such as aspirin or codeine, for discomfort.

If urination is uncomfortable, fill your bathtub with water and sit in it as you urinate.

Except for Zovirax, do not use ointments; they hold moisture against the sores and will make them last longer.

For more information on this subject, call the American Social Health Association's toll-free VD national hotline: 800-227-8922 (800-982-5883 in California). This organization also publishes a quarterly newsletter about herpes, called *The Helper*. This can be ordered from Herpes Resource Center, 260 Sheridan Avenue, Palo Alto, California 94306.

## 1153 How can I keep from catching herpes?

There are two major ways to keep from getting herpes.

First, do not have intercourse with anyone except your own husband, and he only with you.

Second, if you are not married and have intercourse with someone who may have herpes, use contraceptive foam and a condom. Studies have shown that women who use this protection have less chance of getting herpes from their sexual partner. Women can still occasionally contract herpes even if so protected. Remember, anyone who has been exposed to the herpes virus apparently can carry it in his or her tissues for years. People can harbor and shed the herpes virus even when they have never had a sore, and they can also shed the virus between the times of actual outbreaks of herpes sores.

If you are considering marriage, and either you or your loved one has had herpes, you need to tell the other. The one who has not had herpes may develop it after the marriage.

If you or your husband has had herpes or has it at the time of your wedding, I recommend that you not worry about protecting yourselves from each other. If one picks up the infection from the other, it will make no difference in your relationship in the long run since herpes does not actually damage the body. It is better to "share the problem" than to spend years trying to keep the uninfected partner from contracting herpes.

If it is not clear from the foregoing discussion, let me emphasize again that it is in no way dangerous for a person who has an active herpes sore to have intercourse. If the couple is married, they do not even need to use a condom. If they are unmarried, they should use both a condom and contraceptive form to try to prevent passage of the viruses from one to the other, so that the uninfected partner does not get the disease and then pass it on to subsequent sexual partners.

---

**1154** **Why is herpes so feared if it is not dangerous?**

There are many contributing factors to the widespread fear of herpes. One is that as many as ten million genital herpes infections occur each year in the United States, and from 1966 to 1979, the number of consultations with physicians for herpes increased 900 percent. Since that time the number has risen even more dramatically.

Since the only time herpes is dangerous is when a woman is delivering a baby (and that danger can be prevented by cesarean section), there is really no more significance to a herpes infection than to a bad cold, except that a herpes infection indicates that a person has had intercourse with someone else who had herpes, that the first episode of infection can occasionally be quite painful, and that recurrent outbreaks can be aggravating.

In spite of the relative "harmlessness" of herpes, one study showed that 84 percent of people with herpes reported occasional episodes of depression, with half of those describing the depression as being "deep." About 70 percent of people with herpes noted a feeling of social isolation. About 53 percent said that they consciously avoided potentially intimate situations, even during periods free from herpes outbreaks, and 10 percent of this group said that they had stopped having intercourse completely.

The lesson that herpes teaches is that in spite of the fact that we would all like to be able to do anything we want to without any consequences, our actions always do have a result, sometimes an undesirable one. If you have intercourse with someone who has had intercourse with someone else, you can catch herpes.

Once herpes is a part of your life, however, there is nothing to do but accept it. There is certainly nothing to be gained by depression, griping, or complaining. Accept the condition as a natural consequence of the choice you made; realize that it is not going to damage you physically and go on with your life from there.

# Gonorrhea

## 1155 What is gonorrhea?

The late Dr. Herman L. Gardner said, "Gonorrhea is probably the most important bacterial infection in the civilized world." In a book that he wrote with Dr. Raymond Kaufman (*Benign Diseases of the Vulva and Vagina,* Boston: G. K. Hall, 1981), Dr. Gardner states further: "Except for herpes genitalis, gonorrhea is the most prevalent of the major venereal diseases, its occurrence being several times that of syphilis. The incidence has risen steadily since 1958 and has nearly doubled since 1965."

As many as 100,000 women are made sterile by gonorrhea each year in the United States. About 20 percent of women who contract gonorrhea and develop pelvic inflammatory disease (PID) have continuing pelvic pain for years, and there are a million episodes of PID per year in women in this country. It has been estimated that gonorrhea costs the women of our country two billion dollars per year.

Although you may have heard similar facts many times before, let me urge you to consider them carefully. Gonorrhea is not something that "always happens to somebody else."

If you are having intercourse with anyone other than your husband, or if your husband is having intercourse with someone else, you can get this infection—and it can be devastating to your female organs. It was primarily the realization of the effect of this infection on American women that caused William M. McCormack, M.D., of Downstate Medical Center, Brooklyn, New York, to write an article titled "Sexually Transmitted Disease: Women as Victims" (*Journal of the American Medical Association,* July 9, 1982, pp. 177–178). Dr. McCormack states:

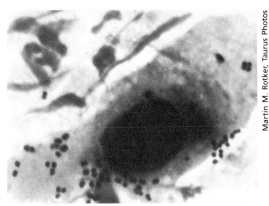

Gonococcus germ, magnified 1475 times

Pelvic inflammatory disease is by far the most important complication of the sexually transmitted diseases in contemporary industrialized societies. The economic costs are staggering. The direct cost of treatment of acute PID in the United States has been estimated to be more than six hundred million dollars annually. The total cost of this disease is upwards of three billion dollars a year.

The human costs, although less easily qualified, are also of enormous importance. Almost one million women are treated for PID in the United States each year, necessitating more than two hundred twenty thousand hospital admissions. Involuntary sterility, ectopic pregnancy, and chronic pelvic pain are important sequelae.

The long-term complications of PID result from the healing process. As the inflamed fallopian tubes heal, they may become completely occluded, resulting in involuntary infertility. The risks are substantial. Patients who have a single episode of gonococcal PID have a six percent chance of becoming infertile. The prospects for future reproduction are even poorer for women who have had multiple episodes.

Partial obstruction of the fallopian tubes predispose to ectopic pregnancies. Women who have had PID are six to ten times as likely to have an ectopic pregnancy as are women who have not had this infection.

Adhesions that occur during the healing of acute PID can result in chronic pelvic pain if the adhesions compromise the ovaries, the bowel, or other tender pelvic structures. Chronic pelvic pain occurs in ten to twenty percent of patients.

All of these complications can result from one episode of exposure to gonorrhea, but what frightens public health officials even more is that penicillin-resistant strains of gonorrhea have developed. This means that by the time an appropriate antibiotic can be found for a woman, her gonorrhea infection may have spread "out of control," perhaps even requiring hysterectomy for abscess formation.

## 1156 What causes gonorrhea?

Gonorrhea is caused by the germ *Neisseria gonorrhoeae*, which was discovered by Dr. Albert Neisser in 1879. This germ lives only in moist, warm areas and is passed only by sexual contact: vaginally, rectally, or orally.

## 1157 Will I know if I have contracted gonorrhea?

The incubation period for a woman exposed to a man with gonorrhea is usually from two to seven days, but it can be much longer than that. *Incubation* refers to the time from exposure to the time when symptoms of an infection appear. Only 20 percent of women with gonorrhea will have definite signs of such an infection; the remainder will not be aware that they have contracted the disease.

The 80 percent of women who carry gonorrhea without knowing it are like human time bombs. The germs can suddenly start proliferating, several months or years after exposure.

One of the major problems of a woman carrying the gonorrhea germ without being aware of it is that she can pass it to any sexual contact that she has.

## 1158 What symptoms might I detect if I have contracted gonorrhea?

*Vague, mild symptoms.* There may be a messy, watery vaginal discharge. Burning with urination may occur. These symptoms may be present without any symptoms of infection of the uterus, tubes, or ovaries.

*Symptoms of significant infection of the pelvic structures.* The first symptoms of a gonorrhea infection one may have often are those caused by inflammation of the pelvic organs: low abdominal pain and fever. Once these symptoms start, they usually get worse and worse, with the pain increasing and the fever going higher until effective treatment is begun. The typical patient with such an infection walks into the doctor's office or the emergency room bent over at the waist because of the pain.

*Combination of symptoms.* A woman who has intercourse with a man who has gonorrhea often develops a vaginal discharge a few days later. This is a symptom of vaginal and cervical infection by the gonococcus organism. When she has her next period, the gonorrhea germs will start growing profusely. They will ascend into the uterus and invade the uterine lining, tubes, and ovaries.

*Pain during the pelvic examination.* Once the pelvic organs are infected, they become tender. This tenderness is especially noticeable during a pelvic exam. When the doctor touches her infected uterus, tubes, and ovaries, a woman feels a great deal of pain. When a doctor does a pelvic exam on a woman with pelvic pain and fever, and finds her pelvic structures very tender, he or she can usually be sure that she has pelvic inflammatory disease caused by gonorrhea, some other sexually transmitted organism, or an IUD.

## 1159 Is gonorrhea really that serious?

Yes, gonorrhea is an extreme hazard to your physical and emotional health. Merely having the germ in your body will not damage you, but as early as two days after exposure the gonorrhea germs can cause pelvic inflammatory disease (PID).

Single people tend to read such warnings and ignore them, laugh them off, or say that somehow they will escape infection. However, infertility is no laughing matter when it happens to you. It can cause great emotional stress and regret.

In addition to the infertility that can result, there may be enough pelvic pain to warrant surgery. This type of persistent pain often is not relieved without a hysterectomy.

Because of the scarring, gonorrhea is also a major cause of tubal pregnancies. (See Q. 344–350.) A woman who has had a tubal pregnancy has only a 50 percent chance of ever becoming pregnant in the future.

Most women do not realize that a gonorrhea infection can spread to other parts of the body. It can cause Bartholin's gland abscesses (see Q. 676–678), infections in the joints (gonococcal arthritis), and skin abscesses.

If a woman delays treatment of a gonorrhea infection, she can develop an abscess which involves her ovaries. If such an abscess does not respond to antibiotics, it can produce a life-threatening situation. When an ovarian abscess ruptures, there is a significant chance of death because of the spread of infectious pus through the abdomen and rest of the body. Treatment for a pelvic abscess that does not respond to antibiotics is surgery, usually requiring removal of the tubes, ovaries, and uterus.

## 1160 Is gonorrhea dangerous during pregnancy?

The gonorrhea germ cannot get into the pregnant uterus, but if the organism gets into the baby's eyes during delivery, it can cause blindness. Fortunately public health laws in most states now require that an antibiotic solution be put in the eyes of all newborn babies to prevent this catastrophe. Since 80 percent of women with gonorrhea are unaware of it, many newborns would be blinded if this law were not in effect.

## 1161 Can gonorrhea be cured?

Gonococci can be killed with antibiotics, but treatment cannot erase any scarring that might have been caused by the infection before the antibiotics were given. Penicillin is normally adequate for gonorrhea, but if a woman is allergic to penicillin, other antibiotics will be substituted. If a woman has been infected with a penicillin-resistant gonorrhea organism, she will need to be treated with a different type of antibiotic, which at this writing is usually spectinomycin (Trobicin).

The first doubly resistant gonococcus (resistant to both penicillin and spectinomycin) was reported in late spring of 1981 in California. This indicates that new gonorrhea strains, which may be difficult to cure, are developing.

It is important that you talk to public-health officials about your sexual contacts if you have gonorrhea, because anyone with whom you have had intercourse while carrying a gonorrhea infection must also be treated. Otherwise the infection will flare up and possibly cause damage to his sexual organs, as well as infect his future sexual contacts. You have broken no law if you contract gonorrhea. Public-health officials are interested in finding people who have been infected only to help stop the spread of this disease.

If you have any reason to suspect that you may have been exposed to gonorrhea, insist that your physician do cultures of the area of your body with which you had sexual contact. You cannot be cured of gonorrhea unless you know it is there, and up to 80 percent of those with gonorrhea are unaware of its presence. If you have intercourse with anyone other than your own "faithful-and-true" husband, you could have come in contact with gonorrhea. In addition, it is also important that you have a culture done a week after your treatment is completed to be sure the disease has been eradicated.

## 1162 Can I get gonorrhea again?

Your body does not develop an immunity to gonorrhea. Therefore, repeated gonorrhea infections are possible. Remember, the more episodes of pelvic inflammatory disease from gonorrhea a woman has, the more likely she is to become permanently sterile.

## 1163 How can I keep from catching gonorrhea?

The most obvious way is not to have intercourse until marriage and then to have intercourse only with your husband, who has intercourse only with you. If you violate this rule of good health, you and your sexual contact can at least try using foam and rubbers in an attempt to keep from passing gonorrhea to each other. There is good evidence that this does decrease the spread of gonorrhea. Women who are taking oral contraceptives are a little less likely to develop gonorrhea. Women with IUDs, however, have an increased chance of developing this infection.

## Chlamydia

## 1164 What is chlamydia?

Chlamydia (pronounced *cla-mid'-ee-a*) is the most common sexually transmitted disease in America. Five to 7 percent of American women and 30 to 40 percent of some groups of teenagers are carrying chlamydia bacteria.

Chlamydia infects at least three million Americans a year and is a major cause of pelvic inflammatory disease (PID), which often results in sterility for women. It is estimated that chlamydia causes 11,000 American women to become sterile each year and produces at least 3,500 tubal pregnancies. As with gonorrhea, about 70–80 percent of women who have the germ have no symptoms.

You may have not heard much about chlamydia. One reason is that cultures for these bacteria in the past have not been reliable. Since new tests are now available, doctors are now beginning to culture women's secretions more efficiently.

Another reason that you may have heard of chlamydia is that the similarities between gonorrhea and chlamydia are so striking that both doctors and patients can confuse the two. When a woman develops a pelvic infection, it is easier for her doctor to tell her that this is "probably gonorrhea" than to say it is "probably chlamydia" because the doctor knows that the patient will have heard of gonorrhea and will know the significance of that.

## 1165 What are the symptoms of chlamydia infection?

As with gonorrhea, a woman may have a vaginal discharge, a Bartholin's gland abscess (see Q. 676–678), or infection in the pelvis which causes pain with or without fever.

A man who has a chlamydia infection, as with gonorrhea, may have a urethral discharge and burning with urination, or he may have no symptoms.

## 1166 What germ causes chlamydia infection?

The bacterium that causes chlamydia infection is *Chlamydia trachomatis*. It is difficult to culture, and culture techniques are still not even available to many physicians in this country.

## 1167 Is chlamydia dangerous?

The major problem of chlamydia infection is that it, like gonorrhea, can cause pelvic inflammatory disease. This germ, however, is even more likely to cause sterility than is gonorrhea. One report says that 25 percent of women who have one chlamydia infection in their fallopian tubes will become sterile; after a second infection, 50 percent of the patients will be sterile; and after a third infection, 75 percent of patients will be sterile. Additionally, 20 percent of women will have pelvic pain that persists for months and even years after only one episode of chlamydia infection. The infection is now considered so dangerous and so rampant that some experts believe that all reproductive age women having extramarital intercourse should have a chlamydia culture each year at the same time they get a Pap smear.

## 1168 Is chlamydia dangerous during pregnancy?

Although this germ does not get into the uterus during a pregnancy, it is a common cause of infection in the uterus after delivery. A woman who has fever and pain in her uterus after delivery may have a chlamydia infection.

Newborn babies can develop an eye infection if their mother has chlamydia in the vagina. In fact, it is the most common cause of eye infection in young babies. It rarely causes blindness, but it can.

Babies can also develop a mild pneumonia from the chlamydia organism. For a normal baby this is not dangerous, but for a baby weakened in some way (for example, prematurity) this infection can be a problem. As many as 30,000 newborns each year develop this pneumonia. Chlamydia can also cause ear infections in infants.

## 1169 Can chlamydia be cured?

As with gonorrhea, the chlamydia organism can be killed with antibiotics, but the scars that have already developed will not clear up after antibiotics have been taken. Antibiotics that kill gonorrhea germs may not kill chlamydia. If chlamydia is suspected, tetracycline is quite effective in curing the infection. If a woman does have pelvic inflammatory disease, even if caused by gonorrhea, she should also be treated for chlamydia at the same time.

## 1170 Can I get chlamydia more than once?

The body does not develop an immunity to chlamydia, so you can get a second or third infection. If this happens, your chance of total sterility in the future is greatly increased.

Normally tetracycline or erythromycin can be used to get rid of chlamydia that has been found on culture of the vagina or cervix, but more intensive antibiotic treatment would be necessary if you have developed chlamydia pelvic inflammatory disease.

## 1171 How can I keep from getting chlamydia?

The best method of prevention is not to have intercourse until marriage and then to have intercourse only with your husband, and he only with you. The use of foam and rubbers every time you have intercourse outside of these guidelines may help prevent your catching this infection, but studies about this are not yet conclusive.

## 1172 Is there anything else I need to know about chlamydia?

This is a confusing infection, both for patients and for doctors, but these recommendations may be helpful:

If a doctor is doing a culture on you for gonorrhea, ask to have one done for chlamydia, if possible. Then you will know whether or not you can get by with the shorter antibiotic therapy adequate for gonorrhea, or whether you should have the longer therapy needed to treat both gonorrhea and chlamydia.

If you have a continued vaginal discharge and have had sexual contact that could have given you a venereal disease, have your doctor culture you for chlamydia, especially if that discharge is not clearing up with use of other methods of treatment.

If you have had three or more sexual partners in the previous year, you are much more likely to have chlamydia than if you have had fewer sexual partners in that period. You should probably be getting not only a culture for chlamydia but also a culture for gonorrhea and a blood test for syphilis every six months, if you continue that sexual pattern.

If you have pelvic inflammatory disease you should be treated as though you have chlamydia since 50 percent of PID episodes in this country are a result of infection by chlamydia rather than gonorrhea.

## Syphilis

## 1173 What is syphilis?

Other than AIDS, syphilis is potentially the most dangerous sexually transmitted disease. Thirty thousand cases of syphilis were reported in 1982, but it is estimated that there were three times that many unreported cases.

Syphilis is acquired only by sexual contact with someone who has syphilis. About 50 percent of those who have such contact with a syphilis carrier will catch it.

Because of the danger of syphilis, it is extremely important that you have a blood test if you had intercourse with anyone who might have a sexually transmitted disease. This test should not be done until twelve weeks after exposure because it is not until then that the test will reliably be positive. If you have the test done sooner and it shows a negative result, you will, perhaps falsely, think you are free of the disease.

## 1174 What are the symptoms of syphilis?

Without a blood test, syphilis is extremely difficult to detect in women. The first sign is usually a painless sore, called a chancre (pronounced "shanker"). This sore is located where the infectious organisms enter the body and usually develops from ten to ninety days after intercourse with an infected person. It may look like a pimple, a blister, or an open sore, and it is usually not tender. This chancre usually goes away in two weeks, causing many people to think, falsely, that they are cured. This is never the case, however. The disease has only gone "underground" in the body to begin its insidious work.

A woman may have a chancre in her vagina or on her cervix where it is not visible. For this reason it is best for a woman to have a blood test twelve weeks after exposure to a sexually transmitted disease. If she has sexual contact with a man who knows he has syphilis, she would need to get immediate treatment and also to be tested twelve weeks later to make sure the medication worked.

Once the primary syphilis stage is past, a woman will not show signs of syphilis for from six weeks to six months. Secondary syphilis then develops, causing fatigue, fever, hair loss, skin rash, a warty-looking growth (condyloma latum) around the vulva or anus, and enlarged lymph nodes in various places around the body. Secondary syphilis can also cause hepatitis, kidney disease, meningitis, changes in the bones of the body, and eye infections.

This process can go on in a woman's body for four years before she enters the third or tertiary stage of syphilis which develops in about 25 percent of patients who have not been treated. Tertiary syphilis is a common cause for aortic aneurisms and disease of the heart valves. It is also a common cause of insanity.

Blood tests can determine the presence of syphilis, or a smear of the secretions from a chancre can show if syphilis germs are present. If either test is positive, a person has syphilis and must be treated.

## 1175 Which organism causes syphilis?

*Treponema pallidum*, a spirochete-type microbe, causes syphilis.

## 1176 Is syphilis dangerous?

Syphilis is a horrible, destructive disease. Untreated, it can cause insanity, nerve damage, blindness, deafness, and heart disease. It can also cause miscarriage, stillbirth, congenital abnormalities of a newborn, and

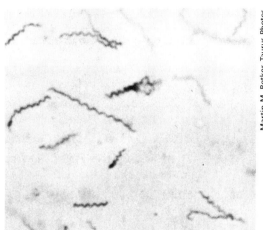

Martin M. Rotker, Taurus Photos

Syphilis spirochetes, magnified 1000 times

even death to both mother and child. (See next question.)

## 1177 Does syphilis affect pregnancy or the newborn?

If a woman has untreated syphilis while she is pregnant, she can have a miscarriage. If she does carry the pregnancy to term, the baby can be so badly infected that it is stillborn. Even if this does not happen, the baby may be born with bone deformities, tooth abnormalities, or blindness. A baby can be born looking normal but with the syphilis organism in its body. If untreated the baby can later become blind, deaf, paralyzed, insane, or have an early death.

There is one note of assurance, however: if you discover that you have syphilis before the eighteenth week of your pregnancy, you can be treated and the baby will almost certainly not be affected. Syphilis organisms generally cannot cross through the placenta from you into the baby until after the eighteenth week of pregnancy. It is for this reason that most states require a blood test for syphilis early in pregnancy. An untreated mother has only one chance in six of delivering a healthy baby. If your state does not require syphilis testing in pregnancy and your doctor does not order it, say that you want it done anyway. (See Q. 532–535.)

## 1178 Can syphilis be cured?

Yes. Antibiotics will always kill the germ that causes syphilis, although they will not reverse any damage that might have already occurred in a woman's body if treatment has been delayed.

If you have had intercourse with someone with syphilis, it is best to go ahead and have a dose of antibiotics (4.8 million-unit shot of procane penicillin with one gram of probenecid by mouth to make the penicillin more effective). There is no need to wait for a blood test to see if you have syphilis before you get treatment since there is a 50-percent chance of your contracting the infection. If you get treatment the syphilis infection would be cured before it could cause any damage to your body.

## 1179 Why take probenecid?

Probenecid keeps the body from getting rid of the penicillin as fast as it would otherwise. This delayed excretion of penicillin keeps the blood levels of the antibiotic higher than they would otherwise be, allowing the antibiotic to be more effective in killing the organisms of sexually transmitted disease.

## 1180 Can I get syphilis more than once?

Yes, you can. Any time there is a possibility of your having contracted this disease you should get tested and/or treated.

## 1181 How can I keep from getting syphilis?

As with other sexually transmitted diseases, the way to prevent infection is to refrain from intercourse before marriage and then to have intercourse only with your husband, who has intercourse only with you.

If you do have intercourse with someone else, use foam and rubbers. There is some indication that this might keep you from catching a venereal disease, but you must use these items every time you have intercourse.

## 1182 Is there anything else I should know about syphilis?

If a person has untreated syphilis, that person can infect sexual partners for up to four years. After that a person with syphilis cannot usually infect anyone else, but the damage from syphilis continues in that person's body for as long as he or she lives.

A syphilis test is required before marriage and when a woman becomes pregnant (in most states) because people can have syphilis and not know it.

Syphilis is totally responsive to penicillin if treated early enough. If it is neglected, the damage from the infection cannot be reversed by the penicillin, even though the progress of the disease can be stopped.

If you have syphilis it is extremely important that you talk to someone from your local health department. Their goal is to stop the transmission of syphilis and to try to eliminate the horrible effects of this disease from society. You should cooperate freely with this organization.

## Other Sexually Transmitted Diseases

## 1183 Are there other STDs?

Yes, there are. Three of these "minor" venereal diseases are: chancroid, lymphogranuloma venereum, and granuloma inguinale. They are considered "minor" for two reasons. One is because they occur so much less often than any of the STDs mentioned previously, and the other is because they are confined locally to the area where the infection starts and grows, rather than affecting the rest of the body. Because of this they are not usually life-threatening.

*Chancroid.* This infection is a highly contagious infection caused by a bacterium called *Hemophilus ducreyi.* It has been described as a "relative medical curiosity in the United States," and is a disease of the sexually promiscuous. It is more common in underdeveloped countries of the world, and a lack of personal cleanliness seems to be a major factor in developing the infection. The disease is first seen as a small bump (in women this is usually located on the labia, most often near the clitoris), which turns into an abscess, and finally into a tender ulcer. The ulcer is shallow and looks infected. If neglected it can spread to the inner thighs and groin areas and can be present for years.

*Lymphogranuloma venereum (LGV).* This infection produces enlarged lymph nodes in the groin and a rectal infection that causes a discharge of mucus and pus from the rectum. Enlarged lymph nodes around the anus may be present as the first sign of infection in a woman. This is especially so in patients practicing rectal intercourse. Occasionally these lymph nodes can break open and produce draining ulcerations. The agent that causes LGV is thought to be a form of chlamydia, but the usual chlamydia organism does not cause this disease.

*Granuloma inguinale.* This sexually transmitted disease is only mildly infectious and is extremely rare in the United States where fewer than one hundred cases are reported each year. The infection is most commonly reported among black people in the southeast United States.

This infection starts as a small, painless bump on the genitals. If it is not treated, it gradually enlarges over a period of months, finally developing a velvety, beefy-red growth.

Since a cancer of the vulva can look much like this infection, it is important that the doctor do a biopsy to make sure that the problem is not cancer. Enlarged lymph nodes are not usually present with this infection, making it different from the previous two STDs. Granuloma inguinale is caused by a microorganism called *Donovania granulomatis.*

Chancroid, granuloma inguinale, and lymphogranuloma venereum are not often seen in this country. However, since these infections can be dangerous and destructive, they should not be taken lightly. They can cause enlargement of the sex organs, stricture of the intestines with blockage of the intestinal tract, and even, rarely, death. A person with one of these diseases will know it and should see a doctor for diagnosis and treatment.

---

# 1184   What are "crabs"?

Unlike most of the other STDs, this condition is not dangerous, but it certainly can be disconcerting. Pubic lice ("crabs") are small parasites that can be seen without magnification. They live in the hairy areas of the body and most commonly occur in adults in the genital hair. Pubic lice are usually passed by direct contact with the pubic hair of an infected person. These organisms can, however, be picked up from bed sheets, clothing, or towels.

This infestation usually causes extreme itching in the area where the lice are present, but some people have no symptoms at all.

The treatment for pubic lice is a shampoo such as Kwell, which contains a lice-killing medication that will get rid of the organisms. Fortunately the treatment is easy and always works. The treatment should be repeated one week after its first use. Also all underwear, bedclothes, and pajamas should be washed at the same time during that week. It is important that both you and your sexual contact be treated.

The lice that live in a person's pubic area are different from those which infest the hair on the head. Generally pubic lice stay in the pubic hair and head lice stay in the area of the head. If a woman has pubic lice, she does not need to wash her hair with the same medicated shampoo that she uses in her pubic area.

## 1185 What is scabies?

Scabies is a condition caused by a mite, a parasite which burrows under the skin and causes itching. The infestation can exist in the skin folds of the body, and on the genital areas, on the fingers, wrists, and nipples, and even in the navel. The primary problem associated with scabies is severe itching wherever the mite is present in the skin.

When a doctor is examining a patient who has itching and small bumps in the areas of skin typically infested by scabies, he or she will examine the skin with a magnifying lens. If the doctor finds the burrows caused by the presence of the mites, a definite diagnosis of scabies can be made.

Several types of medication can be applied to the skin to kill these parasites. This infection is not dangerous, only very annoying.

## 1186 Is hepatitis a venereal disease?

Most of us do not think of hepatitis as a venereal disease, but one of the major ways in which it is spread is by sexual contact. The increased significance of sexual contact and its relationship to hepatitis is linked to the growing incidence of sexually transmitted disease in our entire society. Since any disease that can be spread sexually is becoming more common, hepatitis (which falls into this category), is also becoming more prevalent.

All three types of hepatitis are transmitted sexually, as far as researchers know now, but hepatitis B is the type that seems most likely to be transmitted in this way. The hepatitis B virus can be present in saliva, blood, urine, stool, menstrual blood, vaginal secretions, and other bodily secretions. It has been shown that in a group of people who have hepatitis B, one-third of their spouses will develop hepatitis, while only 2 percent of the other household contacts will develop it. There is also more hepatitis B among prostitutes, homosexuals, and patients attending venereal-disease clinics. A mother can pass hepatitis to her unborn child or to her baby during delivery. (See Q. 365.)

The course of hepatitis in a person's body is the same, no matter how a person contracted the infection.

A person who is exposed to hepatitis can receive gamma globulin to help decrease the chance of their developing the disease.

## 1187 Can vaginitis and vaginal yeast infections be sexually transmitted?

These problems can be sexually transmitted. (See Q. 689–693.)

*Yeast infections (monilia vaginitis).* Monilia vaginitis can be passed from a woman to her husband. It is rare for a man to be the first to develop this infection and then transmit it to his wife, and it is unlikely for a man to reinfect his wife unless he is uncircumcised and uses poor hygiene.

When I treat a patient who has a monilia infection, I encourage her to continue having regular intercourse. As she uses her medication, some of it will get on her husband's penis and treat him at the same time.

Monilia infection in the man can produce an irritation on his genitalia, of his groin areas, and of his inner thighs ("jock itch"). A man can use the same medicine that his wife uses for her infection. All he needs to do is rub this cream on himself two times a day. He will normally get well sooner than his wife because his genitalia are not so moist as his wife's vulvar and vaginal tissues.

Monilia vaginitis is not dangerous, but it is irritating. The primary problem a woman will have with monilia vaginitis is itching on her vulva.

*Trichomonas vaginalis vaginitis.* If a woman develops trichomonas, she and her husband must both be treated with Flagyl because if a woman has "trich," her husband also has it. If she is treated and her husband is not, he can give the infection back to her as soon as she stops her antibiotics.

Though trichomonas is normally passed by intercourse, it is quite common for a woman to get this germ on her hands from someone else and then transfer it to her vagina by touching her vulvar tissues.

The important thing is that once a woman develops trichomonas, she *and* her husband be treated in order to get rid of the problem.

The primary symptom of trichomonas vaginitis is vulvar itching.

*Gardnerella vaginalis vaginitis (Hemophilus, or H.V.).* Infection by the gardnerella organism is, like trichomonas, not transmitted only by intercourse, but once a woman has the infection, her partner has it too. When a woman has the typical odorous discharge (this infection does not cause itching), she needs to be treated. First, of course, she must be seen by her physician. Once the diagnosis is made, treatment is given to both her and her partner.

## Acquired Immunodeficiency Syndrome

### 1188 What is AIDS?

AIDS stands for "acquired immunodeficiency syndrome." It is a disease of previously healthy (and often young) people that begins with such nonspecific signs and symptoms as feeling listless, fever of unexplained cause, marked weight loss, diarrhea, and enlarged lymph nodes in several areas of the body. In this weakened state the body is susceptible to diseases that usually occur only in older, debilitated people or in people whose immunity is otherwise altered, such as transplant recipients who are on immunosuppressive drugs.

AIDS, therefore, is a collapse of the body's immune defense system, resulting in death by rare forms of cancer, pneumonia, or other overwhelming infections. This collapse is due to a virus that actually destroys the body's immune system, making it vulnerable to a wide range of other diseases. AIDS appears to be caused by a virus called the HTLV-III or lymphadenopathy-associated virus (LAV).

Some researchers believe that AIDS has existed for a long time in the African green monkey and in the past twenty to forty years it spread to men, possibly from monkey bites. Then there was a gradual migration of the residents from the rural area in which AIDS was prevalent into more populated areas. According to this theory, the virus spread from urban Africa to France and Belgium, and finally to other areas of the world.

### 1189 Who in the United States is most likely to have AIDS?

The disease strikes most frequently in male homosexuals (78%), intravenous drug users

(15%), women and babies of victims (5%), and recipients of blood transfusions (2%). From first reports in 1981 to mid 1985, more than 12,000 AIDS cases and more than 5,000 deaths caused by AIDS were reported in the United States, according to the Center for Disease Control in Atlanta. AIDS is already ten times more common in single men aged twenty-five to forty-five in San Francisco than all cancers combined.

The homosexuals who seemed to have the biggest risk of developing AIDS, according to first research, are those who have a large number of sexual contacts. One study of a group of early AIDS victims showed that they had an average of 120 different sexual partners during the year before they developed symptoms of AIDS. One man had had up to 250 different sexual partners in each of the three years before he developed symptoms.

These early studies of AIDS victims suggested that a very promiscuous homosexual sex life or a contaminated blood transfusion was necessary for a person to acquire AIDS. We now know this is not the case. In early 1985 it was estimated that more than one million Americans were infected with the AIDS virus and that 5 to 20 percent of those infected would develop AIDS in the next five years. This suggests that at a minimum 50,000 men and women who are presently infected with the AIDS virus will die of this disease in the next few years unless some treatment is found. This does not take into account the additional number who will become infected during the next few years. The number of AIDS victims can become astronomical.

We now know that this is not only a disease of homosexual men. Heterosexuals do acquire AIDS from sexual contact. Women do acquire it from men and they in turn can transmit it to their babies during pregnancy. Women can also pass it to men, and it does appear that prostitutes can be a source of AIDS infection. Prostitutes are more likely to have AIDS than other women because more of them are intravenous drug users and also because they are more likely to be exposed to men with AIDS.

If you are in any of the high-risk categories mentioned above and become sick, be sure to tell your physician. There is no definite diagnostic test for AIDS, but tests of a person's immune system (tests of T-helper and T-suppressor cells against T4 and T8 antigens) can suggest AIDS. Your doctor would suspect AIDS if you seem to have poor body defense against infections and contracted any one of several serious infections that usually occur only when a person's body defenses are low.

For instance, if a young woman develops Kaposi's sarcoma or pneumocystis carinii pneumonia, she probably has AIDS, unless there is some other reason for poor body defense against infection, such as being on immunosuppressant drugs as a transplant recipient would be.

In early 1985 Abbott Laboratories received the first United States license for a test that evaluates blood-bank blood or plasma for AIDS. One of the most frightening aspects of AIDS is that it could be passed in blood transfusions. At the time of this writing, it was felt that this test is accurate, sensitive, and also specific for detecting blood that contains antibodies against the AIDS virus. It is reassuring to know that such testing is becoming available to protect people who otherwise have not been exposed to AIDS. It is possible, however, for a person to develop AIDS soon after he or she donated blood. Even though that blood tested as free of the AIDS antibodies because the antibodies were not increased in the donor's bloodstream, the AIDS virus would be passed on to the recipient of the transfusion.

Anyone who has been told that his or her blood shows AIDS antibodies should consult a physician who deals with the syndrome to determine the significance of such a finding. A large number of such tests will falsely indicate the presence of AIDS antibodies. One study indicates that only 6 percent of those who show a positive initial response to the tests will actually develop AIDS.

Other information about AIDS can be obtained from various AIDS hotlines that have been established around the country. One of these is in New York. That phone number is 800-462-1884.

## An Afterword

Whether or not we accept the fact that God created our bodies or that he has anything to say about how we use them, it seems reasonable to learn how our bodies function best. One way to do this is by observing what happens to other people. When we do this, we can develop guidelines for our own activity.

Let's review a few of the things that have been discussed.

AIDS is a frightening new disease. It has no cure and results in death. It would not exist except for sexual promiscuity in our world and infects more heterosexual men and women every month.

Precancerous and cancerous growths of the cervix are now epidemic in our society. They almost never occur in virgins or in married women when neither husband nor wife has ever had intercourse with anyone except each other. The virus that causes venereal warts seems to cause precancerous and cancerous changes of the cervix; and spread of this virus is primarily by sexual intercourse.

One of the most common causes of infertility in our society is PID (pelvic inflammatory disease), usually caused by gonorrhea or chlamydia. People who get these infections are permanently sterile 10–20 percent of the time after only one infection.

Syphilis, if untreated, can lead to multiple and severe health problems. Worse, if a woman's syphilis has not been treated, it can lead to severe congenital abnormalities in any baby she might deliver.

STD infections are often present without symptoms. One can have intercourse with a person who has not had intercourse with anyone else in years and still catch a sexually transmitted disease from that sexual partner.

If the pattern of sexual activity we engage in has the potential for cutting out from under us the basics of life itself—health, fertility, and longevity—it seems reasonable to reevaluate that pattern.

I hope the facts discussed in this chapter will help you to be more confident of your sexual lifestyle if it is healthy and reevaluate and change that pattern if it is destructive. I hope you can learn from these words and not have to experience an irreversible process in your body that can affect you for the rest of your life.

If you contract one of these diseases, you can survive. Perhaps you can live with the infertility that you might experience from an episode of PID, but the regret and frustration of such an experience can affect you for the rest of your life.

Do not expect to hear much about this problem from your physician. Most physicians are afraid of sounding moralistic to their patients. They are so reluctant to come across this way, in fact, that they do not treat sexually transmitted disease as they do other infectious processes. For other infectious diseases for which there is no immunization, doctors quarantine patients so that they stay out of contact with other people. There are laws, for example, in most states that force a person to be quarantined if he or she has infectious tuberculosis.

Most doctors treat STD differently, however. They almost never recommend that an infected person stay away from others so that the disease spread can be stopped. The emphasis is usually on treatment of the disease rather than on prevention.

It seems reasonable to me that physicians should at least warn patients that sex outside marriage can cause their bodies and emotions irreversible harm.

The one practice that will absolutely stop the spread of sexually transmitted disease is for men and women to have intercourse with no one until they are married, and then only with their husband or wife. Of course, remarriage increases a person's sexual contacts, but this would be minimal when compared to the general sexual exposure in our society today.

Perhaps we need some motivation other than fear of damage to our bodies from sexually transmitted disease to accept the validity of reserving sex for marriage. Could it be that the motivation we need to help us treat our bodies right might come from the One who made our bodies in the first place: God? I personally think so.

I believe that God made me and therefore knows how I will function best and how I will be happiest. To this end he has written an "Owner's Manual" for the human being: the Bible. Just as I look in my Buick's owner's manual when I want to know how my car will function best (because it was written by the people who made my Buick), so I look into the Bible to see how my psyche and my body will work most efficiently.

The Bible has some specific guidelines about sexual function:

A man will leave his father and mother and be united to his wife, and they will become one flesh (Gen. 2:24).

Marriage should be honored by all, and the marriage bed kept pure, for God will judge the adulterer and all the sexually immoral (Heb. 13:4).

Therefore what God has joined together, let man not separate (Mark 10:9).

Husbands, love your wives, just as Christ loved the church and gave himself up for her ["died for her" would be my addition] (Eph. 5:25).

You shall not commit adultery (Exod. 20:14).

> The wife's body does not belong to her alone but also to her husband. In the same way, the husband's body does not belong to him alone but also to his wife (1 Cor. 7:4).
>
> God gave them over in the sinful desires of their hearts to sexual impurity for the degrading of their bodies with one another (Rom. 1:24).

God knows what will provide us with the happiest, healthiest life. His guidelines concerning sex say that we will enjoy sex most if we reserve it for marriage. In spite of that, some of us will try to use sex in ways outside God's guidelines. If we do, not only will we eventually have greater emotional instability and problems than we might otherwise have had, but we may also contract disease.

If we do become temporarily involved in sex outside marriage, it is important that we recommit ourselves to sex only in marriage. We will then be ultimately happier and, of course, physically healthier.

To ignore the warnings of sexual encounters that lead to STD can also cause us further physical damage because of the natural laws of infectious disease. Other laws illustrate that principle. If I try to ignore the natural law of gravity, for instance, because I feel that it restricts me too much, I will damage or kill myself. I cannot walk off the top of a building without suffering the consequences!

It is important to remember that God loves you more than you love yourself. He wants the best for you now and in the future. He did not design your psychological make-up or the physical laws of the universe for any reason other than for your ultimate benefit.

God knows we have a need for intimacy—he created us with it. But we will not find that intimacy by engaging in sexual intercourse. As a matter of fact, Dr. J. Dudley Chapman of Ohio University College of Osteopathic Medicine recently pointed out that "the sexual revolution with its emphasis on performance has caused some people to shy away from intimacy." We can enjoy true intimacy only by developing a loving relationship with a person of the opposite sex, by becoming committed to him or her, and then becoming intimate with him or her in marriage, the environment God planned for this intimacy.

This is what God meant when he said, "A man will leave his father and mother and be united to his wife, and they will become one flesh" (Gen. 2:24).

# 14
## Marital and Sexual Relationships

Although this book is concerned primarily with the physical aspect of a woman's body, the sexual and relational aspects of a woman's life are discussed in this chapter. My patients confront me every day with concerns about marital and sexual relationships: frustrations with their husbands, a recent divorce, or their children's marital problems. Many of these women are literally dying emotionally. You may be experiencing some soul-wracking emotions in your personal life. If you are, you need to seek the cure for that "emotional cancer," just as you would search diligently for treatment of a physical malignancy.

If you have a good marriage, do not blissfully assume that you will live happily ever after. If you are wise, you will do the things necessary to keep future problems from developing in your relationship with your husband. A good marriage takes a lot of work, sacrifice, and tender loving care. Such a marriage is worth the work, however, because the satisfying, harmonious, and secure relationships that characterize it encourage all members of the family to develop to the maximum of their God-given potential.

Those who are trying to decide whether or not they want to be committed to marriage may argue that—since there are so few happy marriages in our society—they would be better off not getting married at all. I feel that just as a woman should not get married only because society expects her to, so she should not avoid marriage because she fears the problems that society says exist in marriage. If she lives her life based on fear of what "might happen," she would never move away from home, never drive a car, never get married, never have children, and never do anything worthwhile.

It is important that if a woman does choose to get married, she not do it expecting her husband to fulfill all her needs completely. In her book *The Joy of Being a Woman*, Ingrid Trobisch says (p. xiii), "No man will ever be able to satisfy completely the innermost desires of a woman's heart for love, beauty, and shelteredness. I believe it is possible to live a full life, whether single or married, in spite of unfulfilled desires. We can only look to the One who says: 'My purpose is to give life in all its fullness' (John 10:10)."

Marriage can never be "perfect" since it reflects the imperfect natures of the men and women who make up the union. It can, however, provide the stage and the raw materials for the emotional and spiritual growth of a man and woman who are part of it.

## Some Basic Marital Principles

**1190** **What can I do to help make sure I develop a good marriage or to improve the marriage I have?**

My wife, Marion, and I have read and studied about marriage extensively through the years of our marriage. We have discovered some general principles that seem to recur in any discussion on the subject of developing and maintaining a healthy marriage. In addition to this, although I am not a marriage counselor, I do a lot of marriage and sexual counseling. All gynecologists do. Many women do not have a clergyman they can talk to, and many couples do not feel that their problems are bad enough to warrant a formal appointment with a psychologist or psychiatrist. Consequently the gynecologist often ends up being the profes-

sional who is first approached with a problem. The suggestions that follow are not all inclusive, but they do address areas of need that my patients often express. You may not agree with all of these suggestions. They are, however, principles that many counselors who deal with marriage problems see couples frequently violating. I hope this discussion can help you avoid some common problems in marriages. They may improve your marriage if you use them as a pattern to change things that need changing.

*Never consider divorce as an option.* Most problems that occur in life can be solved. Present-day technology has shown us that solutions can be found to seemingly impossible problems. This holds true for marriage, and yet we tend not to believe it. If we enter marriage considering divorce as an eventual option, when we encounter problems, which we definitely will, divorce will seem to be the only solution. Leaving even the possibility of divorce at the marriage altar will free our minds to find other solutions to the problems that will inevitably surface.

There is no question that there will be times when you will want to bail out of your marriage. If you and your husband deny yourselves the option of ever considering divorce, you will not incubate thoughts about separation but will spend your intellectual and emotional energy in working out your problems. This will greatly increase the chance that you and your husband will enjoy the treasure of a long and happy life together.

*Realize that no two people are perfect for each other.* I am not saying that God has not chosen two people to be man and wife, but rather that those two people are neither perfect in themselves nor perfect for each other. Marion and I have often said that without our commitment to each other and to our God, we could have easily ended up in the divorce courts. Although our personalities are totally different, with the help of God we have been able to work out our differences and build a happy home and marriage.

*Expect—but don't push—change.* You should never enter marriage planning to make changes in your husband later. You should realize, however, that neither you nor he will stay the same person you were when you married. You will both change. You must marry your husband (and he you) for all the different people that each of you will be in the future. If you have been married for a long time, you are probably quite aware that you are not the same person you were on your wedding day. Marriage is a constant process of adaptation to and acceptance of each other, and this flexibility is one of the things that adds spice and life to the marriage relationship.

*Learn to love.* Amazingly, many marriages in the world are still arranged by the parents. In many of these marriages the couples learn to live together and to love each other. Although most of us would probably deny it, we still have a Hollywood approach to love in our society, characterized by talk such as "falling in love" usually "across a crowded room." There will be times in your marriage when you do not feel love for your spouse. It is important that you know this beforehand, so that you will not think that all hope is gone and fear that you can never have a healthy emotional relationship with your husband again. You can learn to love again, even when you feel that you have lost the spark that you had when you got married. In fact, it is only when you come to the point of losing the short-lived, emotional spark that you can start developing the deep, abiding, warm, and mature love that characterizes the sound marriage we all desire.

*Sacrifice and compromise.* Marriage is not a fifty-fifty proposition. It is a ninety-ten arrangement whereby the husband and wife both must give 90 percent and expect only 10 percent in return. I believe that this is one of the key elements in having a happy marriage. To be willing to give more than you get requires discipline, and both discipline and giving are completely opposite to the values society seems to be teaching us today. It is impossible for a person to be happy without giving and sacrificing and compromising. If we try to find fulfillment by "getting," we will find that the more we receive, the more we want, and that there is no end to that cycle. Our only hope for happiness is in "giving," and our only hope for a good marriage is in being willing to sacrifice and give for our spouse. Amazingly, with that attitude, both partners usually end up receiving more than they expected!

*Don't misuse pride.* Pride is one of the most damaging forces in a marriage. Men in particular often find it difficult to say, "I'm wrong," or "I'm sorry." That attitude is caused by pride. Likewise, women are being told that if they "give in" to their husbands they are retreating from their rightful position as modern women. This too is a problem of overblown pride. Neither husbands nor wives can afford to tolerate unbending pride in themselves if they are to have a good marriage.

*Never entertain the thought of being unfaithful.* Most husbands or wives do not wake up suddenly one morning and say, "Today I am going to destroy my life and my marriage and have an affair." They are more likely to allow dissatisfaction to incubate, then to grow, then to produce the action that tears their homes apart. Once planted, the seeds of lust or desire toward someone other than a mate can grow by leaps and bounds, nurtured by feelings of injustice, frustration, and self-pity. It soon becomes a full-grown plant, choking out any good fruits of the marriage and ultimately destroying the whole with its clutching, tearing tentacles. Just as the tallest mountains are moved one shovelfull at a time, so adultery becomes reality one thought at a time. An improper thought rejected, however, will be quickly replaced by a better thought, and those of us who truly desire a good marriage ultimately learn that truth. We deliberately refuse the luxury of planting the seeds of self-indulgence, and choose instead to nurture the growth of our marriages. It is a matter of conscious choice.

*Treat your mate as your best friend.* Sadly, the people we love the most are often the people we treat the worst! We would never treat the people we work with, or strangers on the street, the way we all too often treat our families. Not only should the Golden Rule be in effect in our homes, but we should handle with tender care the relationships that are of utmost importance to us.

*Leave mother and father.* A marriage in which either partner is still emotionally dependent on a parent is headed for trouble. A healthy marriage requires emotionally mature people. If a husband or wife is still dependent on his or her parents, that person is functionally immature and childlike. Any person in a marriage who has this type of dependency should get counseling imme-

diately if the problem cannot be solved by the partner.

*Have a spiritual commitment together.* A spiritual commitment creates a lasting foundation for the home. A mutual commitment to God gives the family security and a common purpose. God instituted marriage and the home, and on this foundation we can be assured of being in a God-ordained institution from which we can work out his will in our lives.

*Realize the importance of sex.* A marriage is not just a spiritual, emotional, or friendship partnership. Marriage is also quite definitely a physical relationship. The Bible reveals how God integrated the physical aspect of marriage (including nakedness) into the sanctity of the home:

> A man shall leave his father and his mother, and shall cleave to his wife; and they shall become one flesh. And the man and his wife were both naked and were not ashamed (Gen. 2:24–25, NAS).

And from the Song of Solomon 7:10–12 (NAS):

> I am my beloved's,
> And his desire is for me.
> Come, my beloved, let us go out into the country,
> Let us spend the night in the villages.
> There I will give you my love.

It is sometimes easy to focus on improving communication and solving problems and to forget about the importance of working on improvement of the sexual relationship in marriage.

*Communicate.* In his book, *Why Am I Afraid to Tell You Who I Am?* (Allen, Texas: Argus, 1969), John Powell shares the following tremendous insight (pp. 43–44):

> Harry Stack Sullivan, one of the more eminent psychiatrists of interpersonal relationships in our times, has propounded the theory that all personal growth, all per-

sonal damage and regression, as well as all personal healing and growth, come through our relationship with others. There is a persistent, if uninformed, suspicion in most of us that we can solve our own problems and be the masters of our own ships of life, but the fact of the matter is that by ourselves we can only be consumed by our problems and suffer shipwreck. What I am, at any given moment in the process of my becoming a person, will be determined by my relationships with those who love me or refuse to love me, with those whom I love or refuse to love.

It is certain that a relationship will be only as good as its communication. If you and I can honestly tell each other who we are; that is, what we think, judge, feel, value, love, honor and esteem, hate, fear, desire, hope for, believe in and are committed to, then, and then only, can each of us grow.

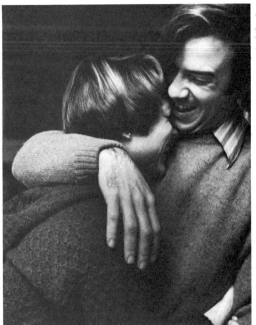

A relationship is only as good as its communication.

These words eloquently emphasize the importance of communication in marriage. They also explain why destructive, unproductive, or nonexistent communication in a marriage can become intolerable and damaging. We would all agree that talking with a spouse is of a higher priority in life than watching TV, but we sometimes find it hard to make the decision to cut off the TV to talk about a problem or just to "visit" with each other. When we compare the ultimate value of TV with talking together as husband and wife, it is incredible that there is any difficulty in making the right decision.

*Be willing to get help.* From the day a couple is married, they need help, and there are many sources of outside support. Don't be afraid to learn from parents, trusted friends, or your pastor. If you and your husband develop some knotty problems you cannot untie, don't be afraid or ashamed to go to a psychologist, psychiatrist, or a member of the clergy for counsel. If your pastor, priest, or rabbi does not feel competent to counsel you, he or she will probably be able

to suggest a psychologist or psychiatrist. It is important that you like your counselor and that you share a mutual value system. If a counselor suggests activities or solutions that offend your morality or values, you should find another source of counsel.

Remember, it is much better to go to a counselor for solutions to a problem when it starts than to wait until it has become ingrained.

*Invest time and work.* It is hard to overemphasize the importance of this particular aspect of marriage enrichment, yet it is one of the most neglected areas. Husbands and wives seem to feel that a good marriage should exist without working at it—but it will not. Men and women work at their jobs, in their homes, and at clubs or schools. It seems that we are willing to work at everything except our marriages and families. It is small wonder that there are more divorces than marriages in some cities.

Unfortunately, it is easier to pretend that a marriage is good than to spend time and effort fixing it. Yet couples must allow adequate time for the marriage relationship, even if it requires turning down a higher-paying job, or social and club activities. This "sacrifice," in the long run, will make for a happier life and marriage. Money cannot produce happiness in our later years, nor can fame. In fact, they seem merely to complicate life.

*Envision the future.* Each of us needs a vision of the years ahead and a willingness to invest whatever it takes to insure as happy and peaceful a future as possible. Much time, work, and dedication must be expended on a marriage today, to make it "profitable" in the future. It is nice to know, as the years go by, that our investment will pay rich dividends in a deep, close relationship with another human being who loves us and whom we love in return, who needs us and whom we need, and who is our best friend.

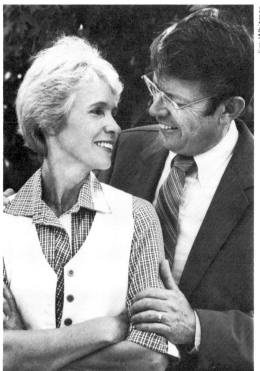

It is the joy of a loving relationship with someone who understands and accepts us and whom we understand and accept that will produce the peace and contentment that will make us feel that our life has been a success.

---

**1191** **When you say, "Realize the importance of sex," does that mean you believe that a couple's sexual relationship is a primary factor in marriage?**

Yes. As a matter of fact, it is important enough to spend most of the rest of this chapter discussing it.

Obviously one of the primary functions of a woman's body is sexual activity. This is evident not only by the way that the body is made, but also from statements in Scripture in which sexuality is discussed. Many sections of the Bible point out the importance of the physical/sexual aspect of married life, and it is important for women to understand this.

There is no foolish naivete about a woman's body, about marriage, about sexuality, or about sexual intercourse in the Bible. God did not design one part of the body to be more important than another, nor

did he create "good" body parts and "bad" body parts. Every part of a woman's body is important and was designed to be properly used.

Sexual intercourse is one of the most intimate forms of communication between husband and wife. Physical intimacy should communicate the love, emotion, and commitment that each has for the other. Sexual intercourse is an almost unbelievable combination of emotional and physical communication between two people. Even more marvelous than this is the fact that such a union can produce a baby who is, in a true sense, the "one flesh" that two people become when they have intercourse.

It seems clear that from the beginning God created us as sexual persons with the ability to have intercourse as a way to express and experience the deepest form of personal relationship with each other. In addition, and just as important, is the ability to reproduce ourselves by that act. Because of this, it seems clear that no marriage can reach its highest potential for a loving, happy relationship between a husband and wife without a healthy, fulfilling sexual compatibility. It may also be true that—if a couple is able to have children—their marriage may not reach its highest potential until a child has resulted from their union.

## Preparing for Marriage

### 1192 What do I need to know about sex if I am about to get married?

Contrary to prevailing modern opinion, if you have not had intercourse before marriage, you have a headstart in your marital sexual relationship over the woman who has already had intercourse. It is even better if neither you nor your husband has had intercourse before. You will be able to develop patterns of sexual activity together, unhindered by "comparisons" to former partners, sexual hangups carried over from past experience, guilt from former sexual activity, or physical problems (including possible infertility) that may have resulted from sexually transmitted disease or abortion.

I encourage you to read books about sexuality and sexual intercourse. A list of books I have found helpful for patients is included in Q. 1221. One particularly good book is *The Joy of Being a Woman* by Ingrid Trobisch. In this book the author says, "The secret [to sexual fulfillment and happiness] lies in the self-acceptance of the woman as a woman and especially in saying Yes to her body with its special ways of experiencing life." (p. 7). In other words, the way that a woman can most enjoy her body is to accept her sexual nature and allow herself to experience sex.

Trobisch's discussion of the wife's sexual involvement in marriage includes this statement: "This confidence in herself and complete trust in the sheltering love of her husband will enable her, figuratively speaking, to be able to jump off a cliff without any doubt in her heart that her husband will be there to catch her." It is important to develop that type of trust in your husband and acceptance of yourself as a woman that will enable you to have this abandonment of yourself to your husband in sexual intercourse. The end result is not self-deprecation in "giving yourself" to your husband, but rather the total fulfillment that comes with your emotional and physical immersion in a relationship with someone whom you love and trust implicitly.

If you have had sexual intercourse before marriage, it is best to try to put behind you any past experience and preconceived ideas about intercourse and enter marriage with an open mind. This will allow you and your husband to develop your own personal approach to your sexual interaction.

One of the most pleasant surprises about sex is that a husband and wife never achieve perfection. There is always an improvement or variation that can become a part of sexual relations that makes it different, even when a couple has been married fifty or sixty years!

### 1193 Is it important to have a physical examination before marriage?

Yes. Consulting your doctor before marriage is a good idea for several reasons. If you are a virgin, a pelvic examination will reveal any abnormalities you may have: a hymen that might be too tight for intercourse (see Q. 17, 687), a growth on an ovary or the uterus, or a major abnormality that might signal an infertility problem. If you have had sexual intercourse before, the physician can perform tests to see if you have any detectable sexually transmitted disease. In most states a blood test for syphilis is required before you can get a marriage license. The physician cannot tell just by the physical exam whether or not you have a venereal disease. If you think that there is any possibility that you might have a sexually transmitted disease, tell your physician so appropriate testing can be done.

A major reason women see a doctor before marriage is for counsel and advice concerning contraception. You might find it helpful to read chapter 12 before seeing your doctor for a premarital exam. Being knowledgeable and prepared for your appointment will allow you to utilize your time with the doctor much more effectively. If you have a good idea beforehand what kind of contraceptive you want to use, your doctor can tell you more about it and give you a prescription if one is necessary.

In addition to performing the physical examination, most doctors will encourage you to discuss your attitudes concerning sexuality. If you are aware of having any hang-ups, say so. Your doctor can answer your questions and will refer you to a counselor if you need further information or advice about marital and sexual relations.

If you do have sexual problems or hang-ups, you should not feel guilty about this. Our personal perception of sex is a result of input from our families, our peers, what we read, movies we have seen, and so on. In one sense we are not really responsible for the way we feel, but we are responsible for allowing distorted views and misinformation to persist in our minds.

## 1194 Is premarital counseling really important?

Because there are so many strikes against marriage today, if I were getting married now I would avail myself of some good premarital counseling.

In the early 1980s there were about 2.5 million marriages per year and about 1.1 million divorces per year, almost a 50-percent divorce rate. Among people who have had one divorce, there is a 60-percent divorce rate for later marriages. These statistics reflect only those who believed that divorce was the answer and do not show how many more couples are living in unhappy situations because they do not choose divorce. Obviously there is a need for marriage counseling.

Good premarital counseling can help a couple be aware that marriage is not the ethereal, live-happily-ever-after life that they had expected. It will underscore the truth that marriage takes hard work, sacrifice, and letting go of pride.

## 1195 Is a good knowledge of male and female sexual anatomy important to marriage?

It is vital that you know about your own sex organs and their function, and it is just as important to know about your husband's sex organs. This information is important not only for the actual sex act, but for sex-related matters such as contraception, pregnancy, delivery, and so on.

In a wonderful little book, *Better Is Your Love than Wine*, by Jean Banyolak and Ingrid Trobisch (Downers Grove, Ill.: InterVarsity, 1979), this intuitive statement appears (p. 19): "The act of love is an intimate encounter of the whole masculine person with the whole feminine person. It is the total union of body, soul and spirit." If you are going to have this type of intimate contact with another person, you need to know what that person looks like naked and what he looks like sexually aroused.

It is each partner's responsibility to caress and stimulate the other in the foreplay that is so important to arousal in the sex act. You must, therefore, know what parts of your husband's body are sexually sensitive, where those parts are, and what they look like.

(See chapters 1 and 10 for complete information on the female body and female organs. See the next question for a brief discussion of the male organs.)

## 1196 What are the male sex organs and how do they function?

To help you understand the male genital organs, two illustrations are provided. Using these illustrations you can see where the sperm are produced and can follow their course from origin in the testicles (testes) through the internal and external male genitalia to the outside of the body.

The scrotum is the sack of skin that holds the man's two testicles. If a man has only one testicle, he generally still has more than enough sperm for fertility and more than enough testosterone production to be a totally normal male. Both testosterone and sperm are produced in the testicles. Testosterone, a male hormone, is secreted into the veins of the scrotum and distributed through the man's body by the blood-vessel system.

The man's seed (sperm) is produced continuously by the testicles, but the same amount of sperm is not produced each day. A few years ago, an eminent urologist did a study in which he counted one man's sperm every few days for more than a year. There were days when the man's sperm count was very low and days when it was very high. This is one reason a couple does not achieve pregnancy every time they have intercourse during the woman's fertile period.

The sperm produced by the testicles are passed into a collecting system called the epididymis. Each testicle has an epididymis contained entirely inside the scrotum.

The vas deferens is the tube that passes up from each epididymis, out of the scrotum, over the pubic bone, and back down into the man's pelvis to connect with a storage chamber for sperm, the ampulla, which is located just above the prostate gland. The ampulla penetrates through the prostate gland to connect to the urethra, the tube from the bladder that carries urine and sperm to the outside through the penis.

Just before the ampulla connects to the urethra, the seminal vesicles open into the ampulla. The seminal vesicles are glands that produce seminal fluid which carries the sperm down the urethra and out of the penis. If all the sperm in a man's ejaculate were concentrated, there would be only a small mass of cells. Without the seminal fluid, they would not make up enough volume to leave the man's penis. Most of the material that comes out of a man's penis with ejaculation is, therefore, the mucus produced by the seminal vesicles and the prostate gland.

Just below the bulb of the urethra are two pea-size tubular glands, called Cowper's glands, which discharge a mucus secretion into the urethra.

The urethra serves two functions: it is the tube through which urine is passed from the bladder and it is also the tube through which the seminal fluid is ejaculated. When ejaculation occurs, the semen is squirted forcefully and quickly through the urethra to the outside. Simultaneous with this event, the base of the bladder clamps down, preventing the flow of semen back through the urethra into the bladder at the time of ejaculation.

The penis is an ingenious organ, carefully created to perform three intricate functions: the first is the passage of urine from the bladder; the second is erection, which allows the penis to be inserted into the woman's vagina; and the third is the passage of semen from the ampulla.

The foreskin of the penis is merely loose skin which covers the head of the penis (the

# Adult Male Internal Sex Organs

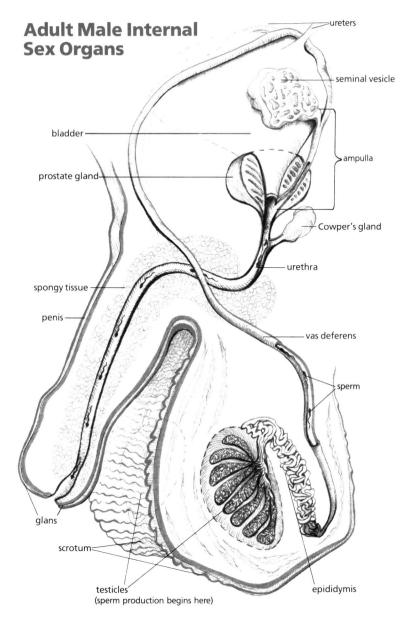

ureters

seminal vesicle

bladder

ampulla

prostate gland

Cowper's gland

urethra

spongy tissue

penis

vas deferens

sperm

glans

scrotum

testicles
(sperm production begins here)

epididymis

glans penis). When a man's penis is erect, the foreskin pulls back away from the glans. If a man has been circumcised the glans stays exposed all the time. If a man is not circumcised, he should retract the foreskin from the glans daily and wash under it.

A man's penis becomes erect when blood flows into the spongy tissue of the penis. Valves in the veins that flow out of this spongy tissue keep the blood from flowing back out as fast as it flows in. It is interesting that a man's erection can become slightly flaccid and then rigidly erect again. Since an erection is emotionally controlled, a distraction can cause an erection to be lost or weakened.

An erect penis is important for pleasure and for conception. Intercourse would be

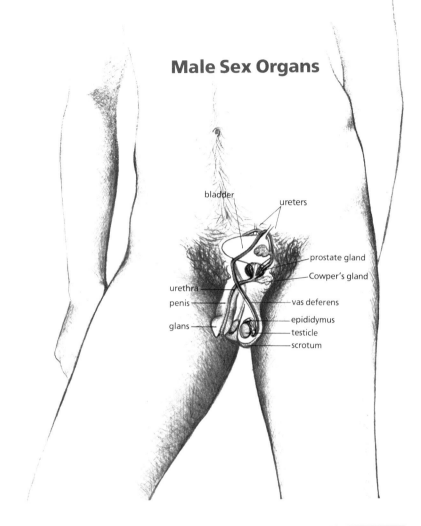

## Male Sex Organs

bladder
ureters
prostate gland
Cowper's gland
urethra
penis
vas deferens
glans
epididymus
testicle
scrotum

impossible without it. Without a firm penis, the deposition of semen inside the woman's vagina against her cervix would be impossible. Incidentally, the force of the ejaculate does not push the semen up inside the woman's uterus, but merely deposits it high in the vagina, where the sperm have the best chance of swimming out of the semen into the cervical mucus. (See the complete discussion on conception in chapter 6.)

God ingeniously designed the female and male bodies to fit together perfectly. In doing this, he not only provided for procreation but for pleasure as well.

**1197** **Which areas of a man's body can be used to stimulate him sexually?**

A sensitive partner can arouse her mate by touching him almost anywhere, but there are some areas that are more sexually sensitive than others. Most of these erogenous zones are in the genital area. A general rule for both men and women is that the closer the stimulation is to one of the openings of the body, the more arousing it is.

A man's nipples, like a woman's, are often sexually sensitive, and his scrotum can be gently touched to produce erotic stimulation. The closer to the urethral opening at the end of the penis a man is stimulated, the more likely he is to be sexually aroused. Often the area on the underside of the glans penis (where the glans attaches to the shaft of the penis) is one of the most sensitive areas of a man's body.

The area around the anus is often sexually sensitive, and the armpits and the inside of the thighs are areas that can often be used to arouse either a man or a woman.

In stimulating these areas, it is important to realize that the more sexually excitable an area is, the more likely it is to be delicate and sensitive. Stimulation should be gentle.

## 1198 Where are a woman's erogenous zones?

You will probably find that your areas of sexual sensitivity are much like those of the man. Stimulation of your mouth and ears and the areas around them will probably be pleasant to you, and sensitive stimulation of your breasts will probably be erotic. Just as a man's scrotum is sexually sensitive, so are both the labia minora and majora when touched carefully and stimulated gently. Just as a man's penis is his most sensitive area sexually, so your clitoris is your most sexually responsive area. As a matter of fact, the clitoris is the only organ in either the male or the female body that is made only for sexual pleasure!

## 1199 What premarital suggestions do you have for a couple who is nervous about beginning sexual relations?

These suggestions may help you and your husband become relaxed with each other sexually.

*Premarital counseling.* Be sure that you

have taken advantage of any counseling available and have read some pertinent books, so that you thoroughly understand what your bodies and sex are all about.

*Talk with each other.* If you have embarrassment or hesitation about the importance of sex in your life as a married couple, talk about this, both before and after marriage. Share openly with each other. Be gentle with each other, and try to be understanding. Realize that you will not experience all there is to sex on the first night of your honeymoon. Sex is something that develops over your entire life together as you work at it and allow it to grow.

*Wedding night bubble bath.* The wedding day can be exhausting. To help you both unwind and to start the physically intimate part of your relationship in a relaxed way, try the following: slip into a warm bubble bath while your new husband undresses in the bedroom. Then call him into the tub with you. Rub and caress each other. When you are ready, get out of the tub and gently dry each other off. From there, progress to doing what comes naturally—you will both be a lot more relaxed than you were. This suggestion comes from the excellent book by Clifford and Joyce Penner, *The Gift of Sex: A Christian Guide to Sexual Fulfillment* (Waco: Word Books, 1981.)

*Explore.* Exploring each other's bodies is a good way to become comfortable about sex. You may not want to do this type of exploration immediately after you are married, but after a few weeks or months you may find it helpful to check each other out carefully.

You can explore each other, both visually and with your fingers. Your husband can show you, and let you touch and feel, his penis and scrotum. He can show you areas of his body that he particularly likes you to touch. You can prop up on the bed in a semi-reclining position, spread your legs, and point out your labia majora and minora to your husband. You can guide his hand to your clitoris and show him what it looks like. Show him the areas of your genital region that are most sexually exciting for you. Then guide his fingers into your vagina to show him what it feels like and what areas of it are particularly comfortable for him to touch and manipulate. While his fingers are still inside your vagina, you can tighten your pelvic muscles, squeezing his fingers the way you would his penis, to show him that you do have some control of your vaginal muscles.

## Maximizing Your Sexual Pleasure

### 1200 What is the best environment for sexual activity?

Both you and your husband will enjoy love play more when you know that you will not be interrupted. You need to be sure that the phone is covered with a pillow or disconnected. If there are other people in the house, make sure that the door is locked and that they will have no reason to knock on the door.

Personal hygiene on the part of both you and your husband is important. Just as you will not appreciate his body odor, he will not want your breath to smell of onions! Be sensitive to each other; learn what things are likely to make your total environment conducive to sexual arousal.

From the beginning it is important that you and your husband vary the place, atmosphere, and method of your sexual activity. Since sameness and routine become boring and unexciting, it is important to change some aspect of the circumstance in which you make love as often as you can.

Some couples have the mistaken romantic notion that sexual activity should take place only when there is complete unity of desire, intensity, and setting. This implies that each sexual experience is a perfect sexual experience and places unnecessary restraints and constrictions on your lovemaking. Sexual pleasure is elastic and as a couple spontaneously explores the range of sexual responsiveness, their enjoyment of each other intensifies. Don't wait to initiate sexual activity until both spouses seem to be equally interested. If you do, you will cheat yourselves out of a broad range of interesting and exciting activity.

### 1201 What are the phases of sexual responsiveness?

Masters and Johnson, well-known researchers in the area of human sexuality, describe a "sexual response pattern" (see diagram) in their book, *Human Sexual Response* (Boston: Little, Brown & Company, 1966). They identify four phases through which a couple normally passes during sexual excitement.

*Excitement phase.* It is during this phase that foreplay should occur. You should gently stimulate your husband, and he should gently stimulate your sensitive areas. As you become sexually aroused, your labia majora and a minora will swell, and lubrication of your vaginal opening will occur. Your breasts and nipples will also become engorged and somewhat swollen. In addition, both your heart rate and your breathing rate will increase. As you stimulate your husband, his penis will become erect and hard. The skin around his testicles will become thickened, and the testicles themselves will seem to be drawn up against his body more tightly.

The amount of time that you and your husband spend in foreplay is a completely personal matter. The key is that you allow enough time for each partner to become fully aroused. If you feel that your husband is

# Sexual Response Pattern

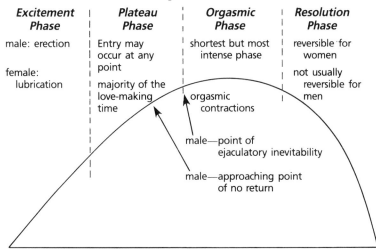

| Excitement Phase | Plateau Phase | Orgasmic Phase | Resolution Phase |
|---|---|---|---|
| male: erection | Entry may occur at any point | shortest but most intense phase | reversible for women |
| female: lubrication | majority of the love-making time | orgasmic contractions | not usually reversible for men |

male—point of ejaculatory inevitability

male—approaching point of no return

Adapted from Masters and Johnson, *Human Sexual Response* (Boston: Little, Brown, & Co., 1966).

rushing you, let him know. Likewise, if he feels that you are rushing him, he should tell you.

**Plateau phase.** Once you have stimulated each other into the "plateau phase," both will be ready for entry of the penis into your vagina. During this interval, the changes that occurred during the excitement phase will continue, but with greater intensity. This phase should last long enough to bring you both to orgasm, usually simultaneously. If your husband experiences premature ejaculation, he will lose his erection. In that case, the way for you to reach orgasm is for him to stimulate you manually or orally.

A husband can learn to hold back his orgasm for at least fifteen minutes of continual thrusting, and he can also learn to keep his erect penis in your vagina for thirty minutes. Probably neither you nor he would want to have intercourse for this long every time, but it is possible. (See Q. 1207.)

**Orgasm.** You may not always have an orgasm with intercourse and yet feel quite fulfilled with the lovemaking experience. It is important that you let your husband know that you can be satisfied with his love-making even without having an orgasm. Women occasionally tell me that they are not sure whether or not they have an orgasm, but most women definitely know when it occurs. If you are satisfied and relaxed after intercourse, you have probably had a climax even though it may have been a quiet one.

Orgasm for a woman involves involuntary contractions of the muscles surrounding the outer portion of the vagina, which includes a thrusting of the pelvis. Contractions of other muscles of the body may also occur. A woman may perspire and salivate, and her increased heart rate will peak. The feeling is one of intense pleasure and relief, unlike any other sensation a woman will ever experience. For a woman, orgasm is an all-encompassing event involving the whole body. A man's orgasm is much more localized, as the majority of his intense feelings are directed toward his pelvis and penis.

A woman can have repeated orgasms. For some women this is a regular occurrence; for others it is rare. You may find that your husband will ejaculate after you have had one orgasm, but that he can continue to stimulate you and bring you to orgasm repeatedly. If you want him to do this, guide his hand to your clitoris or other erotically sensitive parts of your body and move his hand around in such a way that he brings you to climax again.

A man's orgasm occurs only once during an episode of sexual excitement, but it involves multiple contractions of the prostate gland, the ejaculatory ducts, and the penis. These contractions usually occur five or six times and at tenth-of-a-second intervals. A man ejaculates about one teaspoon of seminal fluid, which contains an average of 350 million individual moving sperm.

***Resolution phase.*** During this time, engorgement of a woman's pelvic structures and of her breasts gradually returns to normal. If she has had an orgasm this engorgement diminishes more quickly than if she has not been brought to climax. During this phase of resolution, a woman can sometimes be brought to orgasm again by stimulation.

Most of the time a man cannot immediately have another erection and orgasm and will relax and go to sleep more quickly than his wife. If your husband does this and it bothers you, ask him if he will stay awake with you a little while and hold and caress you until your resolution phase is complete. Some men can have an erection and ejaculation again in an hour or two. If your husband can do this, a little closeness can turn into more than that if you both want it to. However, many men must wait several hours or overnight to develop another erection.

---

## 1202 How often is "normal" for couples to have intercourse?

The frequency of intercourse that satisfies you and your husband is the "normal" frequency for you. Some couples have intercourse only once a month; others have intercourse every day. Either one of these habits of intercourse—and anything in between or beyond—is normal if the couple is happy with it.

Most young to middle aged couples, however, want to have intercourse about two or three times a week unless there is a medical or emotional problem. For the purpose of fertility, couples who have intercourse three to four times a week are the most likely to get pregnant during a one-year period.

One of the clearest directives to married couples concerning frequency of intercourse is in 1 Corinthians 7:3–5 where the apostle Paul states: "The husband should fulfill his marital duty to his wife, and likewise the wife to her husband. The wife's body does not belong to her alone but also to her husband. In the same way, the husband's body does not belong to him alone but also to his wife. Do not deprive each other except by mutual consent and for a time, so that you may devote yourselves to prayer."

If you or your husband is extremely dissatisfied with the frequency of your intercourse, don't pretend there is no problem. Get sexual counseling if you cannot work it out on your own. Too often a husband or wife will tolerate the frustration related to frequency of intercourse, suffering in silence until he or she is filled with anger and resentment, finally "bursting out" and saying and doing things that would never have been necessary if the dissatisfied partner had been more open earlier.

In most such cases the wife is satisfied with the frequency of intercourse, but the husband wants to have relations more often. He may need to adjust his demands to some extent, but the wife may also need to modify her willingness to satisfy his needs and desires. Compromise on both parts is the ideal, and communication is usually the key.

It is best to remember that you and your husband have promised yourselves to each other. You will want to enter into intercourse with your husband frequently enough to relieve the emotional tension which sexual need produces in him. Although he does not want to cheat on you in order to meet his needs, he can become filled with a great deal of resentment and anger if you habitually avoid having intercourse with him as frequently as he feels the need for it. He can feel trapped, caught between your resistance to his advances and moral values that deny him sexual release with anyone else. A situation like this can affect not only his happiness but your own as well.

---

**1203** **Will it hurt my husband physically if he does not have intercourse frequently enough for his needs?**

Refraining from intercourse is often necessary for a variety of reasons, and this practice will not hurt a man physically. Nature has a way of providing the release of the sperm and seminal fluid that are continually produced by the testicles and prostate glands: nocturnal emissions, or "wet dreams."

A nocturnal emission is simply an ejaculation that occurs while a boy or man is asleep. When there is a buildup of sperm and semen, these secretions distend the internal genital organs, stimulating an ejaculation.

Nocturnal emission is a normal event for boys and men who do not have intercourse or who are prevented from having it for a period of time, although it is also just as normal for them not to have nocturnal emissions. It seems quite obvious that God has provided nocturnal emissions for the relief of the sexual tension that men might otherwise feel drives them toward extramarital sex.

---

**1204** **Is the desire for oral sex normal?**

Oral sex, which refers to the stimulation of the sexual organs of either partner with the mouth or tongue of the other, is ultimately a matter of personal preference. The best discussion I have seen concerning oral sex is in the book, *The Gift of Sex*, by Clifford and Joyce Penner (Waco: Word Books, 1981). I encourage you to get a copy and read this discussion.

The Penners point out that in the Bible's Song of Solomon, reference seems to be made to the lovers stimulating each other with their mouths. If this is so, it would seem to indicate that from God's perspective there is nothing wrong with the practice of oral sex (Song of Sol. 4:16–5:1). The authors do stipulate, however, that although there is nothing unnatural or wrong about oral sex, it would be wrong if it "violates" one of the partners. They state: "It does not violate anyone to *avoid* oral sex, but it certainly *may* violate someone to be pushed into it" (italics mine).

The Penners feel that there are three questions that should be answered concerning this subject.

*Is it natural?* A body part is still a body part, no matter where it is located. Oral stimulation of the genitals, therefore, can be accomplished as "naturally" as can oral stimulation of the breasts, the mouth, and the ears. What would make oral sex and other sexual variations "unnatural" would be in insisting that a partner participate against his or her wishes. Having intercourse should be an act of love, and it is unnatural to intentionally violate the one you love.

*Is it right?* Although the Penners use the Bible as their authority and refer to the passage in Song of Solomon, they point out that Scripture is not really clear on the matter of oral sex, and the Bible cannot be used to either support or incriminate it. They conclude: "The principle of what is loving and caring for the other person must be addressed; on the other hand, the teaching that our bodies are each other's to enjoy must also be incorporated."

*Is it clean?* There are three conditions that can exist in the bodily systems related to sexual relations: sterile, clean, or contaminated. The urinary system is normally "sterile" (it has no bacteria); the reproductive system, which includes the penis and the vagina, is "clean" (normally free of any disease-producing organisms; the rectal area and the mouth are "contaminated" (have disease-producing microorganisms). If the body is washed and there are no infections present, the mouth would not be contaminated by the genitals. If any contamination did take place it would be from the mouth to the genitals, but this is unlikely.

It is important to remember that just because something is not clearly wrong or dirty or unnatural does not necessarily make it right, natural, or necessary for you. The factual data in this section is intended merely to clear up some myths and distortions concerning oral sex.

In conclusion the Penners make this statement: "To the one who desires oral activity but is inhibited by the hesitancy of your spouse, we offer encouragement. Many couples change over time, and what was uncomfortable for one becomes more natural as that one is cared for and loved without judgment and without demand."

---

## 1205 Is it normal for intercourse to be so messy?

Yes, it is. Some couples who have not been forewarned of this are surprised to find that there is such a mess after intercourse. Although your husband's ejaculate amounts to only about one teaspoon of semen, it may seem to be a gallon! Your body, too, contributes to the mess, since moist secretions come from your own vaginal and vulvar areas during sexual excitement.

The secretions that result from intercourse are normal body fluids and will not cause irritation or infection. If you do not wash them off, they will dry on your body without harm. There is no medical reason to douche after intercourse.

Most couples, however, prefer some degree of cleaning up after intercourse. You may want to keep some towels or tissues at your bedside, or you may prefer to go to the bathroom and wash off after intercourse before you go to sleep or dress for the day. You may find it helpful to insert a tampon to absorb these secretions.

Don't let the "untidiness" of intercourse bother you. Think of the secretions as not only "life-giving," but also as a by-product of the most intimate relationship that a man and a woman may have.

---

## 1206 Is it all right to have intercourse during my period?

Although most couples do not choose to do so, there is nothing wrong with having intercourse during the wife's menstrual period. Intercourse during menstruation is the safest, in terms of avoiding pregnancy, and is not harmful to the woman in any way. Unless normal menstrual cramping interferes with their pleasure, many women find intercourse at this time satisfactory.

The major disadvantage to this practice, of course, is that it can be extremely messy. Towels positioned under the couple during intercourse will help alleviate that problem.

God told the Israelites (Lev. 18:18) to avoid intercourse during the woman's menstrual period. Couples must decide for themselves if they feel they must observe this portion of the Mosaic law.

---

## 1207 What can be done about the problem of premature ejaculation?

When a man ejaculates before, or soon after, his penis enters his wife's vagina, a great deal of frustration can develop for both the husband and wife. Fortunately there is help.

Joseph Dillow, a former marriage counselor, offers the following advice from his book, *Solomon on Sex* (Nashville: Nelson, 1982):

**STEP 1 Eliminate past myths.**

There are two main myths that hinder solution.

First, it has been taught that because men reach orgasm more quickly, the wife should refrain from direct stimulation of the husband prior to intercourse. The contrary is usually true. A man is more likely to reach orgasm prematurely when he goes **unstimulated** through a long period of preparatory arousal for the woman. Because he becomes too preoccupied with the time for intercourse, anticipation builds to an unbearable degree. Furthermore, through stimulation, the wife can bring him to a sexual peak prior to orgasm that actually reduces the need of climax immediately. Of course, for the wife to refrain from full participation removes the sense of physical intimacy and mutual experience. The whole experience is reduced to getting her ready, entering her, and ejaculating immediately. There is little opportunity for intimacy.

Secondly, the myth that the man is supposed to put his mind on other things needs to be rejected. I've seen Christian books in which the man is instructed to mentally recite Bible verses to get his mind off the pleasure he is experiencing! Others counsel him to worry about business problems. There are two basic downfalls to this "solution." It doesn't work, and it spoils the sense of enjoyment!

**STEP 2 Commit your situation to the Lord as a couple.**

Ask one another's forgiveness for any hurts that may have developed in your marriage because of this problem, then join together in prayer asking the Lord to give you the wisdom and unconditional acceptance necessary to implement these steps. If you are unable to pray about it openly in front of each other, you do not have the necessary acceptance and freedom level to solve the problem. If you can't pray about it, there are some things in your relationship that need to be resolved before you'll be able to work at this. Most sexual problems are either caused by spiritual and relationship problems, or they are made more complicated by these factors.

**STEP 3 Employ the "squeeze technique."**

Agree on a session of sexual stimulation with no goal orientation. There will be no intercourse and no "failure," just mutual sharing of love. The wife should sit at the head of the bed with legs spread. The husband lies between her legs on his back with his head pointing toward the foot of the bed. His genitals are now close to those of his wife. The wife lovingly and gently caresses her husband's genitals, especially the head of the penis or wherever her husband directs her, to encourage him toward orgasm.

As soon as he approaches orgasm, he gives the signal and she applies the "squeeze technique." She places her thumb on the underside of the penis just where the shaft ends and the head begins (the frenulum). She also places the first two fingers of that same hand on the opposite side of the penis, then squeezes her thumb and first two fingers together with very hard pressure for at least four seconds. She should squeeze as hard as she can. (On an erect penis this will cause no pain.) This pressure will immediately make him lose his desire to ejaculate, and he will lose some of his erection. After fifteen to thirty seconds, she repeats the procedure, manipulating him to full erection again and repeating the squeeze.

**STEP 4 Intercourse in the "woman above" position.**

After learning some control, the husband lies on his back and the wife uses the squeeze technique two or three times: she then straddles him and, leaning forward about 45 degrees, very gently and slowly inserts the penis in her vagina. She should remain motionless—giving her husband a chance to achieve control. If he feels he is going to ejaculate, she merely raises her body and repeats the squeeze procedure, then gently reinserts the penis. After a few sessions of practice in this position, the husband is to thrust just enough to maintain his erection until they can stay in this position for fifteen or twenty minutes before ejaculation. The "male above" position is the most difficult in which to maintain control.

**STEP 5 Intercourse in lateral coital position.**

After control increases, the couple is encouraged to move from this female superior position to the lateral coital position (sideways). Lying on her right side, she leans forward to lie against his chest as she extends her right leg behind her. He bends his left knee, keeping it under her leg and flat against the bed. This position leaves both partners with the greatest freedom and comfort as well as the best ejaculatory control. It has been found that couples who have tried this position use it (by choice) about 75 percent of the times they have intercourse.

**STEP 6 Repetition once a week for six months.**

You should use the squeeze technique at least once a week for the next six months and practice it for about twenty minutes at some time during each of the wife's menstrual periods. Complete ejaculatory control is usually attained in six to twelve months. By this we mean the husband develops control to the point where he can restrain ejaculation indefinitely.

While the couple is learning these steps, it may be necessary for the husband to use manual stimulation or other agreeable means to give the wife sexual fulfillment.

It must be noted here that there often is temporary impotence after the premature ejaculation problem is solved, primarily due to increased frequency of the sex act.

Researchers tell us the squeeze technique is never effective if done by the husband on himself—the wife must be involved.

Even if you are not having problems with premature ejaculation, but you don't have sufficient control to maintain continuous thrusting for fifteen minutes, this technique can be used to build your control up to as long as your wife desires. By making sideways motions with his hips the husband can stimulate his wife's clitoris without bringing any friction on the penis, significantly lengthening the time of intravaginal containment (pp. 162–165).

If you are embarrassed or uncomfortable in performing the squeeze technique on your husband, there may be some false modesty on your part, and this is something you can and should overcome. Inhibition of this type can have a restrictive and oppressive effect on your entire sexual relationship. In this case the squeeze technique may not only have an advantage for you in prolonging intercourse time with your husband but also in improving your freedom to experience fully the relationship between the two of you.

---

**1208** **Can drugs taken for a medical problem affect sexual responsiveness?**

Yes. Drugs can definitely affect sexual responsiveness in both men and women. Unfortunately many people and many doctors do not associate drugs with sexual problems.

Men and women can lose their sexual desire because of certain drugs, and men may lose their ability to have an orgasm or their ability to ejaculate. Some drugs cause men to have persistent erections (called priapism), and others cause men and women to become sleepy and lose their energy, which can alter their desire for intercourse. Testosterone, occasionally used in ointments for postmenopausal women who have vulvar irritation, can cause vulvar and pelvic discomfort and distorted sexual interest. More information is given in the accompanying chart.

Alcohol also can negatively affect sexual

# Drugs and Their Effects on Male Sexual Response

| Name/Trade Name of Drug | Libido Decreased | Loss | Impotence | Ejaculation No | Delayed | Dysfunction | Other Problems |
|---|---|---|---|---|---|---|---|
| **Heart and Blood Pressure:** | | | | | | | |
| Acetazolamide (Diamox) | | • | | | | | Decreased potency |
| Atenolol (Tenormin) | | | • | | | | |
| Chlorthalidone (Hygroton) | • | | • | | | | |
| Clofibrate (Atromid-S) | • | | • | | | | |
| Clonidine (Catapres) | | | • | | | | |
| Digoxin | • | | • | | | | |
| Disopyramid (Norpace) | | | • | | | | |
| Guanethidine (Ismelin) | | | • | • | | | |
| Hydralazine (Apresoline) | | | • | | | | |
| Phenoxybenzamine (Dibensyuline) | | | | • | | | |
| Prazosin (Minipress) | | | • | | | | |
| Propranolol (Inderal) | | • | • | | | | |
| Reserpine (Ser-Ap-Es, Regroton, Salutensin) | • | | • | • | | | Decreased ejaculation, breast enlargement |
| Spironolactone (Aldactone, Aldactazide) | • | | • | | | | |
| Thiazide diuretics | | | • | | | | |
| Timolol (Blocadren, Timolide) | • | | • | • | | | |
| **Psychoactive:** | | | | | | | |
| Amitriptyline (Elavil, Endep) | | • | • | • | | | Breast enlargement, swelling of testicles |
| Aoxapine (Asendin) | | • | • | | | • | |
| Butaperazine (Repoise) | | | | • | | | |
| Chlorpromazine (Thorazine) | • | | • | • | | | Priapism |
| Diazepam (Valium) | • | | | | • | | |
| Doxepin (Sinequan) | • | | | | | • | |
| Haloperidol (Haldol) | | | • | | | | Painful ejaculation |
| Imipramind (Tofranil) | • | | • | | • | | Painful ejaculation, delayed orgasm |
| Isocarboxazid (Marplan) | | | • | | • | | |
| Lithium (Eskalith) | • | | • | | | | |
| Nortriptyline (Aventyl, Pamelor) | | | • | | | | |
| Pargyline (Eutonyl) | | | | • | | | |
| Perphenazine (Trilafon) | | | | • | | | Decreased ejaculation |
| Pheneizine (Nardil) | | | • | • | • | | Difficulty achieving orgasm |
| Thioridazine (Mellaril) | | | • | | | • | Priapism |
| Thiothixene (Navane) | | | | | | | Spontaneous ejaculation |
| Tranylcypromine (Parnate) | | | • | | | | Spontaneous erections |
| Trifluorperazine (Stelazine) | | | | | | • | |

| Name/Trade Name of Drug | Side Effects | | | | | | |
|---|---|---|---|---|---|---|---|
| | Libido | | | Ejaculation | | | Other |
| | Decreased | Loss | Impotence | No | Delayed | Dysfunction | Problems |
| **Gastrointestinal:** | | | | | | | |
| Chlodiazepoxide (Librax) | • | | | | | | |
| Cimetidine (Tagamet) | • | | • | | | | |
| Dicyclomine hydrochloride (Bentyl) | | | • | | | | |
| Methantheline bromide (Banthine) | | | • | | | | |
| Propantheline bromide (Pro-Banthine) | | | • | | | | |
| **Hormonal:** | | | | | | | |
| Estrogen | • | | | | | | |
| Hydroxyprogesterone caproate (Delalutin) | | | • | | | | |
| Methandrostenolone (Dianabol) | • | | | | | | |
| Norethandrolone | • | | • | | | | |
| Norethindrome (Norlutin) | • | | • | | | | |
| Progesterone | • | | • | | | | |
| **Others:** | | | | | | | |
| Aminocaproic acid (Amicer) | | | | • | | | |
| Fenfluramine (Pondimin) | | • | • | | | | |
| Homatropine methvibromide (Homapin) | | | • | | | | |
| Metronidazole (Flagyl) | • | | | | | | |
| Naproxen (Naprosyn) | | | • | • | | | |
| Phenytoin (Dilantin) | • | | | | | | |

responsiveness. Although a small amount of alcohol can reduce tension from the day's activities or from anxiety about the sexual relationship, larger amounts of alcohol decrease libido and sexual interest in both men and women. For example, about 40 percent of alcoholic men are impotent and about 40 percent of alcoholic women have poor response to sexual stimulation. If either partner drinks excessively, the sexual relationship will suffer. Other drugs such as marijuana and cocaine may also affect sexual responsiveness.

---

## 1209 What can be done to enliven and strengthen a "too routine" sexual relationship?

The fact that you want to improve your physical relationship indicates good emotional health. Too many couples become bored with their relationship and with each other, a problem which can fester and finally explode, damaging their marriages even more.

Some suggestions I offer my patients include:

*Improve your spiritual relationship.* If you and your husband have entered a period of sexual drought, the solution may lie in improving your spiritual relationship with God and in improving your personal relationship with each other. In an excellent little book, *Better Is Your Love than Wine* (Downers Grove Ill.: InterVarsity, 1979), Jean Banyolak says (p. 42), "Human power alone is not enough for a successful marriage. We would be lost if God Himself were not willing to give us His power in order to put this counsel into practice. In order to be able to understand each other and to love each other intimately in the way I have described, it is necessary for each one of us to have a personal relationship with God."

*Communicate with each other.* Couples frequently fall into a routine sexual pattern and are embarrassed to tell each other that they want to change it. You may think that your husband ought to realize that you are dissatisfied with your sexual relationship, but he cannot know unless you tell him. Likewise he may feel that your sexual relationship needs change, but asking you to do something different makes him feel like a little boy begging a favor—his pride prevents his doing this. If you sense dissatisfaction on the part of your mate or if you are vaguely discontented, communicate! Talk with each other in an open-minded, accepting way, then initiate some changes to improve the relationship.

*Spend more time together.* Sexual problems often develop in midlife marriages. By this time in life you and your husband can literally be too busy. Overfilled schedules can make unhurried, relaxed, first-class lovemaking an impossibility. Although there is no perfect answer to this problem, the beginning of the solution is the realization that you have fallen into the habit of being too busy for each other. Perhaps you can spend a night at a local hotel or motel once a month, or maybe you can schedule being together at a certain time during the week when no one else is at home. The possibilities are as extensive as your imaginations. Use them to improve your marriage.

*Be willing to change.* Almost everyone is uncomfortable with change. Even if we are not totally happy with a situation, it often seems "safer" than the risk of trying something new and different. If you or your husband become dissatisfied with your love life, however, you cannot afford *not* to change. In the past few years, too many patients have come to my office for annual exams and told me that their husbands left them for younger women during the previous year. I think many of these men found themselves in a marriage relationship that had lost its spark. They began looking for something different,

especially in the sexual area. It is possible that they might have constructed a new and exciting sexual relationship with their wives if they had expressed their dissatisfaction to them or if the wives had not been too busy or too "set in their ways" to change.

It is possible, therefore, for you and your husband to modify your sexual pattern so that he (and you) can say, "Hey, I have a new sexual partner right here at home! Why should I leave home for satisfying sex, with all the heartache that would bring, when we have developed a new and exciting sex life right here?" Don't wait until there is boredom in your relationship. Make some changes, starting tonight.

*Have fun!* If you and your husband have settled into a routine that has lost some of its zip, experiment with some techniques and atmosphere that make it fun for you again. This may involve getting rid of some of your embarrassment and preconceived notions about propriety. Be creative in planning variations. Wear a sexy gown or negligee, plan intimate dinners for two. Be spontaneous. Pick unusual times and places to have sex. It doesn't always have to take place in the bedroom.

In addition to these creative techniques, it may be that you and your husband need to have shared fun and spend time together apart from sexual intercourse. If this is true, you need to schedule times to just be together "for the fun of it" and not "for the sex of it."

*Please your husband.* In one of the best books I have found concerning sexual fulfillment, *The Gift of Sex* by Clifford and Joyce Penner, there is a section concerning ways to increase the pleasure of being together. The authors describe many techniques for expanding constricted and limited pleasure in the sexual relationship. The summary of their chapter on "pleasuring" (p. 149) pretty much says it all: "You will learn sensuous touching as you are free to flow with the pleasure from your inner self and as you are open to learning to touch in a way that is pleasurable to your partner. These two factors, plus the ability to allow variation and experimentation, can keep a relationship exciting for a lifetime."

*Change positions for intercourse.* Many couples fall into a habit of using only one position for intercourse. Although other positions may not be as comfortable for you or for your husband, using them occasionally can make you enjoy your old, familiar way more.

## Problems that Hamper Sexual Enjoyment

**1210** **What are the most common problems relating to sexual intercourse?**

Although there are many problems that can hinder or limit a couple's enjoyment of sex, three of them seem to be most commonly mentioned.

*Pain.* If you have recurrent pain with intercourse, you almost certainly need to see a gynecologist for an examination to determine if there is a physical abnormality causing the pain. Reading Q. 719–729 which discuss problems of the vagina, including painful intercourse, will increase your understanding of this problem.

*No orgasm.* If you are newly married and have not yet had an orgasm, you are probably normal, since many women do not have an orgasm for many months after getting married. Worrying about not having orgasms can turn you into an "observer" of your sex act and further inhibit your ability to come to climax. For now, just enjoy the warmth and closeness of intercourse and don't strive to

have an orgasm, as you will almost certainly be surprised by one when you least expect it.

If you have been married for several years and have not begun having orgasms, consulting a sexual counselor can be beneficial for you and your husband.

*Guilt.* For years secular writers have tried to make those of us who are committed to a religious faith feel guilty about having what they call a "puritanical view toward sex." A survey taken by *Redbook* magazine (September, 1970), however, reported that "sexual satisfaction is related significantly to religious belief. With notable consistency, the greater the intensity of a woman's religious convictions, the likelier she is to be highly satisfied with the sexual pleasures of marriage."

As a matter of fact, Fred Belliveau and Lin Richter in their book, *Understanding Human Sexual Inadequacy,* state (p. 192) that of 193 women treated by Masters and Johnson at their Reproductive Biology Research Foundation in St. Louis for primary orgasmic dysfunction, 41 were from rigidly religious families. The homes of these 41 people were described as being filled with denial and repression, backed by religious sanctions. This is not the type of faith that the Bible teaches. The Bible says that "God is love," and the New Testament points out that the mark of a Christian is love. The emphasis on love in Scripture explains why those who strongly hold a religious faith are more likely to have a healthy sexual relationship than those who do not. Distortion of this aspect of true faith may explain why some so-called religious people have problems with sex.

**1211** **Are there other sexual-relationship problems besides the ones you have mentioned?**

Sexual dysfunction covers a broad field and is extremely diverse. Obviously such a large subject cannot be dealt with in its entirety in a book such as this.

Sexual problems occur frequently. In their book, *Human Sexual Inadequacy,* Masters and Johnson state that "a conservative estimate would indicate half of the marriages [in this country] are either presently sexually dysfunctional or imminently so in the future." These researchers are talking about problems such as so-called frigidity on the part of a woman, about women who find it difficult to be aroused, and about men with premature ejaculation and impotence.

In their research, Masters and Johnson found that they could help about 75 percent of people with such problems using a two-week therapy program. Since many of their patients had experienced difficulty for years, this is an astoundingly short treatment period to produce such success and is certainly worth the investment.

If you are experiencing a sexual problem in your relationship with your husband, don't tolerate it any longer. The longer the problem exists, the more difficult it will be for you to correct.

If your problem requires professional help, I would suggest that you see a counselor who employs the techniques espoused by Masters and Johnson. These counselors do not go into deep psychotherapy; they go directly to the problem and solve that problem for most people with short-term therapy.

Remember that the choice of a counselor is a very personal thing; if you find that the personality or morality of the one you have chosen bothers you, change. Do not, under any circumstances, cooperate with a "counselor" who suggests that sex with him will cure your problem, or that an affair with another man will help you. This is unsound and unethical counsel and can lead you into even more problems and guilt.

## 1212 What can I expect from sexual counseling?

If a counselor recommends prolonged therapy for a sexual problem, be sure that your problem demands such a long period of therapy. Most problems of sexuality can be cured within a few short weeks. Compare the program your counselor recommends with the one outlined below. In *Understanding Human Sexual Inadequacy* by Fred Belliveau and Lin Richter (New York: Bantam, 1970), is an excellent summary (pp. 87–110) of the Masters and Johnson treatment program.

***Day One:*** The couple and the co-therapists, usually a male and a female meet together for the initial interview, then they separate. The male co-therapist goes with the husband and the female co-therapist goes with the wife for a history-taking session. These interviews involve thorough questioning about the specific sexual problem(s) and about each person's past life, including a social, sexual, and medical history. At the end of the session the couple is asked not to have any sexual activity until told to do so by the therapists.

***Day Two:*** On this day the husband is interviewed by the female co-therapist and the wife by the male co-therapist. Masters and Johnson have found that a person being interviewed will often tell something to a therapist of the opposite sex that he or she would not tell to a therapist of the same sex. The second-day interview concentrates on the motivation of the patients for coming to therapy and includes a more relaxed discussion of the problem that brought the couple for therapy in the first place.

***Day Three:*** Complete medical histories are taken, physical examinations are done, and diagnostic laboratory tests are performed. Following these procedures, a round-table discussion with the four people takes place. At this session the co-therapists share what they have found from the two history-taking interviews and the physical examinations. The patients are given the opportunity to discuss situations that the therapists seem not to understand thoroughly and to disagree with the therapists if they wish. Masters and Johnson say "the marital partners must continue while in therapy to represent positively their own social and sexual value systems and their preference in lifestyle."

At the round-table discussion the co-therapists give their ideas of what is probably causing the problem. At the end of this discussion the patients are given "physical direction." In essence this physical direction, or "sensate focus," relies on the principle that, for a couple to achieve fullest sexual expression, they must touch each other in a communicative way. Sensate focus is a concept devised by Masters and Johnson to help people learn to communicate by touching. They are told to choose two periods of time between the end of the round-table on Day Three and the therapy on Day Four, during which they will practice sensate focus.

Sensate-focus activity primarily involves pleasurable touching of the husband by the wife or the wife by the husband. The goal is for the person who is touching the other to discover what type of touching his or her partner finds the most pleasant. During this time the couple is not to have intercourse or touch each other's genitals or the woman's breasts.

**Day Four:** A therapy session is held to review the couple's experience with sensate focus. Further discussion is held, with instructions given for changing the sensate-focus technique slightly. On Day Three the one who received the touching was to be passive, doing nothing but keeping the other from doing anything that was unpleasant, distracting, or irritating. On Day Four the one who receives the touching is to participate actively by putting his or her hand on the hand of the one who is doing the touching to show the toucher which places to touch, how hard to touch, and in what direction to move his or her hand. In this session

pleasurable stimulation is applied to all parts of the body, including the genitals and breasts, but without the demand of sexual response.

**Day Five to End of Therapy:** On this day in therapy the therapists start working with the patients on their specific problems, such as painful intercourse, premature ejaculation, and so on. This therapy continues to the end of the treatment program. During the entire treatment program, the couple may spend between twelve and thirty hours with the therapists in addition to the hours spent doing their "homework." Masters and Johnson have found that the results come quickly, and the patients themselves report rapid response to therapy.

For a more complete discussion of this mode of therapy I suggest that you get the excellent book *Understanding Human Sexual Inadequacy* by Fred Belliveau and Lin Richter (New York: Bantam, 1982). (This book is basically a lay interpretation of Masters and Johnson's book *Human Sexual Inadequacy* which was written for the medical profession.)

The reason I recommend counseling that has some resemblance to this technique is that the cure rate is good (about 75 percent) and the time it takes is short.

There is no accrediting organization for sexual-dysfunction clinics in the United States, and the only list of these clinics that I know of is published annually by a magazine mailed to physicians, *Sexual Medicine Today.* The list is not all-inclusive, but it can give you the name of an organization in your area that could refer you to a local sexual dysfunction clinic or physician. For a copy of this list write to *Sexual Medicine Today,* 257 Park Avenue South, New York 10010.

---

**1213** Is it normal for my husband and me to enjoy physical closeness without it culminating in sexual intercourse every time?

Not only is it normal, but it is good—and often necessary.

Most women like to be held and cuddled, and many times they need the comfort and security of their husband's arms around them: with a freedom that allows sex to be the furthest thing from their minds. Unfortunately, many women find that any attempt to have physical closeness is perceived to be a "come on" for sex. A husband should be sensitive to the needs of his wife in these cases, as should a wife be when her husband just "needs to be held."

There are times when one or the other of you cannot have intercourse—because of illness or pregnancy, for example—and there are times when one or the other of you will be too tired, disinterested, or distracted to have intercourse. A relationship that *must* always result in intercourse whenever there is private, physical intimacy is usually not a healthy relationship and can become confining. Usually one person or the other will begin to feel used, because closeness seems only to lead to the other's personal sexual gratification.

A husband and wife need to be able to express love and affection for each other without the feeling that it must always lead to intercourse. This can be a wonderful part of marriage. Such closeness can include massaging each other's backs, kissing, holding each other close, and going to sleep in each other's arms. The variety can be as endless as your love for each other.

This type of relationship assures your partner of your love for him (and you of his love for you) that is not dependent on intercourse each time there is any display of intimacy. Such a relationship is quite helpful if one of you develops a medical problem that makes intercourse impossible for a time, because you will know that you can still enjoy physical closeness.

Arousal, especially of the man, will occur occasionally when neither of you intends it to happen. This does not mean that your husband must have intercourse, or that you need to feel guilty if you do not want to have intercourse at that time. It will not hurt his body to let the arousal pass, any more than it hurts a person's body to feel hungry and let the hunger pass without eating for a while.

## Sexual Function and the Age Factor

### 1214 At what age does sexual function diminish?

Masters and Johnson were the first to show that men and women in good health should be able to continue to function sexually for as long as they live. In a study done in 1983, Consumer's Union (well-known evaluators of everything from cars to toasters) interviewed elderly people concerning their sexual activity. The majority of respondents reported that they were leading happy sexually active lives. A large number of them claimed that although frequency and passion were diminished somewhat, the overall quality of sex had improved as they got older.

A study done at Duke University Medical Center in 1982 revealed that of 278 married couples over forty-six years of age, 52 percent reported having intercourse at least once or twice a week, and 9 percent had intercourse three times a week. Only 38 percent had intercourse less than once a week.

### 1215 What is the key to enjoying sexual activity past the age of menopause?

There are four keys to enjoying sexual activity during the years from menopause on.

*A healthy relationship.* If you and your husband have not established a good marital relationship with each other over the years, you probably have already had sexual problems by the time you reached middle age.

The time to work things out is when the problems surface. If you and your husband are having difficulties now, work together on some solutions immediately so that you can enjoy each other emotionally and physically as the years go by.

If you cannot solve your problems alone, go to your pastor or a counselor for help. The postmenopausal years can be some of the happiest of your entire life if you can develop and maintain a happy and healthy relationship with your husband.

*Healthy sex.* Just as it is important that you have a good overall emotional relationship with your husband, so it is important that you have a satisfying relationship with him sexually if the many years of life you have left after menopause are to be fulfilling.

Most authorities who write about "over fifty" sex say that if a man has an enthusiastic and willing sexual partner, he can usually respond in a healthy and normal way sexually. It seems, therefore, that part of the success of your future sexual happiness depends on your being highly motivated and involved, so that your husband will continue to be sexually responsive. (See the next three questions for possible changes in responsiveness after midlife.)

*A Healthy Body.* In chapter 5 on menopause and chapter 15 on general health, we emphasize the fact that you can probably keep your body functioning in a relatively normal way, right on into old age. This has more reward than just keeping you out of a nursing home; it can also keep you functioning sexually in a normal, active, and healthy way. If you let yourself become fat, tired, and out of shape, you will not perform as well sexually, because sex is a physical activity.

If you or your husband has developed arthritis or some other medical problem that limits your general physical activities, you can usually continue to have sex. Find a position that is comfortable. You and your husband should be open and frank about the problems and solve them together. If you need more help, see your gynecologist, your husband's urologist or other specialist, or talk to a sexual counselor.

*A healthy mind.* If you have allowed your mind to grow old and lazy, your sexual function will probably diminish also. The saying, "You are as young as you feel," is tried and true. If you begin feeling that you are old and cannot perform sexually, you will actually talk yourself into becoming sexually unresponsive. If this attitude creeps into your mind, put some of the suggestions in this chapter and chapter 5 to work.

---

**1216** **What changes in sexual function occur in postmenopausal women?**

There are subtle changes that occur in the sexual function of both men and women from midlife on. Although some of these changes can be bothersome, most of the resulting problems can be solved. Many of the changes are positive ones that actually enable a couple to enjoy sex more than they did when they were younger.

Sexual changes for the woman include:

*Sexual responsiveness.* The four phases of the sexual response are excitement, plateau, orgasm, and resolution. For the woman past menopause there are mild changes in each of these phases. The excitement phase, or the period of foreplay, must last longer to bring the woman to sexual excitement and lubrication. Instead of sexual arousal's development in less than a minute, it may take four or five minutes of sex play to achieve adequate lubrication. The plateau phase, which normally includes the insertion of the man's penis into the vagina, may be less intense than it was when a woman was premenopausal. Periods of orgasm are likely to be shorter. Because there is less intense response to sexual stimulation, the period of resolution will probably be quicker. There is less swelling to diminish as a postmenopausal woman relaxes after intercourse.

*Thinning of the vulvar and vaginal tissues.* After menopause, if a woman does not take estrogen the tissues of her vulva and vagina can become very thin because they lose the stimulation of the estrogen that the body produced before menopause. Because of this it is important that a vaginal lubricant be used. I recommend Maxilube because it does not leave the skin or bed clothes greasy and is absorbed into the body.

If a lubricant is not adequate to prevent painful intercourse, estrogen, either by mouth or as a vaginal cream, is helpful. (See Q. 266, 279, 284.)

I believe that every postmenopausal woman should take estrogen, so for most of my patients a dry, sensitive vagina due to lack of estrogen does not become a problem. If your doctor will not prescribe estrogen and you have no medical problem that makes estrogen dangerous, I encourage you to see a physician who will give you estrogen. Not only does it help you stay sexually responsive and comfortable, but it will also help prevent your developing osteoporosis and bone fractures later. In addition, a Consumer's Union report showed that postmenopausal women who took estrogen were more sexually active than those women not taking estrogen. Finally, it has been shown that postmenopausal women who have regular intercourse have a healthier, stronger, and thicker vaginal lining than women who have infrequent intercourse after menopause.

*No general decline in sex drive.* Studies have shown that many women have no decline in their sex drive as they get older. Some women may have an increased sexual interest after the menopause. This may be partly due to social changes and to the new sense of freedom, now that the children are no longer in the home and the fear of pregnancy is gone.

A sophisticated study done in 1984 which measured spontaneous vaginal contractions while women were exposed to erotic stimuli showed that the postmenopausal woman's vagina was only a little less responsive to erotic stimuli than the vagina of the premenopausal woman. The difference was not significant and was not in a range that would produce sexual dysfunction in the postmenopausal group. It seems obvious that a woman's body is made to continue normal sexual function until the day she dies.

---

**1217** **What changes in sexual responsiveness occur in men as they get older?**

Masters and Johnson found that the four phases of sexual responsiveness change in men as they get older. If a man understands that his sexual function will undergo changes at about the age of fifty, he will take this into account and change his lovemaking accordingly. If he is not prepared for these changes in responsiveness, he can become so scared that he becomes impotent on a purely emotional basis.

The excitement phase of intercourse, which is the phase during which foreplay occurs, usually takes longer from middle age on. The man takes longer to develop an erection, and the erection is not as hard when it first develops. The actual likelihood of a man's developing or not developing an erection remains the same, no matter what his age (unless there is an unusual medical problem).

During the plateau phase, which is the period during which the husband usually inserts his penis in the vagina, he will often find that he is able to maintain an erection without the need to ejaculate for a much longer time than when he was younger. It is the discovery of this fact which allows many couples in their midlife period or beyond to have more satisfactory sex than they have ever had.

Orgasms for the man of fifty years or older are usually shorter and produce less semen volume than ejaculations of previous years. The expulsion of the seminal fluid is also less forceful for the older man than for the younger man. As a man gets older, he may even find that he does not need to ejaculate to be satisfied and can therefore bring his partner to satisfaction and then stop the sex act.

The phase of resolution is usually much shorter for a man from fifty on. After ejaculation his penis usually becomes totally flaccid within a few seconds. He also may not be able to have another erection for many hours; whereas when he was younger he was able to develop another erection, either immediately or within an hour or two.

Obviously a man's body is designed to have intercourse until the day he dies. If he will realize that slower arousal during foreplay allows the advantage of better control during intercourse, he will not begin to question his ability to achieve an erection. Once he begins questioning this ability, he becomes a mere observer of his own performance, watching to see whether or not his penis will erect. When he becomes a spectator he has taken the first step on the road to impotence.

It is important that a man accept the changes in his body as improvements and recognize that for the last half of his life he will probably find it easier to satisfy his wife, especially if her response has always been slower than his own.

---

**1218**  **What if my husband and I have reached midlife and are having sexual problems?**

I suggest a thorough review of this chapter, plus a reading of some of the books mentioned in Q. 1221. If you continue to have problems in spite of trying some of the suggested techniques, see your gynecologist and urge your husband to see a urologist. For example, if a man develops prostatitis, it can affect his sexual responsiveness. If both you and your husband are healthy and normal and yet are not able to make love physically to your mutual satisfaction, see a sexual counselor to get things straightened out. Then you can get on with a healthy sexual relationship.

---

## Choosing a Sexual Lifestyle While Single

---

**1219**  **Is celibacy by choice for a single woman normal and healthy?**

Yes. There is no physical or mental danger to celibacy by choice. Domeena C. Renshaw, M.D., professor of the department of psychiatry and director of the sexual dysfunction clinic of Loyola University of Chicago states: "Many persons handle voluntary celibacy healthily and quite happily. Sexual feelings occur naturally and recur cyclically, regularly, including during sleep. Even when the fact that it is natural to have sexual feelings is recognized, accepted, and understood, the individual may still choose a lifestyle in which physical expression is controlled" (*The Female Patient*, Vol. 8, October, 1983, pp. 38, 55).

Many women who have been in the habit of "sleeping around" often find great freedom when they decide to stop this type of sexual activity. The following excerpt from a booklet by V. Mary Stewart called *Sexual Freedom* (Downer's Grove, Ill: InterVarsity Press) expresses such feelings:

I began to see that the need to be always in a sexual relationship with someone really did not have that much to do with the release of sexual tension. Rather, it was a desperate fight against a rarely admitted loneliness and isolation; it was the best (or only) way I knew how to approximate some reassurance that somehow, for a little while anyway, there was a semblance of commitment, caring and communication. Very simply, it was an attempt to fill that "God-shaped void" of which Pascal wrote. Over the weeks and months that I still tried to get the best of both worlds, that is, tried to be a Christian and still sleep around, I reached two conclusions. The first was that while I had never had any trouble *attaining* that desired commitment and communication, I was never able to *maintain* it. It was always the same way: A fellow and I would start out with a tremendous euphoric closeness which sooner or later became empty and ritualized. We would go along playing the game for a while, but finally one or the other of us would pull out, determined that next time it would be different. It never was.

The second thing I learned was that feeling isolated has little to do with whether or not one is sharing a bed with someone, or even trying to share a life. I cannot count the nights I have lain awake, sometimes muffling sobs in a pillow, beside a satiated, soundly sleeping male, wondering why I was feeling so alone. It was not that the men in question were doing all the taking and not giving—I did not specialize in relationships like that. Mostly they were people who themselves wanted a real and pretty total relationship. But somehow, just because we were trying to get it all from each other, we ended up having even less than we started with, feeling only constraint instead of communication. Somehow we were running the relationship on the wrong fuel.

On the other hand, I will never forget the tremendous liberation I felt the first night I had enough strength in the Lord to say No and not feel any need to apologize for it or rationalize it. I remember how good it felt to fall asleep alone, in my own bed, by my-self, and how overjoyed I was to wake up in the morning and confirm that no one was there beside me. I have never felt *less* isolated in my life—then, or ever since.

It is healthy and normal for a single man or woman to be celibate if he or she so chooses. Some doctors do not understand that choice; others make it a practice to question all female patients, married or single, about the use of contraceptives. If you are single and celibate, do not be offended if your doctor questions you about birth-control practices; it is merely a routine question and you should treat it as such.

---

## 1220 Why not just live together without the entanglement of marriage?

There are some basic problems with a nonmarital union of a man and a woman. If you are thinking of entering such a relationship, you might consider the following.

*Too little investment.* Anything that is of any value has a price. If a relationship with a person of the opposite sex costs little, it is probably worth little. It may be physically pleasant for a time or emotionally comfortable to some extent, but to compare this kind of relationship with one in which you have invested a great deal of time and effort is like comparing a pond to an ocean.

*Lack of commitment.* Living together without being married is a relationship founded on a lack of responsible commitment. Obviously there is enough commitment to live together, but not enough to say, "No matter what it costs me, I will help you and be with you." The nonmarital relationship, therefore, is one that most individuals enter into only for what they can get out of it, with minimal commitment to the other person. It is essentially a selfish arrangement.

*Loneliness.* In spite of all the recreational

and social opportunities available in our society, loneliness is epidemic. Daily I find patients crying out for friendship and understanding. A relationship in which there is no sense of lasting commitment can neither meet a woman's needs nor soothe the loneliness she feels. Dr. Paul Tournier, a Swiss psychiatrist and author, said, "No one can develop freely in this world, and find a full life, without feeling understood by at least one person." This relationship can best evolve in a marriage where two people are committed to each other for life. In a relationship lacking this commitment, such fulfillment is unlikely to develop.

*Unfaithfulness.* Most of my patients who have lived in a sexual relationship with a man without benefit of marriage have experienced unfaithfulness on the part of their partner. Infidelity is an extremely common problem in such relationships. This occurs in marriages, of course, but at least a married person considers being unfaithful "breaking a promise," whereas such a promise is not an important part of a nonmarital union.

*Children.* No contraceptive is perfect. Any fertile woman living with a fertile man may become pregnant. If she chooses to have the baby, the couple has the problem of raising a child in a situation where the parents themselves have minimal commitment to the family unit. Studies have shown that one of the most important factors in the healthy emotional development of a child is knowing that his or her parents are committed to a permanent union and love each other and their child in that framework.

For further information on this subject, read the small booklet *Sexual Freedom* by V. Mary Stewart (Downer's Grove, Ill.: InterVarsity Press). It discusses this subject better than any other book I have read.

---

**1221** **What books do you recommend on marriage and sexual relations?**

There are many excellent books on both these subjects. These five books are from InterVarsity Press (Downer's Grove, Ill.):

*Love Is a Feeling to Be Learned*, Walter Trobisch

*Better Is Your Love than Wine*, Jean Banyolak

*Learn to Be a Man; Learn to Be a Woman*, Kenneth and Floy Smith

*Free to Do Right*, David Field

*Sexual Freedom*, V. Mary Stewart

These books give sexual guidance:

*The Gift of Sex: A Christian Guide to Sexual Fulfillment*, Clifford and Joyce Penner (Waco, Tex.: Word Books, 1981).

*Intended for Pleasure: Sex Technique and Sexual Fulfillment in Christian Marriage*, Ed and Gaye Wheat (Old Tappan, N.J.: Fleming H. Revell, 1977).

*Solomon on Sex*, Joseph C. Dillow (Nashville, Tenn.: Thomas Nelson, 1977).

*The Joy of Being a Woman and What a Man Can Do*, Ingrid Trobisch (New York: Harper & Row, 1975).

*The Marriage Builder*, Lawrence J. Crabb, Jr. (Grand Rapids: Zondervan, 1982).

---

### Afterword

In conclusion I quote Ingrid Trobisch: "Marriage is not a destination, but a journey. As husband and wife make this journey together, growing and maturing and learning how to love, they will reach sexual harmony as a ripe fruit of their marriage." (*The Joy of Being a Woman and What a Man Can Do*, p. 30).

# Part Four

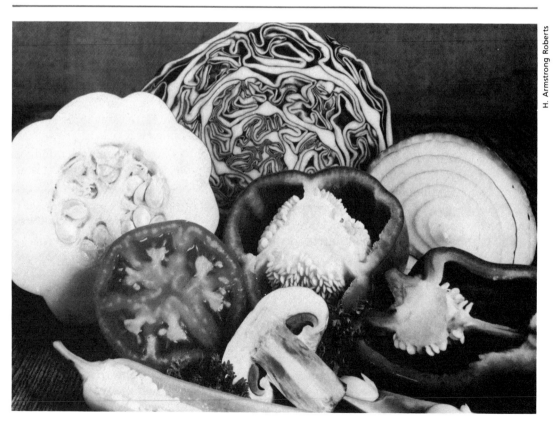

H. Armstrong Roberts

# A Healthy Lifestyle

**15   Sound Habits for Lifelong Well-Being**

# 15
## Sound Habits
## for Lifelong Well-Being

An annual check-up no longer is limited to a Pap smear, breast exam, and the other things usually associated with a yearly physical. Increasingly conscientious doctors are practicing preventive medicine and now routinely provide patients with information and advice that will help them stay out of wheelchairs and nursing homes in later life. Likewise, I want to do more for you, the reader of this book, than just explain about diseases or other medical problems you might develop; I want to tell you how to avoid poor health in the future.

There's a catch, however, for nothing worth having comes easily. The key to your present and future well-being is to make some immediate changes in your lifestyle; and change is difficult for everyone. Foresight, right priorities, and discipline are necessary for a person to accomplish these changes, but the rewards of lasting good health are well worth it.

It takes foresight to be able to see that if you do not change some of your health habits, you may spend the last twenty or thirty years of life in a wheelchair, with a colostomy or with some other disabling medical problem. Likewise, right priorities are necessary in order to put important things first, not letting matters that seem immediately urgent crowd out those habits that are truly necessary for maintaining good health.

Of course, you must have personal discipline if you sincerely want to exchange unhealthy habits for sound ones that can insure a healthier future. Many practices detrimental to good health are merely habits to which you have become accustomed, and you will find yourself just as content with their replacements as you are with the status quo.

If you have the foresight, right priorities, and discipline necessary for preserving your good health, you can expect the following rewards:

*A bonus now.* You will feel better right now if you practice good health habits. I recently bought a subscription to *Sports Illustrated* and before I ever received my first copy of the magazine I got a bonus desk clock and calendar. As with many investments, there is an immediate bonus in laying a foundation for your physical well-being.

*Good health later.* Being physically healthy, able to travel and enjoy the things you want to do as you grow older is the goal of good health care. Using my *Sports Illustrated* example, about two months after paying for my subscription, I got the reward, my first issue. Likewise, there is a long-term return for your past investment in good health.

The suggestions for good health in this chapter are those about which there is essentially no argument. They are not gimmicks but are practices that most experts have accepted as improving a person's chances of living a long and healthy life.

My first goal is to convince you that you need to start doing certain basic things that have been found to be necessary for the proper functioning of the human body. My second goal is to motivate you to do them. The argument I hear most often from my patients is that they don't have the time to work at good health habits. My reply is, "There is always time to do the things we consider important."

Research has shown that if we spend time building our bodies and our minds when we are younger, the probability of enjoying good health when we are older is greatly increased. If we neglect our physical and mental resources when we are young, we are more likely to face years of illness and disability later on.

It is a sad woman who suddenly realizes when she is sixty-five years old that she now wants to be healthy but is not. By that time no matter how hard she may try she may have so irreversibly damaged her body by past inattention that she cannot ever again be in good health. Fortunately most of us, no matter what age, can start some sound health habits today and reap significant benefits later.

There are different health patterns suggested for different decades of your life.

*The teens and before.* Teenagers do not normally think much about maintaining a healthy lifestyle, but those who are fortunate enough to be reared in homes where parents have emphasized good health have a head start. They have established wholesome habits and often do not need to change anything about their eating and exercising practices as time goes by. They will grow up to be healthy, alert adults who will live longer and with less pain and problems than most of their peers.

*The twenties.* During this decade there is still an opportunity for a woman to develop sound health habits, and it is during this time that an individual can most easily change her lifestyle accordingly. However, the problem is that most women in their twenties seem to believe subconsciously that they are "immortal" and have no need for changing anything that they are doing, especially if they feel generally strong and healthy. If you are in your twenties, I encourage you to heed the information in this chapter. Change your habits now so that you not only can reap the rich rewards of good health in the future but also will not develop ingrained unhealthy habits that are difficult to change.

*The thirties.* Women in this age group usually notice that they have begun to put on a little weight and do not feel quite as well as they once did. Because of this they usually listen to their doctor when he or she discusses the importance of good health habits. The chief problem is that by the thirties, many people have already developed some deeply entrenched unhealthy practices. Smoking, for instance, may be such an "addiction" by this time that it seems impossible to stop. To avoid many illnesses in the next few years, it is vital that certain health habits be changed during the thirties.

*The forties.* We all hear of people who have heart attacks in their forties and of men and women who develop cancer of the colon and end up with major surgery, colostomies, or death at this age. Had these people practiced a healthy lifestyle when they were in their teens and twenties, they could probably have prevented many of their premature health problems. Fortunately it is probably not too late for most people to begin good health habits in the forties. It is certainly better than continuing bad ones, at any rate.

*The fifties.* During these years the effects of bad health habits of the past really take their toll. Heart attacks in men and women, colon cancer, lung cancer, and cirrhosis of the liver are common in people who are in their fifties. Toward the end of this decade of life many women who did not start taking estrogen after their menopause will start experiencing physical deterioration because of fractures of the vertebrae from osteoporosis, and both men and women who have not been exercising will start experiencing physical deterioration because of poor muscle tone.

*The sixties and beyond.* If a woman who has not been previously practicing sound health care starts doing so in the sixties, she will undoubtedly feel better. However, most diseases that she might have as a result of past poor health habits usually will not go away. I strongly encourage my sixty-year-old patients to improve their lifestyle—which includes stopping smoking, beginning an exercise program, changing their diet, and taking estrogen and progesterone. If the body is not otherwise damaged, these women will feel better, be less apt to break bones, and be more vigorous and alert than if they are not exercising, not eating properly, are continuing to smoke and drink, and are not on estrogen.

Our society has assumed that getting older, feeling badly, and ending up in nursing homes is a normal, inevitable pattern of life. We have also assumed that diverticulitis, heart attacks, strokes, and colon cancer are normal diseases for all human beings. This is not so. Most of these problems are a result of the way we have been living for years and have no relationship to the aging process, except for the length of time we have been mistreating ourselves.

Older people can be healthy and strong. I realized this fact when I read a report about people who were in masters' swimming programs. These men, all over fifty, were swimming competitively. Many of them were swimming distances in shorter times than they did in college. By every measure many of them had bodies that were as healthy as they had been when they were younger: blood pressure, muscle mass and tone, fat content, and lung capacity were sound. These men were not "he-men." They were normal men who were committed to regular exercise.

Joe Bailey, M.D., a colon and rectal specialist in Austin, Texas, pointed out to me years ago that if people would eat more fiber and less concentrated sweets, they would have fewer colon problems. I did not listen at the time. The passing years have proven his insight to be true. Many of the health problems that we have always assumed were part of growing older have been caused by the foods that we eat. If we change our diet early enough in life, we will not be subject to many of these problems.

Lack of good health in one area can affect your abilities in other areas. For instance, if you smoke you may not have the lung capacity to exercise adequately. The limited exercise can then affect your total future health. If you overeat, you may be too heavy to exercise adequately, and this would affect your future well-being. I encourage you to become firmly convinced that good health habits are important for you and to get involved in all of them. Try to realize that success in one of these areas leads to success in another, just as failure in one can lead to failure in another. The key elements to good health are these:

Do not smoke.
Eat reasonable amounts of properly balanced foods.
Exercise regularly.
Do not drink alcohol in excess, if at all.
Have regular exams by your physician.
Wear seat belts in your automobile.
Maintain a manageable stress level.
After menopause take estrogen and progesterone and get adequate calcium.
Avoid extramarital sex.

A discussion of each of these aspects of good health follows, with the exception of the last two which were discussed in depth in chapters 5 and 13.

The following story about George Ford (*TIME*, March 26, 1984, p. 56) aptly illustrates the importance of this discussion.

Everybody knows George Ford. Or somebody like George Ford. There he was, 52, the energetic president of a small Ohio electronics firm who "wouldn't eat an egg unless it was fried in bacon grease." His lunches were executive size. He matched his business cronies drink for drink. He smoked "pretty heavily" and exercised with a knife and fork.

In the winter of 1981, doctors informed Ford that his cholesterol levels were dangerously high; by April, he required a quadruple coronary bypass operation. He emerged from the hospital determined to revise his way radically. Today he does not smoke, he exercises four or five days a week, and he sticks scrupulously to a diet high in fiber and low in cholesterol and fat.

"I haven't had a slice of bacon in three years," he says. He is proud and relieved that his cholesterol level is normal. "Maybe heart disease is God's way of telling us we're living too damn high on the hog," Ford says. "It's hard to practice moderation in this country. We're a nation of excess."

## Stop Smoking

### 1222   Is smoking really that bad?

Many physicians consider smoking to be the major health problem in America. Let's look at some startling statistics about smoking-related problems.

*Cancer.* Smoking causes 30 percent of all cancer deaths in America. These cancers include cancer of the lung, the larynx, the esophagus, the pancreas, the bladder, the cervix, the kidneys, and the mouth. Although you may not die from one of these cancers, surgery to cure them can involve measures such as removal of the larynx, which would prevent normal speech for the rest of your life, and removal of a lung, which could affect the way you feel for the rest of your life. In addition, there would be the lifelong fear of recurrence of the cancer. Recent studies indicate that if someone in the home smokes, the risk of cancer in all body sites of family members increases by 60 percent for children and 50 percent for adult spouses. The cancer risk more than doubles for individuals who were exposed to smoking both as children and as adults.

Women rightfully fear breast cancer and yet, because so many women smoke, the number of women who die from lung cancer will be more than the number of women dying from breast cancer starting in 1985.

*Heart attacks.* Cigarette smokers experience a 70 percent higher death rate from heart attacks than do nonsmokers. Their risk of sudden death from heart attacks is two to four times greater than those who do not smoke. Women who smoke *and* take birth-control pills have a ten times greater chance of having heart attacks than women who neither take birth-control pills nor smoke. It is estimated that cigarette smoking could, because of heart disease alone, be responsible for the premature death of as much as 10 percent of the population of the United States.

*Ill health.* Smoking produces bronchitis and increases the chance of emphysema. Both of these problems cause discomfort and misery and can be life-threatening.

*Hardening of the arteries.* Studies indicate that smoking increases the chance of having hardening of the arteries (arteriosclerosis), a condition that can result in stroke or heart attack.

### 1223   Will it really help to quit smoking?

C. Everett Koop, M.D., Surgeon General of the United States Public Health Service, has reported that when smokers quit they begin to reduce their heart-disease risk almost immediately. Ten years after quitting, those who had smoked less than a pack a day have a heart-disease death rate similar to that of nonsmokers. The best way to eliminate the cancer risk due to smoking is never to smoke at all, but the next best way is to stop smoking. Studies suggest that smoking-related cancers are more likely to occur in people who have been heavy smokers for a long period of time. If a person stops smoking, however, the chance of developing cancer from smoking will be significantly reduced. Like any serious disease, smoking is a grave health hazard and should be treated as such. Just as a woman would go to great lengths to rid herself of any illness, she should also be serious in her attempt to stop smoking.

### 1224   How can I stop smoking?

Some people can stop smoking "cold turkey," but others find that they cannot. The reason is that smoking is as true an addiction as is alcoholism. I suggest using every crutch you can find to stop smoking. Crutches are legitimate instruments for the purpose of helping people do something that they cannot do by themselves. Some of the suggestions that I offer my patients include:

Call your local American Cancer Society or American Lung Association. Both sponsor clinics that help smokers kick the habit.

Call your county health department or local hospital. They too may have classes for those who want to stop smoking, or they may have information about where you can attend a class in your community.

Look up SmokeEnders in your phone directory. They hold seminars that can help you stop smoking.

Find a doctor who will put staples in your ears! This acupuncture-type procedure seems to help some people. In keeping with my recommendation to try anything to stop smoking, I recommend this—though with no promises.

Use WaterPik filters in your cigarettes. These filters decrease the tar and nicotine that come through the smoke, helping you to wean yourself gradually from cigarettes. There are also other commercial products designed specifically for this purpose.

Chew nicotine gum. This is available by prescription and may help with the weaning process. I recommend using it only on the advice of a physician. It must not be used in pregnancy.

One note of encouragement as you try to kick the smoking habit is that many doctors are also stopping. About 64 percent of physicians who formerly smoked have quit. Because of this, the death rate among physicians has dropped. Studies have shown that the difference in death rates between physicians and the general population is caused by the fact that fewer physicians smoke.

## Eat Right

**1225** **What does "eating right" mean, and why is it so important?**

The primary problem with the American diet is that during the past hundred years we have started eating much more animal fat, much less high-fiber carbohydrate foods (such as whole-grain bread and cereals), and more concentrated, nonnutritive sugar. The carbohydrate foods that we normally eat either have had most of their natural fiber content removed or they are "sugar carbohydrates," which are almost completely without fiber.

I picture food as being on a balance scale. Fiber-rich cereals are on one end of the scale and sugar on the other end. In America today sugar weighs far heavier in what we eat than fiber-containing cereals. It should be the other way around. I now think of fiber as being similar to vitamins—an essential element the body continually needs to maintain health.

The human body was designed to function on a diet high in fiber and low in sugar, just as your new car engine was designed to run on gasoline high in octane and low in lead. If you run it on leaded gasoline, the engine will become gummed up and start functioning poorly. In the same way your body will function poorly and deteriorate if you persist in eating a diet that is low in fiber and high in sugar.

It now seems quite certain that many of the common diseases and health problems that we have always thought to be a natural part of growing older are due to the foods we have been eating rather than to the aging process. This is exciting news, because it means that if we establish new habits of eating we can eliminate many of the diseases always assumed to be part of old age.

---

## 1226 Is a high-sugar, low-fiber diet really harmful to a person's health?

In his book *Eat Right—To Keep Healthy and Enjoy Life More* (New York: Arco, 1979) Dr. Dennis Burkitt points out the absence of a certain group of diseases in Third-World countries where a high-fiber, low-sugar diet is the norm. He contrasts that with the astoundingly high incidence of this same group of diseases in the Western World. The author makes these observations as a researcher who worked for twenty years as a surgeon in Africa. Dr. Burkitt found several interesting facts about the following problems.

*Heart attacks.* This is one of the most common diseases in America, killing about one man in four and becoming more common in older women who are no longer protected by natural estrogen. This health problem is almost completely unknown in rural areas of Third-World countries.

*Gallstones.* The operation for removal of the gallbladder is one of the most common operations in America. Gallstones almost never occur in rural areas of Third-World countries.

*Diverticulitis of the colon.* This problem causes untold misery and pain for older people, necessitating operations for removal of parts of the colon and often mandating colostomies. It occurs in our country in about one in ten people over the age of forty and one in three over the age of sixty. This disease is almost unknown in Third-World communities. (See next question for a discussion of diverticulitis.)

*Appendicitis.* An appendectomy is the most common emergency operation done in the United States. Appendicitis almost never occurs in rural countries.

*Hiatus hernia.* The herniation of the stomach up through the diaphragm causes burning, indigestion, and discomfort in the upper abdomen. It is quite common in the United States, and it can be so severe that major surgery is necessary. It almost never occurs in rural Africa.

*Varicose veins.* Most women naively assume that varicose veins are a result of having been pregnant, and it is reported that as many as 44 percent of women between the ages of thirty and fifty have varicose veins. In rural societies, however, varicose veins occur in less than 5 percent of the population.

*Hemorrhoids.* The American who does not have hemorrhoids is fortunate. At least 50 percent of the people in the United States do, and many of those victims have had surgery because of this problem. Although it is assumed by most American women that hemorrhoids occur only as a result of pregnancy and labor, this problem almost never is seen in rural parts of Third-World countries.

*Cancer of the colon.* This cancer is the most common cause of cancer deaths in the Western World, but it is unusual in rural and agrarian societies.

*Diabetes.* Diabetes is quite common in our society, occurring in as many as 15 percent of adults over the age of fifty. This disease is very uncommon in all rural and agrarian societies.

*Obesity.* This is an extremely common problem in this country, where at least 40 percent of middle-aged adults are overweight. Yet obesity is almost never a problem for rural people who feed themselves by growing their own food.

History indicates that these diseases occurred infrequently in the Western World until the last hundred years, and that they all seem to be associated with the change in our dietary habits. One of the examples that Dr. Burkitt uses is that although all these diseases are rare among black South Africans, they affect white South Africans to approximately the same extent as they do Americans—and in the United States they affect blacks and whites alike. His explanation is that in South Africa the blacks still exist on an agrarian diet, while the whites eat the traditional over-refined Western foods.

## 1227 How does a high-sugar, low-fiber diet harm the body?

Fiber is the part of food which is not digested. It passes right through the small intestines without being changed, and it contributes no calories at all to our body. Because of this passive role, fiber has been ignored by most nutritionists until recently.

We know now that fiber is extremely important for the body's health because it adds bulk to the contents of the colon, making it possible for the intestines to function in optimum fashion. Just as it would be difficult to hold on to a tennis racquet if the handle were as thin as a pencil, so it is hard for your colon to squeeze down on its contents if those contents are small in volume. When this happens the colon may allow its contents to accumulate until there is a large enough bulk to be squeezed out; or it may try to eliminate the hard, small-volume stool it contains by working harder. This is constipation, which necessitates harder contractions by the colon and more abdominal straining and pushing with bowel movements by the individual involved. These harder colon contractions can cause the colon wall to pouch out and form "diverticuli," producing the diseases called diverticulosis and diverticulitis. The increased straining and pushing can also result in hemorrhoids, varicose veins, and hiatus hernia.

Research is not complete as to the exact mechanism by which fiber exerts its effect on the human body or exactly what all its effects are. However, in addition to increasing the bulk of the stool, fiber appears to be beneficial in the following ways.

Fiber allows a person to increase the amount of food he or she eats without increasing the caloric intake. (High-fiber foods are usually lower in calories than low-fiber foods.)

Fiber slows down the absorption of starch and sugar from the intestinal contents. This not only decreases the calorie intake and helps with weight control but also decreases the body's demand on the pancreas for insulin.

Fiber absorbs or in some way interacts with the cholesterol and bile salts that the liver secretes into the intestine, decreasing cholesterol levels in the blood stream and making heart disease less likely.

Fiber seems to absorb "poisonous" substances from the stool so that they are not rubbed or held against the intestinal wall. This decreases the chance of colon cancer. Since fiber increases the bulk of the stool and produces more frequent bowel movements, it keeps the stool from being so concentrated and from being retained in the colon so long. This reduces the length of time that toxic substances are in contact with the colon wall.

Fiber increases the bulk of the stools, making them easier for the colon to expel and eliminating straining with bowel movements. It is this straining with bowel movements that seems to produce hiatus hernia, hemorrhoids, and varicose veins.

## 1228 How do I go about changing my diet and the diet I feed my family?

Read all you can on the subject. For years I have recommended the book *The Save Your*

*Life Diet* by Dr. David Reuben (New York: Bantam, 1976) but I do not suggest it as the only book to read since his emphasis is mainly on adding bran to your diet. I believe that Dr. Dennis Burkitt's emphasis in *Eat Right—To Keep Healthy and Enjoy Life More*, (New York: Arco, 1979) is more balanced, as he suggests a change in the whole dietary pattern, which might include adding bran. Ted L. Edwards, Jr., M.D., has an excellent discussion of this same subject in his book *Weight Loss to Super Wellness* (Austin: The Hills, 1983).

Talk to yourself and to your family. Old habits do not die easily. Dr. Joe Bailey talked to me for several years before I understood what he was saying about the importance of dietary fiber in the diet. When I did, I talked to my wife and daughters for several years before they were convinced. As a result of reading and talking over a period of years, the foods that our family eats have changed dramatically.

Make a plan for the way you are going to eat. Many families never change because they do not have a definite diet plan. Decide, for example, how often you are going to eat desserts and whether or not you are going to have soft drinks in the house. Decide if you are going to eat miller's bran and how much each of you will eat.

When you have decided what you think is best, serve it to your family. This may not be easy if you have older children and a husband who are not interested in changing. If you have young children, however, and a husband who sees the importance of improving his diet, you have a great opportunity for decreasing the chance of illness for your whole family.

An additional advantage of starting this eating pattern while your children are young is that it will become habitual for them, making their future lives healthier. Even if you have an uncooperative family, there are ways you can unobtrusively increase the fiber content of the foods that they eat. As previously mentioned, I picture fiber as balancing out sugar. If you cannot decrease the amount of sugar that your family is eating, at least you can increase the amount of fiber and attempt to "neutralize" the sugar in their diet.

The way you eat is probably as much tradition as it is habit. Most of us eat the way our parents did, and there are "warm fuzzies" when we have a special food now that we remember eating when we were children at the table with our parents. I do not belittle the tumult that usually accompanies the change in a life habit as basic as diet. All I can say is that for most of us, the change is necessary and important.

---

**1229** **What changes in dietary habits are most important if I am eating the typical American diet?**

There are three basic principles.

Increase the amounts of carbohydrates consumed, to the point where you have doubled the amount of calories you get from carbohydrate foods, especially those rich in fiber and low in refined sugar.

Simultaneously reduce the amount of fat in your diet so that you have decreased the amount of calories from fat by at least one-third.

Decrease the amount of sugar in your diet by at least one-half or more.

---

**1230** **What practical suggestions do you have for changing our diet?**

Eat bread that is made from whole-grain flour. This bread has four times as much dietary fiber as white bread does.

Eat high-fiber cereal for breakfast. For example, All-Bran cereal has 27 percent fiber;

Puffed Wheat has 15 percent fiber. Shredded Wheat has 12 percent fiber, and Corn Flakes has 11 percent fiber. Many new high-fiber cereals are being marketed today.

Wheat bran (miller's bran) has 44 percent fiber. Because of its fiber content, I recommend adding miller's bran to cereal or other foods you eat during the day.

The general recommendation is that a person take in about twenty-five grams of fiber every day. Two heaping tablespoons of miller's bran provide seven grams of fiber; you can decide on the basis of your diet how much you should use. Use the chart on p. 677 to determine your daily fiber intake. You may wish to read *Plant Fiber in Foods*, which gives figures on fiber content of over 300 foods (Diabetes Foundation, P.O. Box 22124, Lexington, Ky. 40522).

Eat more vegetables and fruit. Peas, beans, and nuts are richer in fiber than most fruits and leafy vegetables. Lettuce has almost no fiber (1.5%) while spinach is quite high in fiber (6.3%). Eating a lettuce salad may keep you from eating more fattening foods, but it does not add significantly to the amount of fiber that you take in.

Cut down on foods containing refined sugar and get all sugar-containing soft drinks out of the house. Americans consume in soft drinks more than 50 percent of the sugar produced here or imported into this country. These drinks are insidious. Because they contain a great deal of sugar, they taste good. They are convenient and easily become habit-forming. A large part of the dietary change you and your family might make, if you drink soft drinks, is to have absolutely no sugar-containing ones in your house.

Eat meat sparingly and no more than once a day. Cut out the fatty parts of the meat. The leanest animal proteins are chicken, turkey, and fish, especially white fish. Red meat, such as beef, lamb, and pork, should be drastically reduced in your diet.

You should consider changes in your diet as being permanent rather than temporary, and you should not think of the new diet plan as denying yourself or your family things. Once you have made the change you will find that your new dietary habits include foods just as tasty and appealing as the former ones, and they are certainly more healthful.

## 1231 How will I know if I am getting enough fiber?

If you are getting enough fiber, you will have a bowel movement daily and the stool will be eliminated without your having to strain. You will also notice that your stools are lighter and softer, perhaps even floating on the water. Your stool should not have nearly as much odor as it may have had prior to the change in diet. You should continue adding more fiber to your diet until you accomplish these things.

## 1232 What are some benefits of eating a high-fiber diet?

*Probable weight loss.* First of all, if you are eating reasonable amounts of the proper

### Desirable Weights for Women Age 25 or Over

| Height (with shoes) | | Weight in Pounds | | |
|---|---|---|---|---|
| Feet | Inches | Small Frame | Medium Frame | Large Frame |
| 4 | 11 | 95–101 | 98–110 | 106–122 |
| 5 | 0 | 96–104 | 101–113 | 109–125 |
| 5 | 1 | 99–107 | 104–116 | 112–128 |
| 5 | 2 | 102–110 | 107–119 | 115–131 |
| 5 | 3 | 105–113 | 110–122 | 118–134 |
| 5 | 4 | 108–116 | 113–126 | 121–138 |
| 5 | 5 | 111–119 | 116–130 | 125–142 |
| 5 | 6 | 114–123 | 120–135 | 129–146 |
| 5 | 7 | 118–127 | 124–139 | 133–150 |
| 5 | 8 | 122–131 | 128–143 | 137–154 |
| 5 | 9 | 126–135 | 132–147 | 141–158 |
| 5 | 10 | 130–140 | 136–151 | 145–163 |
| 5 | 11 | 134–144 | 140–155 | 149–168 |

For girls between 18 and 25, subtract 1 pound for each year under 25.

foods, your weight will most likely decrease, or at least be easier to control, because you are eating less sugar. This is a wonderful side benefit of a high-fiber diet. Eating less sugar is healthier, and your weight is decreasing too.

*Less weakness and tiredness.* Hypoglycemia seems to be epidemic in our society. A great deal of this is because individuals eat so many sweets that their pancreas just cannot keep up in its production of insulin. People who reduce sweets in their diet and start "eating right" usually have less hypoglycemia and have an increase in their energy level.

*Less disease.* This factor would not be noticed immediately, but in comparing your overall well-being with that of your friends who have not made any changes in their diet and lifestyle, you will probably gradually notice that you are having fewer hospitalizations, fewer medical problems, and a general feeling of robust good health.

---

## 1233   Is it necessary to take vitamins to be in the best possible health?

No one knows the complete answer to this question. If you eat healthy, well-balanced foods, you may not need any vitamin supplements, but you should not assume that you follow this type of diet. Most of us do not eat as adequately as we think we do. Reading books on nutrition will help you determine how adequate your diet is in meeting the established daily requirements for the essential vitamins and minerals necessary for good health. If you are not eating well, your first change should be to improve your diet, not to start taking supplements.

I feel that it is fine for women to take a good multivitamin-with-iron tablet once a day. Because of loss of iron in their menstrual flow every month, most reproductive-age women are a little more anemic (have a lower red blood count) than they should be.

Replacing iron loss by a multivitamin-with-iron supplement can make many women have a healthier blood count and therefore more energy and less tiredness. Whether the vitamin part of the pill is important for this purpose is unknown.

Dr. Ken Cooper, author of *Aerobics*, while admitting that scientific evidence is scanty, seems to recommend that an athletic person take 1,000 mg of vitamin C a day. (*The Aerobics Program for Total Well-being*, New York: Bantam Books, 1982).

Vitamin B6 has been found helpful with premenstrual syndromes. (See Q. 204.)

Vitamin E is often helpful for women who have tender breasts. (See Q. 881.)

One thing authorities know is that excessive vitamin intake can be harmful. Vitamins that are absorbed by the body's fat can be accumulated in the body in such large amounts that disease may result. It is important, therefore, to avoid excessive doses of vitamins A, D, E, and K.

Water-soluble vitamins can be toxic if taken in such large doses that the body cannot get rid of them fast enough. Dr. Herbert Schaumberg, a neurologist at New York's Albert Einstein College of Medicine, has found a group of patients whose neurological symptoms were due to the intake of massive doses of vitamin B6. These patients were taking a minimum of 4,000 mg of B6 a day. At this level B6 is no longer a vitamin; it is a dangerous drug. As low a dose as 500 mg per day may cause these symptoms.

In his book *Vitamins and Minerals: Help or Harm?* (Philadelphia: Stickley, 1983), biochemist Charles W. Marshall advocates vitamin supplements only for premature infants, elderly persons, and people with specific diseases that make vitamin intake necessary. If you are interested in this topic, you might want to read his book.

Vitamins and iron can be expensive, but low-cost vitamins seem to be as effective as the expensive, so-called natural brands. If

## Fiber Content of Major Food Items

| | Fiber Content per Serving (grams) | Size of Serving | Calories per Serving |
|---|---|---|---|
| *Vegetables* | | | |
| asparagus | 3.5 | ½ cup | 18 |
| bean sprouts | 1.5 | ½ cup | 13 |
| beans | | | |
| navy | 8.4 | ½ cup | 80 |
| kidney | 9.7 | ½ cup | 94 |
| lima | 8.3 | ½ cup | 63 |
| pinto | 8.9 | ½ cup | 78 |
| string | 2.1 | ½ cup | 10 |
| broccoli | 3.5 | ½ cup | 18 |
| brussels sprouts | 2.3 | ½ cup | 20 |
| cabbage | 2.1 | ½ cup | 10 |
| carrots, raw | 1.8 | ½ cup | 15 |
| cauliflower | 1.6 | ½ cup | 14 |
| celery, raw | 1.1 | ½ cup | 8 |
| corn | 2.6 | ½ medium ear | 72 |
| eggplant, raw | 2.5 | ½ cup | 16 |
| kale greens | 1.3 | ½ cup | 15 |
| lettuce | .8 | 1 cup | 5 |
| onions, raw | 1.2 | ½ cup | 14 |
| peas, canned | 6.7 | ½ cup | 63 |
| potatoes | | | |
| white, baked | 1.9 | ½ medium | 72 |
| sweet | 2.1 | ½ medium | 79 |
| radishes | 1.3 | ½ cup | 7 |
| squash | | | |
| acorn | 7.0 | 1 cup | 82 |
| zucchini | 2.0 | ½ cup | 8 |
| tomato, raw | 1.5 | 1 small | 18 |
| turnip | 2.0 | ½ cup | 12 |
| *Fruit* | | | |
| apple | 2.0 | ½ large | 42 |
| apricots | 1.4 | 2 | 32 |
| banana | 1.5 | ½ medium | 48 |

| | Fiber Content per Serving (grams) | Size of Serving | Calories per Serving |
|---|---|---|---|
| blackberries | 6.7 | ¾ cup | 40 |
| cherries | 1.1 | 10 large | 38 |
| grapefruit | 0.8 | ½ | 31 |
| grapes, white | 0.5 | 10 | 36 |
| orange | 1.6 | 1 small | 35 |
| peach | 2.3 | 1 medium | 38 |
| pear | 2.0 | ½ medium | 44 |
| pineapple | 0.8 | ½ cup | 41 |
| plums | 1.8 | 3 small | 38 |
| raspberries | 9.2 | 1 cup | 42 |
| strawberries | 3.1 | 1 cup | 45 |
| *Grain Products and Others* | | | |
| bread | | | |
| french | 0.7 | 1 slice | 71 |
| rye | 0.8 | 1 slice | 62 |
| white | 0.7 | 1 slice | 64 |
| whole wheat | 1.3 | 1 slice | 59 |
| cereal | | | |
| All Bran® (100%) | 8.4 | ⅓ cup | 70 |
| Corn Flakes® | 2.6 | ¾ cup | 70 |
| Wheaties® | 2.6 | ¾ cup | 73 |
| Shredded Wheat® | 2.8 | 1 biscuit | 70 |
| crackers | | | |
| graham | 1.4 | 2 squares | 53 |
| rye | 2.3 | 3 wafers | 64 |
| saltine | 0.8 | 6 crackers | 76 |
| popcorn | 3.0 | 3 cups | 62 |
| rice | | | |
| brown | 1.6 | ⅓ cup | 72 |
| white | 0.5 | ⅓ cup | 76 |

Adapted from *Diabetes: A Practical New Guide to Healthy Living,* Dr. James W. Anderson, Arco Publishing, Inc., 1981.

you are going to take vitamins or iron, I recommend that you ask your druggist for a reputable but inexpensive variety that you can take once a day. Apparently this will do as much good for your body as a high-priced kind.

It is wise for most women over thirty-five to take extra calcium every day. From the age of thirty-five until menopause, most women need 1,000 mg of calcium a day. After menopause, they need 1,500 mg a day. If you eat or drink an average amount of calcium-containing foods (milk, yogurt, cottage cheese, and cheese), you get about 500 mg of calcium a day in your diet. You would then need an additional 500 mg a day before menopause and an additional 1,000 mg a day in tablet form after menopause.

If you get out in the sun at all, you do not need a vitamin D supplement. If you never get any sun, allowing the body to make its own vitamin D, you should take calcium pills containing this vitamin, since vitamin D makes the body's absorption of calcium possible. (See Q. 274.)

## Exercise Regularly

### 1234 Is exercise an important part of good health?

Yes. It is quite clear that exercise is a most important habit for those who want to be healthy now and avoid disease in the future. This seems to be supported by statistics that show that ever since more and more of our population started exercising, there has been a decrease in the number of deaths from heart disease.

Since 1968, when Dr. Kenneth Cooper first published *Aerobics*, there has been a gradual decline in the number of deaths from heart disease. As of 1980, there was a 27-percent decrease in the number of people dying of heart disease in our country as compared to 1968, although most experts had predicted an increased incidence of heart disease during these years. During this period of time the number of adults in our population who exercised regularly increased from 25 percent to 50 percent. I mention these figures in association with Dr. Cooper's book because his book and his influence seem to have been the impetus that started Americans exercising.

These facts alone should encourage everyone to start active exercise, but I have found that many women, especially those who are fifty and over, tune me out when I talk to them about increasing their physical activity. They seem not to believe me when I tell them that there will be advantages now as well as in the future.

### 1235 What are the immediate benefits of exercise?

There are several direct rewards for anyone who starts a regular program of exercise.

*Feeling better.* When patients complain to me of feeling tired and of not having much energy, I assure them that if they will begin exercising, within two weeks they will feel like different people. When they return to my office, they almost always say that they did start feeling better almost immediately. The only way for you to know if this would be true for you, however, is to try it for yourself.

*Increase in mental alertness.* Many people who feel mentally lethargic find that exercise seems to increase alertness.

*Weight is easier to control.* Although the best way to control weight is by eating properly, regular exercise supplements and "encourages" a weight-loss program. If you are depending on exercise alone for weight control, a great deal of fairly strenuous activity will be necessary, such as jogging four or five miles a day.

*Less illness and fewer accidents.* Studies have shown that if employees exercise and keep physically fit, there is an increase in productivity as a result of a decline in absenteeism and accidents. This translates into money savings for businesses. Companies with employees who exercise and stay in good physical shape have one-half of the insurance-premium costs of companies whose employees are not staying fit.

## 1236 What are the long-term benefits of exercise?

The long-range positive expectations for maintaining a regular program of exercise are equally important.

*Less heart disease.* Studies are beginning to show that a person who exercises has less chance of a heart attack. Exercise appears to increase the high-density lipoproteins (HDL) in the blood stream, and HDL seems to protect the body from hardening of the arteries (arteriosclerosis).

*Less hypertension.* People who exercise generally find that their blood pressure decreases. Lower blood pressure is associated with decreased chance of stroke or heart attack.

*Fewer accidents in later life.* Studies have shown that older people suffer fractures from falls for two reasons: they cannot see well, and they are in poor physical condition. The first can usually be treated by an ophthalmologist, but the second must be taken care of by the person herself before she gets to the point where she is so "out of shape" that she can no longer exercise and then falls and breaks her bones.

*Increased chance of independence and good health in later life.* Women who exercise can continue to be active and healthy as they grow older. It is true that some people seem to inherit "healthy genes," but you cannot count on that in your own particular situation. You have to assume that you will grow old and debilitated unless you take care of yourself now.

*Less pain from job-related demands.* Many working Americans develop back, neck, and eye pain that has been assumed to be job-related. Denise Austin, a Los Angeles-based exercise specialist, has discovered that most of these pains are due to lack of exercise rather than to any of the machines that people use in their workday. She has found that by working some easy-to-do exercises into the daily work schedule the problems

that employees develop either disappear or are prevented. Some of these problems are stress-related, and others are due to the positions assumed in front of computers, word processors, and typewriters. In spite of this, however, exercise helps.

## Calories Burned by Physical Activities

| Activity | Calories Consumed in Twenty Minutes of Vigorous Exercise |
|---|---|
| Badminton | 115 |
| Bowling | 90 |
| Brisk walking (4.5 mph) | 100 |
| Brisk jogging (5.5 mph) | 210 |
| Bicycling (13 mph) | 220 |
| Heavy gardening (digging, etc.) | 140 |
| Gymnastics | 140 |
| Golf (flat course) | 90 |
| Football | 180 |
| Horseback riding | 115 |
| Square dancing | 115 |
| Lawn mowing (power mower) | 80 |
| Ice skating | 160 |
| Skiing (cross-country) | 180 |
| Skiing (downhill/water) | 160 |
| Handball/racquetball | 200 |
| Rowing | 180 |
| Swimming | 240 |
| Tennis | 160 |

## 1237 How do I begin an exercise program?

I suggest to my patients that they first get a copy of *Aerobics for Women* by Mildred Cooper and Kenneth H. Cooper (New York: Bantam Books, 1973). I believe this is the best exercise book for women of any age.

Then pick an exercise that you think you can enjoy and will be able to do from now on. Start slowly—the level at which you start exercising will depend on your present state of conditioning and your age. Checking this out with your doctor is a good idea.

Be sure to arrange your schedule so that

you can exercise regularly for the rest of your life. By the way, if at all possible, start exercising with someone else. This will help your discipline in maintaining regular exercise, especially in the beginning.

Studies have shown that twenty minutes of active aerobic-type exercise three times a week is enough for proper body conditioning. The important thing is that the exercise be done strenuously enough to produce a heart rate that is 70–80 percent of a person's predicted maximum safe rate. The calculation is quite simple. You should subtract your age from 220 and multiply that by .7 or .8. This gives the rate (beats per minute) at which you should keep your heart going for twenty minutes of exercise.

The mistake that most people make, which often leads to failure, is choosing an exercise that they do not like. Very few people have the discipline to spend from one to three hours a week doing something that they do not enjoy when they do not have to do it. As far as exercise is concerned, there is no need for this to happen, because a person may choose from so many different types of good exercises. Find something you like and do it from now on.

Another mistake made when people start a fitness program is that they forget to plan a realistic schedule for exercise because they fail to make exercise a top-priority activity.

I believe "priority" may be the most important factor for a woman to consider as she thinks about exercise. I still feel guilty when I rush out of my office to keep my racquetball date three times a week, even though I am committed to exercise and enjoy racquetball. The guilt comes because I know there are always other things that I could be doing during those hours.

My system of priorities, however, says that if I do not stay in good physical condition, I will gradually become less healthy, will miss work, and will be less efficient—as physician, husband, and father.

You should consider a reasonable amount

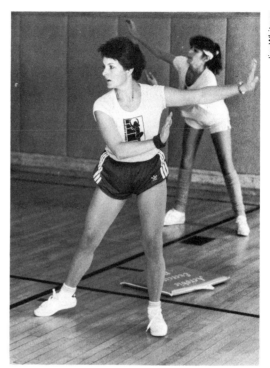

Jim Whitmer

Twenty minutes of active aerobic-type exercise three times a week is enough for proper body conditioning.

of exercise an absolute priority in your life. Sit down with your husband and children and plan a schedule that allows you this time. You will need to use your ingenuity to decide how you can do it, but it is possible. My wife finally settled on Jazzercise and walking. She thoroughly enjoys her exercise program and is in better shape than she was when she was in college. She also looks and feels terrific.

## 1238 Are there age limitations on beginning an exercise program?

No. Whatever your age, you should start an exercise program of some sort. Dr. James M. Hagberg of Washington University in St. Louis found that he could successfully "rehabilitate" people over sixty years old. He has them start their program by walking for half an hour every day for six months before beginning a more vigorous activity, including bicycling. These patients were able to tolerate this exercise program, and their heart performance improved by as much as 30 percent as time went by.

If you are over forty years of age and have been sedentary, you should see a physician for a check-up before beginning an exercise program. If you are thirty-five and have any health problem, such as hypertension or heart disease, or if you are a smoker, you should have an examination before you start exercising.

## 1239 Will exercise keep me young?

We are all going to grow old—if we don't die first. The real question should be, "How do I want to grow old?" Do you want to become gradually debilitated, or do you want to stay in the best physical condition you can for as long as you can, enjoying life with the freedom that goes with good health?

The older you are, the more rigid you must be in maintaining your exercise program. The older you are, the faster you lose your body conditioning when you stop exercising. Also, the older you are, the longer it takes to regain your conditioning once you have lost it.

A downward spiral can often start in the forties if a woman has not yet acquired an interest in or the habit of exercising. This spiral starts as a woman in poor shape does some physical activity (as simple as lifting a large flower pot) and, in so doing, sprains a ligament or strains a muscle. She will then say, "I am getting too old to do this sort of thing" and becomes even less physically active. The ligaments and muscles get still weaker, and the next time she does anything physical, she will pull a muscle again. This time she will say, "Well! I need to do even less physical activity because I am getting even older."

This downward spiral can lead a woman to a state of mind that convinces her that she needs to keep slowing down and that she is, indeed, getting older. Instead, it is the fact that she is so sedentary that is causing her body to conform to the stereotype that an "older" person cannot do anything physically demanding.

The right course to follow when you pull a muscle or ligament is to redouble (or start) an exercise program. Use that injury as a sign that you are not as physically fit as you should be and that you must improve your exercise plan.

A few years ago my knees started swelling when I played racquetball. This was before I understood the concepts I just described. I thought that I might be too old to play the game. An orthopedist explained to me, however, that I merely needed to do "straight leg" lifts to strengthen the ligaments and muscles around my knees. After doing this for a while, I found that my knees improved and I now play racquetball vigorously with no knee pain.

The cardinal rule is: Never let aches or pains keep you from persisting in a regular exercise program. See your regular doctor or an orthopedist to make sure nothing is wrong, and exercise that particular area of your body according to his or her recommendations. After a while you will probably find that the pain goes away.

## 1240 Should I exercise if doing so makes me sore?

As you grow older, normally around the age of forty-five, you will find that exercise leaves you more achy than it did in the past. This should probably be ignored, unless it is extremely uncomfortable. Such soreness is probably just the price you must pay for maintaining good health (and may diminish as you continue your program). It certainly is a cheaper price to pay than the price of not exercising, which is ill health and debilitation.

---

## 1241 Will exercise cause vaginal relaxation?

There have been some articles in the past few years stating that if women exercise strenuously, they are more likely to develop vaginal relaxation. This is a condition in which the support of the vagina is lost and the bladder and rectum bulge down into the vagina. Occasionally the vagina may even begin to turn inside-out. A variation of this problem involves loss of support of the uterus, sometimes referred to as a "fallen uterus."

Exercise does not cause either one of these problems. I find that if patients have been exercising, their vaginal strength and tone is better than before they began exercising. I strongly encourage you to exercise and not worry about this problem.

However, if you have already lost the support of your vaginal tissues and physical activity causes a "bottom falling out" feeling, see your doctor to determine if exercise is aggravating a condition that already exists. Even with this situation, my experience is that a patient's vagina often tones up when she is exercising regularly. If this does not happen and you continue to be uncomfortable, it would be better for your health to have vaginal repair surgery so you can continue to exercise than to let your vaginal problem stop your fitness program. (See Q. 699–704.)

---

## 1242 Will exercise keep me from getting pregnant?

The type of exercise done by most women will not change their hormone systems at all and therefore will not affect their fertility. However, if a woman exercises excessively,

she may stop having menstrual periods. In this situation she will usually not ovulate and will therefore be unable to become pregnant. Studies have shown that exercise can cause a woman to stop having periods because of the weight loss often associated with continual vigorous exercise. It has been found that if a woman's body fat drops to less than 22 percent of her body weight, she is likely to stop menstruating. Since this varies a great deal from individual to individual, some women would have to lose a great deal of fat before this would happen. Anorexia, bulimia (see Q. 149) and stress are other factors associated with a cessation of periods. However, when a woman's body fat is below 22 percent and she is not having periods, if she has been a competitive athlete, her menstruation may return when she stops competition.

Certain women are more likely to develop this problem than others. A woman who normally weighs less than 115 pounds and loses more than 10 pounds from exercise may stop having periods. Even a woman of average size who loses 10–15 percent of her weight from exercise may stop menstruating. Either one of these conditions results in a body-fat level of less than 22 percent.

A situation like this does not permanently change a woman's hormone system. When she gets out from under the stress of competition and/or when she gains some weight, her menstruation will almost always return. Therefore, when such a woman wants to become pregnant, she must do those things necessary to let her menstrual cycle resume. If you are having no periods and want to become pregnant, it would be best for you to talk to a doctor informed about problems of infertility. (See Chapter 11.)

When weight loss so affects a woman's cycle, there can be one additional problem if she goes a long period of time with no menstruation. Her bones can become very thin, a condition called osteoporosis. Such fragile bones can fracture more easily than normal. Therefore, if you are having no periods for more than a few months, you need to see a gynecologist familiar with this situation and discuss the advisability of taking some estrogen and progesterone hormones to replace those not being produced by your own body.

No one knows exactly why loss of body fat plays these tricks on the hormone system, but we do know that it is almost never irreversible.

## Alcohol and Other Addictive Drugs

**1243** **What are some of the physical and psychological problems associated with the use of alcohol and other drugs?**

*Decreased energy.* Alcohol consumed to any significant extent decreases a person's energy level, causing drinkers to exercise less than they should. This can become part of a downward health spiral, causing eventual sickness and debility.

*Weight gain.* Even moderate drinking stimulates appetite, resulting in consumption of more calories than are necessary for good health. Weight gain results. In addition, alcohol itself is a high-caloric substance, adding more than its share to the number of calories consumed.

*Impairment of intellectual judgment.* Alcohol, like other drugs, can affect one's thought processes, causing poor judgment, bad decision making, faulty reactions, and impaired comprehension of a situation.

One of the saddest effects of alcohol is the debilitation of intelligent, apparently successful men and women. Clinical experience shows that success and alcoholism often go hand in hand. Although alcohol does not contribute to success (an individual becomes successful because he or she is talented, dedicated, and bright), successful people often allow social drinking to become a way of life and therefore a vicious destroyer of all that is bright and beautiful in their lives. A woman who is professionally successful but begins drinking too heavily may coast on her career reputation for a while, or seem to still be doing an excellent job because of bright and loyal co-workers, but eventually her inability to continue to produce will take its toll. If such a woman had to enter the job market with her current alcohol intake, she would probably be unable to get or keep a job.

A full-time homemaker may also be susceptible to alcoholism. Easy access to alcohol and the possibility of concealing drinking habits may develop "closet alcoholic" tendencies. Initially alcoholism may be kept from family members but in time the effects of alcohol will impair a wife's or mother's ability to care adequately for her home, her family, and herself.

*Accidents.* Drunk drivers are a leading threat to public safety in America. Although drivers who have been drinking make up a small percentage of all the drivers on the road at any one time, they are responsible for over 50 percent of all fatal automobile accidents. Few drivers who were involved in an accident after drinking thought they had had enough alcohol to cause their accident, and they certainly did not think they were drunk. The lesson from this is that the effect you may feel from your drinking can be subtle, yet enough to cause you to have an accident that can make you an invalid or a guilt-ridden person for the rest of your life because of hurting or even killing someone else.

*Attitude.* Drinking affects a person's attitude, which can affect one's interaction with a spouse, children, friends, or co-workers. Doing and saying things that a woman will later regret can produce a downward spiral in her self-esteem and sense of self-worth, and in her relations with the important people in her life.

*Cirrhosis and general health problems.* Cirrhosis of the liver is usually a problem of those who drink heavily. Alcohol damages not just the liver, however, but other body tissues as well. It is not known at what level of drinking a body will be seriously damaged, although most likely any level of drinking over the years will ultimately produce a health problem.

*Cancer.* Excessive amounts of alcohol intake are associated with an increased cancer risk. Cancers of the mouth, throat, esophagus, and liver occur more frequently in people who drink alcohol to excess.

---

## 1244 How much alcohol is safe to drink?

The specific effect of a given amount of alcohol on an individual's body is not known. Although there is a certain blood-alcohol level that defines a person as "legally drunk," not reaching this level does not guarantee that alcohol has no effect. For several years it had even been widely reported that *moderate* alcohol use can decrease the chance of heart disease, but this has been disproved. In general the effects of long-term moderate drinking have been proven negative rather than positive.

The following chart shows how much alcohol consumption will produce various percentages of alcohol in the blood. Most law enforcement authorities consider a blood-alcohol level of more than .10 percent to be legal intoxication. For women, driving would usually be impaired after drinking three beers in a two-hour period. If a woman weighs over 160 pounds, it would take four beers in a two-hour period to produce this blood alcohol level.

## Number of Drinks (Two-hour Period)

1½ ozs. 86° liquor or 12 ozs. beer

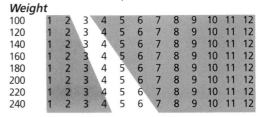

| Weight | | | | | | | | | | | | |
|---|---|---|---|---|---|---|---|---|---|---|---|---|
| 100 | 1 | 2 | 3 | 4 | 5 | 6 | 7 | 8 | 9 | 10 | 11 | 12 |
| 120 | 1 | 2 | 3 | 4 | 5 | 6 | 7 | 8 | 9 | 10 | 11 | 12 |
| 140 | 1 | 2 | 3 | 4 | 5 | 6 | 7 | 8 | 9 | 10 | 11 | 12 |
| 160 | 1 | 2 | 3 | 4 | 5 | 6 | 7 | 8 | 9 | 10 | 11 | 12 |
| 180 | 1 | 2 | 3 | 4 | 5 | 6 | 7 | 8 | 9 | 10 | 11 | 12 |
| 200 | 1 | 2 | 3 | 4 | 5 | 6 | 7 | 8 | 9 | 10 | 11 | 12 |
| 220 | 1 | 2 | 3 | 4 | 5 | 6 | 7 | 8 | 9 | 10 | 11 | 12 |
| 240 | 1 | 2 | 3 | 4 | 5 | 6 | 7 | 8 | 9 | 10 | 11 | 12 |

Blood-Alcohol Content

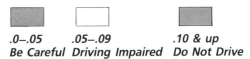

| .0–.05 | .05–.09 | .10 & up |
|---|---|---|
| Be Careful | Driving Impaired | Do Not Drive |

Further facts that relate to this subject are:

- A cold shower and/or black coffee will not sober up a person. Only time will lessen the effect of alcohol in a person's body.

- Spreading the length of time between drinks will decrease the effect.

- A 12-ounce mug of beer is just as intoxicating as a 6-ounce glass of wine or 1½ ounces of 86-proof liquor.

---

## 1245 Is it safe to drink while pregnant?

It has been found that babies of alcoholic women invariably have congenital abnormalities when they are born. The severity of the abnormalities varies and is seemingly related to the degree of alcoholism. But it is not only confirmed alcoholics who hurt their babies by drinking; almost all but the lowest levels of alcohol intake have been shown to produce some bad effect on unborn babies. A study reported in 1984 showed that a pregnant woman who has one drink daily will definitely hurt her baby's growth during pregnancy. Since the "lower limit" has not been determined, most obstetricians advise women to abstain or to drink no more than an occasional small glass of wine during pregnancy. (See Q. 474, 475.)

## 1246 How can I know whether or not I am an alcoholic? Is total abstinence the best practice?

Alcoholics Anonymous offers the following guidelines for determining whether or not you have a serious drinking problem. (Answer "yes" or "no" to these twelve questions.)

1. Have you ever decided to stop drinking for a week or so, but only lasted for a couple of days?

2. Do you wish people would mind their own business about your drinking?

3. Have you ever switched from one kind of drink to another in the hope that this would keep you from getting drunk?

4. Have you had a drink in the morning during the past year?

5. Do you envy people who can drink without getting into trouble?

6. Have you had problems connected with drinking during the past year?

7. Has your drinking caused trouble at home?

8. Do you ever try to get "extra" drinks at a party because you do not get enough?

9. Do you tell yourself you can stop drinking any time you want to, even though you keep getting drunk when you don't mean to?

10. Have you missed days of work because of drinking?

11. Do you have "blackouts"?

12. Have you ever felt that your life would be better if you did not drink?

According to AA, if you answer "yes" to four or more questions, you are in trouble with alcohol. Contact your local Alcoholics Anonymous office, or call a psychiatrist for a private consultation.

Total abstinence is probably a wise course, if only for our children's sake. There are many influences on our children that aggravate the growing alcohol problem among young people. Peer pressure and school pressure are major factors. But a major cause of the problem is us: their parents. If we drink, no matter what we say, we give our children our stamp of approval for their drinking for the rest of their lives. We may argue that they should not drink when they are "too young," or that they should not drink "so much," but those are only peripheral issues. The fact is, they suppose that if we drink, it is okay for them to drink.

I cannot see how we parents can afford to set this kind of example for our children, not when we see the statistics on teenage alcoholism.

About 15 percent of high-school students are heavy drinkers or have a problem with alcohol. More than 3.5 million teenagers in the United States are actually addicted to alcohol, and 31 percent of high-school students are considered to be alcohol abusers, drinking at least once a week with five or more drinks per drinking occasion. In addition to this, 41 percent of high-school seniors had taken five or more drinks in a row in the two weeks prior to the survey from which these statistics were compiled by the National Council on Alcoholism Prevention and Education Department, and it has been shown that teenage girls drink almost as much as teenage boys.

The average age at which kids begin to drink is thirteen. In a booklet, *Alcohol and Adolescents,* by Margaret Bean, M.D., and published by the Johnson Institute, Dr. Bean points out that teenagers who become alcoholics have their emotional development arrested at the age their drinking becomes a problem. An additional devastating result of teenage drinking is the high auto accident rate among teenagers.

I became aware of another reason for total abstinence as a result of research I did for this chapter. Recent studies have shown that even small amounts of alcohol can produce some damage to the liver. While it is true that the damage appears to heal within a few weeks, no one knows for sure that the human body is safe from any amount of alcohol.

Liver disease due to alcohol consumption is one of the fastest-growing disease problems in the United States. For every person who is ill because of known liver disease from alcohol, there are probably hundreds who do not feel well because their bodies are mildly affected by their drinking—yet do not even know it or refuse to believe that alcohol is the culprit.

I believe total abstinence is the safest course. You must decide for yourself. As you do, please carefully consider all the issues.

### 1247 What about other drugs?

I have singled out alcohol in this section because it is the major drug problem in the United States. I could just as well have been talking about marijuana or any of the other addictive drugs, such as cocaine or amphetamines. All these are hazardous to your health. There are other and more subtle drug problems rampant in our country. Thousands of women and men are addicted to prescription drugs, such as Valium, codeine, and Darvon. Almost every month I discover that one of my patients has been lying to me about her actual need for a prescription drug and has been using it to feed her drug habit. These drugs can be destructive, not only to a woman's body but also to

her mind and her interpersonal relationships with her husband, her children, and her friends. If you know you are misusing drugs, please admit it to yourself and get help.

For further information about drugs, contact The National Clearinghouse for Drug Abuse Information, P.O. Box 1701, Washington, D.C. 20013. Not only can this organization provide information about various drugs, it can also help you find help in your local community for yourself or a loved one.

## Handle Stress Properly

### 1248 Is stress really a health hazard?

Yes and no. Stress is like fire; whether it is helpful or destructive depends on how it is handled.

Some stress is necessary and productive, since almost any responsibility involves some pressure. This book, for instance, would not have been written if I had not been willing to endure a certain amount of stress. If a woman's stress level is excessive, however, it stops being a beneficial force in her life. If she finds that tension and pressure in her life are beyond her ability to cope with them, she can develop emotional and physical problems as a result.

### 1249 How can I know if I am handling stress poorly?

If you find that you are constantly feeling pressured or overburdened and are becoming anxious or depressed, you may be handling stress poorly. This is particularly true if you are becoming dissatisfied with yourself or feel that you cannot cope with life as it is today. If you are handling stress poorly, you may experience physical and mental problems such as these described in a 1984 article in *Philadelphia Magazine* (the Los Angeles Times Syndicate):

*Motor tension.* Shakiness, tension, aching muscles, inability to relax, jumpiness, or fatigue.

*Uncontrollable body sensations.* Sweating, pounding heart, clammy hands, dry mouth, dizziness, light headedness, hot or cold flashes, upset stomach, lump in the throat, diarrhea, pallor or flushed face.

*Apprehensive expectation.* Fear, worry, rumination, anticipation of misfortune to self or others.

*Constant hyperattention.* Difficulty with concentration that leads to irritability, impatience, insomnia, and the feeling of always being on the edge of panic.

*The sudden onset of explosive, overwhelming feeling of terror:* This is as if the body's alarm system were ringing for no apparent reason.

*Unreasonable fear.* Fear of flying, fear of closed spaces, fear of getting up in the morning.

## 1250    What are the results of poorly handled stress in a person's life?

Dr. Holly Atkinson, former medical reporter for "CBS Morning News", was quoted in the *Dallas Times Herald* (March 12, 1984) as saying that today's women are revealing the effect of stress in a variety of ways:

They are developing more gastric ulcers.

They are becoming alcoholics from excessive drinking.

They are developing lung cancer from excessive smoking.

They are gaining weight because they deal with stress by eating.

They are remaining childless because they feel they must choose between having a career or having a family.

The sad thing is that although stress has caused these problems to develop, the way such women deal with stress will cause even more stress.

## 1251    How can stress be handled properly?

Dr. Atkinson (see above) recommended that women "take a lesson from men who have learned about the health dangers of their lifestyle. Give up smoking; quit eating and drinking to excess; and learn to go to the gym and exercise to reduce stress. For women, exercise is seen as just one more thing on their list of things to do. Learn to treat exercise as a reward. Learn that when you are under mental stress, doing something physical helps." She adds, "We must choose our priorities. We cannot be Super Woman."

Many of my patients seem to be trying to be that "Super Woman." Those who do not work outside the home are often involved in so many community, social, or child-related activities that they do not have time to take a deep breath. Women with careers are often trying to balance doing well on the job with being a good wife and mother, which obviously includes attending all the Little League games, all the piano recitals, and all the plays in which their children participate.

Women often experience stress when the following things are neglected:

*Time alone.* Every woman needs some time just for herself.

*Time alone with her husband.* Every couple needs regular time together to maintain an abiding relationship.

*Time with her family.* A woman who has family responsibilities but does not find time to fulfill them adequately can feel a great deal of guilt about it.

*Time with God.* There are some fantastic promises in the Bible to the person who will develop a personal relationship with God. He helps us deal with the stresses of life as we learn to know and trust him.

## 1252 What should I do if I feel that my stress is getting out of control?

If you experience any of the symptoms listed in the previous two questions for more than a month or two, and stress-control techniques you are trying are not working, you should get help. That help may be found in reading books on the subject of handling stress, or you may need to see a doctor, psychiatrist, psychologist, your pastor, or a good friend for counsel.

Another source of help available in some communities is a local workship or clinic on stress. If you are referred to one of these places you may receive expert assistance for coping with your stress problem.

Books can be a great help with handling the pressures of daily life. They often provide significant insight into specific stressful situations. Two excellent books on this subject are *Stress/Unstress* by Keith W. Sehnert (Minneapolis: Augsburg Publishing House, 1981) and *Living with Stress* by Lloyd H. Ahlem (Ventura, Calif.: Regal Books, 1978).

## Wear Seat Belts

## 1253 Why is "wearing seat belts" included in this chapter on maintaining good health?

If you question my reason for including such a "mundane" suggestion as wearing seat belts in this chapter, you do not understand the significance of traffic accidents in our society. Wearing seat belts is the single most important health measure to keep you alive and well into old age, other than not smoking.

Traffic accidents steal more total years of life than any other cause of death, because auto accidents affect so many young people. Each time a twenty-year-old dies, fifty years of life expectancy are wiped out. Motor vehicles constitute the Number-One killer of people between the ages of one and thirty-eight, and more than 37,000 drivers and passengers are killed each year in auto accidents.

In the light of such devastating statistics, one important fact stands out: it has been proven that using seat belts can significantly reduce fatalities and serious injuries by from 35 to 60 percent, depending on the research source.

For every person killed in an auto accident, however, there are many more who are temporarily disabled or disfigured or crippled for life. Millions of Americans are coping with permanent injuries caused by automobile accidents.

The importance of the use of seat belts cannot be overemphasized. Please buckle up!

## An Ounce of Prevention

## 1254 Is a yearly physical examination important?

Yes. It is important for every adult woman to have a physical examination each year from the time she becomes sexually active, or from the age of twenty, for the rest of her life. More frequent examinations are necessary if there is a problem that requires close watching or treating. (See Q. 151–153).

## 1255 Is taking estrogen an important health factor for postmenopausal women?

Definitely. No matter how carefully you follow the suggestions given in this chapter, if your skeleton deteriorates, causing bone fractures, you cannot be healthy.

Estrogen will keep your bones strong after menopause, so that you can benefit from practicing all the health hints that we have given in this chapter. (See Q. 265–280.)

## 1256 How are sexual practices related to good health?

Sexually transmitted disease is a major health problem in our society. It causes bad health, infertility, sterility, insanity, and death.

There is a method of prevention, however. Stated in the simplest manner, the way to avoid STD and related problems is this: have sex only with your husband, who has sex only with you. (See Q. 747.)

## An Afterword

Although it may appear from this chapter that I feel the ultimate goal in life is good health, that is not so. My relationship with God, my wife, and my daughters is a priority that rises head and shoulders above the health of my own body.

I do believe, however, that God has given us our bodies and expects us to take care of them. To enable us to do this, he has given us minds to use for that purpose.

With our God-given intelligence, it is possible for most of us to sit down with our spouses, children, and others who are involved in our everyday lives, do some brainstorming, and come up with a way to have time to eat right, sleep enough, exercise properly, and have our annual examinations. With that same mindset we can find the means to stop the cigarette habit, to cut alcohol intake to a minimum, and to manage stress. Likewise our intellects can lead us to truly intimate relationships—without the complications and dangers of premarital or extramarital sex.

The rewards for such changes in your lifestyle can be enormous. You can feel better now and have more energy, less depression, and less illness. You can look better; eating wisely and exercising can make you more trim, whether or not you lose weight—and it can make you look younger. Beneficial changes in your lifestyle can enable you to be healthier in the future. It seems fairly certain that what you do now does dramatically affect your health in later life. If you choose a healthy pattern of living today, you will almost certainly have less disease and have better general health tomorrow and beyond. I encourage you to think through these things and start making necessary changes now.

# GLOSSARY

**abdomen**  The portion of the body, below the chest, which contains the stomach, intestines, gallbladder, liver, spleen, pancreas, lymph glands, kidneys, bladder, and, in a woman, the female reproductive organs.

**abortion**  The loss of a pregnancy before the twentieth week of pregnancy. An abortion may be spontaneous or induced.

**abscess**  A collection of pus surrounded by an inflamed area.

**actinomycosis**  A relatively uncommon fungus infection. It can develop in the uterus of a woman who has an IUD (intrauterine contraceptive device) in place for an extended period of time.

**acute illness, acute pain**  "Acute" indicates a relatively sudden onset of pain or illness, with definite symptoms and limited duration, as opposed to "chronic" pain or illness, which is a recurring illness or pain of indefinite duration and less intensity.

**adenoma**  Noncancerous (benign) tumor composed of glandlike tissue.

**adenomatous hyperplasia of the endometrium**  Overgrowth of the uterine lining. Not malignant at this point.

**adenomyosis**  Endometriosis that is present in the muscular wall of the uterus. This condition exists when tissue like the uterine lining is present in the muscular wall of the uterus.

**adenosis**  A condition in which areas of the vaginal lining (squamous epithelium) are replaced by tissue that is like the cervical lining (columnar epithelium). Often caused by exposure to DES (diethylstilbestrol) in the mother's womb.

**adhesion**  Scar tissue binding together structures of the body that are not ordinarily attached to each other. This may result from surgery, inflammation, or injury. (See Q. 923.)

**adolescence**  The period of human life between puberty and adulthood.

**adrenal glands**  Part of the endocrine system. These glands, one located on top of each kidney, produce hormones that control defense mechanisms, regulate the supply of water and salt, and help maintain correct blood pressure.

**AIDS**  Acquired immunodeficiency syndrome. A collapse of the body's immune defense system, usually resulting in death by rare forms of cancer, pneumonia, and overwhelming infections. Appears to be virus-caused and contagious.

**albumin** A protein found in egg whites, in plants, and in animals. When found in the urine, it may indicate the presence of kidney disease.

**allergy** A reaction to a substance (called an antigen) by a person sensitive to that substance. Symptoms may be so mild as to go unnoticed or may be severe enough to produce death.

**amenorrhea** Absence of menstrual periods. Primary amenorrhea means that a woman has never had a period. Secondary amenorrhea means that a woman has had one or more periods and then stopped having them for a length of time equal to three or four menstrual cycles.

**amniocentesis** Removal of some of the fluid that surrounds the unborn baby during pregnancy, usually for testing purposes. This is done by insertion of a needle into the pregnant uterus through the skin of the abdomen.

**analgesic** A drug which reduces pain.

**androgen** A male hormone that produces and controls the secondary male sex characteristics, such as the beard, muscles, and deep voice. Testosterone, the male sex hormone is the primary male hormone (androgen). Normal women secrete androgens in small amounts from their ovaries and adrenal glands.

**anemia** Low concentration of hemoglobin (oxygen-carrying material) in the red blood cells. A "blood count" tells if a woman is anemic.

**anesthesia** The absence of pain sensation, with or without a loss of consciousness. *General anesthesia* involves loss of consciousness. *Regional anesthesia* produces loss of pain sensation in a particular area of the body by the use of caudal, spinal or other nerve block. *Local anesthesia* is produced by injection of an anesthetic agent into localized tissue. *Topical anesthesia* is a lack of pain on a surface area from direct application of an anesthetic agent.

**angioma.** *See* vascular spider.

**anorexia nervosa** A condition most often found in young women, characterized by amenorrhea (absence of menstrual periods), by a loss of appetite, and by an aversion to food. Death may result if the problem is not treated. Another re-

lated eating disorder is bulimia, a condition in which young women overeat and then cause themselves to vomit. An aspect of this problem is that they often develop severe dental decay because of the effect of stomach acid on their teeth from the repeated vomiting. Bulimarexia is a condition that combines aspects of both diseases. Bulimia, bulimarexia and anorexia nervosa all require psychotherapy.

**antibiotics** Drugs that kill or inhibit the growth of bacteria.

**anticoagulant** A drug that hinders clotting (coagulation) of the blood.

**antihistamine** Drugs which oppose the effects of histamine in the body. Used in allergic conditions, such as hay fever and serum sickness, and also for alleviation of cold symptoms.

**anus** The opening at the lower end of the bowel canal; the opening of the rectum through which bowel movements are eliminated from the body.

**Apgar score** A rating system used to document a newborn's condition after birth. Includes heart rate, muscle tone, respiration, color, and response to stimuli. It is normally used to evaluate the infant one minute after birth and again five minutes after birth.

**appendicitis** Inflammation of the appendix, a small organ (three to six inches long) that projects from the lower bowel in the lower right part of the abdomen. A potentially fatal condition, appendicitis must be treated with immediate surgery.

**areola** The ring of darkly pigmented skin around the nipple of the breast.

**arteriosclerosis** Hardening of the arteries, a condition in which the walls of the arteries become coated with deposits of a cholesterol-containing material. The resulting degeneration of these blood vessels causes a loss of resilience often resulting in hypertension. The obstruction that develops can result in heart attacks, strokes, and gangrene of fingers and toes, arms and legs.

**artificial insemination** Instillation of sperm into the vagina or uterus by medical technique rather than by intercourse. Husband's sperm may be used (AIH), donor's sperm may be used (AID), or the insemination can involve putting washed sperm into the uterus (intrauterine insemination—IUI). Washed sperm may be from a woman's husband or from a donor. (See chapter 11 regarding this technique.)

**aspiration**   A procedure in which fluid or material is drawn out of a cyst, growth, or body cavity with a needle or tube. Suction is usually applied with a syringe.

**atypical endometrial hyperplasia**   A precancerous form of endometrial hyperplasia (overgrowth of the uterine lining). Not malignant, but 80 percent of women who have it will develop cancer if it is not treated.

**augmentation mammoplasty**   An operation, performed by a plastic surgeon, in which an implant is put into the breast to make it larger or more shapely.

**axilla**   The underarm or armpit.

**Bartholin's glands**   Vulvar glands that secrete a clear, thin mucus to lubricate the vulva during intercourse. They increase their output of mucus during sexual excitement, adding to the lubrication for intercourse. One gland is located on either side of the lower part of the vulva, with an opening just inside the labia minora.

**basal body temperature**   Body temperature immediately on awakening in the morning, before any daily activity (including getting out of bed) has begun.

**benign**   Not malignant, not cancerous.

**bilateral salpingo-oophorectomy**   Surgical removal of both fallopian tubes and both ovaries.

**biopsy**   Surgical removal of portions of the body's tissue for microscopic study and diagnosis.

**birth control pills ("OC'S", "the Pill")**   A pill containing synthetic estrogens and progesterones. Use of such pills produces an artificial menstrual cycle that prevents the release of the egg from the ovary each month.

**bran**   Ground husks of cereal grains. A convenient source of fiber, useful for increasing the amount of bulk in a person's diet. *See* fiber.

**Braxton-Hicks contractions**   Sometimes called "false labor pains." The uterus contracts all the time, even when it is not pregnant but the contractions are made more obvious by the enlarged uterus of pregnancy. Braxton-Hicks contractions do not prepare the uterus for labor, nor cause labor to start.

**breast reconstruction**   Rebuilding the breast after surgical removal or deformity. Such plastic surgery can involve augmentation with implants and remodeling using other body tissue and skin.

**breech birth**   A delivery in which a baby's bottom end (buttocks or feet) comes first, rather than its head.

**BSE**   Breast self-examination.

**bulimia or bulimarexia**   *See* anorexia nervosa.

**carcinoma**   A technical word for cancer. It is important to remember that a growth can be a cancer (carcinoma) and, in its early stages, not be dangerous for an individual if proper treatment is obtained. Skin cancer is a good example of this.

**carpal tunnel syndrome**   Pain or numbness of the hands, produced by swelling in the wrists. This is often seen during pregnancy.

**caruncle**   A condition in which the lining of the inside of the urethra seems to protrude from the urethral opening. This is not a malignant growth.

**catheter**   Any of the variety of tubes for insertion into the body.

**caudal anesthesia**   Often given during childbirth, it numbs a woman from the waist down but usually allows her to move her body and to push, assisting in delivery. Injected in the lowest end of the spinal column, just above the tailbone, it differs from an epidural only by where the needle is inserted into the body. It is not the same as a spinal. *Compare* epidural and spinal anesthetic.

**celibacy**   The state of remaining single, but the term is most often used to define a voluntary abstinence from sexual relations.

**centimeter**   A unit of measurement; .3937 inch; cc—cubic centimeter, there are about 30 cc in a fluid ounce.

**cerclage operation**   An operation in which a suture or band of material is put around the cervix to strengthen it so as to prevent miscarriages or premature deliveries.

**cervical cap**   A "miniature diaphragm" that fits

over a woman's cervix and acts as a barrier between the sperm and the cervix.

**cervical erosion**  Properly termed *ectropion*. A reddish discoloration immediately around the opening of the cervix caused by the lining of the inside of the cervix extending from the cervical opening to cover a part of the external cervix. It is not an "erosion" of tissues. That term was applied to this condition many years ago before careful study showed that it is a normal condition.

**cervical intraepithelial neoplasia (CIN)**  Precancerous cells of the cervix. Graded by physicians as to severity and extent:

CIN I—cells are mildly precancerous

CIN II—cells are moderately precancerous

CIN III—cells are severely precancerous

This is the new terminology that most gynecologists are now using instead of "dysplasia."

**cervical nabothian cyst**  Small hard nodules on the cervix caused by clogged mucus glands. Not precancerous, dangerous, or painful. Does not usually need treatment.

**cervix**  The lower part of the uterus that includes the mouth of the uterus. It is about two inches long and one inch wide in an adult.

**cesarean section**  Surgical operation for delivering a baby through an incision in the abdomen when normal vaginal delivery is dangerous or impossible.

**chancre**  A hard ulcer, usually painless, that is the entry site of syphilis into the body. *See* syphilis.

**chancroid**  A STD (sexually transmitted disease) caused by *Hemophilus ducreyi* bacteria.

**chemotherapy**  The administration of medications for the treatment or prevention of a disease. Although this term usually refers to the treatment of cancer, technically it can apply to the use of antibiotics and other drugs for any disease.

**chlamydia**  The most common sexually transmitted infection (STD) in the United States. A major cause of PID (pelvic inflammatory disease) and sterility. Caused by the bacterium, *Chlamydia trachomatis*.

**chloasma**  "Mask of pregnancy." Various-sized brown patches that occasionally appear on the face of a pregnant woman as a result of hormonal effect on her skin. Birth-control pills may also cause these discolorations.

**choriocarcinoma**  *See* malignant molar pregnancy.

**chorionic villi sampling**  A procedure in which an instrument is inserted through the cervix into a pregnant uterus for the aspiration of some of the placenta. This placental tissue is then tested to determine whether or not the unborn baby has a genetic abnormality. This procedure, which is new, can cause miscarriage.

**chromosome**  A microscopic piece of protein, several of which are present in the nucleus of every living cell. Each chromosome is made up of hundreds of smaller units called genes, which carry the genetic material that transmits physical traits from generation to generation.

**chronic**  Long-continued or of long duration. A chronic disease is one that is prolonged, or one that progresses slowly, as opposed to "acute," which denotes a sudden onset and limited duration.

**cilia**  Small, hairlike structures. In this book the term refers to cilia that line the inside of the fallopian tubes and are also on the tubes' fimbriated ends. Cilia beat constantly, sweeping the egg (ovum) into and through the tubes.

**circumcision**  Surgical removal of the foreskin, the loose fold of skin that covers the head of the penis.

**clinical pelvimetry**  Physician's examination of a pregnant woman's pelvis. This is done to determine if her pelvic bones are normal and large enough to allow the vaginal delivery of her infant. The physician does this through the vagina by feeling her bone structures with his or her hand.

**climacteric**  The period of life (usually about age 40) when the ovaries begin having decreased estrogen production. Includes the menopause and ends when all estrogen sensitive tissues have thinned out and lost all the effect that estrogens have had on them.

**clitoris**  A highly sensitive organ, consisting primarily of erectile tissue, which is located above the urethra in front of the vulva. It is one of a woman's external sex organs and corresponds to the male penis.

**coccyx**   The vertebral bones at the lower end of the spine. The tailbone.

**colitis**   Inflammation of the colon.

**colon**   The large intestine, the part of the intestine that extends from the end of the small intestine to the anus.

**colostomy**   A surgically constructed opening of the large intestine to the outside, usually through the lower left side of the abdomen, which allows evacuation of stools through that opening. A colostomy may be temporary or permanent.

**colostrum**   A thin, bluish fluid produced by the mother's breasts after childbirth. Often precedes the true milk by two or three days. It can also be secreted by the breasts during pregnancy. Such production can start months before delivery and is totally normal.

**colposcopy**   An examination of the vulva, vagina, or cervix by magnification of these areas by a colposcope. This is done primarily to detect precancerous or cancerous growths.

**colpotomy**   An operation in which the abdomen is entered through an incision in the upper back part of the vagina. This procedure is not often used, having been replaced by another technique. *See* laparoscopy.

**conception**   The union of sperm and ovum, the male and female sex cells, which leads to the development of a new life. It is sometimes called fertilization or impregnation.

**condom**   A contraceptive used by the male. A rubber sheath that covers the penis and prevents the sperm from being deposited in a woman's vagina.

**condyloma acuminata**   *See* venereal warts.

**congenital**   Existing at birth.

**conization**   An operation in which the doctor removes a cone-shaped piece of tissue from the portion of the cervix that can be seen through the vagina.

**contraception**   A method, device, or substance used to prevent conception.

**contraceptive foam**   A barrier-type contraceptive that coats the cervix and vagina with a sperm-killing agent. The same type of agent is used, in jelly form, with a diaphragm.

**contraceptive shots**   Injections of 150 mg of Depo-Provera (a long-lasting progesterone) which prevents pregnancy for about three months. Not yet FDA-approved.

**contraceptive sponge**   A sponge made of soft polyurethane material that contains a sperm-killing chemical. When inserted in the vagina, the sponge acts as a barrier between the cervix and penis but produces its contraceptive effect primarily by absorbing the sperm and killing them with the chemical it contains.

**contraceptive vaginal suppository**   A suppository which contains a sperm-killing chemical and is inserted into the vagina prior to intercourse. It is a relatively unreliable method of contraception.

**corpus luteum**   The structure left in the ovary after ovulation has occurred, formed from the follicle in which the egg developed. The corpus luteum is actually a short-lived gland. After ovulation, it begins producing progesterone and continues this for two weeks, unless pregnancy occurs. If pregnancy does occur, the corpus luteum continues to produce progesterone for a few weeks longer.

**counterfeit contraception**   Ineffective methods of birth control, which include douching, withdrawal, feminine-hygiene products, breastfeeding, intercourse during a menstrual period, plastic wrap and similar products used as condoms, and so on.

**couvade syndrome**   Symptoms of pregnancy experienced by the male. May mimic all symptoms of pregnancy, including nausea, abdominal pain, vomiting, diarrhea, burning with urination, and blood in the urine.

**"crabs" (pubic lice)**   Small parasites that live in body hair. Treatment is with medicated shampoo. Pubic lice are a different parasite from the head lice that so often occur in children. Usually passed by sexual contact, pubic lice are found primarily in pubic hair.

**CT (computerized tomography) scan**   A sophisticated technique for taking an X-ray across a portion of a person's body instead of in the usual manner. The typical X-ray view is much like a photograph. The CT scan is done as though a part of the body were cut through with a knife and a cross-sectional picture made of the severed end. A computer is used to put together several X-ray exposures for the final result.

**curettage** The scraping of a body cavity with an instrument to remove tissue and secretions. *See* D&C.

**cyst** A sac containing fluid or semisolid material. Some cysts are present in the body as a normal part of its function (i.e., follicle cysts of the ovary which release an egg each month). Some cysts in the body are abnormal growths.

**cystitis** Inflammation of the bladder caused by infection or irritation.

**cystoscopy** An operation in which a physician looks into the bladder with a lighted telescope called a cystoscope.

**D&C** Dilatation and curettage. An operation performed on a woman's uterus through the vagina. General anesthesia is usually required. The cervix is dilated with a series of larger and larger round dilators. When the cervix is dilated enough, a scraping instrument is inserted into the uterus and is used to scrape (curette) the lining of the uterus. Occasionally, a hollow scraping instrument, through which suction can be applied, is used for doing the curettement.

**dermoid cyst** Benign cystic teratoma, a tumor of the egg cells of the ovary. This tumor develops when an unfertilized egg begins growing. It is capable of developing any of the tissues that a human body contains. Typically, such tumors can contain hair, teeth, oil and sweat glands.

**DES (diethylstilbestrol).** A synthetic compound that produces the same effect in a woman's body as estrogen. Formerly prescribed to prevent miscarriage, it can cause sexual organ abnormalities and cancer in the offspring of women who take this drug while pregnant.

**diaphragm** A dome-shaped rubber cup with a flexible spring rim. When inserted in the vagina, this device holds contraceptive jelly against the cervix so that sperm are killed before they can enter the uterus and cause pregnancy.

**diagnostic ultrasonography** *See* ultrasound.

**dilatation and curettage** *See* D&C.

**diuretic** Medication that causes the kidneys to withdraw more fluid from the blood stream than they normally do, causing decrease in fluid retention (swelling) in the body and an increase in frequency of urination.

**douche** A method of cleansing or treating the vagina by irrigating it with water or a water-based preparation.

**Down's syndrome** Often called mongolism. Caused by an abnormality in the chromosomes that can produce mental retardation, a large tongue, cardiovascular abnormalities, and other physical abnormalities.

**dry labor** A nonmedical term that is often incorrectly used to describe the type of labor a woman will have if her "bag of waters" breaks several days or weeks before labor and delivery. This does not usually happen, however, because the amniotic fluid can be replaced completely by the body as often as every three hours. If all the fluid were lost and not replaced, the baby would die almost immediately.

**dysmenorrhea** Painful menstruation, menstrual cramps.

**dyspareunia** Painful intercourse.

**dysplasia of the cervix** *See* cervical intraepithelial neoplasia.

**eclampsia** A very serious toxic disorder of late pregnancy. Preeclampsia becomes eclampsia when a woman develops convulsions. This abnormality can cause death of both the mother and the baby. It is characterized in a pregnant woman by protein in her urine, high blood pressure, and generalized swelling. *See* toxemia of pregnancy.

**ectopic pregnancy** A form of pregnancy in which the embryo begins developing outside the uterus. It is considered an ectopic pregnancy whether the pregnancy is in the fallopian tubes (tubal pregnancy), in the ovaries, or in the abdominal cavity.

**ectropion** *See* cervical erosion, for which ectropion is the correct medical term.

**edema** Increased amounts of fluid in body tissues.

**effacement**   Shortening and thinning of the cervix, a process associated with pregnancy and with labor. The cervix is usually about one inch long. Late in pregnancy or in early labor, the cervix can become shorter than one inch (partially effaced). Labor completes the effacement process as the contractions of labor cause the cervix to totally thin out (100 percent effacement).

**ejaculation**   The ejection of seminal fluid through a man's urethra to the outside. *See* semen. Women do not have a true ejaculation, although some women excrete fluid from their urethras at the apex of sexual excitement. Whether or not this is the equivalent of a male's ejaculation, no one knows for certain.

**embryo**   An organism in the earliest stage of development. A human is considered to be an embryo through the first six weeks of life in the uterus. *See* fetus.

**endocrine glands**   Any of the ductless glands, such as the adrenals, the thyroid, the pituitary, the ovaries, the testes, whose secretions pass directly into the blood stream. The secretions they produce are called hormones.

**endolymphatic stromal myosis**   An overgrowth of the connective tissue of the uterus that causes uterine enlargement and bleeding. It may have a semimalignant effect on the body.

**endometrial biopsy**   A procedure in which a doctor inserts an instrument into the uterus and scrapes out a portion of the lining of the uterus (endometrium) for evaluation.

**endometrial hyperplasia**   Overgrowth of the tissue of the lining of the uterus that is not malignant.

**endometrial polyp**   An overgrowth of the lining of the uterus (endometrium) which develops as a projection from the wall of the uterus.

**endometrioma (chocolate cyst)**   Endometriosis (see below) that results in the collection of enough blood, scar, and tissue to form a cystic mass. When opened, an endometrioma will drain a chocolate colored fluid that is a result of the monthly bleeding of endometriosis tissue. These accumulations are most often found in ovaries, but can be present wherever endometriosis is growing.

**endometriosis**   The lining of the uterus is called the endometrium. When this tissue is present anywhere else in the body (even in the uterine muscular wall), it is called endometriosis. It can be found on a woman's intestines, in abdominal skin incisions, and in other parts of a woman's body. Surprisingly, it has even been found in men, one example being in the lungs of a seventy-year-old man.

**endometrium**   The membrane that lines the inner surface of the uterus.

**endorphins**   The body's own natural, opiatelike hormones. These hormones are used by the body to relieve pain.

**epidermal inclusion cyst**   Small harmless vulvar bumps that may appear on the outer surface of the labia majora.

**epididymis**   The accumulation of sperm-collecting ducts that are present on the back of each testicle.

**epidural**   An anesthetic given through a needle in the lower back, sometimes used during delivery. This anesthetic numbs a woman from the waist down but still allows her to move her legs and to bear down, assisting in the delivery of her infant. Although the needle is put into the back in the same place as the needle for a "spinal," it is not a spinal. For an epidural, the needle is not inserted as deeply as that for a spinal and does not actually penetrate the fluid sac that surrounds the spinal nerves. *Compare* spinal anesthetic.

**episiotomy**   A surgical incision in the outer end of the vagina that allows more room for delivery of the baby. This procedure is used to prevent tearing of the vagina during delivery.

**epulis**   Swelling of a person's gums in such a way that the enlargement resembles a growth.

**estriol test**   A diagnostic evaluation of an unborn baby based on the amount of estriol (a form of estrogen) present in the mother's blood or urine. Estriol is produced in large quantities by the baby if it is healthy. If the baby becomes unhealthy inside the uterus, it will begin producing less estriol. Since this hormone is present in both blood and urine of the mother, the test can be performed on either of these fluids.

**estrogen**   The primary female sex hormone. A woman's estrogen is principally produced in her ovaries. When the ovaries stop working at menopause, a woman's body will contain very little natural estrogen.

**external cervical os**   The portion of the cervix that opens into the vaginal canal.

**fallopian tubes**   Structures attached to the upper corner of the uterus on either side. They are about the same shape and size as a normal sized earthworm. The outer ends of the fallopian tubes are open, and it is through them that an egg passes from the ovary to the uterus. *See* fimbriae.

**fascia**   Sheets of fibrous tissue which hold muscles and various body organs in place.

**fertile**   Able to conceive.

**fertilization**   The union of the male sperm and the female egg (ovum).

**fetoscope**   A stethoscope-like instrument which allows a listener to hear a baby's heartbeat while that baby is still inside its mother's uterus.

**fetus**   A term used for the unborn baby from the start of the seventh week of pregnancy until it is delivered. *See* embryo.

**fiber**   The part of food that is not digested. Fiber adds bulk to the stools and is an essential part of a healthy diet.

**fiber-optic light**   This light has made it possible for physicians to brightly illuminate cavities of the body so they can be viewed with small "telescopes." The light bulb is outside the body and is projected at one end of a bundle of flexible glass fibers. This special fiber bundle carries the light to the inside of the body for laparoscopy, hysteroscopy, and other procedures, such as arthroscopy, cystoscopy, and so on. The advantage of this procedure over the old technique of using a light bulb at the end of the telescope is that the light can be much brighter, but without the telescope getting too hot. *See* laparoscopy.

**fibroadenoma**   A benign growth of the breast that comes from the lining of the gland tissue inside a woman's breasts.

**fibrocystic disease**   Used here as it applies to the breast. An overreaction of breast tissue to normal female hormones. Causes pain and lumpiness, and a slightly increased risk of cancer.

**fibroid tumor**   A common benign growth of smooth muscle fibers of the uterus. Since fibroid tumors almost never become malignant, they are surgically removed for reasons other than the chance of malignancy.

**fibromas**   Tumor composed of fibrous connective tissue that does not become malignant but can get quite large.

**fimbriae**   Small tentacles on the end of the fallopian tube that sweep over the surface of the ovary to capture the released egg.

**fissure**   A slit, break, or crack in a part of the body. An example is a crack in the nipple of a nursing mother.

**fistula**   An abnormal, usually narrow passage from the body cavity to the outside skin or from one cavity to another. A more common fistulae of the female organs is an opening from the rectum into the vagina as a result of child-birth.

**follicle stimulating hormone (FSH)**   A female hormone released from the pituitary that is responsible for the development of the egg-containing follicles of the ovaries.

**follicular phase**   The part of a woman's monthly cycle during which her egg is developing. When the woman ovulates (releases the egg from the ovary), the follicular phase is ended and the luteal phase has begun. *See* luteal phase.

**forceps**   Instruments which fit around an infant's head and assist in its birth. Obstetrical forceps are designed so that they do not squeeze the baby's head. Pulling pressure is applied to the strongest part of the bones of the baby's head.

**gardnerella (hemophilus)**   Vaginal infection. The most commonly transmitted infection of the vagina. This infection is characterized by a discharge that is watery, often heavy, with a fishy odor. This vaginal infection does not cause burning or itching of the vulva.

**Gartner's duct cyst**   The most common vaginal cyst. These cysts arise from tissues that lie in the walls of the vagina on either side. Gartner's duct cysts do not become malignant, are usually not painful and do not need treating unless they become bothersome because of their size.

**gastroenterologist**   Medical specialist who diagnoses and treats intestinal problems. Gastroenterologists do not perform surgery. They refer patients who need intestinal surgery to a general surgeon.

**gene**   Part of a chromosome, a basic unit that determines hereditary traits.

**general anesthesia**   An anesthetic that puts a person to sleep. General anesthesia is normally started with Pentothal in the veins and then continued with a gas administered with a mask or with a tube into the lungs. General anesthesia given today has an astounding safety record because of new developments in the field.

**gestation**   *See* pregnancy.

**gestational diabetes**   Diabetes that develops during pregnancy but was not present before the pregnancy started. It usually ends when the pregnancy is over. If it does not, the mother is then a true diabetic.

**GIFT (gamete intrafallopian transfer)**   An adaptation of the IVF procedure in which eggs and semen are injected directly into the fallopian tubes by means of a thin tube threaded through an incision made during a laparoscopy or mini-laparotomy.

**glans penis or glans clitoris**   The head of the penis or head of the clitoris.

**gonad**   Sex organ in which the reproductive cells develop and sex hormones are produced. Ovaries are female gonads; testes are male gonads.

**gonadotrophin**   A hormone produced by the pituitary gland capable of promoting ovarian or testicular growth and function. *See* follicle stimulating hormone (FSH) and luteinizing hormone (LH).

**gonorrhea**   A contagious venereal disease, characterized by inflammation of the internal genitalia and caused by a microorganism known as the gonococcus.

**gossypol**   Discovered in the People's Republic of China, this substance is a male contraceptive that is made from an extract of cottonseed. It is not approved for use in the United States.

**graafian follicles**   The tiny sacs, each containing an egg, that are present in the ovaries of even newborn baby girls. Starting at puberty, one follicle generally matures and ovulates each month, making it possible for pregnancy to occur.

**grade**   When applied to cancer, this is a technical term used to describe the aggressiveness of the cancer cells.

**granulation tissue**   "Proud flesh." Red sensitive tissue that often forms in the vagina after a hysterectomy, which can cause bleeding, spotting, discharge, and pain with intercourse. This tissue may remain for months or years unless a doctor destroys it by cauterizing it. This type of tissue can develop at the site of an injury of the skin, mouth, or vagina.

**granuloma inguinale**   A venereal disease whose main symptom is ulceration of the external genital organs. It is rare in the United States.

**granulosa-theca cell tumor**   Nonmalignant, ovarian tumor. Produces increased amounts of female hormones and, occasionally, malelike hormones.

**gynecology**   The branch of medicine dealing with diseases of women, particularly those of the reproductive organs and the breasts.

**hemangiomas**   Benign accumulation of blood vessels.

**hematoma**   Mass of clotted blood present in a person's tissue. If it is present under the skin, it is seen as a bump, with bruising around and over the area. A hematoma that develops inside a person's body from a severe injury or from surgery can contain from a small amount of blood to several pints of blood and can cause a person to become so anemic that transfusion is necessary.

**hemophilus**   *See* gardnerella.

**hemorrhage**   Excessive bleeding from the body. Hemorrhage can be internal or external. If not controlled, hemorrhage can lead to shock and even death.

**hermaphrodite**   A person who has both testicular and ovarian tissue present in the body, with ambiguous genitalia.

**herpes**   Virus-caused infection of two types. Herpes simplex virus type I produces fever blisters; herpes simplex virus type II is the sexually transmitted form of herpes. Both types of herpes are characterized by small blisters that break open, leaving small, shallow, sensitive ulcers.

**hormone**   A substance, produced by specialized body tissue called an endocrine gland, that is carried by the blood stream to another part of the body. It has a specific effect on hormone-responsive cells, thereby exerting its effect on the body. Hormones can also be manufactured synthetically. *See* endocrine glands.

**human chorionic gonadotrophin (HCG)**  A hormone produced by the placenta in pregnancy that is necessary for the maintenance of pregnancy. Because HCG has an effect in the body similar to a luteinizing hormone, it is often given by injection to make the ovary release its egg at the appropriate time in the monthly cycle.

**hydatid cysts of morgagni**  Small, grapelike structures usually found near the open end of fallopian tubes. About one-fourth to one-half inch in diameter, they are fairly common, nonmalignant, and do not need to be removed unless they seem to be distorting the open end of the tube because of their size or position. Occasionally a hydatid cyst will grow large enough that a doctor will be able to feel it during a pelvic exam. Surgery may be necessary to make sure that the growth is not a tumor on the ovary.

**hydatidiform mole**  An abnormal pregnancy in which the placenta has developed as a mass of grapelike cysts. *See* molar pregnancy.

**hymen**  The membrane at the opening of the vagina that partially blocks the entrance to the vagina. Lay people have named this the "maidenhead."

**hyperthyroidism**  Overactivity of the thyroid gland, producing weakness, heat sensitivity, sweating, weight loss despite increased appetite, restlessness, heart palpitation, staring, tremor, and protrusion of the eyes.

**hypoglycemia**  A condition of the body in which a person's pancreas does not control the level of sugar in the blood properly. Because of the resulting low blood sugar, a person will often feel badly experiencing headaches, hunger, trembling, dizziness, and weakness.

**hypothalamus**  A portion of the brain at its base, just above and attached to the pituitary gland. The hypothalmus is the "master control unit" for the female hormone cycle, but also controls the body's other glands and their hormone production.

**hypothyroidism**  The underfunctioning of the thyroid gland. The condition may produce dry cold skin, puffiness of the hands and face, slow speech, weight gain, mental apathy, con-

stipation, hearing loss, and memory impairment.

**hysterectomy**  Surgical removal of the uterus.

**hysterosalpingogram**  An X-ray procedure in which dye is injected through the cervix into the uterus and out through the fallopian tubes. As the dye is injected, X-rays are taken to facilitate evaluation of a woman's uterus and fallopian tubes. The evaluation is very reliable for the uterus but not quite so reliable for the fallopian tubes.

**imperforate hymen**  A hymen that has no opening. If this condition is not found before a girl starts her menstrual periods, it can cause problems with the female organs. The hymen is normally open enough to allow the menstrual flow to exit from the body through the vagina.

**impotence**  A man is impotent when he cannot develop an erection that is adequate for penile entry into the vagina or when he cannot maintain an erection long enough after entry for ejaculation to occur there. A woman is not considered impotent unless she has a physical condition or emotional problem that prevents the entry of a man's penis into her vagina.

**incompetent cervix**  A cervix that is too weak to hold a pregnancy.

**incontinence**  Leakage of stool or urine. Women may leak urine with an occasional hard cough or vigorous laugh, and such occasional episodes of soiling are not abnormal. If they occur often enough to be embarrassing or bothersome, however, treatment may be necessary. Any persistent leakage of stool is abnormal and should be evaluated.

**infertility**  A condition in which a supposedly fertile couple does not achieve pregnancy after twelve to eighteen months of regular, normal intercourse. "Sterility" is a condition in which factors exist in either male or female that prevent pregnancy from occurring.

**inguinal hernia**  Protrusion or bulging of a body organ through the tissues that normally contain it.

**intraductal papillomas**  Small, tumorlike growths of the ducts of the breast. May cause oozing of fluid (sometimes bloody) from the nipples.

**intrauterine growth retardation (IUGR)** A condition in which the fetus is not growing as rapidly as it should inside the mother's uterus. This problem may be due to many factors, and may or may not be a cause of abnormalities in the newborn.

**invasive molar pregnancy (chorioadenoma destruens)** Pregnancy in which the very abnormal placental tissue grows into (invades) the uterine wall. *See* molar pregnancy and malignant molar pregnancy.

**in vitro (test tube) fertilization (IVF)** A technique whereby a woman's egg is taken from her body and placed in a culture dish to which sperm are added. When fertilization has occurred, the embryo is placed in the woman's uterus, where it develops as any normal pregnancy would.

**IUD** (intrauterine contraceptive device) A small device that is inserted into a woman's uterus to prevent conception. It normally remains in place until removed by the physician.

**IUGR** *See* intrauterine growth retardation.

**Kegel's exercises** Exercises of a woman's pelvic muscles to increase vaginal support and thereby reduce vaginal looseness.

**labial agglutination** A condition in which the edges of the two labia majora stick together, making the vagina appear closed. This is usually due to minor inflammation and is not dangerous, since the labia do not actually grow together.

**labia majora** The large outer lips of the vulva. Normally covered with hair in adult females.

**labia minora** The small folds (lips) within the larger labia majora that surround the vaginal opening.

**lactation** Production and secretion of milk by the female breast following childbirth and during the months of nursing.

**lactiferous sinus** The widened part of the milk ducts in the breast, just under the nipple, that act as a reservoir for milk during the nursing process.

**laparoscopy** An examination that allows the physician to view the female organs and the abdominal cavity with an optical telescope that is passed through a small incision in the abdominal wall (usually through the lower edge of the navel). Some procedures, such as sterilization, laser operations and cutting apart adhesions can be done at laparoscopy.

**laparotomy** An operation on a person's abdomen in which the abdominal cavity is opened. For example, an appendectomy is a laparotomy done for removal of an appendix.

**leukoplakia** White patches on the "skin" of the vulva, the vagina, or the cervix. Not malignant, or premalignant, as was thought in the past.

**leukorrhea** A discharge from the vagina due to an infection or growth.

**libido** Sexual drive.

**lichen sclerosus et atrophicus (LS&A)** A condition in which the skin of the vulvar tissues becomes thin and somewhat shrunken. Vulvar itching often accompanies the condition. (The name for this problem has recently been changed to *lichen sclerosus*, leaving off the *et atrophicus*.)

**linea nigra** A dark line that appears on the abdomen of pregnant women from the navel to the pubic hair.

**lipoma** Painless, nonmalignant tumor made up of fatty cells. Since lipomas rarely become malignant, they generally do not need to be removed unless a doctor is unsure of what they are or if they are in some way bothersome.

**local anesthetic** An anesthetic administered by injecting an anesthetic agent directly into the tissues that need to be made painless.

**lumpectomy** A nonmedical term which refers to breast surgery in which only the cancerous lump—not the entire breast—is removed.

**lupus erythematosus** Disorder which occurs most often in young women. May be limited to the skin, producing a butterfly-shaped red rash on the nose and cheek. In its more serious form, it may affect joints, lungs, or kidneys, producing fever and muscle/joint pain. The cause is unknown.

**luteal phase** The part of a woman's monthly cycle which lasts from the moment she ovulates (releases an egg) until her menstrual period starts, (usually fourteen days.) It is called the luteal phase because, as soon as ovulation occurs, the ovary is left with a small cystic structure, called the corpus luteum, which produces both estrogen and progesterone until menstruation starts. *See* follicular phase.

**luteinizing hormone (LH)** A hormone produced by the pituitary that stimulates the ovary to release its egg.

**lymphogranuloma venereum (LGV)** A sexually transmitted disease (STD) that produces enlarged lymph nodes in the groin and a rectal infection with discharge of mucus and pus from the anus and from the open sores that develop.

**magnetic resonance imaging** *See* MRI.

**malignant** Cancerous.

**malignant molar pregnancy (choriocarcinoma)** A condition of the uterus containing highly invasive and malignant tissue developing from placental tissue. Choriocarcinoma can occur after a normal, a tubal, or a molar pregnancy.

**mammography (Xerogram, Xeroradiography)** A special X-ray of the breast for detection of malignancy or to help in the diagnosis of breast lumps.

**mastectomy** Surgical removal of the breast. *See* radical mastectomy, simple mastectomy, subcutaneous mastectomy, lumpectomy, and resection.

**mastitis** The precise definition of mastitis is "breast infection," which occurs most commonly either immediately after the delivery of a baby or during the nursing of a baby. Mastitis is also used in reference to women who have tender, cystic breasts (cystic mastitis). *See* fibrocystic disease.

**meconium** Material that is passed from the bowels of an unborn baby into the fluid surrounding it. This can be a normal occurrence, but it is frequently an indication that the baby is under stress. This term also applies to the stools that normal newborn babies pass before they have had anything to eat. Such stools are dark green, very sticky, and without odor.

**Meig's syndrome** A condition in which an ovarian tumor, called a fibroma, is associated with fluid in the chest cavity (around the lungs) and excessive fluid in the abdominal cavity.

**menarche** The term used for the first menstrual period.

**menometrorrhagia** Excessive loss of blood with the menstrual period combined with bleeding between the menstrual periods.

**menopause** The term used for a woman's last menstrual period.

**menstruation** The periodic (monthly) flow of blood and debris from her uterus during a woman's reproductive years.

**menstrual extraction** A smoke-screen term used by some people to refer to a very early abortion. A small suction apparatus is used to remove the uterine lining and the embryo if it is present immediately after a woman has missed a period.

**metrorrhagia** Bleeding between menstrual periods.

**miscarriage** *See* abortion.

**mittelschmerz** "Mid pain." Discomfort at the time of ovulation.

**molar pregnancy (hydatidiform mole)** A pregnancy in which an abnormal placenta is produced. The abnormal placenta is characterized by the presence of multiple, grapelike cysts. *See* invasive molar pregnancy and malignant molar pregnancy.

**molluscum contagiosum** An infection caused by a virus which is mildly contagious. This infection is characterized by small, dome-shaped bumps that grow primarily on the inside of the upper thighs. It is not dangerous and can be cured by scraping away the small, pearly-appearing center of each bump.

**mongolism** *See* Down's syndrome.

**monilia vaginitis** Also called fungus or yeast infection, this is the most common vaginal infection. Characterized by itching, vulvar redness, and a cheesy, white discharge.

**mons pubis, mons veneris** The pubic mound, or fatty pad overlying the pubic bone and over which the pubic hair grows.

**mucous cystadenomas** Nonmalignant ovarian tumors which contain mucuslike material. If left alone, they can grow and rupture, or can become malignant.

**mullerian duct cells** The cells in a female embryo that develop into the fallopian tubes, the uterus, and the upper portion of the vagina.

**MRI (magnetic resonance imaging)** A technique for taking pictures of the inside of the body, much like a CT scan but without ionizing radiation (X-ray). Formerly called NMR. This technique, which uses a large magnet rather than an X-ray machine, is more accurate than even the CT scan. *See* CT scan.

**myomectomy** A surgical procedure in which fibroid tumors of the uterus are removed but the uterus itself is preserved.

**natural family planning** Sometimes called the "rhythm method." With this contraceptive technique, which involves no devices or medications, a couple will avoid intercourse around the time of ovulation, when there is an egg present for fertilization. The same principle may be used in reverse by a couple wishing to increase the chance of pregnancy, by scheduling intercourse around the probable ovulation time.

**neural tube defect** A congenital abnormality of a baby, characterized by abnormalities of the central nervous system. An example of this type of defect is *spina bifida*, a condition in which the spinal cord can be exposed because of a defect in the bones and skin overlying it.

**nevus** *See* vascular spider.

**nipple** The small protuberance on the breast from which, in females, the milk glands discharge milk. Contains erectile tissue and is surrounded by the areola, a darker-pigmented circle.

**nodule** A small, hard lump.

**nonstress test (NST)** A diagnostic evaluation of an unborn baby, based on the heartbeat of the baby as recorded by a fetal monitor. When a healthy fetus moves, its heartbeat increases (just as yours does when you exercise). The nonstress test records the baby's heartbeat to see if it increases with movement as is normal.

**obstetrics** The branch of medicine that deals with pregnancy and childbirth.

**oophorectomy** Surgical removal of the ovaries.

**orgasm** The climax of sexual excitement.

**osteoporosis** Weakened and brittle bones, most common in women after menopause. When osteoporosis is present, the bones are weak and can easily break. When postmenopausal women break a bone, it is usually because they have developed osteoporosis. The "dowager's hump" and loss of height that are sometimes seen in postmenopausal women are caused by recurrent fractures of the vertebrae.

**ovaries** Two sex glands, located in the lower part of the abdomen on either side of the uterus. Their primary function occurs between menarche (first menstrual period) and menopause. During this time, they release an egg each month, making pregnancy possible if the egg is fertilized. The ovaries also produce the female hormones responsible for changing a girl's body into that of a woman and preparing the body for the occurrence of pregnancy.

**ovulation** The process in which the egg (ovum) is released from the ovary. In sexually mature females, ovulation usually occurs every twenty-eight days, halfway between the menstrual periods. Ovulation usually starts a fourteen-day chain of events that ends with a menstrual period if pregnancy does not occur. *See* follicular phase and luteal phase.

**ovum** Egg cell. When fertilized, it is capable of developing into a person similar to its parents in traits that are hereditary, or transmitted by the genes of the chromosomes.

**oxytocin challenge test (OCT)** Also called "stress test." A diagnostic evaluation of an unborn baby's condition. This evaluation is different from a "non-stress test" in that Pitocin is given intravenously to cause the uterus to contract. Since an unhealthy baby cannot tolerate the normally decreased blood flow through the uterus that results from a contraction, its heartbeat will drop, indicating a problem.

**papilloma** A small tumorlike growth that may or may not be malignant. Papillomas may be present in the breast or in other parts of the body.

**Pap smear** In gynecology, the term *Pap smear* refers to a smear of scrapings from a woman's cervix or vagina that is transferred to a glass slide. After being stained, the cells in the scraping can be viewed by pathologists to determine whether or not malignancy exists. Such a smear may also show infection, though it is not widely used for that purpose. Pap smears can be taken from other parts of the body and are helpful in determining if there is cancer in the lungs, in the breasts, and other parts of the body.

**paracervical block**   An anesthetic technique in which anesthetic drugs are injected into the tissues on either side of the cervix at the top of the vagina. Paracervical block is very useful for procedures done on the cervix or uterus in a doctor's office. It is rarely used during labor because it often causes a baby's heartbeat to slow down.

**PCOD.**   *See* polycystic ovarian disease.

**pelvic congestion syndrome**   A condition in which the pelvic tissues become swollen, boggy, and congested. Because of these changes in the tissue, women will often feel pelvic discomfort and pain.

**penis**   The male organ of copulation. Also contains the urethra, which carries urine from the body.

**perineum**   The part of the perineum that a woman can see is the tissue between her vulva and her anus. The woman's perineum is actually a much more extensive structure than this, including the muscles and tissues of her lower pelvis, through which the vagina and rectum exit to the outside. It is the tissues of the perineum that hold the intestines and internal organs inside a woman's body.

**peristalsis**   Rhythmic contractions of tubular structures in the body that propel their contents. The intestine's peristalsis, for example, propels food through the intestines; and the fallopian tubes have rhythmic peristaltic contractions that propel the egg down the tube.

**peritoneal fluid**   The fluid that bathes the internal organs and is contained inside the peritoneal cavity (the space between all the organs inside the abdominal cavity).

**peritoneum**   The membrane that lines the internal abdominal wall and all the internal abdominal organs.

**peritonitis**   An infection or inflammation of the peritoneal cavity (the space between all the organs inside the abdomen). Such a condition causes a great deal of pain. Peritonitis may be caused by infections of the female organs, appendicitis or a ruptured gallbladder. This condition must be accurately diagnosed and quickly treated, because death can result.

**placenta**   An organ through which the fetus is fed and provided oxygen while in the mother's uterus. The placenta also removes waste from the amniotic fluid; it filters out germs, keeping them from getting into the uterus; and produces the hormones necessary for maintaining the pregnancy in a healthy condition. The placenta is a temporary organ that develops upon fertilization of an ovum and is delivered soon after the baby is born. *See* umbilical cord.

**placenta previa**   A term applied to a placenta that is located completely or partially in the lower part of the uterus. Because the cervix tends to stretch during the latter part of pregnancy, a placenta previa will often bleed. If the placenta previa is too low in the uterus, a woman must deliver her baby by cesarean section, since death from blood loss can result for both mother and baby if a vaginal delivery is attempted.

**PMS (premenstrual syndrome)**   This term is applied to the symptoms a woman may experience prior to her menstrual period. They may begin at ovulation and last until the period begins, approximately fourteen days. May include cramps, backache, tension, depression, irritability, mood swings, swelling, breast tenderness, and so on.

**polycystic ovarian disease (PCOD; Stein-Leventhal Syndrome, sclerocystic ovaries)**   An abnormality of the ovaries which produces irregular periods and can result in infertility.

**polyp**   Nonmalignant tumor that hangs by a pedicle, or stalk, from a body cavity. Polyps are often found hanging from the cervix. They may be present in the uterine cavity itself.

**postmature syndrome**   A term used to describe the condition of a baby who is born more than two weeks past the due date and who has been affected by that situation. For example, weight loss may have resulted because adequate nutrition has not been able to pass through a placenta that has been gradually deteriorating because of the length of the pregnancy.

**postpartum sterilization**   Sterilization procedure done immediately after delivery or during the next few days. *See* sterilization procedure.

**precocious puberty**   Sexual development before the age of eight. If a girl has menstrual periods before the age of eight, she has precocious puberty. If she has significant breast or sexual hair development much before that age, she may have precocious puberty and should be evaluated by a physician.

**preeclampsia** *See* eclampsia.

**pregnancy** The state of a woman from conception of a child to delivery of that child, usually 280 days.

**premature menopause (premature ovarian failure)** Cessation of ovarian function before age forty.

**premenstrual syndrome** *See* PMS.

**presacral neurectomy** This procedure, often associated with infertility treatment, involves cutting the sympathetic and parasympathetic nerves that spread out inside the abdomen to the uterus and tubes. The theory is that such an operation relieves any uterine and tubal spasm that might be inhibiting fertility. This procedure does not affect sexual feeling at all. Most women are aware of having had this procedure only because they have less menstrual cramps and often will not feel any pain with labor.

**progesterone** A female hormone produced by the ovaries after ovulation.

**prolapsed uterus** A condition in which the uterus loses its support and falls down into the lower vagina, or even out of the vagina. If the uterus protrudes from the vagina, it can cause a great deal of discomfort, but if it is only down into the lower vagina, it may cause no discomfort at all. If a woman has no discomfort with a prolapsed uterus, she need not have surgery done; if she does, surgery will usually eliminate the discomfort.

**puberty** The period of life during which a person becomes capable of reproduction and manifests such secondary sex characteristics as growth of pubic and underarm hair, and development of breasts in the female.

**pudendal block** An anesthetic procedure in which the anesthetic agent is injected through the wall of the vagina, about halfway up on either side, producing anesthesia of the pudendal nerves and numbing the lower half of the vagina and the vulvar and anal areas.

**pulmonary embolism** A blood clot that breaks loose and is carried by the flow of blood to the lungs. It results in chest pain, a cough, and la-bored breathing. This is a critical problem that can result in death. Very specialized medical care is required.

**radical mastectomy** Removal of the entire breast, the underlying chest muscles (pectorals), and the lumph nodes under the arm (axilla).

**rectovaginal fistula** A hole from the vagina into the rectum. A fistula of this type will usually allow stools to pass from the rectum into the vagina. This condition can almost always be successfully repaired surgically.

**rectum** The lowest segment of the digestive tract. Terminates in the anus, through which solid waste is evacuated from the body.

**resection of breast tissue (segmental or quadrant)** Surgical procedure involving excising as much as one quarter of the breast tissue and, usually, the lymph nodes in the axilla, or underarm.

**Rh factor** A hereditary factor in the blood that can cause complications if the mother is Rh negative and the fetus is Rh positive.

**rhythm method** *See* natural family planning.

**round ligament pain** Pain during pregnancy caused by stretching or pulling of the round ligaments of the uterus. These ligaments are located on each side of the uterus and help hold it in position. Such pain is not dangerous, but it can cause as much pain as appendicitis and last for several days.

**salpingitis isthmica nodosa** Nodular thickening along the course of the fallopian tubes. This condition usually results in infertility. It can occasionally be diagnosed by a hysterosalpingogram, but will often require a laparoscopy or laparotomy for diagnosis.

**scabies** Infection caused by mites, parasites which burrow under the skin.

**scan** Often used by obstetricians and gynecologists to refer to an ultrasound study.

**scrotum** The sac of skin that holds the male's testicles.

**semen** The material which is expelled from a man's penis at ejaculation. The largest component of semen is mucus, the result of secretions from the prostate gland and seminal vesicles. In the mucus of the semen is contained the sperm, the most "important" element but the smallest in volume. If all the sperm from a semen specimen were gathered together, they would amount to only a small pellet of material, no more than one-sixteenth of an inch across.

**septate uterus**  Incomplete fusion of the two halves of the uterus, resulting in a wall or division in the uterus.

**serous cystadenomas**  Nonmalignant ovarian tumors which contain cystic areas of fluid. If left alone, they can grow and rupture or become malignant.

**severe atypical endometrial hyperplasia**  The most extremely abnormal form of uterine hyperplasia (overgrowth of the uterine lining.) Considered malignant, but it is confined to the surface of the uterine lining. Continued change will result in true invasive cancer.

**sexually transmitted disease**  *See* STD.

**silicone plugs**  When inserted in the fallopian tubes with instruments put through the cervix into the uterus, these plugs prevent the passage of an egg into the uterus. A contraceptive technique; but not yet approved by FDA except as a research procedure (at time of writing).

**simple mastectomy**  Removal of the entire breast, leaving the pectoral (chest) muscles.

**Sims-Huhner Test (SHT)**  A diagnostic procedure used to evaluate the receptivity of a woman's cervical mucus to her husband's sperm. It is normally done a day or two before ovulation and two to four hours after intercourse. It is painless and is much like a routine Pap smear.

**skin tags**  Small, skin-colored projections of skin, about the size of small ticks, that often proliferate during pregnancy. Such growths most often occur on a woman's neck and upper chest. They generally, but not always, disappear after pregnancy.

**smegma**  Secretions that may accumulate either where the labia minora overlie the clitoris or under the foreskin of the male penis.

**sonogram, sonography**  *See* ultrasound.

**sperm**  The male reproductive cell. *See* semen.

**spinal anesthetic**  A technique in which the an-

esthetic agent is injected through the lower back into the spinal fluid. This produces dense numbness and paralysis of the muscles from the waist down, stopping both pain and movement. If a woman has a spinal for delivery, the baby must be low in the birth canal before the spinal is given because she cannot effectively push the baby out while so anesthetized. Using today's improved technique, a spinal is an extremely safe form of anesthesia, both for the baby and the mother. *See* epidural.

**stage (of cancer)**  Technical term used to define the extensiveness of cancer in the body, whether it is just in the organ where it started or has spread to other parts of the body.

**STD (sexually transmitted disease)**  This is the new and modern term for venereal disease. This type of disease is passed almost exclusively by sexual contact.

**Stein-Leventhal syndrome**  *See* polycystic ovarian disease.

**sterility**  Incapacity to produce children, in either the female or the male. *See* infertility.

**sterilization**  A procedure whereby permanent birth control is provided. Such a surgical operation may involve surgery to the fallopian tubes in the female (tubal ligation) or surgery on the vas in a male (vasectomy). A sterilization may be reversible, except in the case of a hysterectomy.

**stress test**  *See* oxytocin challenge test.

**striae gravidarum**  "Stretch marks." Pinkish lines, resembling scars, that appear on the abdomen, breasts, and thighs of some pregnant women, and usually remain after pregnancy.

**subcutaneous mastectomy**  Removal of most of the breast tissue while leaving the surface skin and nipples intact.

**supracervical hysterectomy**  Removal of only the upper part of the uterus, leaving the cervix in place.

**surgical menopause**  Cessation of ovarian function due to removal of the ovaries by surgery.

**syphilis**  If untreated, a most dangerous STD. Caught only by sexual contact with a person who has it. Caused by the germ *Treponema pellidum*, syphilis is a horrible, destructive disease. *See* chancre.

**telangiectasia**  *See* vascular spider.

**teratomas (dermoids)**  *See* dermoid cyst.

**testicles, testes**  Two male sex glands which hang outside the body in a sac called the scrotum. They produce sperm and testosterone, the male sex hormone.

**testosterone**  The primary male sex hormone.

**thermography**  A method of measuring skin temperature of the body. For women, this procedure is used primarily in an attempt to help diagnose breast cancer.

**thrombophlebitis**  Blood clots with resulting inflammation in a person's vein or veins.

**toxemia of pregnancy**  "Poisoning" of pregnancy. A disorder of pregnancy characterized by hypertension (high blood pressure), edema, swelling, and albuminuria (protein in the urine). Doctors use the term *preeclampsia* for toxemia without convulsions and *eclampsia* for toxemia with convulsions *See* eclampsia.

**toxic shock**  A condition caused by the *Staphylococcus aureus* bacterium. Affects both men and women, but sometimes associated with use of high-absorbency tampons. Symptoms may be mild or severe and include any or all of the following: fever, chills, vomiting, diarrhea, dizziness, fainting, sore throat, sunburnlike rash.

**translumination of the breasts**  "Light scanning." A new diagnostic technique for the breasts. Involves no radiation and little discomfort. Accomplished by projecting light through the breast.

**trichomonas vaginitis**  An infection of the vagina caused by a microscopic organism called trichomonas. This infection is usually characterized by a frothy, green discharge that causes significant itching. It can be transmitted sexually, and, if a woman is treated for it, her husband should be treated also. This is not a true venereal disease, as it can be contracted without having sexual intercourse with someone who has trichomonas.

**trophoblastic cells**  Cells which contribute to the formation of the placenta and make up much of the tissue of the placenta.

**tubal ligation**  Tubal sterilization. A procedure which blocks the fallopian tubes by cutting, clamping, cauterizing or (occasionally) tying them, making it impossible for an egg to pass through.

**tubal pregnancy**  *See* ectopic pregnancy.

**tuberculosis**  Infectious disease characterized by tubercles, small, round nodules that may appear on various parts of the body, especially the lungs. Symptoms include weight loss, appetite loss, persistent fever and cough (with expectoration), nausea, and spitting up of blood. This infection is caused by the tubercle bacillus *Mycobacterium tuberculosis*.

**tumor**  A growth. A mass of cells that may or may not be malignant.

**twilight sleep**  Childbirth anesthetic which alleviates pain and erases memory of the birth process. Rarely used today.

**ultrasound (diagnostic ultrasonography, sonogram, sonography)**  Diagnostic tool based on the use of high-frequency sound waves, radiated into the body by a hand-held transmitter, "bounced back" to the transmitting device, and projected onto a screen for evaluation.

**umbilical cord**  The connection of the fetus with the placenta through which blood flows back and forth between baby and mother. This blood, of course, carries the baby's oxygen and nutrition. *See* placenta.

**umbilicus (navel)**  The depressed scar in the abdomen where the umbilical cord was attached to the baby while in the mother's uterus.

**ureter**  The tube through which urine moves from the kidney to the bladder.

**urethra**  The tube through which urine moves from the bladder to the exterior of the body.

**urologist**  Bladder and kidney specialist. These physicians treat kidney or bladder problems. They also treat men for problems of male infertility.

**uterus (womb)**  Hollow, pear-shaped organ in the female pelvis that carries an unborn child for nine months. It is from the uterus that the menstrual flow originates. When the uterus is removed, there will be no more menstrual flow, even though a woman's ovaries may still be functioning normally and producing hormones and an egg each month.

**uterus didelphus**   A congenital abnormality in which the two halves of the uterus failed to fuse together during intrauterine life. In this condition, a woman has two partial uteri. Such a uterus can produce a normal pregnancy and the condition does not usually cause infertility.

**vagina**   Female genital passage which extends from the vulva to the uterus.

**vaginal discharge**   A woman may have various types of secretions from her vagina. Mucus secretions that occur just before a period or ovulation time are usually totally normal, even though they may at times be somewhat heavy. Secretions that smell or cause itching, or are discolored, are often a sign of infection. For such discharge, a woman should see a physician. *See* gardnerella; monilia vaginitis; trichomonas vaginitis.

**vaginitis**   Inflammation of the vagina, usually characterized by discharge.

**vaporization conization**   Laser treatment of the cervix involving vaporization of the tissue of the center portion of the cervix as seen by the doctor through the vagina. The portion of tissue that is evaporated by the laser is similar to the cone-shaped tissue that is removed at a conization done with a surgical knife. *See* conization.

**varicocele**   An accumulation of veins around the testicle that can occasionally result in a man's sperm count or sperm quality being lower than normal, with resulting fertility problems. Such a condition can usually be cured with a minor operation.

**varicose veins**   Veins which become so dilated that they can be seen and felt above the surface of the skin. They appear most frequently in the legs. Women often confuse small spiderlike veins or bluish discolorations of their legs with varicose veins. However, varicose veins are usually as large as a person's little finger lying under the skin. Smaller visible veins are not varicose veins and, most of the time, do not have the potential for becoming varicose veins.

**vascular spider (nevus, angioma, telangiectasia)**   Small red discolorations of the skin which may appear in pregnant women, most commonly on the face, neck, upper chest, and arms. Red lines extend outward from their center. They are not dangerous, and, after pregnancy, will often become much less numerous.

**vas deferens or "vas"**   The narrow tube through which sperm travel from the testes of the male to the seminal vesicles.

**vasectomy**   Sterilization surgery on the male accomplished by cutting the vas, the tube that carries the sperm from the testicles to the internal sex organs.

**venereal disease (sexually transmitted disease)**   Any disease that is contracted through sexual intercourse or intimate contact. *See* STD.

**venereal warts (condyloma acuminata)**   Virus-caused warty growths on the external genitalia, anus, urethra, vagina, or cervix. These may occur in both men and women and are not cancerous. Venereal warts can be spread by sexual contact, but that is not always the case. Special attention is required if they are present during pregnancy.

**vernix**   The white greasy film which covers an unborn child. Composed of secretions from oil glands of the body, hair that has fallen from the skin, and other secretions.

**vesicovaginal fistula**   A hole from the vagina into the bladder. Such an opening allows constant drainage of urine. This drainage of urine causes a woman's vulva to be constantly wet, irritated, odorous, and uncomfortable. This problem usually results from vaginal surgery or from hysterectomies. It can be surgically repaired.

**vulva**   External sex organs of the female.

**vulvectomy**   Surgical removal of the labia majora and minora and, often, of the clitoris, to remove premalignant or malignant tissue of the vulva.

**wedge resection (of ovary)**   Surgical removal of a segment of the ovary in an effort to establish regular menstrual periods and thus fertility. It should be suggested and performed by a gynecologist or other specialist experienced in caring for women with infertility problems. Inexperienced physicians might recommend this procedure when it is unnecessary. It is rarely done today. If it is not done with careful technique and using fine suture, it can result in adhesions of the tubes and ovaries that can result in worse infertility.

**wolffian duct cells**  Cells in the body of the male fetus that will become his vas deferens, epi-didymis, and seminal vesicles as development proceeds.

**womb**  *See* uterus.

**Xerogram, Xeroradiography** *See* mammography.

# Index

*Senior Editor and*
  *Production Coordinator*                Betty De Vries

*Designer*                                Dan Malda

*Artists*
  *Drawings on pages 44, 45, 268, 269, 272,*
  *273, 276, 277, 280, 281, 285, 345, 349, 352*    Richard Bishop
  *Line drawings*                         Dwight Baker
  *Other illustrations*                   Pat Adamik, Dan Malda

*Composition*                             Bailey Typography, Inc.
                                          Nashville, Tennessee

*Printing and Binding*                    Arcata Graphics Group
                                          Kingsport, Tennessee